System of Physic
(GUL MS Hunter 509, ff. 1r-167v)

Late Middle English Texts

3

LMET

Laura Esteban-Segura

System of Physic
(GUL MS Hunter 509, ff. 1r-167v)
A Compendium of Mediaeval Medicine Including the Middle English Gilbertus Anglicus

PETER LANG
Bern · Berlin · Bruxelles · Frankfurt am Main · New York · Oxford · Wien

Bibliographic information published by die Deutsche Nationalbibliothek
Die Deutsche Nationalbibliothek lists this publication in the Deutsche Nationalbibliografie; detailed bibliographic data is available on the Internet at ‹http://dnb.d-nb.de›.

British Library Cataloguing-in-Publication Data: A catalogue record for this book is available from The British Library, Great Britain

Library of Congress Cataloging-in-Publication Data

Esteban-Segura, Laura
System of physic: a compendium of mediaeval medicine including the Middle English Gilbertus Anglicus / Laura Esteban-Segura. – 1st ed.
p. cm. – (Late Middle English texts; v. 3)
Includes bibliographical references.
ISBN 978-3-0343-0077-3
1. Gilbertus, Anglicus. Compendium medicinae. English (Middle English) 2. Medicine, Medieval–England. 3. English language–Medical English 4. English language–Middle English, 1100-1500. I. Title.
R144.G5E88 2012
610.942'0902–dc23

2011052288

This book stems from research project FFI2008-02336, entitled "Development of an Electronic Corpus of Middle English Scientific Manuscripts from the Hunterian Collection (University of Glasgow)" and funded by the Spanish Ministry of Science and Innovation, and from research project PO7-HUM-02609, entitled "Reference Corpus of Late Middle English Scientific Prose" and funded by the Autonomous Government of Andalusia.

ISBN 978-3-0343-0077-3
ISSN 2235-0136

Hochfeldstrasse 32, CH-3012 Bern, Switzerland
info@peterlang.com, www.peterlang.com

Printed in Switzerland

Contents

Introduction

Edition

Preface

This edition of the late Middle English treatise *System of Physic*, held in GUL MS Hunter 509 (ff. 1r–167v), by Laura Esteban-Segura belongs with the larger research projects "An Electronic Corpus of Mediaeval English Manuscripts: Scientific and Technical Texts" and "Development of an Electronic Corpus of Middle English Scientific Manuscripts from the Hunterian Collection (University of Glasgow)", both funded by the Spanish Ministry of Science and Innovation (HUM2004-01075 and FFI2008-02336, respectively). The main objective of these projects is the edition, in electronic or printed format, of the hitherto unpublished mediaeval manuscripts (fourteenth to fifteenth centuries) belonging to the Hunterian collection at Glasgow University Library. This is a large gathering of 10,000 printed books and 650 manuscripts, over 250 from the mediaeval period, bequeathed to the University by William Hunter (1718–1783), who, after studying Divinity at Glasgow and Medicine at Edinburgh, enjoyed a reputation as doctor in London and became Physician Extraordinary to Queen Charlotte, consort of George III. In the course of his career he collected an amount of coins, medals, paintings, anatomical and natural history specimens – shells and minerals – as well as books and manuscripts, mostly related to medicine (<http://www.gla.ac.uk/services/specialcollections/>).

In addition to editing this collection of manuscripts, the projects contemplate two supplementary objectives: (1) the compilation of an annotated corpus derived from the editions, including relevant information of a morphosyntactic and semantic kind (lemma, word-class, accidence, and meaning); and (2) the implementation of a tool – *Text Search Engine* (Miranda-García and

Garrido-Garrido forthcoming) – wherefrom the occurrences of particular items (both words and lemmas) may be automatically searched. A team of scholars from a range of Spanish and British universities, including Málaga, Murcia, Oviedo, Jaén, and Glasgow, under the leadership of Drs Miranda-García and Calle-Martín, have already compiled a corpus consisting of one million items from the manuscripts listed below, the first six of which are already available on the webpage *A Corpus of Late Middle English Scientific Prose* (<http://hunter.uma.es/>).[1]

- GUL MS Hunter 95, *Book of Operation*
- GUL MS Hunter 497, Macer's *The Virtues of Herbs*
- GUL MS Hunter 503, *De probatissima arte oculorum*
- GUL MS Hunter 509, *System of Physic*
- GUL MS Hunter 513, *De probatissima arte oculorum – Antidotary*
- GUL MS Hunter 328, Corbeil's *Treatise on Urines*

- GUL MS Hunter 104, Palladius' *Practice of Husbandry*
- GUL MS Hunter 117, *Medical Receipts*
- GUL MS Hunter 185, *Medical Receipts*
- GUL MS Hunter 307, *System of Physic*

1 Funding has also been obtained from the Andalusian Regional Government (Consejería de Innovación, Ciencia y Empresa), particularly for the projects "A Middle English POS-Tagger" (P09-HUM-4790) and "Reference Corpus of Late Middle English Scientific Prose" (P07-HUM-02609); the latter focuses on the edition of other Middle English medical texts such as MS 404 '*Leechbook*', MS 397 '*Treatise of Powders*', MS 542 '*Miscellanea Medica*', MS 799 '*Treatise of Surgery*', and MS 5262 '*Medical Recipe Collection*', all from the Wellcome Library in London; MS Rylands 7 '*Forme of Curie*' and MS Rylands 1310 '*Treatise on Urines*' from Manchester University Library; MS Rawlinson 7 '*Dome of Urines*' from Oxford University and, finally, MS Sloane 2463 '*Antidotary*', housed in London at the British Library.

- GUL MS Hunter 328, *An Alphabetical List of Remedies and Medicines*

Besides the publication online, printed editions, diplomatic and/or critical, have also been accomplished (Marqués-Aguado, Miranda-García and González 2008; Miranda-García and González 2011) or are being prepared for the brand new Late Middle English Text Series at Peter Lang publishing house. The decision on the part of the series editors – Drs González and Miranda-García – to add this edition of *System of Physic* to this editorial project must be welcome, since it facilitates access to a most popular medical treatise written in a European vernacular of the late Middle Ages. As a matter of fact, the text is one amongst several Middle English adaptations from the Latin *Compendium medicinae* by Gilbertus Anglicus, which survives in thirteen manuscripts dating from its probable composition around 1240 to the first printed version in 1510, as well as in numerous excerpts appended to medical compendia.

GUL MS Hunter 509 is a first-class witness to the outburst of adaptations of Latin scientific texts which accompanied the rise of vernacular languages in Europe from the fifteenth century (Taavitsainen and Pahta 1998; Burke 2004). In fact, it is one of the seventeen Middle English versions of the *Compendium medicinae* that survives nowadays, disregarding excerpts and fragments. Other features of the manuscript, particularly touching on its editorial context and history, make this edition worthy of attention. Hunter 509 was copied in the second half of the fifteenth century (ca. 1460) by Thomas Westhaugh, who was Confessor General of Syon Monastery (Middlesex) by 1472, and possibly relied on a previous Middle English prose version from 1400. Esteban-Segura makes reference to other witnesses closely related to Hunter 509, such as GUL MS Hunter 307 (edition in preparation) and a Latin original – Cambridge, Pembroke College, MS 228 – likely to have been used by the scribe. Comparing the treatment of the contents in all these related sources makes scholars aware of the way scribes adapted earlier versions to the needs of potentially (and relatively) large audiences consisting of both medical practitioners and educated readers competent in the subject. As Esteban-Segura points in her complete introduction to the edition, Hunter 509, for instance, includes information on female 'diseases' which is certainly lacking in other versions, like MS Wellcome 537, possibly addressed to males. Apart from that, Hunter 509 contains an encyclopaedic introductory text on the theory of humours, elements, qualities, and urines (ff. 1–14r), totally spurious to the original Latin *Compendium*. The inclusion of this material is an asset to the present edition and enhances it in comparison to a previous edition of the Middle English Gilbertus Anglicus (Getz 1991), which is in fact the first and only one published of the text hitherto.

Laura Esteban-Segura purports to offer the reader a compromise between a diplomatic and a critical edition. In fact, the digitised images and diplomatic transcriptions of Hunter 509 are already available on the project's website, and therefore undertaking a printed edition that repeats these contents would be pointless. Thus, editorial intervention is not absent from this printed version, where, for instance, the layout has been modified and modern punctuation supplied. Furthermore, despite relying on a single exemplar, this edition is accompanied by an introduction to the history of the manuscript and its contents, by a wealth of comments of a textual, philological, historical and medical character, and by a glossary of Middle English terms. These critical tools ensure that the edition is intellectually profitable to readers with different academic backgrounds: mediaevalists at large, scholars interested in the history of books and manuscripts, philologists and historical linguists, historians of science and medicine, etc.

I would like to finish this presentation by complimenting the author on her most suitable training for the task of editing this treatise. Dr Esteban-Segura has been trained as a philologist and a translator at the Universities of Málaga and Glasgow and she already has an ample experience as editor of mediaeval manuscripts, having accomplished the edition of the West-Saxon Gospel according to St John for her MA dissertation. She has published extensively on philology and the history of English in internationally acclaimed journals, such as *SELIM*, *Neuphilologische Mitteilungen*, *English Studies*, and *Atlantis*, amongst others, and has contributed chapters to volumes published by Peter Lang, Wiley-Blackwell, or Cambridge Scholars. Her research on manuscripts from the Hunterian Collection is also extensive, having finished work on Hunter 503 and Hunter 513 (2011c), as well as on diverse aspects of Hunter 509, such as palaeography (2008b; 2011a; forthcoming), punctuation (2009a), word formation (2009b; 2011b), or dialect (2010). This academic experience ensures that readers will enjoy a comprehensive and wholly reliable edition.

Juan Camilo Conde-Silvestre
Murcia, 12th May 2011

Acknowledgements

I am grateful to the University of Málaga, the Autonomous Government of Andalusia (research project P07-HUM-02609), and the Spanish Ministry of Science and Innovation (research project FFI2008-02336) for funding to publish this book. I would like to thank my colleagues from the research group HUM-497 at the University of Málaga, especially Drs Antonio Miranda-García and Javier Calle-Martín, for their continuous help and wise advice, and Mr Joaquín Garrido-Garrido for technical assistance. Grateful acknowledgement is made to the Keeper of Special Collections at Glasgow University Library, Mr David Weston, for kindly permitting the reproduction of images of the manuscript. Thanks are also due to Ms Ursula Rettinghaus from Peter Lang for her invaluable help and patience throughout the publication process. Last but not least, I wish to thank my parents, Juan and María, and my sisters, Carolina and Natalia, for being unfailingly supportive and encouraging.

List of Abbreviations

adj.	adjective
adv.	adverb
ag.	verbal adjective
ALCH.	alchemy
ANAT.	anatomy
c.	century
canc.	cancelled
COOK.	cookery
corr.	corrected
exp.	expunged
fam.	family
f(f).	folio(s)
follow.	followed
GUL	Glasgow University Library
interl.	interlined
l.-h.	left-hand
MED.	medicine
MED	*Middle English Dictionary*
MS(S)	manuscript(s)
n.	noun
ng.	verbal noun
oblit.	obliterated
OED	*Oxford English Dictionary*
PATHOL.	pathology
PHARM.	pharmacology
phr.	phrase
PHYS.	physics
PHYSIOL.	physiology
ppl.	past participle
prec.	preceded
r	recto
r.-h.	right-hand
sg.	singular
sup.	superlative
SURG.	surgery
underl.	underlined
v.	verb
v	verso
ZOOL.	zoology
|	start of new line or folio

Introduction

The Middle English Gilbertus Anglicus

In the second half of the fourteenth century, there was an urge for scientific and practical writings in English, which had its main impulse in clerical and aristocratic spheres and gave rise to the creation of a wide corpus of works. English versions were rendered out of Latin or French originals, mainly in religious houses. Thus, the remarkable adaptation of Gilbertus Anglicus' *Compendium medicinae* (ca. 1240) seems to be a monastic production (Keiser 1998a: 3595). In monastic scriptoria and academic circles, it was usual for books of the twelfth and thirteenth centuries to circulate as working copies. Mediaeval scholarship ensured the durability of texts and their utility was more important to their owners than the age or material aspect of the manuscript containing them (Harris 1989: 173). This is particularly true of the text under consideration, of which numerous copies were produced and whose medical content bears witness to its practical usage.

A large part of GUL MS Hunter 509 (hereafter *H509*) is based on the Middle English Gilbertus Anglicus, an adaptation written in prose around 1400 of the above-mentioned *Compendium medicinae.* This is amongst the major works of early mediaeval medicine, representing the oldest complete treatise on general medicine written by an English author which has survived to the present day. It also attests the state of medical science at that particular time in England. Although little is known of Gilbertus' life, he was unquestionably one of the most famous physicians of the time as well as the first important medical author of the country (Handerson 1918 [2005]: 17). He is mentioned as one of the authorities of Chaucer's *Doctour of Phisik* (Benson 1987: 30):

> 'Wel knew he the olde Esculapius
> And Deyscorides, and eek Rufus,
> Olde Ypocras, Haly, and Galyen,
> Serapion, Razis, and Avycen,
> Averrois, Damascien, and Constantyn,
> Bernard, and Gatesden, and Gilbertyn.'

Gilbertus is frequently quoted with respect by medical writers of later times and the *Compendium*, printed for the first time in 1510, enjoyed the honour of a second edition as late as the seventeenth century (Handerson 1918 [2005]: 17). It was one of the established references for physicians until that century; in fact, the *Compendium medicinae* was alongside *De proprietatibus rerum* of Bartholomaeus Anglicus, the *Thesaurus pauperum* of Petrus Hispanus, or the *Lilium medicinae* of Bernard Gordon, the standard academic or encyclopaedic text, and all these authors were recognised as academic authorities. These texts were frequently the source for collections of recipes (Jones 1998: 156). In the library of the Faculty of Medicine in the University of Paris between 1395 and 1516, for instance, there were 26 books including the works of Alexander of Tralles, Aristotle, Averroes, Avicenna, Constantin Africanus, Galen, Gilbertus Anglicus, Hippocrates, Rhazes, and Simon of Genoa (Calman 2007: 79).

The works of Gilbertus were also popular both in Latin and in translation, and were widely copied and adapted; Getz (1991: lvi) argues that they had 'a popular appeal', rather than pertaining to part of a popular tradition. Gilbertus holds the seventh position in the list of the fifteen authors or attributed authors appearing most often with Middle English scientific and medical texts, just after Macer and before Albertus Magnus, Galen, or Guy de Chauliac (Voigts 1995: 189).

Amongst the authorities named by Gilbertus, the following are found: Pythagoras, Hippocrates, Plato, Aristotle, Galen, Rufus, Macrobius, Boethius, Alexander of Tralles, Theodorus Priscianus, Theophilus Philaretes, Stephanon, the Arabians Haly Abbas, Rhazes, Isaac Judaeus, Joannitius, Janus Damascenus, Jacobus Alucindi, Avicenna and Averroes, the Salernitan writers, especially Constantin Africanus, Nicholas Praepositus, Romoaldus Ricardus and Maurus, and two unknown authors, Torror and Funcius, labelled by Gilbertus as "antiqui". This list suggests a fine medical library for a thirteenth-century practitioner (Handerson 1918 [2005]: 25).

Gottfried (1986: 197–198) establishes the possibility that the *Compendium* might have been written by a doctor who had never seen a patient, as Gilbertus accepts without questioning the opinion of earlier authorities, and provides cures through exposition and syllogism. The career of Gilbertus is obscure. The same author remarks that it is unlikely that he ever practised medicine, and certain that he was not a surgeon. From documents, it may be inferred that he was a cleric in major orders and physician to the king by 1207. It can also be gathered that he was educated abroad, since English universities were unable at that time to completely educate a medical doctor (Getz 1991: lv). Talbot (1967: 73) suggests the possibility of him being 'a product of Salerno and Montpellier'.

As for the main manuscripts containing the *Compendium*, Getz (1991: liii–liv) provides the following list: TK[2] 3: Bruges, Bibliothèque Publique, MS 469, 244 ff. (dated 1271); Cambridge, Pembroke College, MS 169, ff. 1–233v (13th/14th c.); Cambridge,

2 L. Thorndike and P. Kibre. *A Catalogue of Incipits of Mediaeval Scientific Writings in Latin*. New York: Mediaeval Academy of America, 1963.

Peterhouse, MS 52, ff. 1–92v (13th/14th c.); London, British Library, MS Sloane 272 (named *Laurea anglicana*), 262 ff. (14th/15th c.); TK 380: Oxford, Bodleian Library, MS Bodley 720 (SC 2634), ff. 1–156v (early 14th c.); Florence, Biblioteca Riccardiana, MS 731, ff. 1–231v (14th c.); TK 881: Cambrai, Bibliothèque Publique, MS 906, 247 ff. (14th c.); Vienna, National-Bibliothek, MS 2279, ff. 1–239v (14th c.); TK 1115: Rouen, Bibliothèque de la Ville, MS 984, 225 ff. (14th c.); Oxford, Merton College, MS N. 3. 9. (MS Coxe 226), ff. 207 (14th c.), begins like the 1510 printed edition with the incipit *Incipit liber morborum.*

In Beaujouan (1972: 185), there are references to two manuscripts in Spain: Madrid, Biblioteca Nacional, MS 1199 and Madrid, Biblioteca Universitaria, MS 120. This reference is correct with regard to MS 1199, which is held at the Biblioteca Nacional de España with the title *Incipit liber morborum tam uniuersalium tam particularium a inagistro gileberto editus ab omnibus auctoribus practicis magistrorum exceptus que compendium medicine intjtulatur…* It dates from the fifteenth century and it contains 175 folios. MS 120, however, is housed at the Biblioteca Histórica of the Universidad Complutense de Madrid with the signature BH MSS 120 and the title *Liber morborum tam universalium quam particularium.* Its dates from the thirteenth century and it consists of 172 folios.[3]

There seems to be another manuscript containing the Latin Gilbertus Anglicus (or a part of it), which is not listed in TK and is not mentioned by Getz: Cambridge, Pembroke College, MS 228. This manuscript belonged to the scribe who copied *H509* (discussed below), whose name appears at the end ("T. Westhagh"). The manuscript is named *Medica* in the Catalogue of the Library of Pembroke College, and also contains other medical texts, such as *Aphorisms* by Hippocrates, as well as flyleaves from a music book.

3 This follows the modern foliation of the manuscript.

The following are excerpts from the *Compendium* and other works attributed to Gilbertus: commentary on the uroscopy of Gilles de Corbeil, TK 79, 442, 821, 1483, 1588, 1616; *Antidotarium Gilberti*, TK 54; *De febribus*, TK 553; *Practica*, TK 715; *Quedam de lepra*, TK 1086; *Emplastrum magistri Gilberti Anglici* (not in TK), found in London, British Library, MS Royal 12 D xii (15th c.), f. 64. Sections of the *Compendium* were also translated into other languages during the mediaeval period, such as those incorporated into the writings of Ortolf of Bavaria in (New) High German (London, MS Wellcome 120, ff. 18–48); translations into Hebrew and Catalan were also accomplished (Getz 1991: liv).

Keiser (1998a: 3649) comments that in translating and adapting Gilbertus' *Compendium* into English the writer eliminated the opening section on fevers, discussion relating to charms, and the gynaecological material placed near the end. This last material, however, is present in GUL MS Hunter 307 (U.7.1.), henceforth *H307*; in the case of *H509*, information on women's diseases is scattered throughout the text, but the treatise at the end is missing. From this evidence, the text can be viewed as a living work open to modification, change, etc., that is, to scribal interpretation. Thus, the scribe acts as an editor and reviser, adapting the text to the practical needs of the audience; this was a common practice (Getz 1991: xliv–xlviii; Jasin 1993: 314). Keiser (1998a: 3649–3650) also points out that the number of extant copies indicates an ample audience including medical practitioners and other readers interested in medical knowledge. He adds that the Middle English version 'is written in a clear, concise, and competent vernacular prose style and with a tone of confidence in the translator's understanding of the source and of medical knowledge'.

There are other extant manuscripts based on the Middle English Gilbertus Anglicus. One of them is the previously mentioned *H307*, which includes the text *System of Physic* (with the gynaecology text on the diseases of women) in folios 1r–166v (the Middle English Gilbertus is held in folios 13r–145v). *H307* also contains a pharmacopoeia (ff. 167r–172v). The rest of witnesses, listed in Keiser (1998a: 3834), are the following: Oxford, Bodleian Library, MS 2073 (Bodley 178), ff. 51r–140v (15th c.); Oxford, Bodleian Library, MS 21878 (Douce 304), ff. 2r–103r (ca. 1450); Cambridge, Trinity College Library, MS 1449 (O.9.37), ff. 36r–122r (ca. 1500); London, British Library, MS Harley 3407, ff. 68r–79v (1450–1475; fragmentary); London, British Library, MS Sloane 5, ff. 61r–157r (ca. 1460); London, British Library, MS Sloane 442, ff. 38r–40v (15th c.); London, British Library, MS Sloane 1388, ff. 56r–232r (ca. 1500); London, British Library, MS Sloane 2394, ff. 3r–138r (1450–1500); London, British Library, MS Sloane 3486, ff. 25r–26r, 91r–139r (ca. 1460); London, British Library, MS Sloane 3553, ff. 21r–95v (ca. 1450); London, British Library, MS Additional 25589, ff. 1r–73r (ca. 1450); London, British Library, MS Additional 30338, ff. 11v–151r (15th c.); London, Wellcome Historical Medical Library, MS 537, ff. 48r–310v (ca. 1460); London, Society of Antiquaries, MS 338, ff. 7v–76v (15th c.); San Marino, Huntington Library, MS HM 19079, ff. 27v–32r (1400–1425).

In addition to this, Getz (1991: lxv, n. 90) provides a list with manuscripts containing fragments of the Middle English Gilbertus. Some of the manuscripts listed above share material other than the Gilbertus, which was usually contained in compendia.

When considering textual organisation in late-mediaeval English texts, Keiser (1995: 208–209) discusses San Marino, Huntington Library, MS HM 19079. He dates it ca. 1410 and regards the manuscript as the earliest one of a learned medical treatise. The scribe apparently copied the work in a monastic setting and was very careful to provide a clear, practical, and precise text, succeeding in this task, as the information was organised in a compact manuscript. The treatise follows the same textual order as

H509 (see next section), but it also includes a table of contents at the end, a textual marker lacking in *H509*. Keiser remarks that the device seems to have become an established feature of the text since, in even a later copy such as London, Wellcome Historical Medical Library, MS 537 (ca. 1460), which keeps an abbreviated and inaccurate version of the text, parts of this structure are found intact.

As for the textual type of *H509*, the views on book production held in classical tradition made a distinction between the *scriptor*, someone who reproduces the words of others without any addition or change; the *compilator*, someone who writes the words of others, gathering and joining material, but not their own; the *commentator*, someone who writes mainly the words of others, but also their own to clarify the argument; and the *auctor*, someone who writes the words of others and their own, the latter forming the major part and those of others being appended as a way of confirmation (Minnis and Scott 1991: 229). From this classification, it could be argued that the producer of *H509* would be a *compilator* or compiler, as material is gathered from different sources; this feature is typical of medical texts. Thus, Gilbertus Anglicus states in the opening words of his *Compendium medicinae*: 'Here begins the book of diseases, particular and universal, written by master Gilbert, extracted and excerpted from all the authors and from the practical manuals of the masters' (Calman 2007: 77–79). As pointed out before, he quotes from a very wide range of authorities.

For a deeper insight into the life and work of Gilbertus Anglicus, see Handerson (1918 [2005]) and Getz (1991: liii–lvi; 1998: 39–42). As for the works which analyse English medicine in the mediaeval period, those by Rubin (1974) and Talbot (1967) are still amongst the most representative and basic ones. For a fuller account on medicine in later mediaeval England, see Gottfried (1986), Rawcliffe (1995), and Getz (1998).

The Manuscript: GUL MS Hunter 509

H509 is housed in the Hunterian Collection at Glasgow University Library (press-mark V.8.12).[4] Its main content is the text *System of Physic* (ff. 1r–167v), largely based on the Middle English Gilbertus Anglicus.[5] The first part, however, comprises a treatise on the four humours and their properties, elements, qualities, complexions, ages of man, seasons of the year, types of wind, and division of hours between day and night (ff. 1r–3v). This is followed by a discussion on uroscopy and a further exposition of humours and complexions, as well as the doctor's arrangements before visiting a patient (ff. 3v–14r). The knowledge derives from the Greek tradition in medicine where diet, climate, place, the patient's physical condition, way of life, pursuits, and age were all important issues to be considered (Calman 2007: 32). The source of this first part of *H509* (ff. 1r–14r) is unknown. Some other versions of the Gilbertus share it, but not all of them. Other works different from the Gilbertus also contain this text.

The Middle English Gilbertus is held in folios 14r–167v. The text covers disorders of the human body and its ordering, or *ordinatio*, follows the usual method of the time, a *de capite ad pedem* structure (from head to foot). Textual divisions are clearly marked. At the top of each folio there is a heading title with the name of the malady or the organ affected by it. Marginalia direct the reader to specific matters. The characteristics and symptoms of each disease, the humours provoking it, and the cures, which include dietary

4 The manuscript is listed in Young and Aitken's Catalogue (1908), although no indication of textual relation to the Middle English Gilbertus Anglicus is made. A codicological/palaeographical description of the book is carried out in Esteban-Segura (2011a).

5 Reference is made to the original foliation of the manuscript.

recommendations, pills, ointments, powders, plasters, and therapies such as baths involving the use of herbs, etc., are conscientiously expounded. The exposition opens with the headache (ff. 14r–16v), which is followed by other diseases of the head and brain (ff. 16v–28v) covering mental illnesses and neurological disorders. Next, aches and maladies of the eyes (ff. 28v–44v), ears (ff. 44v–52v), nose (ff. 52v–57r), mouth (ff. 57r–59v), teeth (ff. 59v–62v), and throat (ff. 62v–69v) are dealt with. The chest and lungs (ff. 69v–88v), heart (ff. 88v–95r), stomach (ff. 95r–115r), bowels (ff. 115r–129v), and the anus (ff. 129v–131r) are considered subsequently; then, the liver (ff. 131r–139r), the spleen (ff. 139v–146v), kidneys (ff. 146v–151v), and bladder (ff. 152r–158r). Finally, sicknesses in the siphac or peritoneum (ff. 158r–161r), the penis (ff. 161r–164v), and the anus (ff. 164v–167v) are described.

At the end of the manuscript, some medical recipes for migraine have been written in a different hand (ff. 168v–169r), as well as an added note (f. 171r), and mixed recipes and annotations in various hands (f. 171v).

The text, which was copied during the second half of the fifteenth century (ca. 1460), shows features of the East Anglian dialect.[6] The copyist was Thomas Westhaugh, Confessor General of Syon Monastery by 1472, as some notes written in the manuscript suggest, and was owned by several people, amongst whom was John Sperhawke, a friend of Westhaugh.[7] The last owner of *H509* was Sir William Hunter (1718–1783), a British doctor, educator, and medical writer, who left by will his private collection and the contents of his museum to the University of Glasgow.

6 The study of the dialect is carried out in Esteban-Segura (2010).

7 Composition and ownership of *H509* are tackled in Esteban-Segura (2008b).

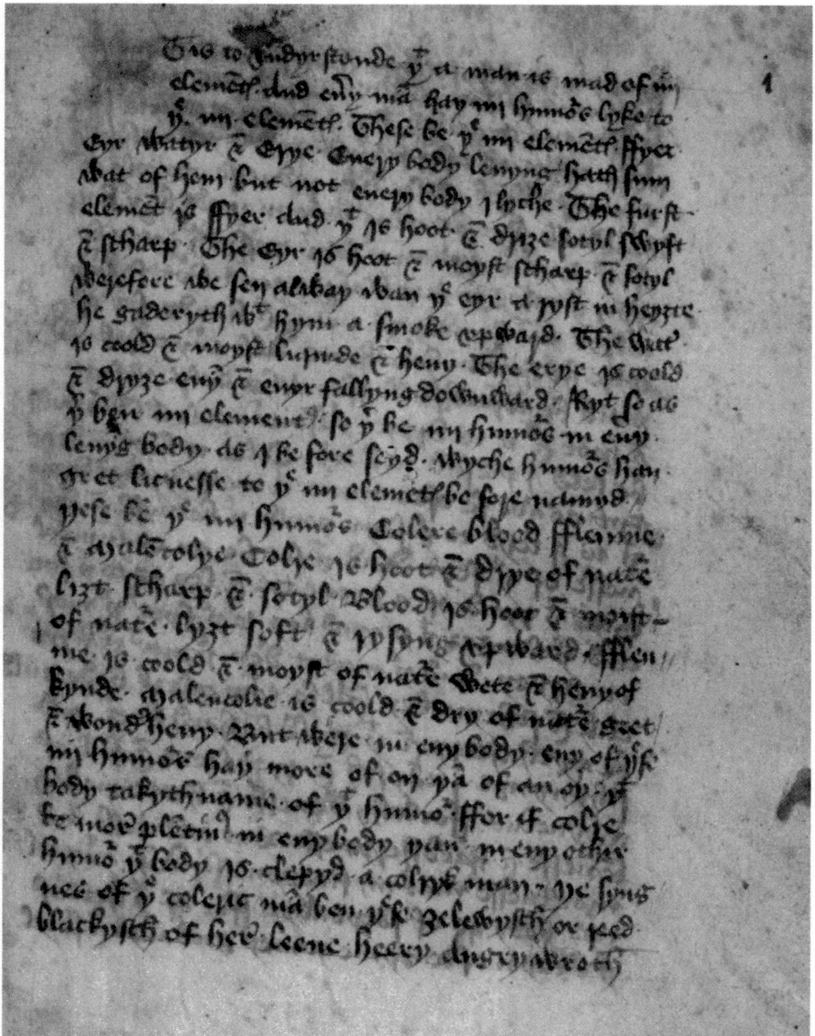

Fig. 1. Digitised image of f. 1r (Reproduced with permission of the University of Glasgow).

Editorial Conventions

Scientific and practical writings in Middle English have received a growing interest over the last two decades (see Pahta and Taavitsainen 2004: 1–9). Keiser (1998b: 110–111) highlights two publications that helped to form a more positive view of this type of vernacular treatises: Robbins' 1970 article "Medical Manuscripts in Middle English" and the 1975–1988 edition of John Trevisa's translation of *De proprietatibus rerum* by Bartholomaeus Anglicus, carried out by Seymour *et al.* These works were followed by editions of several Middle English treatises in the series *Scripta* (Grymonprez 1981; Hallaert 1982), which frequently produced diplomatic or semi-diplomatic editions. The critical edition, however, may furnish a more comprehensive and helpful rendering than that provided by the diplomatic one.

An authorial text can be approached in many ways. As Jacobs (1998: 11) points out, '... there is a range of possibilities running from the reproduction *literatim* of the exemplar to the creation of an entirely new composition only loosely based on it'. With regard to the editorial method followed in the present work, since there is editorial interpretation (for example, in the expansion of abbreviations and in the supplying of modern punctuation), it cannot be regarded as a diplomatic edition. Nor can it be classed as a critical edition, as only one witness of the text is taken into consideration. Thus, the edition is in-between a diplomatic and a critical one; this kind of compromise seems the best editorial method and several reasons can account for this choice.

The first of these is the difficulty in carrying out a critical edition, which would involve the examination of all the extant manuscripts based on the same source as *H509* in order to trace the original text or archetype. Getz (1991: lxv) argues that 'the freedom with which the translator and copyists modified their respective exemplars has made the establishment of common and uncommon texts by critical edition impractical'. She continues to reflect that new manuscripts of the Middle English Gilbertus may be discovered as the nature and scope of Middle English medical literature is progressively updated. Bearing this in mind, the presentation of a single witness appears to be the best option. Apart from the number of copies, the enterprise of collating the texts might be made more difficult or unfeasible by the fact that the treatise is of considerable length.

Second, the edition of one of these manuscripts in particular would place the focus on the scribe and specific readership, rather than on the author. The examination of the text can provide insights into the nature of the treatises and their intended uses. Thus, one of the goals of this edition is to recreate mediaeval culture through a specific text by considering one witness to the Middle English Gilbertus. The edition would then pay special attention to the readership, trying to solve the problems that the manuscript may pose to anyone interested in accessing it. Consequently, the edition takes into account two types of readers, those for whom the text was originally composed, but also a present-day audience.

Editing involves making decisions. The editor has the task of reinterpreting someone else's work with a specific view in mind. Therefore, the final text will depend on this and the editorial choices made will be valid as long as they are well-grounded and justified. For this reason, the editorial procedures that have been followed will be explained next.

The layout of folios has not been kept since the text has been lined to occupy the whole page. This is more convenient both for publishing, as it saves paper, and for readers accustomed to traditional books. The start of a new folio is signalled in the outer margins of the page and with a vertical line within the text. With respect to lines, they do not coincide with those of the original manuscript. All material imported into the text appears in square brackets.

As for letters, ⟨i⟩ is represented as materialised in the manuscript, either ⟨i⟩ or ⟨j⟩. The personal pronoun *I* has not been capitalised. For the *yogh*, the corresponding symbol ⟨ȝ⟩ is used and the *thorn* ⟨þ⟩ has been retained. ⟨Ff⟩ and ⟨ff⟩ have been reduced to ⟨F⟩ or ⟨f⟩, depending on the context in which they appear given that, although they generally stand for a capital letter, it is not unusual to find them in the middle of a sentence, where keeping such a form would not be appropriate; these changes are marked in the apparatus. Letters ⟨u⟩ and ⟨v⟩ are presented as found in the manuscript.

Regarding the different graphs for letters such as ⟨s⟩ or ⟨r⟩, whose use depends on the position that they occupy within the word, the distinction has not been maintained (the transcription is graphemic rather than graphetic).

Abbreviations are very frequent and standard, and are employed throughout the text. They have been expanded and this indicated by means of italics. This method has been preferred since major editions, such as Seymour *et al.* 1975–1988, make use of it. Special signs or brevigraphs are found, for example, for the letters *er*, which may be indicated by a broken stroke above the line (e.g. "feu*er*e", fig. 2), by an upward curve from the end of a letter (e.g. "wat*er*", fig. 3), or by a horizontal stroke over the descender of *p* (e.g. "sup*er*fluite", fig. 4).

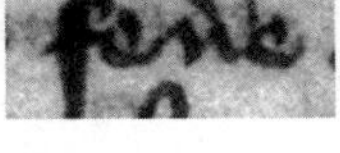

Fig. 2

Fig. 3

Fig. 4

In some words, a letter appears in superscript (for example, ⟨e⟩ in the word "þe", fig. 5), probably in order to save space. In the edition, this type of letter has been silently expanded as it has been considered that, since the letter is actually there, using the italics would not be appropriate (elsewhere in the edition they are employed to mark missing elements). Other editions have been consulted and the problem has been solved in the same way.

Nasal consonants, which are usually abbreviated by means of a straight horizontal stroke over the preceding letter (e.g. "e*m*plast*r*es", fig. 6) and, less often, by a semicircular horizontal curve with a dot beneath (e.g. "sau*n*dres", fig. 7), have been expanded and the expansion indicated by means of italics. Where they seem to have no function, their occurrence is noted in the apparatus reference, but not in the text. During the transcription process, when expansions were ambiguous, attention was paid to neighbouring scribal practice in order to elucidate this ambiguity. For instance, "e*m*plaster" was selected over "e*n*plaster" because, although both words appear in the text, the one having most occurrences is *emplaster*.

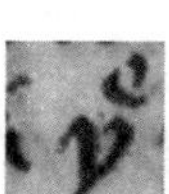

Fig. 5

Fig. 6

Fig. 7

A horizontal stroke through a final ascender or ascenders has been expanded to *e* for consistency's sake, although in some cases it may represent an otiose mark whose only function is decoration. The drawing of a horizontal stroke through or above the *h* in words ending in *th*, *gh*, *ght*, *ch* (e.g. "bladdrisch*e*", fig. 8) had become a well established custom in vernacular writing by the late fifteenth century. The same can be said of the stroke through final double *l* (e.g. "well*e*", fig. 9) and the extension of the last stroke of final *r* (e.g. "mor*e*", fig. 10), *m*, and *n* in a flourish above the line.

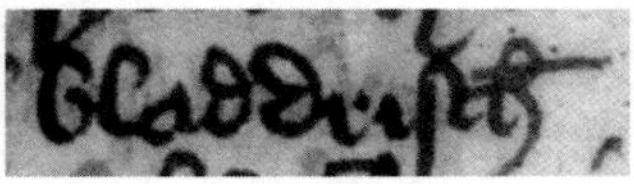

Fig. 8

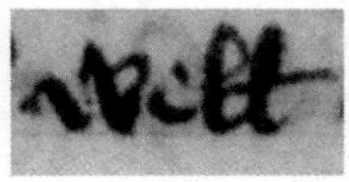

Fig. 9

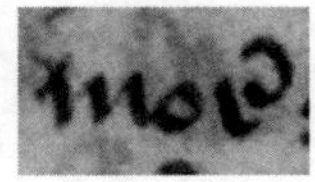

Fig. 10

In some cases, letters are ambiguous and may hinder a correct interpretation. This is especially relevant for minims; the scribe does not always dot letter ⟨i⟩, so different readings may be possible. In such cases, the sense of the word within its context, as well as linguistic information, have helped to make a decision when transcribing.

Symbols for apothecaries' weights have been replaced by the words they denote and this has been conveniently indicated by means of italics. Thus, the symbol which stands for the pound has been transcribed as *pound*, that for the ounce as *ounce* and the one for the drachm, as *dragme*.[8] A long *s* with a backstroke through the centre represents the Latin *semis* (which means a half), whereas when it is preceded by *q* it has been expanded to *quantum sufficit*. A capital *m* has been transcribed as *manipulus*, which refers to "a handful" (this expression is also found in the text to allude to the same quantity). The various ways in which these weights are written in the text are provided next. The pound is represented as shown in figs. 11 and 12; half a pound can be indicated in two different ways: when represented by the abbreviations in fig. 13, it has been expanded to *pound dimidia*, whereas for those in fig. 14, the expansion chosen has been *pound semis*.

8 The word *pound* does not change in the plural, whereas *ounce* and *dragme* have both singular and plural forms.

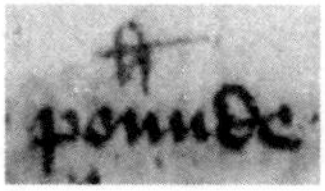

Fig. 11

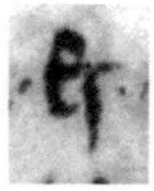

Fig. 12

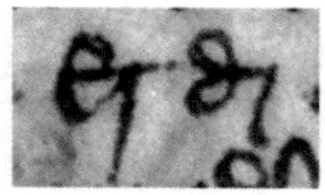

Fig. 13

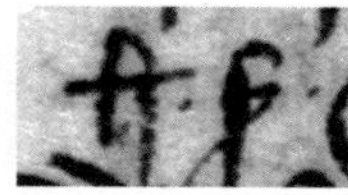

Fig. 14

The symbol used for the ounce is rendered in fig. 15; half an ounce is written as indicated in fig. 16 (*ounce semis*). Those for the drachm and for half of it (*dragme semis*) are presented in figs. 17 and 18 respectively.

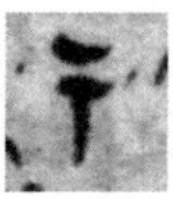

Fig. 15

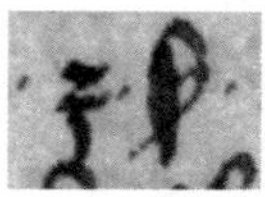

Fig. 16

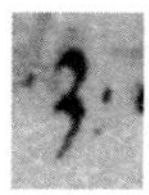

Fig. 17

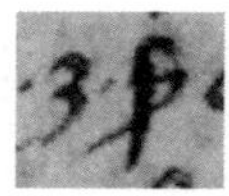

Fig. 18

The *manipulus* or handful is illustrated in fig. 19. There are three different ways to indicate half of a *manipulus* (figs. 20–22).

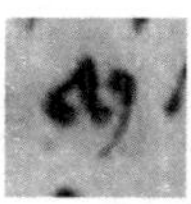

Fig. 19

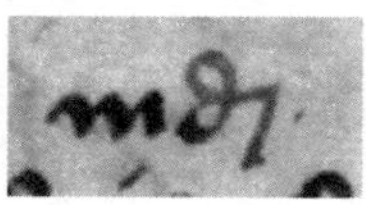

Fig. 20

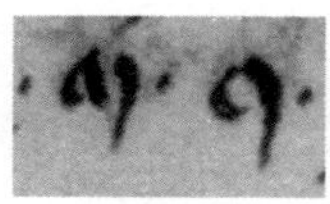

Fig. 21

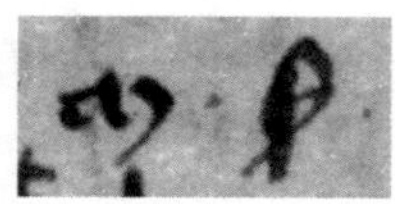

Fig. 22

As far as punctuation is concerned,[9] the system employed throughout the manuscript is somehow systematic (although not always), but it is also complex due to the large number of marks. This fact might prevent a proper understanding of the text and, as a consequence, punctuation has been altered according to modern practice. The main symbols are the punctus, the punctus elevatus, and the virgule; they can also appear combined. Their range of use

9 The original system of punctuation found in *H509* is discussed in detail in Esteban-Segura (2009a).

can vary depending on context. Sometimes, the lack of marks may lead to confusion. In some cases, such as in recipes for preparing remedies or cures, a correct interpretation of punctuation marks becomes crucial. Note, for instance, the following fragment taken from f. 51r:

> 'tak peletre ·of spayne ·& ·of castore ·ʒ ·j ·of mirre ·nytr*e* long/ ·pep*er* ·rwe ·ʒ ·ij ·euforbe ·ʒ ·j ·'

If punctuation is not properly placed, it may be difficult to ascertain which elements go together. The proposed rendering for the previous fragment would be:

> 'tak peletre of spayne, *and* of castore, *dragme* j; of mirre, nytr*e*, long pep*er*, rwe, *dragme* ij; euforbe, *dragme* j.'

In order to regularise the (somewhat chaotic) system of punctuation found in *H509*, each type of mark has been analysed and an equivalent or near equivalent has been provided (often none was needed); context has also been taken into account for this purpose. It has not always been possible to establish a one-to-one correspondence between a mediaeval mark and a modern one. For instance, the punctus has been generally changed for a comma when separating conditional sentences or introducing causal clauses. In other cases, particularly when indicating a medial pause, the punctus has remained as such (a full stop) or has been replaced by a semicolon (or a colon, especially when the explanation of how to make a recipe follows). Nevertheless, in other contexts, it has just been deleted as, for example, when encircling short words to avoid confusion. The punctus elevatus has been usually replaced by a comma. In the manuscript, there are a lot of possible combinations for the virgule, which can be double or be combined with a punctus, etc. Normally, a double virgule and a punctus indicate a long pause, so a full stop and a new paragraph have been inserted.

Capitalisation has also been normalised in line with standard modern usage regarding the first letter of a sentence; however, other letters, although they may have been capitalised by the scribe, are in lower case in the edition in order to conform to modern practice. Capital letters in heading titles, which are provided in the critical apparatus, have been maintained.

The issue of word division is problematic insofar as sometimes a word may occur as just one form or separated with a blank space or a punctus (for example, *a noþer* ~ *anoþer* or *be tymes* ~ *betymes*. The word spacing of the text has been regularised; thus, the elements of what has been regarded as the same word, which in the original text appear separated, have been joined and marked by means of a hyphen (for instance, *with oute* → *with-oute*; *with inne* → *with-inne*; *to gidere* → *to-gidere*). Most of the prefixes of the participles or even compound forms are also split, such as *j medlid*, *j cast*, *j soden* etc., and these have also been united with a hyphen: *j-medlid*, *j-cast*, *j-soden*. For joining or linking words or elements of them, the *MED* has been taken as the main reference. Other types of split forms are those occurring at the end of the line, which are normally followed by a double virgule to indicate that the word has not ended and continues in the next one; occasionally, this double virgule is missing. In both cases, the elements of the word have been joined. Since punctuation has been modernised, no hyphen is provided when there is a mark for the sake of coherence.

Similarly, words which appear combined in the manuscript but are in fact two different terms have been disjoined. Some examples of this are *whitwyn*, *grethete*, or *lytulwyn* (*whit wyn*, *gret hete*, and *lytul wyn* respectively). This type of correction of the original text is always explained in the first apparatus reference.

In connection with the critical apparatus, two apparatus references are given at the foot of the page, and a reference note is provided at the end, following the edited text. In the first apparatus reference, scribal errors and mistakes are included, as well as editorial corrections (marked within the text of the edition by square brackets). They have been corrected when deemed necessary for a proper understanding of the text, but all changes introduced are indicated in both the text and the apparatus. Letters or words which appear above or below the line of writing as a form of scribal correction are treated as interlineation. When cancellation, expunction, obliteration, or interlineation takes place in a letter occurring more than once in a word, the specific letter has been referred to as "first", "second", "last", etc. Running or heading titles found at the top of each folio have also been reproduced in this apparatus reference, in addition to catchwords.

The second apparatus reference comprises the marginalia and glossing; to specify their exact position in the text, the first word of the line in which the marginalia appear is referenced. If the word belongs to the previous line (this would be the case of compounds, for instance), then the next word is provided with a reference. A vertical line in this apparatus means that what follows belongs to a different line.

These two apparatus references do not always appear in every page of the edition, especially the second one, since marginalia are not present in all folios.

The apparatus at the end is a reference note including commentaries on several aspects of the text. Readings taken from parallel manuscripts, which may also have clarified doubts concerning transcription, have also been incorporated here. The explanation is preceded by the page and line where the word(s) or first and last word of the fragment commented occur.

The original foliation, probably mediaeval, is faulty as it starts twice, renumbering folio 3 as "1" and it continues as such until the end, with the following errors: folios 17 and 162 have been numbered twice, and a folio has been omitted between folios 127 and 128. Despite the errors, this foliation has been maintained. As mentioned before, the beginning of a new folio is signalled in the outer margin of the page and the place where it takes place has been marked within the text by means of a vertical line.

As regards scribal mistakes, they have been corrected or omitted in the edition; all material imported into the text has been both enclosed in brackets and indicated in the textual notes. For emendation, any "improvement" that has been made to the manuscript text has tried to keep in accord with the scribe's linguistic habits. For this reason, normalising the spelling variants has not been considered convenient or with a proper justification against retaining the manuscript reading. One of the most remarkable features of Middle English as far as linguistic character is concerned is its variation, which can account for dialectal or idiolectal characteristics. If the spelling were to be standardised, this idiosyncratic and revealing aspect would be lost. In relation to this, Lucas (1998: 174) explains that sometimes editors are tempted to amend unusual spellings of a familiar word even though they are acceptable linguistic forms. Every effort has been made to preserve the manuscript's peculiarities and features, and to produce a consistent and accurate edited text that can be smoothly read.

Edition of GUL MS Hunter 509

[It is] to vndyr-stonde þ*at* a man is mad of iiij eleme*nt*es, and euery man haþ iiij humo*urs* lyke to þe iiij eleme*nt*es. These be þe iiij eleme*nt*es: fyer, eyr, watyr, *and* erþe. Euery body leuyng hath sum-wat of hem, but not euery body j-lyche. The furst eleme*n*t js fyer, and þ*at* js hoot *and* driȝe, sotyl, swyft, *and* scharp. The eyr js hoot *and* moyst, scharp, *and* sotyl. Werefore we sen alway wan þe eyr a-ryst in heyȝte: He gaderyth w*ith* hym a smoke vpward. The wat*er* js coold *and* moyst, liquide, *and* heuy. The erþe js coold *and* dryȝe, [h]euy *and* euyr fallyng downward. f. 1r

Ryt so as þ*er* ben iiij element*us*, so þ*er* be iiij humo*urs* in eu*ery* leuy*n*g body, as j be-fore seyd, wyche humo*urs* han gret licnesse to þe iiij eleme*nt*es be-fore namyd. Þese be*n* þe iiij humo*urs*: colere, blood, fleume, *and* male*n*colye. Colre js hoot *and* drye, of nat*ure* liȝt, scharp, *and* sotyl. Blood js hoot *and* moist, of nat*ure* lyȝt, soft, *and* rysyng vpward. Fleume js coold *and* moyst, of nat*ure* wete, *and* heuy of kynde. Malencolie is coold *and* dry, of nat*ure* gret, *and* wond*er* heuy. But where in eny body eny of þese iiij humo*urs* haþe more of on þa*n* of an-oþ*er*, þ*at* body takyth name of þ*at* humo*ur*.

For if colre be mor*e* ple*n*tiu*us* in eny body þan eny othir humo*ur*, þ*at* body js clepyd a colryk man. Þe syngnes of þe coleric ma*n* ben þese: ȝelewysch*e* or reed, blackysch*e* of her*e*, leene, heery, angry, wroth*e*, | hardy, lyȝt, swyft, drye, *and* of safrou*n* colour*e*. V*ers*us "hirsutus, fallax, irascens, f. 1v

1 It] *3-line space left for initial* **It is]** *corr. from* Tis **3 fyer]** *corr. from* ffyer **5 fyer]** *corr. from* ffyer **10 heuy]** *corr. from* euy*n* **14 fleume]** *corr. from* ffleume **17 Fleume]** *corr. from* ffleume **19 where]** *interl.* h **22 For]** *corr. from* ffor **þan]** *follow. by canc. and exp.* in **26 Versus]** *corr. from* V*ers*er

prodigus, audax, hastutus, gracilis, sicc*us*, crocei-q*ue* coloris”. For-why colere is of þe ferus kynd, wych*e* is hoot *and* dry nat*ur*ellych*e*. Colre haþ rednesse to colo*ur* w*it*h blaknesse, ryt as colys waxyn ryede be þe hete of þe feyr. But wan þe feyr ceesyth*e*, þan be-gyn þe colys to wax blake a-ȝeyn. Ryt so eu*ery* colryk ma*n* kyndly is proud *and* hardy, for of colre he haþ an hoo[t] herte. Also eu*ery* colrik ma*n* xuld be wrathfull*e*, for-why colre is lyȝt *and* hoot, *and* it is dryȝe. Also eu*ery* colrik body xuld be seld j-plesyd in hert. Colre is hoot *and* driȝe, ryt as we se ofte-tyme a moist þynge dryyt þ*at* is j-leyd to þe feyr þorw þe hotnesse *and* drynesse of þe feyr. And þ*at*, see, be an exaumpyl: Tac þe rynd of a grene tre *and* ley jt to þe fyer. And þe lenger þ*at* þe rynd liþ to þe fyer*e*, þe mor*e* it dryeþ. And þe mor*e* it d*r*ieþ, þe mor*e* it wryncli[þ] *and* schrynckeþ. Also eu*ery* colrik body xuld be ryth*e* heery, *and* þ*at* xuld be hard heer*e*, and schynynge reedysch*e*, *and* ryȝt leene, *and* ful of wrynclus, forwhy d*r*ienesse *and* heete maken le*n*nesse *and* hard herynesse. But coldnesse and moistnesse makun smoþenesse. Also eu*ery* colryc body js of sotyl wyt, for of þe hete of þe brayn ofte-
f. 2r tyme comeþ good wyt *and* sotyl, | and of coldnesse comeþ a dul wyt. Also eu*ery* colric ma*n* xuld haue is eyȝen sone meuabyl hidurward *and* ȝy*n*durward, vpward, *and* downward. And also be cause of his heete, he xuld be liȝt *and* nat studefast ne þouȝtful. Also þei xuld be wacful forwhy of þe heete of þe brayn. Þei xuld meche wake *and* litul slepe forwhy coldnesse makeþ on heuy *and* sleepfull*e*. Also eu*ery*

2 For-why] *corr. from* ffor-why **8 for-why**] *corr. from* ffor-why **15 wryncliþ**] *corr. from* wrynclih*e* **17 forwhy**] *corr. from* fforwhy **20 for**] *corr. from* ffor **25 forwhy**] *corr. from* fforwhy **27 forwhy**] *corr. from* fforwhy

colric body xuld, be cause of her*e* hete, be gret lechours. But for as mych*e* as þei ben dry, þei ben sone ou*er*come *and* lytyl mow doon, for heete makeþ þ*at* þei wul mechyl, *and* d*ri*enesse makeþ þ*at* þei ben sone ou*er*-come in þ*at* craft.

Also on þe same maner*e*, where þ*at* blood is regnyng in eny body more þan eny oþ*er* humo*ur*, þ*at* body is clepyd a sanguyn ma*n*. And ȝyf a body be sanguyn, þese be þe tokyns þorow þe wych*e* me*n* may know hym: He is riȝt goold reed or riȝt brown blak; of moistnesse, he is euene fat; and in his face he is ruddy as of heete, for blood is hoot *and* moyst; large in ȝeuyng; louyng; glad of chere *and* reed; *and* moost como*n*ly syngyng; ful of flesch*e*; ful-hardy, *and* riȝt boner*e*, *and* meke. But ȝif he be t*r*oublyd a-ȝens hese lyky*n*g, þa*n* he waxyt to proud, braydyng, wyckyd, hasty, *and* sone for-ȝeu*er*y. Vnde Mac*er*: "largus, ama*n*s, hilaris, ridens, rubeiq*ue* coloris, ca*n*ta*n*s, carnosus, sat*is* audax, valde benign*us*". Also eu*er*y | sanguy*n* body is of good wyt *and* sotyl, *and* liȝt f. 2v to do al man*er* thyng *and* to vndirstondyt longe, for of þe hetnesse of brayn comyȝt a good wyt. And he xuld comely slepe mechil be cause of hese hete *and* be cause of hese moistnesse. Also þei xuld, for hete, be letchours and also, for þei ben moist, þei xuld meche suffyce to þ*at* craft *and* comly be frendful þ*er*-to.

Also wher*e*-so-euyr fleume regneþ in eny body mor*e* þa*n* eny oþ*er* humo*ur*, þ*at* body is clepyd a fleu*ma*tik ma*n*. And kyndly he is coold *and* moist of nat*ure*, for flewme is lycnyd to þe watyr, þe wych*e* is coold *and* moist in kende. Þe signes *and* p*ro*pirtees of a fleumatic body be*n* þese: Þei

3 for] *corr. from* ffor **10 for**] *corr. from* ffor **18 for**] *corr. from* ffor **24 fleume**] *corr. from* ffleume **26 for**] *corr. from* ffor

schullyn be whyth, ȝelwysch*e*, or riȝt whiȝt or palysch*e* lokyng, *and* su*m*tyme brownysch*e*, but seldo*m* whan. But Mac*er* seiþ þei xul be slepy, slowe, riȝt fat, whiȝt colour, *and* dul of wyt. Vn*de* Mac*er*: "hic sompnole*nt*us, pig*er* in sputamine mult*us*, et ebes sensus, pinguis, facie color albus", for-why cooldnesse [haþ] to coloure wiþ v*er*tues *and* eiþ*er*-whyle wiþ blacnesse. Also eu*ery* fleu*ma*tic ma*n* or we*m*ma*n*, be cause of here moistnesse, he xuld be fat *and* nat mych*e* j-heeryd; *and* loþ to be wroth in wraþþe but wan he js j-browt f. 1rbis in wrath sone aft*er* þ*at* he is j-plesyd, he is myld j-now | for þe tendyrnesse of his herte. Þei xul be ferdful *and* dredfull*e*, *and* wene þ*at* eu*ery* man is here enemy. Þei xul ben frendfull*e*, hapfull*e*, *and* nat prowd. Also for cooldnesse of here hert*es*, þei xul be dull*e* of wyt *and* wel slepyng. And by cause of here coldnesse, lytyl þei coueyt to do lecherie. *And* bi cause þ*at* þei ben moist, þei mowe*n* mech*e* þ*er*of. Þei xul be wel wyllyd to werke but þei xul make ofte wo*m*man*us* breidus many thyng*es* to be-gynne *and* few to þe ende. And þei xul be wynfull*e*, *and* coueitouse, *and* bie eu*er* arw, *and* dredfull*e*, *and* schamfull*e*.

Male*n*colie also: Where-eu*er* þ*at* malencolie regniþ in eny bodi more þan eny oþ*er* humo*ur*, þ*at* body is j-clepyd a malencolie ma*n*. And js of þe kynd of þe erþe þ*at* is coold *and* driȝe. Þe signes of þe humo*ur* ben þese: heuy, slow, enuyous, coueitows, hardholdyng*e* þ*at* he haþ falsly get, stameryng, lypschyng, ful of gyle, eu*er* in drede. Vn*de* v*er*sus: "jnuid*us*, *et* trist*is*, cupidus, dextre-q*ue* tenac*is*, no*n* expers fraudis, timid*us*, lutei-q*ue* coloris", selden glad or neu*er* mery, ȝelwysch*e* or whytysch*e*, salewysch or

1 whyth] *interl.* h **2 whan]** *interl.* h **6 for-why]** *corr. from* ffor-why **10 for]** *corr. from* ffor

blacksch*e*, or of cley colo*ur*, eu*er* dredy*n*g or ofte wepyng *and* shyȝynge, *and* ofte repentyng. But be cause þ*a*t þei han meche of þe spleen, þ*a*t is, of þe mylt, þ*er*-fore þei ben eu*er* lawyng, or ellys grenyng, or smylyng. But þ*a*t is nowt in þe hert, but of þe splene. And be cause þ*a*t þei ben dryȝe in kynd, þei xul be lene, ryuelyd, *and* su*m*delle j-heeryd, but nat mych*e*, *and* þ*a*t heer js riȝth hard of d*ri*nesse | of here hertys of malencolie. Þorow malencolie þei xul be slow to werche or to do eny good, but it be selde[n]*e*-whanne. And ȝif þei haue t*re*spasyd, þa*n* he repe*n*teþ sore *and* wexiþ meke *and* hooly, *and* looþ is to take wraþþe. But wha*n* þei haue take wraþþe, þei xul long hold [it] for here coold dredful hert. And bi cause þ*a*t þei [ben] coldere of brayn þ*a*n eny oþ*er* kyndly me*n*, þei be*n* slow, *and* drunklew, feble of wyt *and* riȝt dull*e*, gret-hedid, *and* wel slepyng, but nat mych*e* be cause of here cooldnesse. Þei xul nat wyl to do letchery, *and* be cause þ*a*t þei ben driȝe, lytil or naut þei mown þ*er*-of whan þei come þ*er*-to, for þei coueit hyt nat, ne naȝth*e* mow þ*er*-of. f. 1vbis

Now haue j toold of þe iiij humo*urs* w*ith* here signes *and* w*ith* here p*ro*pirteys þ*a*t longen to he*m*. Þe humo*urs* as j for-seid be lickened *and* taken of þe iiij element*es* a-forn-seid, þe wiche þei ben, j haue schortly wryten hem.

And þ*er* ben iiij ages in þe wyche eu*er*y humour*e* haþ beynge to þorow lycnesse, þ*a*t is, chyldhood, ȝouthe, manhood, *and* elde. Chyldhood is fro þe tyme þ*a*t he is j-bore tyl he be xxv wynt*er* eld, *and* þ*a*t age is hoot *and* moist.

3 spleen] *interl.* last e **9 seldene-whanne]** *corr. from* selder*e* **12 hold it]** *corr. from* holdyd **15 and**[1]**]** *interl.* **18 for]** *corr. from* ffor **24 And]** *2-line space left for initial* **25 beynge]** *follow. by canc. and* **to]** *interl.*

f. 2rbis 3ouþe is fro xxv ȝeer to xxxv | or to xl wynt*er* old, *and* þat age is hoot *and* driȝe. Manhood is fro xxxv or xl wynt*er* tyl he bie fifty or sixty ȝeer*e* elde, *and* þat age is coold *and* driȝe. Elde lastiþ fro fyfty ȝeer*e* or sixty tyl on-to þe lyuys ende, *and* þat age is coold *and* moist. Þese be þe iiij ages þe which*e* be*n* j-lickynd to þe iiij co*m*plexiou*n*s. Jt is to know þat eu*ery* colryc body is su*m*del wel in childhood, more bet*er* in elde þa*n* in ȝouþe, for þei it so be þat eu*ery* colric body be hoot *and* driȝe of co*m*plexiou*n*, nerþeles childhood is hoot *and* moyst. Þe hootnesse of childhood makeþ more þe hete of hys co*m*plexiou*n*. Also eu*ery* colric body is euel in ȝong age, for þat age is hoot *and* driȝe, and colre is hoot *and* driȝe. And þ*er*fore eu*ery* colric body is euyl whan þat so is þat þei comy*n* in-to þe age of ȝouþe, for þe hete of þe colric body is mad moore hoot be þe hete of ȝouþe. *And* þat for drinesse of ȝouþe, eu*ery*ch*e* of hem for-doþ [þe] oþ*er* til þat þe colric body come in-to þe age of ma*n*hood, for þa*n* he is wel *and* ryal in his co*m*plexio*n*; *and* betyr in elde, for colre is hoot *and* driȝe, *and* þat age is coold *and* moist. Sa*n*guy*n* folk, þei be*n* eu*er*mor*e* werst in here childhood *and* su*m*del well*e* in
f. 2vbis here ȝongþe *and* in ma*n*hood, | and in eld [þei ben] riȝt weel. Fleu*ma*tic folk, þei ben wel in childhood *and* in elde, but þei be*n* betyr in co*m*plexion in ȝongþe, but þei ben worst in þe age of manhood.

Riȝt as þ*er* ben iiij ages a-cordyng to þe iiij humo*ur*s of co*m*plexio*n*, riȝt so þ*er* be*n* iiij tymys of þe ȝeer, and iiij man*er* of wyndys, and iiij partys of þe wor[l]d, þe wych*e* ben

8 for] *corr. from* ffor **11 for**] *corr. from* ffor **14 for**] *corr. from* ffor **17 for**] *corr. from* ffor **18 for**] *corr. from* ffor **19 is**] *follow. by exp.* hoot **coold**] *interl.* **21 þei ben**] *corr. from* he is **22 Fleumatic**] *corr. from* ffleu*ma*tic in temprure or in malicie a-cordyng to eu*ery* co*m*plexio*n* for-seyd.

Þese be þe iiij tymes of þe ȝeer: ver, som*er*, heruest, *and* wynt*er*. Ver is hoot *and* moist. Som*er* is hoot *and* driȝe. Heruest is coold *and* driȝe. Wynt*er* is coold *and* moist. Colric folk, þei be*n* wel in ver, euel in som*er*; þei ben wel in heruest *and* in wynt*er*. Sang*ui*n folk ben euele in vere *and* bet*er* in som*er*, *and* wel at ese in heruest *and* in wy*n*t*er*. Fleu*ma*tic folk, þei ben wel in ver *and* in heruest, *and* best in som*er*, *and* werst þei ben in wynt*er*. Malencolie folk, þei ben best in ver, wel in som*er* *and* in wynt*er*, *and* werst in heruest.

Þese be þe iiij wyndys: estwynd þ*at* is hoot *and* moist; souþwynd þ*at* is hoot *and* driȝe; westwynd þ*at* is coold *and* moist; norþenewynd þ*at* is coold *and* driȝe.

Þese be þe iiij parties of þe world: est, souþ, west, *and* north. Est þ*at* is hoot *and* moist; sowth þ*at* is hoot *and* driȝe; | west is coold *and* moist; north*e* is coold *and* driȝe. f. 3r
Colrik folk ben wel whil þe sunne or þe wynd be*n* est, west, *and* north, but þei ben euyl while þe su*n*ne or þe wynd be south. Sanguin folk, þei ben euel if þe su*n*ne or þe wynd be in þe est, and þei be*n* weel j-now while þe su*n*ne or þe wynd be*n* in þe sowth and in þe west, or in þe north*e*. Fleu*ma*tyk folk be*n* wel wha*n* þe su*n*ne or þe wynd be*n* estward, sowthward or toward þe north, but þei ben euele wha*n* þe

9 **Fleumatic**] *corr. from* ffleu*ma*tic **13** **hoot**] *corr. from* hoost **17** **hoot**[1]] *corr. from* hoost (s *exp.*) **23** **Fleumatyk**] *corr. from* ffleu*ma*tyc

7 **wynter**] *in l.-h. margin:* co*m*pleccios acording | to the iiij q*uar*ters of | the yeere

su*n*ne or þe wynd ben northward, but þei ben weele whil it is estward or westward.

Now it is to know þ*at* in day *and* in þe ny3t ben þese iiij humo*urs* regnyng in eu*ery* body. For a day nat*ur*el is of xxiiij hour*es*, but to parte þe day *and* þe ny3t in-to iiij partes to co*n*s*er*ue þe co*m*plexiou*n* w*it*h here humo*urs*, þ*at* is be iiij tymes sexe. Blood haþ sixes houres and colre haþ sixe houres; so haþ fleume *and* so haþ male*n*colie. Blood regnþ fro iij houres aft*er* mydni3t tyl it be ix of þe clook be-fore noon. For-why blood is hoot *and* moist, so is þ*at* party of þe day hoot and moist. And fro ix a-forn noon tyl iij of þe clok aft*ur* noon regnþ colre þ*at* is hoot *and* dri3e, *and* so is þ*at* party of þe day hoot *and* dri3e. And fro iij of þe clok aft*ur* noon tyl ix of þe clok be-for mydnyth regnþ male*n*colie þ*at*
f. 3v is coold *and* dri3e, *and* so is þ*at* party of þe ni3th. And fro | ix of þe clok a-fore mydny3th tyl iij aftyr mydnyth regnþ fleume þ*at* is coold *and* moist, *and* so is þ*at* tyme of þe ni3th. And aft*ur* be-gynnyth blood to reugne a-3en.

Now haue j told of þe iiij humo*urs* w*it*h here p*ro*pirteys. Þ*er*fore, j thy*n*ke to write now how me*n* xal know be þe colo*ur* of þe vrine *and* signys, wych*e* humo*ur* regnþ *and* where he regnþ, and whan he is ful *and* is nat ful. And first at blood j wyl be-gynne.

3yf blood be moost plenteuo*us* in a sik-ma*n*, be þese signys þu xal know yt: The vryn xal be þicke, reed *and* fat, euenly by al þe body w*it*h a derk substaunce; hese pouse swyft, ofte ful, *and* sooft; þe veynys xul be ful in al þe body;

4 For] *corr. from* ffor **6 humours**] *follow. by* to parte þe day *and* þe ny3th in iiij parties **10 For-why**] *corr. from* ffor-why **24 yf**] *2-line space left for initial*

meche hed-ache in þe for-hed or in þe riȝt syde of þe hed. Þe spotel þ*at* þe pacyent spyttyt is swete in þe mowth; þe face reed *and* swollen; þe whyte of þe eiȝen xul be reed *and* blodful. Þe slepe of þe sanguyn bodys arn longe. By al þe body þe heete of nat*ur*el sanguy*n* is a lytil sowr in þe body. And here sorwe is moost aft*ur* mydnyth tyl ix a-fore noon. Þe veynys ben ful betyng. Þese signes be-tokyn þ*at* blood is moost plentiu*us* in þ*at* body þ*at* is of sang*ui*n co*m*plexion, and a-namelyche in ver *and* in som*er*, and in þe howres of blood in vsyng hoote *and* moist dietinges. Þe habundaunce of blood is j-seie also be þe kynde of a sicnesse þ*at* me*n* | f. 4r
clepiþ sinochus þ*at* is a feuer*e* ague for-whi me*n* knoweþ þ*at* blood is plentiuosse in hy*m* þ*at* haþ þ*at* feuer*e*. Also me*n* knoweþ be þese signes: Þe habundaunce of blood as in reed morphees, in reed bylys *and* in pestilence agues. Þese be þe signis of blood.

Þe signes of replecio*n* of all*e* man*er* of colre be þese, to know: Jf þe vrine is reed *and* þinne, w*it*h clere substaunce *and* a schi*n*nyng. But su*m*tyme be cause of indignacio*n* or by disturbacio*n* of humo*ur*s in þe body, þe vrine is mad þicke, oþ*er*-while w*it*h a whit scome, and oþ*er*while w*it*h a ȝelowe co*m*pase; his pouse steryng, swyft, *and* hard; sorwe in þe forheed dou*n* to þe mores of þe eiȝen, jn þe houres of colre moost, a-iij houres a-for noon til iij aft*er* noon. Þa*n*ne hese face wexþ pale as haschen, þe whyte of þe eiȝen ȝelowe *and* al

1 **hed-ache**] *corr. from* hed-age (age *canc.*; ache *interl.*) 7 **ful betyng**] *corr. from* fulbetyng 12 **for-whi**] *corr. from* ffor-whi

12 **for-whi**] *in r.-h. margin:* Sinochus (*underl.*) 15 **morphees**] *in r.-h. margin:* Red morphee (*underl.*)

þe body. For-why þe d*ri*nesse of þe tonge ofte-tyme þirstiþ w*ith* beynge in gret wakyng. Þe spotyl in þe mouþ is bytt*er*, his brakynge or his spewy*n*ge ȝelewe *and* bytt*er* as galle, *and* su*m*tyme grene. His digestio*n* ȝelewe w*ith* defaute of appetit of mete w*ith* gret desyry*n*g of drynk. Þe substau*n*ce of al þe body is dryȝe *and* lene be þe hete of þe wedur þorou f. 4v al þe body. Þese signys ben j-wo*n*t to be*n* of colre. | Jn þo bodys þ*at* ben of colric complexiou*n*, *and* in som*er* namelich*e* þorow vsyng of hoote *and* driȝe diety*n*g of þe kynde of siknesse, we seen þe habu*n*dau*n*ce of colre. Ȝyf it be w*ith* a feuer*e* þ*at* me*n* clepe causon, or w*ith* a t*er*cian, or w*ith* a jaundes jn þese signys, colre is to mych*e* ple*n*tiu*us*.

Þe signys of all*e* man*er* replecio*n* of flewme be*n* þese: Ȝyf it be nat*ur*el fleume, þe vrine is þan thyk, *and* whyt, *and* cremed a-boue. And ȝyf it be salt fleume, þa*n* þe vrine is su*m*del thyk w*ith* comy*n*ly substau*n*ce. Ȝyf it be of ȝelewe fleume or of sowr fleume, þa*n* þe vrine xal be w*ith* an indigestio*n* þ*at* mete is nat kyndly defyyd *and* be þ*at* vrine xal be þi*n*ne. Þese vrinys, jf þei haue spume þ*at* is of ventosite of þe pacient and su*m*tyme trouble be þe ground of þe vessel; here pouse slow, selden softe, *and* empti; greuouste of þe heed in þe nolle or in þe lyft syde for defaut of blood w*ith* a pale face; miche slowþe þorow al þe body; white eiȝen *and* al þe body whith; þe spotyl of hese mouþ nesche as wat*er* of þe nat*ur*el fleume or of þe ȝelewe, but þe spotyl xal be saltysch*e* of þe salt fleume, and of þe swete fleume hit xal be swete, and

1 **For-why**] *corr. from* ffor-why 5 **of**[1]] *prec. by interl.* to **of**[2]] *corr. from* tof (t *canc. and exp.*) 21 **softe**] *corr. from* fsofte (s *interl.*) **and**] *follow. by exp.* e

11 **causon**] *in l.-h. margin:* causo*n* 19 **Þese**] *in l.-h. margin:* no*ta*

it xal be sowr of þe sowr fleume; | *and* mych*e* spyttyng. Þei f. 5r ben slepful folk in dremyng of wyntrys *and* of reyn; *and* bein nat þirsty *and* mow wel ete, but it is longe ar it defiȝe eþ*er* it passeþ vndefiȝed; myche bolkyng, *and* wel farting, *and* gret roulyng i*n* þe wombe, *and* myche strief vnd*er* þe sydes. His ordure is whytisch*e*, wyndisch, *and* bladdrisch*e*. Hys brakyng or hys spumynge xal be watri *and* schyre whyiȝt. Fleume is wont to wexe plentiful in fleu*ma*tik folk *and* in old folk duellyng in colde cu*n*trees, namely in wyntres tyme in vsyng coold *and* moist dietyngis of þe kynde of sicnesse. We ha*n* know fleume by sup*er*fluite as in feuer*e* cotidians, jn apoplexis and paralisis, *and* in siche oþ*er*e.

We mowe know þe vniu*er*sel habu*n*daunce of malencoly þorow hese sig*nifica*ciou*n*s. The toknes of hy*m* be*n* þese: Þe vrine is wyth *and* þi*n*ne w*ith* a schynyng substaunce; and su*m*tyme wan *and* thykke, and ful of fleume or spume þorow þe medelyng of male*n*colys humo*ur*s; also þe vrine is su*m*tyme ȝelewe *and* þi*n*ne w*ith* his spume; his pouse selde *and* late, hard *and* voyd for þe scarsnesse of blood. Þe spotil in his mowth xal be sowr. *And* hese face wan or blackysch*e* and þe whiȝt of þe eiȝen blered; | and febyl of syth; f. 5v þundryng *and* synggyng in his ieeres; *and* al þe body heled w*ith* brownnesse; his digestion hard *and* swart; gnawyng in þe wombe w*ith* mechil wynd. Hys dremyng in hese slep is of dredful þingys and of blake þi*n*ges. Þese ben þe tokens of nat*ur*el male*n*colie. But of vnkyndly malencolie be*n* þese: ȝif

8 **whyiȝt**] *interl.* h **Fleume**] *corr. from* ffleume **fleumatik folk**] *corr. from* fleu*ma*tikfolk 18 **pouse**] *corr. from* poouse (first o *oblit.*; last o *interl.*) **20 mowth**] *follow. by exp.* is **21 þe**[2]] *interl.*

12 oþere] *in r.-h. margin:* Apoplexia

it so be þ*a*t it come of colour newly bre*n*t, þa*n* þe vrine xal be þikke w*ith* a mene substau*n*ce; hete þorow al þe body; blac face and al þe body j-died w*ith* blacnesse, *and* þe white of hese eiȝen; also coueityng to be a-lone; ful of heuynesse *and* of sorow; sour*e* breeþ *and* blac digestio*n*. And ȝif it be of old coloure j-brent, þe vrine is departyd w*ith* a blak face and al þe body is hyd w*ith* blacnesse; his digestio*n* blac; *and* þe oþ*er* sign*us* of male*n*colie. Male*n*colie is wou*n*t to be ple*n*teuouse in leene old folkes in coold *and* driȝe tymes þ*a*t vsen sich*e* man*er* of diety*n*g as coold þi*n*ge *and* driȝe. Be þe kynde of sicnesse, me*n* xal know male*n*colie þ*a*t it wexiþ ple*n*tuouse as in feu*er*e quart*e*i*n*s *and* in sych*e* oþ*er* sicnesse.

And for j haue wrety*n* sufficiently j-now of all*e* man*er* habu*n*daunce of þe iiij humo*urs*, now xal j schewe where eu*er*y humo*ur* haþ his d*omi*nacyon or his lordschipe.

[S]ome humo*urs* regne*n* in þe heed; su*m*me in þe
f. 6r stomac; su*m*me in þe lu*n*gys; su*m*me | in þe lyu*er*e; some in þe galle; some in þe splene; some in þe guttys; some in þe leyndys *and* in þe reynys; some in þe bladdr*e*; *and* some in þe mat*ri*ce of whome*n*. Now wel j telle of þe humo*urs* þ*a*t regne*n* in þe heed. For-soþe in þe heed al iiij humo*urs* han here d*omi*nacion, þ*a*t is to know: blood, colre, fleume, *and* male*n*colie. Ȝif blood be cause of replecio*n* in þe heed, þese ben [here] signes: Þe wo xal be worst be þe morow bifore al þe tymes of þe day; *and* greet hete in-to þe depnesse of þe heed, þe which*e* heete a-boute þe heed þorow þe touchyng of þe veynys may be know as in betyng of þe pouse and in þe veynis of þe tempyls w*ith* al þe toknes of sa*n*g*ui*nite a-for-

4 ful] *corr. from* fful **14 where**] *follow. by canc. twice* n **16 Some**] *2-line space left for initial* **21 For-soþe**] *corr. from* ffor-soþe **22 fleume**] *corr. from* ffleume **24 here**] *corr. from* owr

seid. And ȝif colre regne ou*er* alle oþ*er* humo*ur*s, þorow replecio*n* of hy*m*-self, hys sorow is moost a-bowt noon in þe riȝt syde of þe heed w*ith* alle þe signys of colre as j-seyde be-fore in þe secu*n*de chapitr*e*. Ȝif fleume wexe habu*n*dau*n*t a-boue oþ*er* humo*ur*s of þe heed, þa*n* his sorow *and* his wo is moost at mydnyt and iij houres aft*ur*; *and* þ*a*t sorow *and* wo is in þe lyft syde or in þe nolle of þe hed rysyng vp to molde of þe heed w*ith* þe signes and þe tokyns as j-seid be-fore. And ȝif male*n*colie þorow habundaunce ou*er* all*e* oþ*er* be moost replet, þa*n* his sorow *and* his wo is moost in þe lyft syde of þe heed, *and* namly at euensong tyme fro iij aftur noon tyl ix a-fore mydnyȝt w*ith* þe | signes *and* p*ro*pirtes be- f. 6v
fore told.

Aboute þe lu*n*ges *and* þ*a*t is in þe holownesse of þe lu*n*gys þ*a*t me*n* clepith þe chanel of hem, þ*er* regne iij humo*ur*s, þ*a*t is, fleume, colre, *and* malencolie. Þe habundaunce of eny humo*ur* is know þorow iij weys: Þe letty*n*g of þe spiritual me*m*bris is know as bi kouȝe *and* hoosnesse, *and* be þe man*er* of speti*n*ge, as is ȝelew colowr, blac, whiȝt, or grene; be þe substaunce of spety*n*g, as be þe þicnesse, or þe thynnesse, be þe viscosite; *and* þe slownesse of þe p*ar*ties. Ȝif fleume is moost replet in þe hollownesse of þe lu*n*ges, þese ben þe tokyns: hardnesse in takyng of breeþ, ofte-siþe w*ith* stuth *and* cowȝ; hoosnesse more a-nytȝ þan a-day, more in wy*n*t*er* þa*n* in eny oþ*er* tyme of þe ȝeer, more aft*ur* mete þa*n* by-fore mete, more aft*ur* sleep þ*a*n by-fore

7 **rysyng**] *corr. from* rysynge (e *canc.*) 9 **habundaunce**] *follow. by exp.* of 16 **fleume**] *corr. from* ffleume 22 **fleume**] *corr. from* ffleume 25 **in wynter**] *corr. from* inwy*n*t*er*

22 **fleume**] *in l.-h. margin:* No*ta*

sleep; his spotyl whyt, wat*ery* in þe mowþ, jn þe mowþ þi*n*ne *and* nesche j-teyȝed in þe þrote þ*at* it ne may come owt for viscosite of hy*m*-self w*ith* þe oþ*er* signes be-fore toold. And ȝif colre be moost plente, þa*n* is þ*er* hardnesse or streytnesse of takyng breeþ w*ith* hoosnesse [and] gret hete; and he xal fele hete in þe fundame*n*t of þe breest; þe hoote brestbon is depute dou*n* þorow towchyng; hese breþ hoot; *and* d*ri*nesse of þe mowth *and* harsch*e*; his spotil ȝelwe *and* þicke; *and* al
f. 7r þing to hym is bittyr w*ith* þe signys þ*at* | j haue toold. Ȝif malencolie wexe to habu*n*dau*n*t in þe holownesse of þe lungys, þa*n* is þ*er* streitnesse of þe breeþ, þe driȝe kow, *and* more aft*ur* noon þa*n* a-fore noon. And þ*at* he xuld vnneþe, for driȝe may brynge it forþ. And mychil coold he xal fele in þe depnesse of his lu*n*ges. Þe spotyl þ*at* þei spittyn i[s] bitter w*ith* oþ*er* signes bi-fore-seid of male*n*colie.

Also in some ȝonge folk it is j-seyn þ*at* blood regneþ in here lu*n*ges as be kynd of diu*er*sse syknesse of þe lu*n*ges as diu*er*se docto*ur*s han determynd in here bokys, as in chy*n*nckes postem*us* vnd*er* þe sydys *and* in þe lunges, for þe chynke is a gaderyng of diu*er*se humo*ur*s w*ith*-outen þe vessel of her humo*ur*s wexyng habu*n*daunt in þe vessel bitoknyng postemes. But ȝif blood bie þ*er* habu*n*dau*n*t be þe signes þ*o*u maist knowe: by rednesse in þe visage; grete ful veynys; gret hete in all*e* þe bodys; also his spotyl comeþ su*m*tyme fro þe heed, su*m*tyme fro þe stomac, and su*m*tyme

2 **ne**] *interl.* **9** **þat**] *catchword* (*in bottom margin*): j haue toold **11** **þe**[1]] *follow. by canc.* breest **14** **is**] *corr. from* it **16** **regneþ**] *interl.* last e **19** **for**] *corr. from* ffor **20** **humours**] *follow. by canc.* wexyng **24** **also**] l *interl.*

20 **of**] *in r.-h. margin:* Chynke (*underl.*)

fro*m* þe lungys, and su*m*tyme fro þe breest, and su*m*tyme fro þe sydys, and oþ*er*while fro þe checkys, *and* fro þe þrote. Ȝif þe spitty*n*g come fro þe heed, it comeþ by þe holys of þe palet of þe mowþ w*ith* a drawyng, raskyng, *and* w*ith* a man*er* smytyng fro þe chekys. But fro þe lu*n*gys comeþ no spotyl, but ȝif couȝe make hit. But fro þe stomac *and* fro þe brest | comeþ spotyl *and* spyttyng. f. 7v

Also iij humo*urs* waxen ple*n*tiu*us* in þe stomac: þ*at* ben fleume, colre, *and* malencolie; *and* haue þe same condicions as j haue told here-be-fore in þe ij chapitre of þis tretys.

Also þe same iij humo*urs* ben moost in þe guttys but þe knowyng of hem is be ordur*e*. For ȝif fleume is moost, þa*n* is þ*at* ordure whitysch*e*, wyndysch*e*, *and* bladdrisch*e*, *and* nesch*e*. Ȝif colr*e* be moost, þan is jt ȝelewe as v*er*gyn wax, hard *and* tow. Ȝif male*n*colie be moost, þa*n* is þ*at* ordure swart, hard, *and* blac w*ith* all*e* þe signes a-for-seyd. But of þe hete *and* þe d*r*inesse of colre comeþ a flux þ*at* men clepiþ lient*er*ie. *And* þ*at* is w*ith* mych*e* prickyng *and* gnawyng w*ith*-inne, myche bitternesse *and* þirst in þe mouþ.

Þe mylt is ofty*n*-tyme replet w*ith* iij humo*urs* forseyd, but p*r*incipaly w*ith* malencolye, *and* þa*n* w*ith* fleume, *and* þa*n* w*ith* colre. For þe mylte is a me*m*bir þ*at* is coold *and* driȝe, *and* angry; *and* liþ vnd*er* þe lyft syde; *and* is a receit of þe drastys of blood; *and* ofte is fyllyd aft*er* diu*er*se feu*er*es goyng a-fore, or of his owne febylnesse, or of stoppyng of hys pores, be þe which*e* stoppy*n*g, malencolie is browȝt to þe

12 **ordure]** *interl.* first r **For]** *corr. from* ffor **fleume]** *corr. from* ffleume **20** **with]** *follow. by interl. and canc.* iij *and exp.* humo*urs* **22 For]** *corr. from* ffor

21 and[2]] *in l.-h. margin:* no*ta*

f. 8r stomac | or in-to þe guttes þ*at* þorow his heuynesse is so cast out. Ʒif þe splene be so replet þorow þe humo*ur* of malencolie, þese ben þe signes: Þe vrine is þi*n*ne, *and* whyt, *and* cleer, *and* schynnyy*ng*, *and* ful of beemes; and oþ*er*while þorow his flowyng to þe lyuer*e* *and* þorow his medely*ng*, wha*n* þe þy*n*ne vrine is maad, þa*n* is þere sorow *and* swellyng vnd*ur* þe lift syde w*it*h myche hardnesse; þe disposicio*n* of þe body as it were safru*n* in colowr; w*it*h heuynesse; slombringe; w*it*h febylnesse; of sour bolkyng*es*; mych*e* breeþ as smoke; sour spyttyng; pale visage; þe white of þe eiʒen wan t*ur*nyng in-to an vnnat*ur*el colo*ur*; greuoste aft*ur* mete j-take w*it*h-owte digestio*n*; cryi*n*ge *and* swelly*ng* in his entrailes; his ordure wa*n* *and* bladdry w*it*h mych*e* wynd; mych*e* greuyd in t*ra*uayle *and* moost in goynge weyis *and* in climbynge on hillys or on laddres þ*at* it semeþ þ*at* here leggus woold fayle hem *and* her*e* wynd for þe heuynesse of here spiritual me*m*bris. Ʒif fleume is seyn ple[n]tiu*us*, þ*us* it may be know þa*n* þe vrine xal be whit *and* þicke, oþ*er* whit or þinne, *and* nat clere. And his moost sorow is vnd*er* þe lyft
f. 8v syde w*it*h alle | oþ*er* signes as j now toolde: For þe hiʒe partye is bolkyng þikke; *and* smoke full*e*; hys spittyng wat*ery*; *and* meche hete in hese paume of his hondys *and* in þe solys of hese feet; miche heuynesse a-bowte hese stomac w*it*h all*e* þe oþ*er* signes of fleu*ma*tik a-fore-seyd. To know ʒif þ*at* colre regne in þe splene, þe vrine is lytil *and* þi*n*ne, *and* greuouse of swellyng*es*, and miche hardnesse a-bowte þe splene, w*it*h myche woo in þe depnesse of þe entrailes; drienesse of þe mouþ, bytt*er* *and* þirsti, and oþ*er*-whyle myche brakyng *and* spuynge; þe face *and* all*e* þe body

12 digestion] *follow. by canc.* cry*n*ge **20 For]** *corr. from* ffor **24 fleumatik]** *corr. from* ffleu*ma*tik

3elewysch*e* as virgin wax, *and* lene *and* forwelkyd, w*ith* alle þe oþ*er* signes bifore of colre j-toold. Þat man*er*e of þe splene is but sylda*n* j-holpy*n*, namely 3if it be taky*n* in som*er*-tyme. Oon humo*ur* is wunt to be plentiu*us* in þe galle *and* þ*at* is colre, for þe galle is þe r[e]ceit of colre. Hit falleþ þ*at* þe galle is ofte repleet of to myche diste*m*p*er*aunce of þe lyu*er*e þorow hete, where-of it be-falleþ þ*at* colre bie gendryd in þe more qua*n*tite. And myche of his sup*er*fluite is an vnwurþi norschi*ng* of þe body *and* is sent to þe chest of þe galle of þe stoppyng of þe pores by þe whiche colre is browt to þe stomac *and* to þe entrailes. And to þe stomac colre is browt, þ*at* he xul bre*n*ne þe digestyf v*er*tue. And in-to þe entrailes it is brow3t, þ*at* it xuld brenne þe owt-pyttynge v*er*tue. For-soþe 3if þ*at* colre is plentiuouse in þe galle for þe hoote distemp*er*aunce of þe lyuere, | þis is his tokene: Þe f. 9r
vrine is þy*n*ne *and* reed, w*ith* a 3elewe spume or fatty of hys medlyng; colre is fele vndur þe ri3t syde; þe coloury*n*ge *and* þe chaungyng of þe body *and* of þe whi3t of ei3en in-to 3elewe colour, *and* his ordure al-so. 3if þe ouere poures ben stoppyd bi which*e* colre xuld be brouth dou*n* in-to þe fu*n*deme*n*t of þe stomac, þ*an* xal his body fro þe nauele dou*n*ward bie 3elwe and nat ou*er* þe nauele a-bout þe stomac, [and] noon digestiou*n* ache *and* cry in þe wo*m*be. 3if þe poures bi-neþe bien stopped, bi þe whyche colre xulde be dryue*n* down in-to þe guttes a-boute þe stomac [and] xal be brakyng and spwyng w*ith* alle oþ*er* signes of colre byfor*e*seyd.

2 **Þat**] *follow. by canc. and exp.* ma*n* 5 **for**] *corr. from* ffor 14 **For-soþe**] *corr. from* ffor-soþe

5 **for**] *in l.-h. margin:* no*ta*

Jn þe holownesse of þe lyuere þ*er* regne*n* iiij humours, þ*a*t is, blood, fleume, colr*e*, *and* male*n*col*e*. 3if þe blood be ful mych*e* repleet i*n* þe lyuere, þe vrine is þicke *and* reed w*ith* þe signes a-for-seyd of blood in þe ij chapitre of þ*is* t*re*tys. 3if flewme is ful repleet in þe lyuere, þa*n* is þe vrine whi3t [and] þicke w*ith* all*e* þe signes for-seyd of flewme. And 3if colre be replet in þe lyu*ere*, þa*n* is þe colour of þ*a*t vryne 3elewe *and* þicke, 3elowe as goold puryd, *and* burnyschyd w*ith* all*e* þe o*þer* signes a-for-seid. And ri3t so of male*n*colie.

Jn þe reynys *and* in þe lendus be*n* þese iij humo*urs*
f. 9v repleet, þ*a*t is, flewme, | colre, *and* malencolie, *and* namly in þe we[i]es of þe vrine. 3if flewme be ou*er*pletiu*us*, þese be þe signes: Þe vrine is whi3t *and* fat; but 3if þ*er* be ony o*þer* medelyng of ony o*þer* humours, scales as it were bren or scorff of þe heed, and smale þredis as it were herys; þe goute he xal fele in þe reynys and in þe bac; and coold in þe myd-wardys of þe leendys. 3if male*n*colie bie ou*er*ple*n*tiu*us*, þese been here signes: Þe vrine is swart, *and* þinne, *and* burblyng, and su*m*tyme þicke of þe lessyng of humo*ur* of male*n*colie þorow medlyng w*ith* vrine; w*ith*holdyng; longe resolvyng; w*ith* myche sorow in þe reynys. 3if colre be þ*er*ple[n]tiu*us*, þese be*n* þe signes: Þe vrine is lytyl *and* þi*n*ne or ri3t þicke of medely*n*g w*ith* colerik humo*urs*; þa*n*ne þ*a*t sorowe is scharp a-boute þe reynes *and* p*ri*ckynge.

2 fleume] *corr. from* ffleume **3 ful**] *interl.* **4 of**[2]] *follow. by canc.* þis **5 tretys**] *corr. from* trety*ns* **flewme**] *corr. from* fflewme **9 burnyschyd**] *interl.* last y **12 flewme**] *corr. from* fflewme **and**[2]] *follow. by* þe **13 weies**] *corr. from* weres

Jn þe bledd*er* only be*n* iij humo*urs* as j-seyd of þe reynes: flewme, colre, *and* malencolie. 3if þ*at* flewme be ou*er*plentiu*us* in þe bledd*ere*, þa*n* is þe vrine whi3t, *and* troubly, *and* ful of motus, as it wer*e* swa[r]mes of fysch w*ith* strangury *and* chaudepisse; miche sore in þe pyssyng, nat w*ith* ful streem, but as it were dreppynge; and myche ache *and* wo a-boute þe ers hoole, *and* in þe schaar, and in þe necke of þe 3erde. Ri3t so it is 3if malencolie bie ou*er*-myche r*e*plet | in þe bleddere, but more fretynge *and* p*ri*ckyng xal f. 10r
be twyn þe 3erde *and* þe ers hole goyng vpward *and* dou*n*ward; myche coold a-boute þe schaar *and* þe ers; and þa*n* þe vrine xal be swart *and* þi*n*ne oþur grenysch*e* w*ith* swartnesse þorow medely*n*g of malencolie humo*urs*. 3if colre bie repleet or habu*n*dau*n*t in þe bleddr*e* or a-boute þe bleddere, þese signes schewyn it: Þe vrine xal be ri3t bri3t *and* þi*n*ne w*ith* alle þe oþ*er* signes of flewme *and* male*n*colie, w*ith* gnawyng *and* p*ri*ckyng, but it is mor*e* hatt*ere* þa*n* þe oþ*er* boþ*e*.

Jn þe mat*ri*ce of women, comy*n*ly or su*m*tyme, it is repleet or ful mych*e* habu*n*dau*n*t oon of þese iij humo*urs*, þ*at* is to sey, fleume, male*n*colie, *and* colre. But for it is þi*n*ge of mych*e* p*ri*uyte *and* also for rybawdys, j xal rest at þis tyme to telle þ*er*-of tyl j-come at þe same mat*er* þ*at* j þenke to meue *and* to telle of. Now haue j toold of þe regny*n*g and of þe co*m*plexio*n* of þe iiij humo*urs* co*m*plexif.

J haue rad in diu*er*se bokys of philosophie þ*at* a ma*n* haþ iij man*er* of myst*er*ys w*ith*-i*n*ne hy*m*, þ*at* it to wety*n*, hootnesse, *and* drynesse, moystnesse, *and* cooldnesse þorow þe mynistracio*n* of þe iiij humo*urs*. And hit is knowyn þ*at*

2 flewme[1]] *corr. from* fflewme **9 and prickyng**] *in r.-h. margin*
21 fleume] *corr. from* ffleume **26 J**] *2-line space left for initial*

ʒif colre þ*a*t is hoot *and* driʒe may, þorow hese hete *and* hys
f. 10v d*ri*nesse, ou*er*come in a ma*n* | naturel flewme, þe whiche is
coold *and* moyst, þa*n* þ*a*t body falleþ in-to diu*er*se feu*er*es, as
in-to þe feu*er*e tercyan, symple or dowble, and in-to diu*er*se
maledies þorow retenues or for d*ri*nesse of þe blood in þe
veines for colre. For þe which*e* sicnesse, few þ*er* ben þ*a*t
scape*n* þe bytt*ur*hed, but þe holsomere medicynes be do*n* to
hee*m*. Or ʒif flewme be to-ryf and na*m*ly in an hoold body
þ*a*t haþ moost of þ*a*t humo*ur*, þe wych*e* is coold *and* moyst,
and may ou*er*-come nat*ur*el colre, þe whiche is hoot *and*
driʒe, þa*n* þ*a*t body falleþ in coold feueres cotidianes, and in-
to dropisies, fluxes, lient*er*ies, tooþ-ache, *and* to many oþ*er*
incomodites, as ʒe xul here here-aftur-ward. Riʒt so ʒif þ*a*t
oon humo*ur* may ou*er*-come an-noþ*er* humo*ur*, þa*n* þ*a*t body
falleþ in-to diu*er*se sicnesse. *And* þe sicnesse mou*n* be cause
of gret desesis or of deþ. But ʒif [þe] lechecraft be þe betere
and þe wysere ma*n*, loke to hy*m*, for þ*er* is noo bodyly
sicnesse þ*a*t hit ne mai wel be hoolpyn or ellys esid, ʒif it be
lokyd be tyme þ*a*t is at þe by-gynny*n*g wha*n* it comeþ furst
of a leche þa*n* kan good. But for as miche as many me*n*
f. 11r knowe*n* nat þe feet þ*a*t a leche xulde ku*n*ne, j þenke to | write
þe manere how þ*a*t a lech*e* xal haue hy*m* by-fore þ*a*t he come
to þe seke. Wha*n* þ*a*t he is sent aft*ur* to help þe syk pacie*n*t,
hit behoued þ*a*t þe leche were clene hym-self of gostly
sicnesse *and* of bodyly also, þ*a*t is, þ*a*t he be not in dedly
synne, neiþ*er* no vicyows ma*n*, for wyckyd vicys distreyen
many gode v*er*tues; for godenesse *and* wyckydnesse may not

6 For] *corr. from* ffor **17 for**] *corr. from* ffor **26 for**] *corr. from* ffor
27 for] *corr. from* ffor

24 behoued] *in r.-h. margin:* no*ta*

sta*n*d to-ged*er* for þe oon for-doþ þe oþ*er*. And þ*er*for*e* eu*er*y leche xuld bie a v*er*tues ma*n* and no qweed in hy*m*. And wha*n* he xuld come to þe sike, he xuld prey god in his wey to bie hese help in his ocupacio*n*. *And* þ*at* god wul fowche saf bi þe preieres of sei*n*t Mihel, sei*n*t Gabriel, sei*n*t Raphael þ*at* wery*n* j-sent to hooly me*n*, me*n* in erþe as to Tobie *and* oþ*er* þ*at* þei xulden preie for hy*m* þ*at* he my3te helpe *and* releue þ*at* ma*n* of his sicnesse 3if god wylle.

A ma*n* is maad of iiij eleme*n*t*es* as j haue seyd by-fore. Þ*er*for*e* what man*er* ma*n* wol wite what man*er* of sicnesse he haþ in his body, þ*at* xalt þow know by þe colowr of þe wat*ur* þ*at* comeþ fro þe forseid ma*n*. What man*er* ma*n* xal sye a man*us* wat*er*, he xal take a whi3t glas þ*at* me*n* clepy*n* an vrinal an take no man*er* of vrine of no ma*n* be-fore mydny3t, for þe vrine haþ no | colour tyl it be aft*ur* mydny3t. And þ*at* f. 11v
is kyndly whan þe ma*n* haþ sleped *and* takyn hys rest. Þa*n* tak þe vrine *and* stop þe glas w*it*h a clowth. And let it be schewyd wha*n*ne þe su*n*ne is vppe.

These vrines teche*n* what co*m*plexio*n* a man is of. Wha*n* þe vrine is reed *and* þi*n*ne, jt be-tokynth þ*at* a ma*n* is coleric*us* *and* haþ to mych*e* blood *and* to lytyl moystur*e* of þe wat*er* of kynde. And he moist be kynde [and] be hasty for þe skyl js þis, for in þe galle is a bre*n*nyng heete þ*at* þe moistur*e* haþ no my3th. Wha*n* þe vrine is whit *and* þick, þa*n* is þe ma*n* fleumatic. *And* he haþ to mych*e* spume of þe blood. *And* þ*at* ma*n* law3eþ myche *and* syngeþ gladly. Whan

1 for] *corr. from* ffor **5 fowche]** *corr. from* ffowche **9 A]** *2-line space left for initial* **15 for]** *corr. from* ffor **19 These]** *2-line space left for initial* **22 for]** *corr. from* ffor **23 for]** *corr. from* ffor

22 for] *in l.-h. margin:* no*ta*

þe vrine is þi*n*ne *and* whiȝt, þat ma*n* is male*n*colic*us and* haþ to mych*e* blood. And ȝif he is a blak ma*n*, he is liȝtly wrooþ.

These vrines teche*n* what man*er* sicnesse is in þe heed. Wha*n* þe vrine haþ a þy*n*ng ryng in þe vrinal, þa*n* is a ma*nn us* heed hugely stopped. Wha*n* þe vrine is þi*n*ne *and* cler*e and* þe ryng is reed, þa*n* is þ*er* to mych*e* blood be-fore in þe heed. Wha*n* þe vrine is blw, *and* clere, *and* lytyl, þa*n* is þe heed syk in þe brayn *and* haþ gret sicnesse in þe riȝt syde of þe heed. *And* þat comeþ of colera rubea, for sche liþ on þe same syde. Wha*n* þe vrine is þi*n*ne *and* þe ryng is whiȝt, þa*n* f. 12r is þe syk on þe lyft syde. | *And* þat comeþ of malencolie. Wha*n* þe vrine is whyȝt *and* þicke, þa*n* is þe heed siyk in þe necke. *And* þat comeþ of fleu*ma*tica þat comeþ of cowȝ. Wha*n* þe vrine of þe ryng is blac, þa*n* is all*e* þe heed siyk *and* comyly þa*n* falleþ a ma*n* in-to frenesye. Wha*n* þe vrine is ou*er*all*e* vnsemely *and* felawe lik to a whi*m*man*us* wat*er*, þa*n* is þe heed siyk *and* þa*n* is a ma*n* in gret p*er*ile but ȝif he be sone holpe*n*. Wha*n* þe vrine haþ a þick ryng *and* haþ lytyl foom a-bowte, þa*n* is þe heed siyk *and* þe breest riȝt feble. Wha*n* þ*er* is a ryng in þe vrine, þa*n* is þe heed siyk *and* þa*n* þe ma*n* haþ greet hete in þe body.

These vrines techy*n* what man*er* of feu*er*e a ma*n* haþ. Wha*n* þe vrine is reed *and* þicke, þa*n* [haþ] a ma*n* þe feu*er*es þat he xal wexe feble. *And* hy*m* xal come a sicnesse þ*er*-of þat hiȝt signa febris, ȝif þat feu*er*e come of ou*er*-mych*e* blood þat hatte þe feu*er*e t*er*cian. Wha*n* þe vrine is whiȝt *and* þicke, þa*n* haþ a ma*n* þe feuere cotidian. *And* he comeþ of fleume

3 These] *2-line space left for initial* **9 colera]** *interl.* e **22 These]** *2-line space left for initial*

6 clere] *in l.-h. margin:* no*ta* **25 signa]** *in r.-h. margin:* no*ta*

of coold nat*ure*. Wha*n* þe vrine stondeþ stylle *and* þe ryng quakeþ a-boue *and* is reed, þa*n* haþ a ma*n* to mych*e* moisture; *and* renneþ þorow þe rygge in-to þe heed *and* in-to þe body, þa*n*ne moste a ma*nn*us heed be siyk be resou*n*. Wha*n* þ*er* is mych*e* vrine *and* þi*n*ne, þa*n* begy*n*neþ þe feuere to come. And ȝif þe vrine bicomeþ blac, þa*n* wyl þe cotidian | f. 12v feuere t*ur*ne in-to a tercya*n*. Wha*n* þe ma*n* haþ þe feuere tercia*n*, ȝif his vrine be fyrst reed *and* þicke, *and* wexiþ whyȝt *and* þi*n*ne, and þe sicma*n* be ofte a-þirst, þa*n* xal þe sicma*n* ou*er*come þe feuere þe ij day. Wha*n* a ma*n* haþ a strong feuer*e*, *and* þ*er*e ben in his vrine smale stremys, *and* ȝif þe colo*ur* of þe vrine be blac, þa*n* may þe ma*n* neu*er*e bie hool. Riȝt so ȝif þe vrine be lytyl *and* blac, surely þa*n* is þe ma*n* fey*er*. Wha*n* a ma*n* haþ þe feu*er*e *and* his vrine is grene, in þ*a*t while þ*a*t he haþ þ*a*t feu*er*e, þa*n* comely comeþ þe palesie. Wha*n* a ma*n*nes vrine haþ a reed colo*ur*, þ*a*t is a signe of a feuere cotidian.

Þese vrines techy*n* to know þe sicnesse of þe lu*n*gys. Wha*n* þe vrine is reed *and* þi*n*ne, *and* is mych*e* þ*er*-of, þ*a*t be-toky*n*neþ þ*a*t a ma*n* is syk in þe lu*n*ges. *And* þ*a*t comeþ of g*r*et heete. Wha*n* þ*er* is mych*e* vrine, *and* it be whiȝt *and* þi*n*ne, hit betokneþ þ*a*t a ma*n*nes lu*n*ges be*n* for-frosen. Wha*n* þ*er* is myche vrine, *and* it be reed *and* þicke, þ*a*t be-tokneþ þ*a*t þe lu*n*ges ben broken or brysed. Wha*n* a ma*n*nes vrine is reed, *and* is me*n*gyd w*it*h blac, þ*a*t be-tokeneþ that hese lu*n*ges be*n* to hoote. Wha*n* þe vrine is þicke *and* pale, þa*n* is þe lu*n*ge syk of to myche t*r*auayle. | f. 13r

12 þan] *follow. by canc.* ma*n* y **18 Þese**] *2-line space left for initial*
20 man] *follow. by canc.* nes lu*n*ges ben for frosen (nes *also exp.*)

11 smale] *in l.-h. margin:* no*ta*

Ϸese vrines teche to know al man*er* sicnesse of þe mawe. Wha*n* þe vrine is riȝt þi*n*ne *and* liyk pale, þa*n* haþ þe ma*n* su*m*whatȝ in þe maw þ*at* is to mych*e* defied. Wha*n* þe vrine is whiȝt *and* þi*n*ne, *and* a lytil fatty, þa*n* is þ*er* su*m*whaȝt in þe maw þ*at* is nat defeid.

Ϸese vrines teche to know þe siknesse of þe breest. Wha*n* þe vrine is cleer *and* þi*n*ne in þe ground, *and* þicke in þe mydward, þa*n* is þe ma*n* sik in þe breest. Wha*n* þe vrine haþ a feble colo*ur*, þa*n* is a ma*n* j-stoppyd a-boute þe breeste.

Ϸese vrines teche to know þe stiches in þe syde. Wha*n* þe vrine is þy*n*ne *and* whiȝt of colo*ur*, lyk to a wy*m*man*us* wat*er*, or ellys whiȝt *and* þick, also lick to a wy*m*man*us* wat*er*, þ*at* be-tokneþ þ*at* a ma*n* haþ a stych*e* in þe lyft syde. Wha*n* þe vrine is reed *and* þicke, *and* of heuy cher*e*, þa*n* xal a ma*n* haue styches in þe riȝt syde. *And* þ*at* is mor*e* p*er*ilouse.

Ϸese vrines teche to know þe sicnesse of þe stoon *and* where he lyeþ. Wha*n* þe vrine haþ colo*ur* lyk mylk *and* is lytyl *and* þi*n*ne, þa*n*ne haþ a ma*n* þe stoon in þe bleddere þ*at* me*n* calle*n* oriyn. Wha*n* þe vrine is sondy *and* it semeþ in þe vrine flewme, þa*n* liþ þe stoon in þe fla*n*ke. Ϸis vrine techeþ to know þe sicnesse of þe flancke. Wha*n* þe vrine haþ long f. 13v stremys lyk heer, þa*n* is a ma*n* j-brisud in þe flancke. |

These vrines teche to know where a ma*n* is seke ou*er*-alle. Wha*n* þe vrine is liyk ray *and* smale stremes þ*er*y*n*ne, þa*n* is a ma*n* siyk ou*er*al. Wha*n* þe vrine is ray *and* haþ manye strem*es* or manye man*er*es of colo*ur*s, þa*n* is a ma*n* alle bresyd w*ith*-inne-forþ. Wha*n* þ*er* is mych*e* vrine and is

1 Þese] *2-line space left for initial* **6 Þese**] *2-line space left for initial* **10 Þese**] *2-line space left for initial* **16 Þese**] *2-line space left for initial* **20 flanke**] *corr. from* fflanke **23 These**] *2-line space left for initial* **25 vrine**] *follow. by canc.* haþ

of many man*er* colo*ur*s, þa*n* is a ma*n* syk ou*er*al þe body. Wha*n* þe vrine is pale *and* mylde, þ*a*t be-tokeneþ þ*a*t a ma*n* is not hool.

Þese vrines teche to know þe staat of sicnesse of wy*m*me*n*. Wha*n* a maydy*n* haþ pissed in a glas, þa*n* is þ*er* no corupcio*n* in þe wat*er*. *And* bi reson it xal be soft *and* þ*er*of lytil *and* of cit*ri*ne colo*ur*. Wha*n* a wy*m*ma*n* haþ co*n*seiuyd w*ith*-inne iiij daies or ell*e* w*ith*-i*n*ne iiij monþes, þa*n* xal þe vrine be þy*n*ne, *and* whiȝt, *and* clere, *and* mych*e* þ*er*-of, *and* a glos in þe botme. And wha*n* it is passed iiij monþes, þa*n* xal þe vrine be ou*er*all*e* þy*n*ne, *and* whiȝt, *and* in þe botme a þick glos. Wha*n* a wy*m*ma*n* is seik of me*n*strua, þa*n* is þe colo*ur* of þe vrine pale. Wha*n* a maydenesse wat*er* is drasty lyik a why*m*ma*n*n*us* wat*er*, þa*n* is schie syik of þe mat*ri*ce *and* vulua. Wha*n* þe vrine of a ma*n* is drasty *and* þe mat*er* synckeþ dou*n* to þe ground, jt is a tokeny*n*g þ*a*t he haþ dalt w*ith* a wy*m*ma*n* in schort tyme by-fore. Wha*n* þe vrine is þy*n*ne of colour *and* | lyik to clay or to bren, it be-tokeneþ a fals hert. f. 14r

A ma*n* þ*a*t wole helpe me*n* in here sicnesse hy*m* be-houeþ to know þe enchesou*n*s *and* þe kyndes of þe sicnesse, þ*a*t is to say, wheþ*er* þei ben hoote or coolde, oþ*er* driȝe or moyst. And þis is j-know be many diu*er*se toknes as by þe vrine, by þe pouse, by a ma*n*n*us* colo*ur*, *and* by many oþ*er*e diu*er*se toknes. And w*ith* goddus grace, we wolle*n* wryte of su*m*me sicnessys of þe body, *and* of here toknes, *and* of her*e* cures. And furst we wolle*n* be-gy*n*ne at þe heed, of þe

4 **Þese**] *2-line space left for initial* 6 **soft**] *corr. from* softe (e *canc.*) 15 **vulua**] *corr. from* devulua 18 **lyik**] *prec. by heading* heed-ache 20 **A**] *2-line space left for initial*

sicnessys of þe heed. And furst of þe ache of þe heed þ*a*t may come*n* to a ma*n* of heete, oþ*er* of coold, oþ*er* of d*ri*nesse, oþ*er* of moystnesse. And ȝif it comeþ of heete þese be*n* þe toknes: heete *and* rednesse in þe for-hed *and* a-boute þe eiȝen; and oþ*er*whiles an hoot rewme; reed vrine; *and* a swyft pouse; *and* lytyl sleep. Smoke *and* hoot eiȝyr neyȝen hym, *and* hoote e*m*plast*re*s, and oþ*er* hoote þingys. And coold þy*n*ges co*n*fort hym. And vnneþe he may suffre liȝt oþ*ere* briȝtnesse.

And ȝif it come of coold, he xal fele coold in hese hed, his face wol be pale, and his pouse slow, *and* hys vrine feblysch*e* j-coloured. And he xal slepe mych*e*. And coolde þy*n*ges neyȝen hy*m*.

And ȝif it come of moistnesse þ*a*t bie many sup*er*fluites, f. 14v *and* mych*e* sleep, *and* mych*e* dulschipe of wit. And of clene | moistnesse þ*er* comeþ no gret ache.

And ȝif it comeþ of d*ri*nesse, þe skyn wexiþ driȝe, *and* þ*er* ben few sup*er*fluites, *and* lytel sleep, *and* moiste þy*n*ges doon hym good.

And ȝif þe ache bi of heete, let hy*m* vse coold þy*n*ges, as wat*er* of endyue oþ*er* of rosees, and specialy sugr*e* roset and sugre of violet. And lete hym ky*m*be hese heed w*ith* a[n] yuory combe ofte-syþes, for þ*a*t is good in eu*ery* hedache. And let hy*m* waschyn hese feet w*ith* warm salt-water. And

5 oþerwhiles] *follow. by and* **an]** *in l.-h. margin* **16 moistnesse]** *prec. by heading* heed-ache **23 for]** *corr. from* ffor

1 ache] *in r.-h. margin:* heed-ache (*underl.*) **20 bi]** *in l.-h. margin:* m*anipulum* j **22 kymbe]** *in l.-h. margin:* no*ta* **24 hym]** *in l.-h. margin:* no*ta*

absteyne he hy*m* fro mych*e* waky*n*g, *and* fro mych*e* þow3t, and fro cu*m*peny of wy*m*men, and fro myche baþi*n*ge.

Sugre roset is maad þ*us*: Tak *pound* i of sugre *and* *pound* d*imidia* of te*n*dre rose leues, *and* sta*m*pe he*m* wele to-gedere tyl þei ben smale j-grond *and* wel j-medled w*ith* þe sugre. *And* þa*n* do þ*at* in an erþe*n*ne vessele *and* set it in þe su*n*ne xxx daies aft*ur* mydsomere. And eu*ery* day stere it twies, ones in þe morwetied, *and* ones in þe euetid[e]. But wha*n* xv daies ben passyd, tak *pound* d*imidia* of sugyr nat ful smal jground *and* medle w*ith* þe oþ*ere* w*ith* þi*n* hondes. And wha*n* þe xxx daies ben passyd, pit it in a box, for hit is good for eu*ery* flux of þe womb *and* euelys þat comy*n* of colre, þ*at* is to seie, of hete *and* d*ri*nesse.

And in þe same man*er* is sug*re* of violet maad. And þ*at* is good for al man*er* of vnky*n*de heet*is*, | and for sicnesse of f. 15r
þe breest, and of þe sydes, and of þe lyte, *and* of þe lyuere, *and* for þe cardiacle, *and* for þe feuere tercia*n*.

And 3if þe hedache be of flewme, þ*at* is to seie, of cooldnesse *and* of moistnesse, lat wasche*n* hys fete w*ith* warm salt-wat*er* eu*ery* ny3t. And let hy*m* ofte kembe*n* his heed w*ith* an yuory komb. And of þe askes of heihoue *and* ellerne bowes in grettere q*ua*ntite, *and* of askes of egremony and of betoyne, make li3e *and* wasch þ*er*-wiþ his heed, for it

4 **of**] *follow. by exp.* d*imidia* **8 euetide**] *corr. from* eueteid **9 of sugyr**] *corr. from* ofsugyr **11 for**] *corr. from* ffor **15 heetis**] *catchword* (*in bottom margin*): and for **and**] *prec. by heading* heed-ache **17 cardiacle**] *interl.* r **22 ellerne bowes**] *corr. from* ellernebowes **23 for**] *corr. from* ffor

2 and[2]] *in l.-h. margin:* No*ta* de sugyr | Roset *et cetera* **12 comyn**] *in l.-h. margin:* no*ta* **18 to**] *in r.-h. margin:* M

is good boþe for fally*n*g a-wey of þe heere *and* to do a-wey þe ache. And anoynte his heed w*ith* oile of elerne oþ*er* of seneuey. Also tak galbanu*m* *and* do it on a pece of leþ*er*. *And* lei it to þe place þ*at* akeþ. And mak a plaistere of whete mele, march*e*, wermot, heihoue, rwe, fenel *and* louache. And leue he male*n*coliouse met*es*, as oxe flesch*e* *and* venyson; and fleu*ma*tik met*es*, as whit met*es* [and] pork; *and* salt fysch, and fresch*e* fysch*e* þ*at* is ful fleu*ma*tic, as elys *and* cong*ur*. And ete he no*n* rawe peres ne applys, ne onyons, ne seche oþ*er* rawe þy*n*ges but notes. And vse sause of garlec *and* of pep*er*, gyng*er*, clowes, my*n*ten, peletre, *and* vinegre. *And* good cler*e* whiȝt wyn ben good for hym. And absteyne he hy*m* fro fastyng, fra*m* ydelnesse, fram wraþþe, wakyng, *and* fra*m* coold. Baþi*n*ge is p*ro*fitabyl, but not ofte-syþes.

But ȝif þe ache be of male*n*colie, þ*at* is to seie, of d*ri*nesse *and* of coold, late hy*m* vse al þy*n*ge as þei it were of flewme. But vse he oximel to purge hy*m* of male*n*colie, oþ*er* f. 15v symple | oximel oþ*er* componed.

Simpel oximel is [maad] of hony *and* of vinegre, [b]ut þe twey partes ben of vi*n*egre *and* þe þridde part is of hony. *And* þei xul be medlyd to-gedre ou*er* þe fier.

Oximel co*m*poned is maad on to man*er*es: Su*m* is maad of oximel sympille *and* of an-oþ*er* þi*n*ng j-pit þ*er*-to, as oximel squilytik and oximel of radik. Þe toþ*er* oximel co*m*poned is maad of oximel sympil *and* of many oþ*er* man*er* þi*n*ges.

5 fenel] *corr. from* ffenel **13 fram**[1]] *corr. from* ffra*m* **18 oximel**] *prec. by heading* heed-ache **19 but**] *corr. from* tut

1 fallyng] *in r.-h. margin:* no*ta* **3 Also**] *in r.-h. margin: dragme* M **4 whete**] *in r.-h. margin:* l*ibra* M **6 flesche**] *in r.-h. margin:* no*ta*

Oximel squillytik is þus maad: Tac an oynou*n* of þe see þ*at* is clepyd in Laty*n* squilla *and* do a-wey þe vttere schelles of þe oyno*n*u*n*, for þei be to hoote. And as mony as þ*o*u doost a-wey of þe vtmast, so fele do a-wey of þe inmast, for þei ben to coold. *And* tac he*m* þ*at* be*n* in þe medyl *and* seeþ hem in vinegre. *And* syþþe clanse he*m* *and* cast þ*er*-to þe þryd part of hony, *and* make it vp.

Oximel of radich is þus j-maad: Tac þe rote of radich *and* kyt it in-to smale þy*n*ne rolles, *and* seeþ he*m* in vinegre. *And* syþþe clanse it *and* cast þ*er*-to þi*n* hony.

Oximel co*m*poned is maad of many þi*n*ges. And it defieþ male*n*colie, *and* departeþ it, *and* makeþ it þi*n*ne. And oppeneþ þe weies þ*at* bien stopped of þe liu*ere* *and* also of þe splene. Tac þe rote of march, fenel, p*er*sile, calamyne, thime, rose-marine, sy*n*ngr*e*ne, *and* oþ*er* herbys þ*at* purgyn malencolie. And ȝif þ*o*u wylt haue it strong, do sene þ*er*-to. *And* cla*n*se it *and* siþþe cast þ*er*-to þ*in* hony.

And ȝif þ*o*u wylt | ȝeue a ma*n* oximel co*m*poned, ȝif f. 16r
hy*m* furst oximel symple. But ȝif þe hed-ache comeþ of þe sicnesse of þe stomac oþ*er* of ony oþ*er* sicnesse oþ*er* of ony oþ*er* me*m*bre, hele þ*at* sicnesse *and* þe ache wyl a-wey. And ȝif it come of myche wakyng, make hym to slepe. And ȝif it come of angur, oþ*er* of sorow, oþ*er* [of] mych*e* fasty*n*g, lat hi*m* leue syche þinges and drawe hy*m* to þe co*n*trary þynges.

6 **syþþe**] *corr. from* sy*n*þþe 10 **syþþe**] *corr. from* sy*n*þþe 12 **and**[2]] *interl.* 13 **þe**[1]] *follow. by exp.* veinys 18 **ȝeue**] *prec. by heading* heed-ache 19 **oximel**] *follow. by canc. and exp.* co*m*poned

And ȝif he haue domigrayn þ*at* is þe ache on þe on syde of þe heed, lat hy*m*m vse pullules of arabye, for þei be*n* goode for eu*ery* sicnesse of þe heed, and for eu*ery* ache of þe heed, and pu[r]geþ al noyful humo*urs* of þe brayn, and makeþ a ma*n* glad. *And* doþ a-wey heuynesse, and scharpeþ a ma*n*n*us* wyt *and* a ma*n*n*us* siȝt, and saueþ hese mynde. And suffreþ nat a ma*n* to be hoor ar hys tyme. And helpeþ me*n* þ*at* ha*n* turnyng of here brayn and þe demygray*n*. And þei ben profitabyl boþe to me*n* *and* to wy*m*men.

And þei ben maad on þis wyse: Tac of aloes epatik, *dragme* iiij; of brionye, of mastik, of baies of lorer*e*, of scamone, *and* of clowes, of euerich*e* of þese, *ounce* j. *And* medle þese w*ith* þe iuys of caul oþ*er* of fenel. And do þ*er*-to a lytyl hony for-to sauyn it, for hony wyl kepe alle manere medicinys þ*at* it is pit to fro*m* a-peiryng. And me*n* þ*at* han
f. 16v þe heed-ach*e* of eny humo*ur* in here | heed ne ete þei neþ*er* comyn, nyn anyse, ne oþ*er* aromatik þy*n*ges, for þei wolen heuy*n* vp smokes to þe heed þ*at* scholde encresce þe ache. And ȝif þ*er* be eny enplastre leid to þe hed, it moste be warm, þai it be of coold herbys, to a-bate þe hete of þe heed, for ȝif it bie leid al coold to þe heed it wole do harm to þe brayn.

Jn a ma*n*n*us* heed þ*er* bien many oþ*ere* sicnesses as wele as aches. And su*m*me sicnesses come of fume *and* smokys þ*at* fleen a-boute a ma*n*n*us* brayn, as turnyng of þe brayn *and*

1 syde] *follow. by canc.* onf **14 for**] *corr. from* ffor **17 for**] *corr. from* ffor **21 for**] *corr. from* ffor **23 Jn**] *2-line space left for initial*

2 lat] *in r.-h. margin:* q*ua* iij **4 heed**] *in r.-h. margin:* no*ta* de | pulul*e* | arabie **15 And**] *in r.-h. margin:* no*ta* **25 brayn**[1]] *in l.-h. margin:* Scotomye (*underl.*)

scotomie. Oþere sicnesses ben of humo*ur*s þ*at* ben j-turnyd to postem*us* in su*m*me party of þe brayn, as frenesi [þat] is a posteme of colre in þe furþ*er*e party of þe brayn; and woodnesse *and* liesyng of a ma*n*n*us* wyt *and* his reson þ*at* is a posteme of þe myd-brayn or in þe mydil of þe brayn; and litargie þ*at* is leuyng of a ma*n*n*us* mynde *and* makeþ hy*m* for-ȝytful *and* is a posteme in þe hindre party of a ma*n*n*us* heed; and epilencie þ*at* comeþ of [an] humo*ur* þ*at* filleþ þe parties of a ma*n*n*us* brayn þ*at* scholde be voyid of siche humo*ur*es, *and* makeþ a ma*n* for þe tyme to lesyn his wyt *and* his meuyng; *and* he liþ stille, as þei he were deed. Anoþ*er* euel is clepid apoplexie þ*at* comeþ of humo*ur*es þ*at* stoppy*n* þe pores of þe brayn, *and* makeþ a ma*n* to leue hese wyt for þe tyme *and* alle man*er*e mevy*n*ge, saue only breþi*n*ge. Þ*at* is differe*n*ce | be-twyx it and epilencie. f. 17r

Scotomye is sich a sicnesse of þe brayn þ*at* it makeþ a ma*n* to seme þ*at* he seeþ fliees oþ*er* blake þi*n*ges in þe eir. Turnyng of þe brayn makeþ a ma*n* seme*n* þ*at* al þyng þ*at* he seeþ as it semeþ to dru*n*ke*n* me*n*: Þ*at* þe hows gooþ a-boute hem *and* þ*at* þe wey riseþ vp a-ȝe*n*s he*m*. And þis sicnesse comeþ of þe stomackus greuance, oþ*er* of smokes, oþ*er* of hum*ur*es þ*at* bien a-boute þe brayn. And ȝif it bie of þe stomac, þese ben þe toknes: Þe herte leepiþ *and* haþ gret

2 frenesi] *corr. from* ffrenesi **6 litargie**] *interl.* last i **10 to**] *follow. by canc. twice* s **15 difference**] | *f. 17r* | ce **be-twyx**] *prec. by heading* Scotomye **16 Scotomye**] *2-line space left for initial* **18 he**] *follow. by canc.* seþ

2 to] *in l.-h. margin:* ffrenesi (*underl.*) **3 of²**] *in l.-h. margin:* woodnesse (*underl.*) **6 þat**] *in l.-h. margin:* litargie (*underl.*) **7 of**] *in l.-h. margin:* Epile*n*cie (*underl.*) **10 man**] *in l.-h. margin:* apoplexie (*underl.*)

greuau*n*ce. And aftur mete þe g*r*euance takeþ a ma*n*. *And* wha*n* þei bowen hem down, here brayn turneþ, þ*a*t is to seye, he*m* semeþ þ*a*t þo þinges þ*a*t liȝen stille re*n*nen a-bowten.

But ȝif þis sicnesse come of blood, þese be*n* þe toknes: His te*m*ples meuy*n* faste; heuynesse of hys browes; *and* mych*e* þouȝt of reed þi*n*ges, as of brenny*n*g lampes; *and* bledi*n*ge of þe nose; þicke vrine, *and* reed *and* derk a-boue as blood.

Of colre, þese ben þe toknes: bitt*er*nesse of mouþ, gnawyng at þe hert, þi*n*ne vrine *and* ful reed *and* ful derk a-boue.

Of male*n*colie, þese ben þe toknes: sournesse of þe mouþ, and ȝelewnesse of þe vrine *and* þi*n*ne-schipe, and wiþ-holdyng of fluxes þ*a*t a woma*n* is wont to haue *and* in þe eue*n*tide hir*e* greuau*n*ce is myche.

Of flewme, þese ben þe toknes: greuaunce aftur mete,
f. 17v *and* ache of þe sydys, and meti*n*ge | of wateris, *and* of reynys, *and* of whyte thyngys, and vnstabilnesse of þowt.

And ȝif þe greuance come of þe stomac, it lasteþ whiles þe smoke comeþ fra*m* þe stomac to þe heed, *and* afturward it cesseþ. And þ*er* is ache, *and* greua*n*nce, *and* abhominacio*n* in þe mouþ. *And* me*n* may felen how þe smoke goþ up in-to þe heed. And þe help þ*er*-of is to cast or to spewe. And gret metys þ*a*t vul not bie defied wel, þ*o*u xalt not ete. *And* leef late soperis, *and* grene met*es*, and coole wurtys, *and* strong ale. And benys *and* pesen, þ*o*u xalt not ete. But vse þ*o*u sich*e* met*es* þ*a*t wolle*n* esily be defiȝed.

But ȝif þe greuaunce comeþ of blood, letyng of blood is p*ro*fitabyl on þe hed veyne, *and* so it is in eu*er*y sicnesse of þe

17 of[2]] *prec. by heading* Scotomye

heed þ*at* comeþ of blood. 3if it is so þ*at* he þ*at* is seyk bie repleet of blood oþ*er* of ony oþ*er* humo*ur*, lat diete hym as it was seid of þe heedache. And vse he þese pullulees þ*at* purgen þe heed of euel humo*ur*s *and* profiteþ boþe to a ma*nn**us* si3t *and* to his heringe. And thei be*n* þ*us* j-maad: Tac of aloes þ*at* is wel j-waschy*n* *ounce* ij; of mirab*e* ci[tri], keb*e* indo*rum*, reubarb*e*, mastik, wermod, roses, violet, sene, agaric*e*, cuscut*e*, of eu*er*ich*e* j-lyche myche, *dragme* j. Tempere al þese w*it**h* þe iuys of fenel. *And* 3if þ*o*u wylt make yt scharp, cast þ*er*-to *dragme* vj *and* s*emis* of scamone y-poudered. *And* mak þ*er*-of gobet*es* of þe g*r*etnesse of fuch and 3if hym xj or xiij, [for] þei be*n* ful laxatif. And 3if þ*o*u wilt p*ur*gen hi*m* of colre, dowble or treble mirab*e* ci[tri]. And 3if it be for flewme, double | keb*e* *and* agar[ike]. And f. 17rbis 3if it be for male*n*colie, double ynde *and* sene. *And* þi*n*g þ*at* purgeþ colre, purgeþ blood.

A profitabil salt þ*at* purgeþ al þe humo*ur*s of a ma*n*nus heed, *and* it is good for akyng of ioyntes, *and* for þe podagre, and for þe dropsy, *and* is þus j-maad: Tak of salt armoniac, of cost, xii *ounce*; of blac pep*er*, v *ounce*; of comy*n*, gyng*er*, why3t pep*er*, fenel, canel, of eu*er*ich*e* a-leche mych*e*, *dragme* iij; of clewes, 3oduale, galynggale, quybib[e]s, cardamome, euene, *dragme* iij; of ysope, thime, origane, carwey, anyse, march, p*er*sily, loueache, euene of eu*er*ich*e*, j *ounce and* s*emis*. Mak of all*e* þese a pouder*e* *and* lat he*m* vsen it in stede of salt. And 3if þ*o*u wilt make hym laxatif, cast þ*er*-to

1 **is**[1]] *follow. by canc. twice* soþat **þat**[3]] *follow. by* it **2 humour**] *follow. by* 3if it comeþ of ony oþ*er* humo*ur* **14 kebe**] *prec. by heading* Scotomye **22 quybibes**] *corr. from* quybibos

17 profitabil] *in r.-h. margin:* no*ta*

ij *ounce* of scamone *and* ȝeue it hi*m* to drinke w*it*h meeþ. An-oþ*er* good salt þat purgeþ þe heed, *and* be-nemeþ þe derknesse of þe eiȝen: Tac of salt armoniac, vj *ounce*; of diagridi *and* of euforbe, j *ounce*; of pep*er*, gy*n*g*er*, comy*n*, fenel, anise, march, ameos, louache, cardame, p*er*sili, of eu*er*ich, j *ounce*, *and* make poudere. *And* ȝif hi*m* þ*er*-of a morwetyd iij *dragme* w*it*h wyn or w*it*h meeþ.

And ȝif þou wolt make delicat p*ur*gaciou*n*s for he*m* þ*a*t ben norisschyd in delices, make he*m* in forme of wat*er* *and* ȝif it he*m* to drynke. A[nd] take an herbe þ*a*t hatte eleborus nig*er*, *and* squ*i*naticu*m*, *and* esula, *and* sene, *and* seeþ he*m* in wy*n*, *and* distille þ*a*t into wat*er*, and late a ma*n* vse þ*a*t to purge*n* hi*m* of male*n*colie.

Also sugyr of borage is good in eu*er*y g*r*eua*n*ce of
f. 17vbis male*n*colie, and it is maad of borage floures | as suger roset is maad of roses. And ook apple*n* j-soden in wyn makeþ þe wy*n* medicinable to destreiȝen corupt fumes þ*a*t bien i*n* a ma*n*n*us* heed.

Ffrenesi is a bre*n*ny*n*g posteme in þe forþere party of a ma*n*n*us* brayn oþ*er* in þe skynnes of þe brayn. And su*m* apostym is of corupt blood, and su*m*me of corupt colre, and su*m*me of boþe to-gidere. And comy*n* signes þ*a*t folewen þis sicnesse is: myche wakyng, *and* lackynge of good wyt, wraþþe *and* woodnesse, *and* soden risyng*us* up, *and* sodeyn fallyng*es* dou*n*.

But ȝif it is of colre, þese be*n* þe toknes: gret wil to fyte *and* to smyte, drienesse of þe mouþ, blacnesse of þe tu*n*ge,

2 **An-oþer**] *corr. from* And (d *canc. and exp.*) 10 **And**] *corr. from* As 15 **as**] *prec. by heading* ffrenesye 18 **heed**] *interl.* 19 **Frenesi**] *2-line space left for initial*; *corr. from* ffrenesi 22 **comyn**] *follow. by* sicnesses

mych*e* scharp *and* bytt*er* ache, *and* mych*e* stery*n*ge of þe
hert. And his pisse is swart reed and is eiȝen be*n* to-swolle*n*.
But þe toknes of blood is a clene colo*ur* of þe visage.
And þei be*n* a-bowte to pulle*n* out strees *and* stickes of þe
wowes. *And* þei lacke*n* here wit *and* þreteneþ me*n* *and*
misseieþ he*m*. But ȝif it be nat a verye frenesie but is comy*n*
of su*m*me oþ*er* posteme, as of þe stomac oþ*er* of þe breest
oþ*er* in a wy*m*ma*n* of þe posteme of þ*a*t skyn þ*a*t a child is
co*n*ceyuyd i*n*ne, þa*n*ne þese ben þe tokenes: a gret pouse,
and a swyft, *and* a þick; *and* þe vrine is whiȝt *and* þy*n*ne.
And þe cause þere-of is, for þe | hoote coleric matere þ*a*t f. 18r
xuld make þe vrine reed *and* xuld come downward w*ith* þe
vrine, passeþ vpward in-to [þe] heed *and* makeþ a ma*n*
frentic. And þis sicnesse oþ*er*whiles is a sicnesse bie hy*m*-
seluen, oþ*er*whiles it foleweþ a[n]-oþ*er* sicnesse. Ȝif it be a
sicnesse bi hi*m*-seluen, it may bie þ*us* holpe*n*. Furst late
rubbe softly þe soles of his foote w*ith* vinegre *and* salt *and*
wyn. And ȝif he may not wel take a p*ur*gacio*n* for his heed,
make hi*m* a clist*er*ie on þis wyse: Tac þe hocke *and* þe
holyhocke, flax, sene, fenel, salt, *and* mercurie, *and* seeþ he*m*
in wat*er*. *And* siþþe cle*n*se he*m* *and* cast þ*er*-to hony *and*
oile. *And* lat hi*m* receyuy*n* it by hys fu*n*deme*n*t. Afturward
schaaf hys heed *and* ley þ*er*-to a warm plaastr*e* of coold
herb*e* to driue*n* a-wey þe smoke þ*a*t comeþ to þe bray*n*. And
aft*ur*-ward ȝif it nedeþ, tac a ȝong whelpe *and* slyt hym
a-two. *And* cast a-wey þe guttes *and* ley it al hoot to hese
heed. And wha*n* he is coold, ley þ*er*-to anoþ*er*, for þe moo
þ*a*t þ*o*u hast, þe betere it is. But ȝif þ*o*u haste but on wha*n*

4 **strees**] *corr. from* strees 11 **for**] *corr. from* ffor **hoote**] *prec. by heading* ffrenesye 12 **xuld**[2]] *follow. by interl.* come 16 **Furst**] *corr. from* ffurst 27 **for**] *corr. from* ffor

he is coold, cast hootte wat*er* in hy*m* *and* ley it to eftsones. And aft*er*-ward tac an ou*n*ce of popilio*n*, *and ounce* j of opiu*m*, *and* ij *ounce* of he*n*bane, *and* iij *ounce* of blac popie. And poudere þese *and* medele it w*ith* popilion, *and* wyth þe f. 18v milk of a woma*n* þ*a*t fedeþ a | mayd-chyld, and w*ith* þe iuys of si*ng*r*e*ne. *And* mak þ*er*-of a plast*re* *and* ley it warm on his heed neiȝ hese forheed. And ȝif his sleep a-swage hese foly, it is a good tokne. *And* ellys, it is euel. And wasch*e* hese heed w*ith* þe iuys of march *and* w*ith* vinegre, oþ*er* w*ith* oile of rosees, oþ*er* w*ith* þe iuys of solat*re*, *and* w*ith* þe iuys of march *and* oile of rosees. And lete hym by kept in mych*e* silence. And lat hi*m* be late blood in þe veine þ*a*t is in þe myddele of þe for-heed. *And* lat streyne þ*er*-whyle his nek w*ith* a twaile or a sauenap. And ȝif he blede nat j-now, tac a wat*er*-lech*e* *and* kyt of hese tayl. *And* do hy*m* in þe mydyl of hese for-heed a-boue þe nose oþ*er*e on þe temples be-syde*n* þe eiȝe*n*. *And* lat hy*m* sowkyn owt blood til þei haue sokyn as mych*e* as a blood-letyng is. And ȝif he is not holpy*n* by al þis doyng, tac þe iuys of letuse *and* of portulake, *and* medle he*m* w*ith* þe oile of roses oþ*er* of violet, *and* a dragme *and* an half of opiu*m*. *And* an-oynte þ*er*-wiþ hese temples *and* his forheed. And ȝif litargie comeþ to a fre*n*tik ma*n*, it is a token of deeþ. But ȝif frenesy come to hym þ*a*t haþ þe litargie, it is a good tokne. And it is p*ro*fitabyl to

1 **to**] *follow. by canc. and exp.* so efts 2 **of**[2]] *follow. by canc.* comy*n* 3 **ij**] *follow. by* iij (first i *canc. twice and exp.*) 5 **mayd-chyld**] *prec. by heading* ffrenesye 12 **blood**] *corr. from* bloood 14 **ȝif**] *follow. by canc. twice and exp.* ble 21 **þer-wiþ**] *corr. from* wyȝþ 22 **comeþ**] *follow. by canc. and exp.* of **to**] *interl.*

15 **of**] *in r.-h. margin:* no*ta*

strow his hows w*ith* coold herbys and to make coold wat*er* to renne nyȝ hys chaumbre. And in eu*ery* sicnesse ȝif it be fulgreuous in þe begy*n*nyng, worche w*ith* strong medicines. And ȝif þe sicnesse bie | esy, begyn w*ith* esy medicines. f. 19r

Manya is anoþ*er* sicnesse of þe mydyl parti of þe brayn *and* comeþ of aposteme in þ*a*t party. But oþ*er*while it is a sicnesse hy*m*-self, and oþ*er*whiles it foleweþ a-noþ*er* sicnesse. And su*m* comeþ of blood, and su*m* of colre, and su*m*me of male*n*colie. But of clene flewme, it comeþ neu*er*-more, for flewme is whiȝt as þe brayn is and þ*er*fore it may not a-peyr it. And ȝif it comeþ of blood, þe grewance is w*ith* lawyng. And ȝif it be of colre, it is w*ith* a fers woodnesse. And ȝif it be of male*n*colie, it is w*ith* mych*e* dreed. And ȝif it is of colre *and* male*n*colie j-meynd to-gedere he lauȝeþ *and* fiteþ to-gidere. And so ȝif it is of oþ*er* humours, jt haþ þe p*ro*pirtees of þilke humo*urs*. But comely þo þ*a*t han þese sicnesse of male*n*colie, þei han myche sorow, *and* drede mych*e* of þy*n*g þ*a*t is nat to drede, and þenky*n* of þi*n*g þ*a*t is not to þenkyn on. And he*m* semy*n* þ*a*t þei seen dredful þi*n*ges wha*n* þei seen no þi*n*ges. And he*m* semy*n* þ*a*t þei seen blak deuelus oþ*er* monkes þ*a*t xul slee hem. And su*m* wene þ*a*t heuy*n* wul falle a-dou*n* on he*m* and su*m* þ*a*t þe erþe wul falle vund*er* hem. And þei haue mych*e* desire aft*ur* lechys *and* aft*ur* medicines. And wha*n* þei han he*m*, þei tac lytil feiþ on-to her*e* wurdis. And þei desyr*e* to be in derk places *and* bi he*m*-selfen. But þo þ*a*t ha*n* þis sicnesse of blood loue*n* to walken a-boute ryu*er*es, *and* in þe feeldys, *and* in feyr gardyns, *and* liȝt placys. *And* þei louyn cu*m*pany

4 **esy**[1]] *prec. by heading* Mania **5 Manya**] *2-line space left for initial* **9 neuer-more**] *corr. from* ineu*er* (i *canc. twice and exp.*) **for**] *corr. from* ffor **19 seen**] *in r.-h. margin*

f. 19v *and* myrthe. | And ȝif hem lac sych*e* þinge, he*m* semeþ þ*at* þei be*n* neiȝ deede. But þo þat ha*n* it of colre loue*n* wrastelyng*es*, *and* fytyng*es*, *and* lepi*ngus*, *and* oþ*er*e dedisse of hardinesse, *and* cryyng, *and* mych*e* noyse, *and* sich*e* oþer þi*n*ges.

And ȝif þe sicnesse be of colre or of blood, it is j-holpen as þe frenesie oþ*er* þe heedach*e* þ*at* comeþ of heete. But ȝif it come of male*n*colie, he mote leue male*n*colie met*es* *and* vse met*es* þ*at* bien moist as fisch*e*, and ripe frutys, *and* borage, *and* sych*e* oþ*er* herbys þ*at* bien inscisif as calamy*n*te *and* mynte, and herbys þ*at* bie*n* dissolitif as fenel *and* p*er*sile. But he xal nat eu*er*-mor*e* vse moist met*es*, last his blood bie corupt *and* his co*m*plexion appeirid þ*er*-by. And þese herb*e* bie*n* p*ro*fitabyl for he*m*: arage, letuse, spinage, betes, purslane, oynou*n*s, karses, karlooc, anet, fenel, my*n*te, calamy*n*te. And þese met*es* þ*at* bie*n* moist bie*n* profitable, as lambren, *and* kydes of oon ȝeer, *and* soky*n*ge bestes, *and* he*n*nys, *and* chekens, *and* par*tri*ches, *and* sich*e* oþ*er*; also fisch*e* of ryu*er*es, smale *and* greet, *and* þe fisches þ*at* bie*n* nat ful fat, ne fisch of stony places. And lat he*m* vsen here met*es* j-diȝt w*it*h gyng*er*, *and* cardamomu*m*, *and* safrou*n* *and* clowes, *and* coliaundyr, *and* careawey, *and* comy*n*. And let hi*m* blood in þe neck-piȝt and co*n*forte hy*m* w*it*h m*ur*þe to pitte a-wey his heuynesse. And [if] þei fome*n* at here mouþe
f. 20r as a wood dogge þ*at* were | j-bete, it is a tokne of deeþ w*it*h-i*n*ne vij daies. *And* ȝif he cast miche *and* wlateþ boþe mete *and* drynk, *and* þ*at* lytil þ*at* he reseyuyth standeþ hi*m* but in

1 **myrthe**] *follow. by* And **And**] *prec. by heading* Mania **25 j-bete**] *prec. by heading* Mania

lytil p*ro*fite, ne he may not suffre neiþ*er* heete of þe sunne ne of þe feir, *and* may not slepe but lytil *and* liþ dou*n*-riȝt, þese been toknes of deeþ. And ȝif he haþ not þese signes, ȝif hi*m* pilules jmaad of wyn drestys *and* of whete flo*ur* wha*n* he is fastyng. Also tac of anyse, *ounce* j; of p*er*sily, iiij *ounce*; of pep*er*, iiij *ounce*; of epithime þ*at* is þe flo*ur* of tyme, iiij m*anipulum*, q*uas*i s*emis*; *and* ȝif it hi*m* w*ith* water*e*. And eu*er*y-þi*n*g þ*at* is good for þe feuer*e* q*ua*rteyn is good for þis sicnesse. And in eu*er*y sicnesse *and* liesy*n*g of a ma*nn us* wyȝt, aft*ur* hys p*ur*gacion, lete hy*m* be cuppyd in to þe neþ*er* sydes of þe heed a lytil a-boue þe necke, oþ*er* be-twy*n*ne þe too schuldyr-bladys. And in eu*er*y lesyng of a ma*nn us* wiȝt, make hi*m* a clist*er*ie in þe be-gynnyng of my*n*te, *and* rewe, *and* sich*e* oþer*e* þinng*us*. And it p*ro*fiteþ to sich*e* a ma*n* to bathyn hym oþ*er*whiles, but to dwelle þ*er*-i*n*ne a lytil while. And a special medicine for þis sicnesse is lapis armonic*us* j-ȝeuy*n* in pilulees oþ*er* in decocciou*n*s, j-wasche oþ*er* onwasche, but vnwassch*e* wul make a ma*n* to caste. And ȝif all*e* þese medicinis helpeþ hi*m* nauȝt, þe laste remedie is to sliȝt þe skyn *and* oppy*n* þe skulle. | f. 20v

Ljtargie is a sicnesse þ*at* makeþ a ma*n* so forȝetefull*e* þ*at* wha*n* he haþ j-do a þi*n*g, he ne haþ no mynde þ*at* he dede it. And þis sicnesse comeþ oþ*er*-whiles of to mych*e* corupt flewme in a ma*nn us* heed, oþ*er*wile of aposteme þ*at* is in þe

9 mannus wyȝt] *corr. from* ma*nn us*wyȝt **10 to þe**] *corr. from* þe to **12 And**] *follow. by canc. and exp.* ȝif **13 mannus**] *follow. by canc.* wy*n*ny*n*g **15 man**] *follow. by canc. twice* þat **17 in**[2]] *follow. by canc.* decocci*us* **19 laste**] *follow. by canc.* retme **21 Ljtargie**] *2-line space left for initial; prec. by heading* Litargye

1 þe] *in r.-h. margin:* tokens | of death (*written with pencil*)
18 onwasche] *in r.-h. margin:* no*ta*

he*n*drer*e* party of a ma*nn* *us* heed þ*er*-as his mynde is. And ȝif it is of aposteme, þese bie*n* þe toknes: a continuel feuere, mych*e* sleep, forȝetfulnesse. Wha*n* þei bie*n* j-clepid, vnneþe þei volle*n* answere. And wha*n* here mouþ is opened, vnneþe þei mown clo*n*synd. And þis sicnesse is clepyd a coold frenesie. But ȝif it come of flewme, þese bie*n* þe tokenys: His vrine is turbul as mare pisse; hese pouse is sooft *and* greet; his sleep is dee[p] *and* heuy; his breþi*n*g is slow *and* greuouse. Ȝif it come of flewme *and* colre j-medelyd togid*ere*, þa*n* þe toknes of he*m* bie*n* j-medeled, for his vrine is more reed *and* his pouse is mor*e* swyftt*ere*. Tokenys of deeþ in þe sicnesse bien ȝelwnesse in þe face, *and* qwaky*n*g *and* tremelyng of a ma*n*nys body *and* of hese face, *and* swety*n*g of þe heed wha*n* þe body sweteþ not by-neþen. Also a waterlech*e* wol not cleue*n* on sich*e* a ma*n* to souke*n* owt his blood.

A purgacion to p*ur*ge*n* his heed: Tac of aloes, *ounce* j *and dragme* ij; of agaric, stikades, of eu*ere* eiþ*er*, *dragme* iij; of mastic, spiccassie, canel, clowes, of sq*ui*nantu*m*, gyng*er*, of eu*ery*ch*e*, *dragme* j *and* s*emis*. Mak þereof puleles of þe
f. 21r q*ua*ntite of an ey*n* *and* ȝif | hi*m* þ*er*-of at on*us* *dragme* iij w*it*h warm wat*er*. And mak hi*m* to fnese w*it*h castory, piretre, pep*er*, staphie, nygelle, *and* sich*e* oþ*er*. And let hi*m* chewe þe same þi*n*ges in his mouþ. And mak a plastre on þe mouþ of þe stomac of su*m* hote oile, as oile of rew or sich*e* oþ*er*, *and* schepis wolle þ*at* was j-schor*e* vn-wasch*e*. And

5 clonsynd] l *oblit.*; *in l.-h. margin:* l **8 deep**] *corr. from* deeþ **9 of**] *follow. by canc. twice* l **11 pouse is**] *corr. from* pouseis **21 him**] *prec. by heading* Litargie **22 fnese**] *interl.* first e **23 oþer**] *follow. by canc. and* schepis wolle þ*at* was j-schor*e* vn-wasch*e* and a-noynte hese heed w*it*h oile of rew

anoynte hese heed w*ith* oile of rew, and w*ith* þis oyneme*nt*: Tac of euforbe, piretr*e*, seneuey, affodille, castori, long pep*er*, of eu*er*iche, *ounce* j. Seþ he*m* in þe iuys of rew *and* [in] a good q*ua*ntite of oile til þe iuys bie co*n*sumyd. And cast þ*er*-to a lytyl wex *and* lei it on his heed. Oile of castory is p*ro*fytabyl to he*m*, and oile of peretr*e*, *and* of elerne also. Anoþ*er*: Tac of affodille, piretr*e*, seneuei, of eu*er*iche, *ounce* j *and* vij *dragme*; of castore, *and* euforbe, of eiþ*er*, vij *dragme*. Tempre he*m* w*ith* iuys of wermot *and* of samsuke. *And* anoynte þ*er*-w*ith* þi*n* heed in þe hyndrere p*ar*tie. A-noþ*er*: Tac cley þ*at* is j-bake in a[n] ouene *and* medelyd w*ith* þe iuys of rewe *and* of sich*e* oþ*er*e hoote herbys, *and* ley on his heed. But ȝif his litarge bie w*ith* a feuere, it makeþ hi*m* boþe heuy of sleep *and* for-ȝetful. *And* þ*at* feuer*e* comeþ of aposte*m* in þe hyndrer*e* p*ar*ty of a ma*nnus* heed. And þa*n* þ*o*u xalt legge*n* hym in a liȝt place þ*er*-as he may be-holdyn waky*n*g. And lat hi*m* haue mych*e* | talkyng *and* mych*e* noyse a- f. 21v
bowte*n* hy*m* to lette*n* hym fro sleep. And let his dietyng bie w*ith* coold, þ*at* is to sey, nat to coold. And let hy*m* vse coold surripis, as of violet oþ*er* of roses, *and* sugre roset oþ*er* sug*re* of violet. And late he*m* frote*n* here feet *and* here hond*es* w*ith* vinegre *and* salt. And late he*m* smelly*n* oþ*er*-whiles su*m* stynckyng þi*n*gys, as þe smoke of a que*n*ched candele, oþ*er* ma*nnus* heer j-brent, oþ*er* hert*es*-horn j-brent. And in noon litarge ley coold þi*ngus* to þe heed, but lat schaue þe heed and a-noynt it w*ith* þi*n*ges þ*at* bie*n* te*m*porat, as castore j-te*m*pred w*ith* þe iuys of march oþer of fenel.

10 **anoynte]** *follow. by And* anoynte **16** **be-holdyn]** *interl.* l
17 **talkyng]** *prec. by heading* Litargie **24** **hertes-horn]** hert*es* *follow. by canc.* hor; *in l.-h. margin:* horn

A profitable clistere to make þe mater neisch*e* *and* þe more able to bie j-clensyd: Tac bietes, *and* hockes, *and* m*er*curie, *and* violet, *and* seeþ he*m* wel in wat*er*. *And* siþe cle*n*se it *and* cast þ*er*-to oile of violet oþ*er* oile de olyue, *and* a lytil botyr. *And* lat hi*m* receyue*n* þ*er*-of þe wheiȝte of a pound at oones. And ȝif þ*o*u wult, þ*o*u myȝtest seeþe þ*er*-i*n*ne hocke rootes, *and* femygrek, *and* lynseed.

A clistre mu*n*dificatif: Tak wermod, *and* soþ*er*newode, *and* calamynte, *and* origa*n*, *and* mynte, *and* mercurie, *and* seeþ he*m* in salt-wat*er*. *And* clense it *and* siþþe cast þ*er*-to whete bry*n*. *And* cla*n*se it eft-sonys *and* cast þa*n* þ*er*-to iij *dragme* of hony, *and* ij *dragme* of mete oile, *and* j *dragme* of sal-ge*m*me.

A suppositorie þ*o*u myȝtest make also of hony j-sode til it be þicke. *And* syþþe*n* j-schape*n* as a ma*n*nys lytil fyng*er* and pyt it in at his fu*n*deme*n*t. And for-to make suppositorys esyly to entre in me*n*, vseþ to a-noynte*n* hem f. 22r w*ith* oile or bot*er*e | to make he*m* þe slyderere. Oþ*er* þu myȝtest make þi suppositorys of boles galle, sal-ge*m*me, *and* mouse drit j-medlyd to-gedere. But suppositories for childre*n* xul be maad w*ith* lard, oþ*er* of sugre, *and* salt, *and* oile, *and* vinegre j-sode to-gidere til it be þicke. And þu myȝtest make suppositories for me*n* oþ*er* for wome*n* of hony ysode til it be þicke, *and* siþþe cast þ*er*-to þe galle of su*m* beste *and* namly of a bole. And wha*n* þi hony is ner*e* soden j-now, tac sal armoniac, oþ*er* sal-ge*m*me, oþ*er* nitr*e*, oþ*er* affr[i]cane, oþ*er* euforbe, oþ*er* peletre of spayne, oþ*er* þe

7 femygrek] *corr. from* femy*n*grek **18 botere**] *catchword* (*in bottom margin*): to make he*m* **to**] *prec. by heading* Lytargye

mylk of a fig tr*e*, oþ*er* of [t]itymalle, oþ*er* of scamone, oþ*er* sich*e* oþ*er* thyngis. And a-noynt þi*n* suppositories w*ith* oile.

And vnd*er*stand þ*at* clist*er*ies *and* suppositoris xul be ȝoue*n* to me*n* þ*at* bien costyf oþ*er* ne haue nat good delyueraunce by-neþe. But clist*er*es xul be ȝoue to strong men of co*m*plexio*n*; suppositories a ma*n* may take þouȝ he bie riȝt sike *and* feble. And me*n* þ*at* ha*n* þis sicnesse w*ith*-oute*n* feuere xul be dietid w*ith* þi*n*ges þ*at* bien te[m]p*er*at, þ*at* is, hoot *and* moist.

A good electuarie þ*at* restoreþ a ma*nn*us mende *and* co*n*forteþ hese brayn *and* al his body: Tac of canel, roses, violet, gyng*er*, cardamo[me], of eu*er*ich*e*, ij *ounce*; of dragagantu*m*, anthes, bawme þ*at* is an herbe, maiorane, þe rynde of myrtille, cip*er*i, liquoriys, siler*e*, of eu*er*ich*e*, ij *ounce*; sq*ui*na*n*tu*m*, spik, clowes, q*ui*bibes, folij, galange, aua*n*nce, borage, sene, bren, spodie, coral, mastik, macropip*er*, storax, brend | silk, of eu*er*iche, *ounce* d*imidia*, and *dragme* j; of sirip of roses, *quantum* s*ufficit*. f. 22v

Epilencie is þe fallyng euel, *and* hit comeþ of a moist humo*ur* þ*at* fulfilyeþ þilke places of þe heed þ*at* xuldy*n* bie*n* voide, *and* stoppeþ þe he*n*drere part of þe heed þ*er*-as is þe begynnyng of þe sicnesse, *and* febleþ þe senewes. And þ*er*-fore wha*n* þe accesse of þis sicnese comeþ to a ma*n*, it makeþ hi*m* for a tyme to liese hese felyng *and* his meuy[n]ge. And oþ*er*-while þe sicnesse comeþ of humo*ur*s þ*at* bien in þe heed, and þa*n* it is clepid epilencie. And oþ*er*while it comeþ

1 **titymalle**] *corr. from* citymalle 4 **þat**] *follow. by canc.* capeþ hi*m* **6 suppositories**] *interl.* e **17 silk**] *prec. by heading* Epilencye **18 and**] *interl. dragme* **19 Epilencie**] *2-line space left for initial*

6 men] *in r.-h. margin:* no*ta*

of fumes þ*a*t come*n* in-to þe heed out of a syyk *and* a feble stomac, *and* þa*n* it is clepid analempsie. And oþ*er*-whiles it comeþ of greuances of oþ*er* me*m*bres, *and* þa*n* it is clepid catalempsie.

But of epilencie þ*er* bien to k[i]ndys, þe more *and* þe lasse. Jn þe more epilencie, þe p*ri*ncipal places of þe brayn ben alto-gedere j-stopped. Where-fore in here accesse, þei ne feleþ no-þing, *and* vimeþ at here mouþe, *and* al here body quakeþ, and it is ful hard to hele he*m*. Jn þe lasse epile*n*cie, þe p*ri*ncipal places bien j-stopped but nat alle to-gydere, *and* þ*er*-fore in accesse þei fele*n* su*m*qwhat, and alle þe body ne q*ua*keþ nat, but þe hyndrer*e* party of þe heed. And in epile*n*cie, tre*m*blyng of þe body is an euel signe, but in þe f. 23r palasie it is a good signe. Vomynge here is a good | signe, but in apoplexie it is an euel signe. And þe oft*e* þ*a*t þei falle*n* dou*n* *and* ryse vp sone a-ȝe*n*, þe bet*er* signe it is *and* þe raþere þei mowu*n* bie j-holyd. And ȝif a woma*n* haue þis sicnesse in here ȝouþe *and* bie nat j-heleed, wha*n* sche be-gynnyth to haue here floures xe xal neu*er* bie hool.

And ȝif þis sicnesse bie of humo*urs* þ*a*t bien in þe heed, þese bee*n* þe toknes: heuynesse of þe heed *and* co*n*fusio*n* of here wiȝtt*es*, slouþe, d*ym*nesse of þe eiȝen, bity*n*g of here tu*n*ge, and here pisse, *and* here kynd, *and* here dryȝt passe*n* a-wey fro he*m* a-ȝens here wyl, and so þei falle*n* down *and* mown j-fele no-þing, and namly in þe grett*er* epilencie. And ȝif þe sicnesse bie of flewme, þ*o*u maist know it be þe toknys of flewme, as bi softnesse, *and* whiȝtnesse, *and* slouþe, *and* myche sleep. And ȝif it be of male*n*colie, þ*o*u maist knowe*n* it bi blacnesse, *and* leeneschipe, *and* oþ*er* toknes of

5 **kindys**] *corr. from* kendys (e *exp.*) 14 **signe**[2]] *prec. by heading* Epilencye 22 **wiȝttes**] *follow. by canc. twice* l

male*n*colie. 3if it be of hem boþe to-gydere, þe toknes be*n* j-medlyd to-gedere.

Analempsie comeþ of a fume oþ*er* of a smoke of þe stomac [þat is] male*n*colik. Þe toknes here-of bien: abhominaciou*n* to mete *and* to drynk, tre*m*blyng of þe hert, p*ri*ckyng of þe stomac, and fleu*ma*tic metys *and* male*n*colies doiþ he*m* harm. And oþ*er*-whiles þei falle*n* not, but bie*n* ful feble | a-boute þe tyme of here accesse. And þis sicnesse may f. 23v bie of flewme, of colre, of male*n*colie; and of wych*e* of he*m* it is, þ*ou* maist know bie þe signes of þe humo*ur*s.

Catalempsie comeþ of a venemouse smoke þ*a*t comeþ fra*m* fer in-to þe heed *and* þ*er* he is coold. And þis smoke comeþ of a blood þ*a*t is bri3t *and* bre*n*nyng in su*m*me party of a ma*n*nys body. And þ*er*fore it makeþ a ma*n* ful hoot w*ith*-oute-forþ *and* to haue a swyft breþynge. *And* a-frai3en ful mych*e* here ei3en *and* ofte-syþes make*n* he*m* swonnen. *And* þei han oþ*er*while a feuere þ*er*-wiþ. And þei me clepe he*m* in þe tyme of here accesse, þei 3eue noon answere. And 3if þei speke*n*, þei greue he*m* sore. *And* han an hoot swete in þe deliu*er*aunce of here accesse and here breeþ stinckeþ oþ*er*whiles. And 3if any of þese þre maneris vome*n* myche *and* white [when] þei bie*n* j-falle*n* a-dou*n*, *and* streynen here teeþ to-gedere, þa*n*ne it is of flewme. And 3if he closeþ hese ei3e*n* as þau3 he slepte *and* vomeþ no-þi*n*g, but a-riseþ up sone, þa*n* it is of colre. But 3if he wexeþ blac, and t*ur*neþ a-syde hese mouþ, *and* streyneþ hese hondys to-gedere, *and* liggeþ stille as þau3 he wold bie deed, *and* vomeþ but litil, þa*n* it is of male*n*colie.

4 is] *corr. from* oþer **8 a-boute]** *prec. by heading* Epilencie **25 colre]** *follow. by canc. and exp.* But

Me*n* þ*a*t ha*n* epile*n*cie oþ*er* analempcie xul bie dietid w*ith* met*es* þa*n* bie*n* te*mp*e*r*at j-hoot. But þei þ*a*t ha*n* f. 24r cathalempsie | xul bie dietyd w*ith* met*es* þ*a*t bie*n* te*mp*e*r*ad coold and þese met*es* bien good for hem: hennys, fesauntȝ, part*ri*che, *and* sich*e* oþ*er*e, and scaled fysch, *and* borage, *and* p*er*sile, *and* fenel, *and* good clere wyn. But ȝif it be for þilke þ*a*t han cathalempsie, absteyne þei he*m* fro male*n*colies met*es* as beef *and* alle man*er* of coole wort*es*, biene*n* *and* pesu*n*, mylk *and* oþ*er* whiȝt metis, and fram beetis, *and* march*e*, *and* oþ*er* salt metis, *and* soure met*es* *and* roostid oþ*er* fried, and fram wat*er* foulys, *and* fisches of myry wat*er*es, and fra*m* hert*es* flesch*e*, *and* schepis flesch*e*, *and* swynes flesch*e*, and fra*m* notys *and* applys, *and* barlich*e* breed *and* riȝe breed *and* oote breed, *and* fra*m* baþi*n*ge, *and* fra*m* whome*n* co*m*pany, fra*m* wraþþe *and* fro c*ri*ynge.

And ȝif hi*m* oximel sq*ui*litik, oþ*er* oximel of radich*e*, oþ*er* þis oximel to defiȝe þe mat*er*e of his sicnesse: Tac þe sedys of pyony, *and* sauge, *and* wirmode, netlene, horhowne, laue*n*dre, *and* auence, *and* carses, *and* sene. *And* make w*ith* he*m* oximel *and* cast þ*er*to þe sedys þ*a*t brekeþ þe stoon. But to þe*m* þ*a*t ha*n* catolempsie, pyt borage, *and* yp*er*icou*n*, *and* cuscut*e*, *and* ephitime. And an-othir oximel: Tak þe poudere of heuforbie, *and* s[t]aphie, *and* piretre, *and* piliole, *and* siche oþ*er*e, *and* seeþ he*m* in vinegr*e* *and* in wy*n*. *And* siþe make vp þi*n* oximel.

Aft*ur* þis ȝif hy*m* a p*ur*gacion: Tac aloes, þe wylde gourde þ*a*t is clepyd coloq*ui*ntida in Latyn, bodellie,

3 xul] *prec. by heading* Epilencie **7 cathalempsie**] *follow. by* and **11 myry**] *corr. from* meyry (e *exp.*; first y *interl.*) **15 fram**[2]] *corr. from* ffra*m* **22 poudere**] *follow. by canc.* of eufobie **23 staphie**] *corr. from* scaphie

opoponac, eleborus nig*er*, gu*m*me arabik, of eu*er*ich*e*, *ounce* ij; of euforbe, | *ounce* s*emis*. Mak pillules here-of w*it*h iuys f. 24v of horhoune. Lapis armonic*us* is ful p*ro*fitable her*e*. Aft*ur* iiij daies, let hy*m* blood at þe heed veyne. *And* ȝif he haue myche blood, lat hi*m* bie garsyd *and* j-cuppid in þe necke.

A good pociou*n*: Tak a porcio*n* of sauge, of pyonye in lesse q*ua*ntite, *and* of castorie lasse þa*n* þ*er*of, *and* of antemonye, of eu*er*ich*e* j-lich*e* mich*e*. *And* ȝif it hi*m* in what man*er* þ*ou* myȝt. It is ful good for childru*n*.

Special þi*n*ges for þis sicnesse been: crowes eyren y-eten; antimonye; pionye; þe mawe of a soukyng hare j-dru*n*k in wy*n*, nat þe sky*n* of þe maw but þ*a*t þ*a*t is w*it*h-i*n*ne-forþ; and a wolues herte, and foxis flesch*e* j-ete. And for-to helpe childre*n* þ*a*t ha*n* þis sicnesse, pionie *and* ysope bien moost p*ro*fitable erbys (pionie, to hange*n* a-bowte*n* his necke; jsope, j-ȝeuy*n* hi*m* to ete or to drynke).

Anoþ*er* medicine wha*n* a ma*n* is fally*n* a-down: Slee a dogge *and* ȝif hy*m* þe galle to drynk. *And* he ne xal falle na-more at þ*a*t sicnesse. And it is p*ro*fitable for he*m* to bere rew eu*er*more in here hond *and* to smelly*n* ofte*n*-syþes þ*er*-to. Anoþ*er*: Ʒif hy*m* in drynke antymonye, castorie, olibanu*m*, hou*n*destonge, fenel roote, of eu*er*ich*e*, j-lich*e* mych*e*. Anoþ*er*: Wha*n* he falleþ, furst ȝif hi*m* for-to dry*n*k þe iuys of aq*ui*leie, of valeria*n*, of sanicle, *and* of rewe, *and* he xal neuere haue it mor*e*.

2 ounce] *prec. by heading* Epilencie **15 pionie**] *interl.* last i **24 rewe**] *interl.* first e

13 and[1]] *in l.-h. margin:* no*ta* **17 medicine**] *in l.-h. margin:* no*ta* b*e*n*e* r*e*m*e* **19 profitable**] *in l.-h. margin:* no*ta*

f. 25r A sirrip for þe sicnesse: Tac þe seed of pyonie, | *and* sauge, *and* wermode, *and* netlen, *and* horhowne, *and* seeþ he*m* in wyn. Oþ*er* clarifie þe iuys *and* wyn medelyd to-gedere w*ith* þe white *and* þe schell*e* of eiry*n* ouyr an esy fier. *And* siþþe ȝif hy*m* to drynke. And þus þ*o*u xalt clarefyen alle man*er* iuys of herbys w*ith* þe gleire *and* þe schelles of eiren. And ȝif þei ben costyf, ȝeue he*m* of wat*er* a clist*er*ie þ*at* centorie, *and* anet, *and* camamille, *and* mellilet, *and* siche oþ*er*e bie*n* j-soden i*n*ne, oþ*er* make a byty*n*g suppositorie.

A good oyneme*n*t for his sicnesse (but ȝif a ma*n* haue epile*n*cie, þ*o*u xalt a-noynte hese rigge-boon; and ȝif it bee anale*m*psie, þ*o*u xalt a-noynte hese wo*m*be bi-fore þe stomac; and ȝif it be catale*m*psie, þ*o*u xalt a-noynt þe me*m*bre fro whom þe sicnesse comeþ): Tac castorie, *ounce* ij; of piretre, of oyle de bay, of staphie, of euforbe, of eu*er*ich*e*, *ounce* j *and* d*imidia*; of seneuey, nytr*e*, pep*er*, of eu*er*ich*e*, *ounce* j; of oile *and* of wex, q*uasi* s*emis*.

Anoþ*er* a-noynteme*n*t: Tac hou*n*destonge, plau*n*teyne, bet*es*, souffry wat*er* þ*at* brenston is j-medelyd wiþ, as wat*er* of hote baþes oþ*er* oþ*ur* wat*er* þ*at* me*n* seþeþ i*n*ne, *and* tac þ*er*-to fenel, louage, sisymbre, violet, cent*re* galli, *and* sauge, *and* old sowes grece. And seeþ al þese a good while in wat*er*. *And* siþ gader*e* al þ*at* houeþ a-boue þe wat*er* *and* a-noynte hy*m* þ*er*-w*ith*. And vnd*er*stond þ*at* bitt*er* medicines be*n* p*ro*fitable for þe heed *and* for þe stomac, *and* na*m*lych*e* þilke f. 25v | þ*at* han mych*e* of aloes. And tho þ*at* han þe epile*n*cie lat

1 **þe**[2]] *follow. by canc. twice* se **and**] *prec. by heading* Epilencie **3** **iuys**] *follow. by exp.* in **and**] *in r.-h. margin* **16** **of**[2]] *interl.* **26** **þat**[1]] *prec. by heading* Apoplexie **epilencie**] *interl.* first i

5 **alle**] *in r.-h. margin:* no*ta* ben*e*

he*m* ete by-tymes, for fastyng noiȝeþ hem ful mych*e*, *and* lokyng in a glas, *and* euel smelly*ng*es *and* stynckyng*es*, but it be of rewe, oþ*er* castore, oþ*er* amom*e*, oþ*er* of antymonye. And loky*n*g on gith j-poudrid wul make he*m* falle j-down a-no*n*. But to loke on gith hool doiþ he*m* good, *and* wole make he*m* to ryse vp sone. But to þilke þ*a*t ha*n* anale*m*psie, it is p*ro*fitable to fast, ȝif here heed*es* bie*n* nat feble. And castyng is nat p*ro*fitabyl to he*m* oþ*er*whiles. And it is p*ro*fitable to he*m* þ*a*t ha*n* epilencie to bie late blood on þe veyne þ*a*t is bie-twyn þe thombe *and* þe fyng*ur* þat js nexte hy*m*.

And oile þ*a*t dissolueþ coold humo*ur*s *and* wasteþ he*m* js þus j-maad: Tac a pou*n*d of lorer*e* leuys, *and* stamp he*m* in a pownd of wy*n* *and* a pound of oile, *and* seeþ he*m* so longe til þ*a*t þe wyn bie wasted a-wey. Jn epile*n*cie, a-noynte here-w*it*h hese heed; jn anale*m*psie, þe stomac; jn catalempsie, þe place þ*a*t þe siccnesse comeþ fro. And þis oile is good for akyngge of þe heed þ*a*t comeþ of coold, and for þe palesie, and for þe cra*m*ppe þ*a*t comeþ of ple*n*te of humo*ur*es a-boute þe senewys, and for coold gout*es*.

Apoplexie is a sicnesse þ*a*t comyþe of stopynge of þe places pri*n*cipal þat bien in a man*us* brayn þorow su*m* | f. 26r
corupt humo*ur*. *And* þis sicnesse by-nemeþ a ma*n* his wyt *and* his felyng for þe tyme *and* alle man*er* mouy*n*g w*it*h oute-forþ, saf oonly breþi*n*g. And þ*a*t bie*n* iij ky*n*des of þis sicnesse, a more, *and* a lasse, *and* a mene be-twyn hem to. Þe more sleeþ a ma*n* þe furst day *and* is vncurabyl. Þe meene sleþ a ma*n* w*it*h-i*n*ne iij days, or ellys he turneþ in-to a

3 **amome**] *corr. from* amom*er* 15 **þat**] *follow. by canc. twice* he
21 **Apoplexie**] *2-line space left for initial* 23 **corupt**] *prec. by heading* Apoplexie

palesie; þe lasse w*ith*-i*n*ne vij daies, oþ*ur* t*ur*neþ in-to a palesie. And þ*us* sicnesse comeþ of mych*e* flewme oþ*er* of myche corupt blood þ*at* filleþ þe p*ri*ncipal places of a ma*n*n*us* brayn. And ȝif it bie in so g*re*t plente þ*at* it filleþ al þe brayn, þa*n* it makeþ a ma*n* to lese hese wytt*es*, as his siȝt, heryng, *and* oþ*er* wytt*es* w*ith*-i*n*ne-forþ, *and* hese meuy*n*g also. *And* þis is þe mor*e* apoplexie. But ȝif þe humo*ur* ne stop nat but þe hyndrer*e* place of þe brayn þ*er*-as þe senewys ha*n* here begy*n*ni*n*g, þa*n* it be-nemeþ nat a ma*n* his wytt*es*, but hese meuy*n*g. *And* þ*i*s is þe lasse appoplexie. Þe mene js þe mor*e* violent þa*n* is þis, but nat so viole*n*t as þe grete. And þis sicnesse falleþ to fleu*ma*tic me*n*, oþ*er* to me*n* þ*at* ha*n* to myche blood, *and* lyueþ in mych*e* ese *and* eteþ mych*e* *and* drynkeþ mych*e* and waischeþ mych*e* *and* kembeþ mych*e* heer*e* heed. And þis sicnesse is know by certeyn signes as oþ*er* sicnesses bie*n*, as bi heuynesse of þe heed, *and* stro*n*g breþi*n*g, *and* akyng of þe heed w*ith*-outy*n* eny encheson, a
f. 26v feuere, slouþe, turny*n*g of þe brayn, | derknesse of siȝt. And ȝif it is of blood, þe visage is rody, *and* pale ȝif it is of flewme; ȝelewe or blac, ȝif it is of male*n*colie. In myst*ur*ny*n*g of þe visage, also fally*n*g down to grou*n*d ys a gret toky*n*. But þ*at* comeþ in epile*n*cie, *and* in sicnesse of þe hert þ*at* is j-clepid sincopis, and in wy*m*men*us* sicnesse wha*n* þei be*n* stopped and j-let of here purgaciou*n*s þ*at* þei xulde*n* haue. But þei fallyng a-down bie a tokne of alle þese sicnesses, it is nat in oon maner*e* in he*m* alle. For in apoplexie, a ma*n* wexeþ reed wha*n* he is j-falle *and* his veinys swelle*n* a-boute hese te*m*plis *and* his eiȝen. And þei hese eiȝen bie*n* opene, he ne seeþ noþi*n*g. And he vomeþ at his mouþ, but þ*at* it is a tokne

18 derknesse] *prec. by heading* Apoplexie **26 For**] *corr. from* ffor

of deeþ. And here accesse dureþ long, as a day or tweyne. Jn epilencie, su*m* part*es* of þe ma*n* ha*n* þe cra*m*p *and* is j-t*ur*nyd a-syde. *And* hese body tre*m*bleþ *and* quakeþ, and oþ*er*whiles he vomeþ, *and* þ*a*t is a good tokne, *and* þ*a*t his accesse is nei3 j-doon. Fallyng in sincopis is w*ith* discolori*n*g of þe face. And li3e as þei he were deed, w*ith*-outyn cra*m*pe or tre*m*blyng *and* vomy*n*g also. *And* sone he riseþ up. Jn wy*m*me*n* þ*a*t bie*n* j-stoppid here fallyng is w*ith* mych*e* ache fra*m* þe nauele downward, *and* w*ith* mych*e* heuynesse in here leggis bi-fore þat þei fallen dou*n*. And þei streyne here wombys w*ith* her*e* arm*es*, | and boweþ here heed to here f. 27r knees, and gry*n*teþ w*ith* here teeþ for þe gret ache þ*a*t þei han. And wha*n* þei falle*n* down, su*m*me bieten þe erþe w*ith* here hondys *and* here feet. Su*m*me ligge*n* stille as þei were dede and all*e* here body is ful coold. And su*m*me ryse up sone. And su*m*me liggen in here accesse a day or ij.

Apoplexie þ*a*t comeþ in þe wexyng of þe mone is incurable, and na*m*ly 3if it bie þe mor*e* apoplexie. But 3if it come in þe wany*n*g of þe mone, it is nat so greuous. And 3if he desyre diu*er*se met*es*, *and* as sone as he seeþ he*m*, he haþ abho*mi*n*a*cio*n* of he*m*, it be-tokeneþ deeþ. And 3if he haþ no sich*e* p*er*ilouse toknes, he may bie holpe*n* bie medicines. And 3if it be of blood, let hi*m* bledy*n* in þe hed veyne of þe arme 3if he be of stro*n*g co*m*plexio*n*. And þ*a*t is a souereyn medicine in eu*er*ich*e* apoplexie, of what humo*ur* þ*a*t he bie. 3if þe body bie ful of humo*ur*s and 3if it bie of ony oþ*er* humo*ur* þa*n* of blood, lat purge hese body w*ith* stro*n*g medicinys, as yeralogodio*n*, or ierapigra, theodorico*n*, or

5 Fallyng] *corr. from* ffallyng **11 and**] *prec. by heading* Apoplexie

17 comeþ] *in r.-h. margin:* no*ta*

stomatico*n*, or w*ith* þese pillulees ȝif it bie of flewme oþ*er* male*n*colie: Tac of aloes *and* of euforbe j-lych*e* mych*e*, *and* medle he*m* w*ith* þe iuys of leek. *And* mak pillulees *and* ȝif it hy*m*. And ȝif he bie feble þ*at* he ne may bie late blood ne f. 27v haue no*n* sich*e* stro*n*g p*ur*gacions, | lat schaue hese heed. *And* make a plastre of seneuey *and* of vi*n*egre, *and* medle þ*er*-w*ith* castore *and* euforbe, *and* ley it on hese heed.

Anoþ*er* good plastre: Tac femygrek *and* whete bryn, *and* seeþ he*m* in a lytil wyn. Anoynte also þ*in* heed w*ith* hote oyneme*nt*es j-mad of euforbe, castorie, piretre; oþ*er* of iuys of march*e* *and* euforbbe j-medlyd to-gedere; oþ*er* þe iuys of rewe, of carses, *and* of sauge j-medlid w*ith* þe oþ*er*e. And ȝif þe g*r*euau*n*ce falle a-down in þe chyne, waisch*e* hy*m* w*ith* þe wat*er* þ*at* camamille, mellilet, anet, sansuke, bien j-sode*n* i*n*ne. *And* lat a-noynte hy*m* w*ith* þe onyme*nt*es forseid vp-on þe chyne as j-seid here next be-fore to a-noynte þe heed. Also mak a plastre of þe iuys of ce*n*torie, *and* of netle*n*, *and* of salt, *and* lei to þe hy*n*drer*e* pa*r*ty of þe heed.

And ȝif he bie costyf, mak hy*m* a clyster*e* þ*at* bie scharp *and* bytynge, of hocke leues j-soden in wat*er*, *and* betys, *and* hony, *and* oyle. *And* lat a-noynte hese fu*n*deme*n*t w*ith* boles galle. Oþ*er* mak hy*m* a suppositorie of *dragme* ij *and* d*imidia* of nitr*e*; *and dragme* ij of castore; *and ounce* s*emis* of scamone, *and* hony þ*at* suffisiþ þ*er*-to. Oþ*er* mak a suppositorie of whiȝt hard sope, *and* a-noynte it w*ith* bolys galle *and* w*ith* salt. And her*e* vnd*er*stond þ*at* þer*e* bien ij manere sopees: blac *and* whiȝt. Blac sope is maad of capitelle

5 lat] *prec. by heading* Apoplexie **12 ȝif**] *follow. by canc. twice* hy*m*

26 bien] *in l.-h. margin:* No*ta* for*mam* faci*en*di

and oile j-soden | to-gedere. Capitelle is a liȝe þ*a*t is maad of f. 28r askys of been, halm *and* vnslecked lym, but þe askys schulle*n* bien double to þe lyme. And it xal be maad in þe man*er* of lyȝe. But aft*ur* þ*a*t it haþ þe strencþe *and* þe þrist of þe furst askys þ*a*t þ*o*u heldist it on, þ*o*u xalt helden it on new asky*n* tyl it be weel j-maad. Jt mote bie clere as liȝe, *and* so strong *and* þicke þ*a*t it wole bere an ey þ*a*t it synke nat to þe ground. But whiȝt sope is j-maad of ij partis of þe capitelle *and* þe iij is schepis talowe. And it xal bie maad aft*ur* mydsom*er* in þe caniculer*e* daies bi hete of þe su*n*ne w*it*h-outyn fere. And þese sopys bie*n* good for bre*n*ny*n*g oþ*er* scaldyng, and xal lygge þ*er*-on iij houres or iiij a-noon aft*ur* þe hyrty*n*g. Þei bie*n* good also for scabbys *and* oppeneþ þe pores of þe skyn, *and* makeþ þe skyn whiȝt, *and* for many oþ*er* thyng*es* þei be*n* ful p*ro*fitable.

And in þi worchyng of þis sicnesse, by-gy*n*ne w*it*h esy medicynes *and* siþþe worch*e* w*it*h streng*ur*e. And pit a wegge be-twene hese teeþ to holden hese mouþ open. And siþþe frete his mouþ w*it*h toosted breed þ*a*t is j-wet in þe iuys of mynt. And make hy*m* smelle to a gootus horn j-brent oþ*er* to maiþen. But alle þese medicines xul be doon i*n* þe lasse apoplexie *and* nat in þe mor*e*, for þ*a*t is incurable. And þei xully*n* bie*n* dietyd w*it*h hoote met*es* and | drynkys. And in f. 28v passyng a-wey of þ*a*t sicnesse, good wyn is ful profytabil. And vundyrstand þ*a*t a feuer*e* is p*ro*fitable in þ*a*t sicnesse, and in þe palesie al-so, and in þe cra*m*pe þ*a*t is in replecio*n* of blood. And þ*o*u myȝt make þ*a*t in þ*i*s wyse: Ley þe

1 to-gedere] *prec. by heading* Apoplexie **20 hym]** *follow. by canc.* snel
23 drynkys] *prec. by heading* Sekenesse

11 bien] *in r.-h. margin:* no*ta* **27 þis]** *in l.-h. margin:* no*ta*

syke-ma*n* be-twyne too good feirys *and* ȝif hy*m* to drynk stale ale. And lat hym ete strong garlek and siþþe late hym drynk strong wyn*e*, þ*a*t it bie hoot. *And* do a good q*ua*ntite of pep*er* þ*er*i*n*ne. And a-noynte al his body w*it*h oyle de bay oþ*er* of lorer leu*es*, *and* p*ri*ncipaly vndur his arm-pittys *and* on his reynes.

Jn a ma*n*n*us* eiȝe*n* þ*er* falle*n* many sicnessys *and* g*re*ua*n*ce. Su*m*me comeþ fro w*it*h-i*n*ne-forþ *and* su*m*me fro w*it*h-out-forþ. Fro w*it*h-i*n*ne-forþ comeþ g*re*ua*n*ce, ache, myche re*n*ny*n*g of wat*er*, aposteme in þe whiȝt of þe eiȝe þ*a*t is j-clepyd obtalmie, webbys *and* cloþis also þ*a*t goiþ ou*er* þe eiȝe *and* letteþ a ma*n* to see, and hardnesse of þe eiȝe, and kanker*e* of þe eiȝe. Fro w*it*h-outyn, þe eiȝe*n* bie*n* j-g*re*uyd w*it*h lokyng of þe su*n*ne oþ*er* on a ful whiȝt thi*n*ge, by smoke, dust þ*a*t falleþ in-to a ma*n*nys eiȝen, by wynd, *and* sich*e* oþ*er* thyng*es*.

Ache of þe eiȝen comeþ oþ*er*whiles of smoke oþ*er*
f. 29r poudre þ*a*t noiȝeþ þe eiȝyn, oþ*er* sich*e* oþ*er* þi*n*gys, | and oþ*er*-whiles it comeþ of humo*ur*s þ*a*t falle*n* a-dou*n* in-to þe eiȝen, as of blood, of colre, of flewme, oþ*er* of malencolie. And ȝif it is of blood, þese bie*n* þe toknes: reednesse a-bouty*n* þe eiȝe*n*, *and* heete, *and* swellyng, w*it*h mych*e* heuynesse boþe of þe eiȝe*n* *and* also of þe forheed. *And* þe eiȝen bie*n* moist and wepyng. And wha*n* þe ledys bie*n* j-closed, þei fele*n* myche scharpnesse w*it*h-i*n*ne-forþe, as þow

2 garlek] *corr. from* garleko (o *canc.*) **5 of**] *follow. by* lorer (e *oblit.*) **lorer**] *in r.-h. margin* **6 reynes**] *interl.* **7 Jn**] *2-line space left for initial* **9 Fro**] *corr. from* ffro **13 Fro**] *corr. from* ffro **18 and**] *prec. by heading* of the eiȝen **23 of**[1]] *in r.-h. margin*

25 felen] *in r.-h. margin:* Tokens to | know of what | humor þere wore grauel in here eiȝen. And here visage is ful of blood.

Of colre, þese bie*n* þe toknes: reednesse of þe eiȝen þ*a*t is nat a clere reednesse as þ*a*t þ*a*t comeþ of blood, but a man*er* of brown reed; and þei bie*n* hoote *and* smertyng; g*r*et ache *and* greuau*n*ce w*it*h-owte*n* swelly*n*g of þe eiȝen. But ȝif it bie of flewme, þere is more swellyng *and* lasse ache. And þe wat*er* þ*a*t floweþ a-nyȝt fro þe eiȝyn is viscous as byrdlym *and* makeþ he*m* su*m*what blere-eiȝed. And here eiȝeledys cleueþ to-gidere, and þei felyn mych*e* heuynesse in here eiȝen. And ȝif þe ache come of male*n*colie, þe eiȝe*n* swelle*n* but lytil, ne bur[n] nat ful hoote ne ful reede. *And* þe humo*ur* þ*a*t comeþ fro*m* hem wexeþ harde *and* is of meene colour, nat riȝt whiȝt ne riȝt brown. Oþ*er*while þe ache of þe eiȝen comeþ of þe browes *and* of su*m* humo*ur* þ*a*t is in he*m*. And of what humo*ur* þ*a*t it bie, þ*o*u maist know bi þese for-seid toknes.

Also ache | of eiȝen comeþ oþ*er*while from þe stomac. f. 29v
And þa*n*ne þe ache is grett*er* aft*ur* mete þa*n* bie-fore. And ȝif it come of coold humo*urs* þ*a*t bie*n* in þe stomac, lat hi*m* caste aft*ur* mete and vsen p*ur*gaciou*ns* þ*a*t seruy*n* to þe humo*ur* þ*a*t makeþ þe ache. And oþ*er*while þe greuau*n*ce of þe eiȝen comeþ of rewme of þe heed. And þa*n* hele þe heed of his rewme *and* þa*n* þe eiȝe*n* wol bie hole. And here-fore pylulees of dycastore, of myrab*e*, of eiþ*er dragme* iij; of musk, a greyn *and* an half; of aloes, j *dragme*; of ase, mirr*e*, euforb*e*, *dragme* j *and* vviij greynys; of folii, antymonye,

8 þat] *follow. by canc.* fol **18 of]** *prec. by heading* Jnfirmyte of the eyȝen

7 swellyng] *in r.-h. margin:* no*ta* **19 þe]** *in l.-h. margin:* no*ta* ben*e*

piretre, liquorik, dragag*e*, calamy aromat[ik], nit*re*, galbanu*m*, sq*ui*na*n*tu*m*, spik, oppopanac, reupont*e*, serap[inum], storac, galing*e*, ging*er*, canel of eu*er*ich*e*, *dragme* j; *and* of greynes, staphyne, dauk, fenel, p*er*sili, march, silor*e* mou*n*tayn, petroley, sangedragou*n*, ence*n*ce, cardomome boþe þe more *and* þe lasse, agarik, mastik, sal armoniac, ȝedoare, an*is*, of eu*er*ich*e*, *dragme* j *and* ix greynes; of saturie, ysope, camedreos, piliole, origanu*m*, baume, oȝimi, beet*es*, dyteyn, rewe, sene, aristo[logie] boþe long *and* þe round, aaro*n*, macematico*n*, asari, sauge, bedellie, of eu*er*ich*e*, xviij grei*n*s; alipiades, cap*er*is, xj greyns; anacardy, sauyne, genciane, of ryndys of ma*n*drage, xj greyns; peusadan[um], wermot, vij greyns; yreos, xiij greyns *and* þe iij part of half an ha*n*ful. *And* make here-of pululees
f. 30r of þe q*ua*ntite of a note. | Þese bien good for þe g*re*uau*n*ce of þe heed, *and* for þe palasie, *and* for þe lyu*er*e, *and* for þe splene, *and* þe reynys, *and* for alle coold sicnesses. But for greuance of þe eiȝen þ*at* comeþ of þe rewme, þ*ou* xalt castyn of þe pilulees in wyn *and* cast þat in þyn nestrilles. And poudre piretre, *and* staphiȝag*re*, *and* mastik *and* chew it. Oþ*er* melt it w*ith* wex and ley it on a clooþ to þi foreheed, for it dissolueþ þe flewme, *and* drieþ þe brayn, *and* cleriþ þe siȝt. And a-noynte þe foreheed w*ith* oyle of lorer*e* oþ*er* of piliole, or make a cyred clooþ of poudre of mastik, *and*

1 **aromatik**] *corr. from* aromat*e* 3 **serapinum**] *corr. from* serap*er* 9 **aristologie**] *corr. from* aristob*e* 13 **peusadanum**] *corr. from* peusadan*er* **vij**] *corr. from* vijj (last j *canc. twice*) 15 **note**] *catchword* (*in bottom margin*): þese bie*n* goode **Þese**] *prec. by heading* ffor the eiȝen 22 **for**] *corr. from* ffor

18 **xalt**] *in r.-h. margin:* no*ta* b*e*n*e* no*ta*

olibanu*m*, *and* wex j-cast þ*er*-too *and* hony. Oþ*er* let hi*m* blood up þe coppe of þe nose. Oþ*er* lat hym baþe hy*m*, oþ*er* han a stewe w*it*h hote herbis. *And* haue a purgacio*n* þ*a*t wery*n* j-toold in þe sicnesse of þe heed.

But ȝif þe ache of þe eiȝen bie of blood, lat hy*m* blede*n* at þe heed veyn of þe arme, oþ*ur* bie cuppid oþ*er* bie garsyd in þe necke-pyt, oþ*er* be-twyne þe two schuldres. And ȝif it is of colre, ȝif hi*m* a colo[go]ge, þ*a*t is to seie, a medicine þ*a*t wol cle*n*se hi*m* *and* purge*n* hi*m* of colre, as mirab*e* ci[tri], oþ*er* oximel maad w*it*h coold herbis, oþ*er* electuare maad w*it*h þe iuys of roses *and* oþ*er* coold þi*n*ges, oþ*er* pilulees þ*a*t bie*n* j-maad of þe fyue kyndes of mirabol*e*. And aft*ur* his p*ur*gacio*n*, þ*o*u xalt legge þ*in* medicines to his eiȝe*n*.

Dieti*n*ge of sich*e* me*n* xal bie as me*n* þ*a*t ha*n* þe | feuere f. 30v tercia*n*. And absteyne þei algatys fro wy*n* and fryed met*es*, *and* rostyd metys, *and* salt metys, and bytyng metys, *and* sowre. And lat hy*m* bie in derk places. Wha*n* þei slepy*n*, lat here heed leggy*n* hey. And here mete xal by sich*e* þ*a*t wole esyly be defiȝed, and here drynk clene, cleere, *and* smal as wat*er* oþ*ur* smal ale.

Special medicines for ache of eiȝen þ*a*t comeþ of heete, as of blood þ*a*t is hoot *and* moist, oþ*er* of colre þ*a*t is hoot *and* dryȝe, þei mote*n* bie*n* coold for-to bie myt[i]gatifs, þ*a*t is to say, to a-swage þe v[i]ole*n*ce of þe ache. And þei mote*n* bie coold to bie*n* rep*er*cussyues, þ*a*t is to sey, to smyty*n* a-ȝey*n* fro þe eiȝe þe humo*ur* þ*a*t is encheson of þe ache. And þese to kyndes coold medicines ha*n* þei þ*a*t bie*n* mytigatifs

1 **and**[1]] *follow. by and* 14 **feuere**] *prec. by heading* ffor the eiȝen
23 mytigatifs] *corr. from* mytagatifs

8 is[2]] *in r.-h. margin:* no*ta*

and rep*er*cussiues. But me xal nat vse eu*er*more mitigatifs *and* rep*er*cussiues, but oþ*er*-whiles dissolutyues, þ*a*t is to sey, hoot medicines þ*a*t mowe*n* dissolue*n* þe mat*er* of þe sicnesse ry3t as þe heete of þe su*n*ne dissolueþ þis oþur snow in-to wat*er*. And me xal not vse eu*er*-more dissolutiues, but oþ*er*whiles co*n*fortatyues to co*n*forte þe ei3e, for to hoote medicines or to coolde *and* þei weru*n* eu*er*-more j-leid co*n*tin[u]elych*e* to þe ei3e, þei wolde*n* as weel distroy þe ei3e as þe ache of þe ei3e. And so it fareþ of eu*er*ich*e* ach*e* where-
f. 31r eu*er* it bie in | a ma*nn*us body. And þ*er*-fore in þe be-gynny*n*g of þe ache, þu xalt vse co*n*fortatifs to confortyn þe membre þ*a*t akeþ. For but 3if þe me*m*bre bie strong to wretche hi*m*-selue*n*, þe stre*n*cþe of þe medicine ne xal a-vayle but lytil, for þe medicine is but an help and þe p*ri*ncipal is þe me*m*bre þ*a*t is siyk. And þ*er*for*e* it nedeþ to haue co*n*fortatyues in þe be-gy*n*nyng þ*a*t bien neþ*er* ful hoote naþ*er* ful coolde. And in wexi*n*ge of þe sicnesse *and* wha*n* þe sicnesse is moost greuous, let hy*m* vse medicines þat bien co*n*fortatyues *and* oþ*er* dissolutyues j-medlyd to-gedere. And in passyng a-wey of þe sicnesse, þu xalt vse dissolutyues.

But þu xalt vund*er*stonde of þese medicines, su*m*me bie*n* symple *and* su*m* bie*n* co*m*poned. Simple medicines bien as of oon herbe bi hy*m*-self, oon wat*er* þ*a*t is j-maad of oon herbe, oþ*er* hony, oþ*er* oyle de oliue, oþ*er* oon gu*m*me, oþ*er* oon sp[i]c*ery* bi hi*m*-self. Componed medicines þ*a*t bie*n* maad of two þi*n*ges, oþ*er* þre, oþ*er* manye j-medlyd to-gidere. And symple medicines, su*m*me bie*n* hoote *and*

1 **euermore**] *follow. by canc.* mitag 6 **for**] *corr. from* ffor 8 **continuelyche**] *corr. from* co*n*tinielych*e* 10 **a**] *prec. by heading* ffor the ei3en 12 **For**] *corr. from* ffor 14 **for**] *corr. from* ffor

dissolutyues, *and* su*m* bie*n* coold *and* mitigatyues *and* rep*er*cussyues. Of hoote medicynes þ*at* bie*n* dissolutyues, su*m* bie*n* st*r*onge dis[solutyues] *and* su*m* bie*n* feble dis[solutyues].

Strong dissolutyues bie*n* reed netlees, rew, celydonie, baume þ*at* is an oynement, | camfer, aloes, amber, þe galle of f. 31v
eu*er*ich*e* beest, eu*er*ich*e* salt, *and* eu*er*ich*e*-þi*n*g þ*at* is ful corrosyf *and* ful frety*n*g. And siche stronge dissolutiu*us* nyeden bien medlyd w*it*h esy mytigatyues oþ*er* rep*er*cussyues wha*n* þe ache is bowyng a-wey-ward. Feble dissolutyues bie*n* þe ȝelke of an eiȝe, þe iuys of my*n*te, of basilico*n*, of sansuke, v*er*ueyne, endyue, þe leues of madur, hoote cru*m*mes of whete bried j-spreynd w*it*h wyn oþ*er* w*it*h rose wat*er*; also þe iuys of fenel, of eufrace, of heyhoue, liciu*m*, þe iuys of sloon, sarcocolle, acacia, musk, þe wat*er* of a vyne, hony, þe blood of a culu*er*e oþ*er* of an hen [or] cheku*n*, [and] þe lymaile of goold. And wha*n* þe ache sto[n]deþ *and* naþ*er* waxeþ ne abateþ, sich*e* xulle*n* be j-medlyd wiþ esy rep*er*cussyues.

Rep*er*cussyues þ*er* bie*n* also su*m* ful strong *and* su*m*me ful feble. Stronge rep*er*cussyues bien j-clepid stupefactis, for þei a-stoneyen a me*m*bre þorow here coold *and* so þei make*n* a me*m*bre to liese boþe his ache *and* his felyng. And for here gret viole*n*ce, me vseþ hem nat in ache of þe eiȝen ne in noon oþ*er* ache, but ȝif þe ache bie more violent *and* p*er*ilouse. And sich*e* rep*er*cussiues bien þe rynde of ma*n*drake *and* þe fruyt, and he*n*bane, *and* morel, *and* orpy*n*, *and* popy seid, *and* na*m*ly of þe blac popi. Feble repercussyues bien j-clepyd mitigatyues, for þei a-swage*n* þe

1 bien] *follow. by canc.* ho **6 camfer**] *prec. by heading* The eiȝen
10 Feble] *corr. from* ffeble **28 Feble**] *corr. from* ffeble

f. 32r ache *and* co*n*forty*n* þe | membre. And sich*e* bien woma*nn*es meylk *and* asse mylk, þe white of an ey, and oile of roses, *and* of violet, *and* mussilage of salie, *and* lynsed, *and* sich*e* oþ*er*e; portulake, *and* þe iuys of solatre, *and* stancrop, *and* syngrene bien strong rep*er*cussyues.

Of co*m*poned medicines, þ*er* bie*n* many þ*at* bie*n* p*ro*fytable for þe ache of eiȝe*n* þ*at* comeþ of heete. Oon is þis: Take wat*er* of roses, *and* þe whiȝte of eyren, *and* wo*m*man*us* mylk, *and* a lytil whiȝt wyn. And þ*er*-wiþ waisch*e* he his eiȝe*n*. Anoþ*er*: Seeþ fenel rootys, *and* violet, *and* popy seed in wat*er*. *And* þ*er*-w*it*h a-noynte hese eiȝe*n*. *And* p*er*sillie do it on wat*er* of roses *and* ley þ*at* vp-on his eiȝe*n* al nyȝt in þe man*er* of a plastr*e*. And ley þ*is* plastre oon his temples: Tac rosees, anyse, *and* ceruse þ*at* is j-clepyd blank plu*m* *and* whiȝt leed, *and* sancdragou*n*, *and* gu*m*me arabik, of eu*er*ich*e*, j-lych*e* myche. And powne he*m* *and* tempre he*m* w*it*h wat*er* of rosees *and* raw gleir of eyren. *And* lei þ*at* on his for-hed *and* on his te*m*ples. *And* lat it legge þ*er* iij daies. Anoþ*er* plastre: Tac þe iuys of violet, þe gleyre of eyren, *and* wat*er* of roses, barly mele, *and* mak þ*er*-of a plastre, *and* ley on his eiȝe*n*. Oþ*er* tac þe iuys of syngrene, *and* woma*nn**us* mylk, *and* þe whiȝt of an ey, *and* þe iuys of endyue ȝif þ*o*u wolt, oþ*er* wat*er* of rosees, *and* medle he*m* to-gedere. *And* weet a clowt þ*er*-i*n*ne *and* lei it vp-on his eiȝe*n*.

1 **membre**] *prec. by heading* The eiȝen 12 **persillie**] li *interl. and follow. by canc.* and

6 **þat**] *in r.-h. margin:* no*ta* 14 **þat**] *in r.-h. margin:* A plaster foor | the foorehead

Also | in gret ache of þe eiȝen, þ*o*u myȝt wasche he*m* f. 32v w*ith* warm wat*er* þ*a*t femygrek *and* mellilot bie*n* j-sode*n* i*n*ne, ȝif it is soo þ*a*t it flowen nat, for ȝif it is soo þat þei flowen, þei xul haue no wasschyng w*ith* warm wat*er*. But þ*o*u xalt make a strictorie, *and* leie it to hese foreheed, of encense *and* barly mele, oþ*er* whete mele *and* gleire of eiren. But narþelees, ȝif his body bie ful moist *and* his heed bie repleet w*ith* humo*ur*es, ne make hym no st*ri*ctorie, but ȝif hy*m* a p*ur*gacio*n* a-cordyng to þe humo*ur*s þ*a*t make*n* þe ache *and* þe flowyng of þe eiȝen. And wha*n* þe flowyng cesseþ oþ*er* waxeþ lasse þa*n* it was, þa*n* vse rep*er*cussyues *and* mytigatyues. And ȝif þe ache bie ful violent, ne vse nat þer*e* nat oonly coold þinges, but medle he*m* w*ith* hote þi*n*ges so þ*a*t þe hote þi*n*ges mown su*m*wat dissolue*n* þe mat*er* of þe ache, *and* þe coold þi*n*ges mown a-swagyn þe violence of þe hete *and* of þe ache. And in þe ende *and* in þe declinacio*n* of þe ache, vse dissolutyues. And wha*n* þ*o*u vsist to waisch a ma*n*n*es* eiȝen, ȝif hese g*re*ua*n*ce encresceþ, leue hit. And ellys, co*n*tinue it. And in a rootid *and* in an hold greuau*n*ce of þe eiȝen, it is p*ro*fitabil for-to baþe*n* in an hoot baþ, and aft*ur*-ward to drynke a good drawt of wyn *and* tac þa*n* a good sleep *and* a swoot. And þe iuys of chikemete þ*a*t haþ a reed flewr *and* þe iuys of grapys þ*a*t bie*n* not ripe is p*ro*fitabile. | And þe iuys of plau*n*teyne *and* of verueyne j- f. 33r medlyd to-gedere is good also. *And* y-medlyd w*ith* þe gleyr of eyren, it is good for icchyng of þe eiȝen *and* to don a-wey þe blood þ*a*t is in þe eiȝen. And þe same doiþ þe cru*m*mys of

1 in] *prec. by heading* The eiȝen **3 for**] *corr. from* ffor **24 And**] *prec. by heading* The eiȝen

27 And] *in r.-h. margin:* no*ta* per

an hoot loof as he comeþ fra*m* þe oue*n* j-sprent w*ith* þe wat*er* of rosees ȝif þe ache is of hete, and ȝif it is of coold, w*ith* wyn. *And* y-leid on þe eiȝen doiþ a-wey þe ache, *and* þe icchyng of þe blood. A plastre j-maad of þe iuys of radich, of netle seed þ*er* powned, *and* carses, *and* mastik, *and* olibanu*m*, *and* rye mele, ne suffreþ noon hoot humo*ur* flowen at þe eiȝen, ȝif it bie j-plastred on þe for-heed. And ȝif þe eiȝe*n* smerty*n* *and* mou*n* suffre neiþur liȝt ne fier, tak valeria*n*, *and* march*e*, *and* plau*n*teyn, *and* syngr*e*ne, of eu*er*ich*e* j-lych*e* mych*e*, *and* tac þe iuys of he*m* *and* medle it w*ith* sowr*e* wete breed. *And* mak þ*er*-of a plastre, neiþ*er* harde ne neische, *and* ley it coold to hese eiȝen. But ley a þi*n*ne clowt bi-twene þe plastre *and* his eiȝen, and in oon nyȝt it wele hele*n* hy*m*, þei þe eiȝen bie hel[e]d w*ith* blood.

A collirie: Tac of amyde, ceruse, gu*m*me arabik, dragag*e*, of eu*er*ich*e*, *dragme* iij; of opiu*m*, *dragme* j. Te*m*pre it w*ith* þe white of eyren oþ*er* w*ith* þe wat*er* of roses. And loke þ*at* alle þe poudres þ*at* bie*n* doon in colliries bie j-powdred as smale as þ*o*u myȝt, *and* siþþe j-bulted þorow a f. 33v dowble smal clooþ for þe greuau*n*ce of þe eiȝe*n*. And | wasch*e* þe eiȝen w*ith* wat*er* of roses, oþ*er* of eufras, oþ*er* of fenel, oþ*er* w*ith* wyn, ar þ*o*u do þi collire in-to þ*in* eiȝen. But þe ache of þe eiȝen comeþ oþ*er*whiles of coold, as of flewme oþ*er* of male*n*colie, oþ*er* of a pose. Ȝif it comeþ of a pose, hele þe pose as we wolle*n* telle afturward in þe chapetre of þe pose. And ȝif it comeþ of flewme, p*ur*ge hy*m*

14 heled] *corr. from* helod **20 dowble**] *follow. by interl.* a **21 wasche**] *prec. by heading* The eiȝen **22 collire**] *interl.* last l **23 But**] *follow. by* ȝif

12 ley[2]] *in r.-h. margin:* no*ta*

as it was j-told in þe heed-ache *and* oþ*er* sicnesses of þe heed. And ȝif it bie of male*n*colie, p*ur*ge hy*m*. *And* siþþe stuwe hy*m* ou*er* a styue v siþes oþ*er* vij siþes þat is maad of wermot, of beteyne, fenel, sauge, floures of tyme, camamille, mellilot floures, of hockes, *and* march. And alle þese xul bie*n* j-sode*n* in wyn *and* wat*er* j-medlyd to-gedere, so þ*a*t þ*er* bie as mych*e* wyn as wat*er*. And lat hi*m* hange*n* hese eiȝe*n* *and* his heed ou*er* þe stwe. And siþþe weet lynet or cotu*n* in þe wat*er* *and* a-noynte þ*er*-wiþ hese eiȝen. And lat hym bie cuppid in þe neþ*er* party of þe heed by-hynde-forþe oþ*er* bi-twyne hese schuldr*e*-blades, oþ*er* lat hy*m* blood on þe veyne of þe elbow. *And* set an horn al a-bowte þe elbow *and* cuppe hy*m* þ*er*e. But vnd*er*stond þ*a*t alle þese blood-latynges xulle*n* bie raþ*er* j-don þ*er*-as ache comeþ of hete þa*n* of coold. Also tac rewe *and* hete it on an hoot tiylston, *and* mak þ*er*-of a plastre on his eiȝen. Oþ*er* wete lynet in þe iuys of rewe *and* of fenel, *and* ley on his eiȝe. And waisch*e* his eiȝen at even *and* at morow i*n* þe wat*er* of lilye rot*es* oþ*er* whiȝt wyn þ*a*t spicnard is j-sode*n* i*n*ne. | Oþ*er* waisch*e* hym w*i*t*h* f. 34r whiȝt wyn þ*a*t mellilot, *and* popy, *and* comy*n* bie*n* j-soden i*n*ne, oþ*er* w*i*t*h* whiȝt wyn þ*a*t olibanu*m* *and* roses bie*n* j-soden i*n*ne, oþ*er* w*i*t*h* wyn þ*a*t bras oþ*er* goold han ofte bien que*n*chid i*n*ne, oþ*er* w*i*t*h* wyn þ*a*t gyng*er* *and* rwe ha*n* bie soden i*n*ne. Oþ*er* tac p*er*it*er*ie, *and* pyt it in a bagge *and* mak a plastre þ*er*-of aft*ur* þe q*ua*ntite of þe eiȝe, *and* lei it to al coold. Oþ*er* mak a plastre of barly mele oþ*er* bren j-soden i*n* whiȝt wyn *and* j-piȝt in a bagge *and* j-leid on þe eiȝe, for it

4 **fenel**] *corr. from* ffenel **floures**] *corr. from* ffloures (u *interl.*)
5 **floures**] *corr. from* ffloures 18 **whiȝt wyn**] *corr. from* whiȝtwyn
19 **Oþer**] *prec. by heading* The eyȝen 20 **and popy**] *corr. from* andpopy

holeþ þe ache þ*at* comeþ of coold. Oþ*er* seeþ in wyn femygrek meele oþ*er* of lynsed, oþ*er* of mellilot in a bagge *and* ley it on his eiȝe*n*.

A collirie: Tac of liciu*m*, acacie, amyde, sarcocolle, calamyne, ence*n*se, of eu*er*ich*e*, *dragme* j *and* s*emis*; coperose, memythe, ceruse, myrr*e*, aloes, of eu*er*ich*e*, *dragme* j; of opiu*m*, x greyns. Tempre it vp w*it*h þe iuys of fenel *and* of eufrace. *And* siþþe, driȝe it þries or iiij syþes in þe su*n*ne. *And* te*m*pre it aft*ur* his dryi*n*ge in þe same iuys. And siþþe driȝe it vp *and* pit þ*er*-of in his eiȝe a-morowen *and* a-euene. And it doeþ a-wey heed-ache þ*at* comeþ of coold *and* heleeþ blereid eiȝen, but it is su*m*what fretynge, *et* c*etera*.

Obtalmie is a p[o]steme in a ma*n*n*us* eiȝe þ*at* comeþ of corupt humo*ur*s þ*at* fally*n* a-down in-to a ma*n*n*us* eiȝen. And þis posteme is oþ*er*-whiles w*it*h-owte*n*, oþ*er*whiles w*it*h-i*n*ne. And i*n* boþe þe places, it comeþ of blood, oþ*er* of colr*e*, oþ*er* of flewme, oþ*er* of male*n*colie. And ȝif þe posteme
f. 34v | by w*it*h-owtyn, me*n* may sone j-wety*n* of which*e* humo*ur* it is. And ȝif it is w*it*h-inne þe eiȝe, it is drawen a-brood, *and* swelleþ, *and* akeþ, *and* þe siȝte wexeþ derke, *and* þe veines bien fulle. And ȝif it is of blood, þei watteryn, *and* swellu*n*, *and* wexe*n* reede. *And* here fore-heed akeþ *and* here te*m*ples also. Ȝif it is of colre, þei felu*n* gret prickyng *and* smertyng by-neþe in þe depnesse of þe eiȝe. *And* þei ha*n* ful myche hete in here eiȝen. Ȝif it is of flewme, þei bie*n* blere-eiȝed, *and* wat*er*eþ w*it*h viscouse mat*er*. Ȝif it is of male*n*colie, þe eiȝen ne watt*er* nat mych*e*, but þei beyn blerid. And i*n*ne

14 **Obtalmie**] *2-line space left for initial* **posteme**] *corr. from* pasteme **comeþ**] *follow. by canc. twice* þat **19** **by**] *prec. by heading* The eyen

eu*er*ich*e* of þese, þ*er*e is ache, su*m* more *and* su*m* lasse. But oþ*er*wiles þis sicnesse comeþ of þe pose; heele þe pose. And ȝif þe body bie replet, let hy*m* blood in eu*er*y cause. And it is p*ro*fitabil to bie*n* j-cuppyd in þe necke-pyt, oþ*er* be-hynde þe heed in þe two hornes þ*a*t ioyne*n* to þe necke. And ȝif he bie costyf, it is p*ro*fitabil to make su*m* laxe. And baþi*n*ge is p*ro*fitabyl, and good dietyng, as we seyde*n* in þe last chapit*re*. And ne wasch*e* nat his eiȝen w*it*h no warm wat*er* ne warm þi*n*ges ȝif þei bie*n* ful moist, for drawyng of more mat*er* þ*er*-too. But vse strictories *and* rep*er*cussyues to þe heed in þe be-gy*n*ny*n*g, as we told bie-fore. But ley þ*o*u no strong rep*er*cussyues in þe be-gy*n*ny*n*g to þe heed, ne to þe eiȝen. But bie-gy*n*ne w*it*h co*n*fortatyuys, *and* mitigatyues, *and* strictories. And i*n*ne þe | f. 35r encressyng of þe sicnesse, vse co*n*fortatyues *and* feble dissolutyues. And wha*n*ne þe ache *and* þe sicnesse stondiþ stille, naþ*er* wexyng ne decrescy*n*g, and in passyng a-wey, esy dissolutyues. And ȝif þis sicnesse bie of xv dayes, it may lytly bie helyd, oþ*er* of a moneþ. But ȝif it bie of a ȝeer oþ*er* more, vnneþis wole it eu*er* bie hoolyd. For þei þe posteme bie heelyd *and* þe ach*e* also, oþ*er*whiles þ*er* leueþ a lytil web; *and* þ*er*of comeþ a clooþ; and þ*er*-of a nayl. Þese þre bien of oo kynde: Þe clooþ is þicker þa*n* þe web, *and* þe nayl is þicker þa*n* þe clooþ.

A colliry þ*er*e-as þe obtalmye is y-hid w*it*h-i*n*ne-forþ: Tak of þe roses, *dragme* iiij; of acacie, *dragme* ii; of spik, *dragme* j; of opiu*m*, *dragme* s*emis*. Te*m*pre he*m* w*it*h wat*er* of roses, oþ*er* of reyn, oþ*er* w*it*h þe iuys of plau*n*teyn, of violet, of endyue.

5 **heed**] *follow. by* þe heed 6 **make**] *follow. by* su*m* (s *oblit.*) **sum**] *in l.-h. margin* 9 **for**] *corr. from* ffor 14 **encressyng**] *prec. by heading* The eiȝen 20 **For**] *corr. from* ffor

Anoþ*er* þ*a*t is a whiȝt collirie: Tak of gu*m*me arabik, dragag*e*, amyde, of eu*e*rich*e*, *dragme* iiij; of ceruse, *dragme* j; of opiu*m*, *dragme* j. Te*m*pre he*m* w*it*h þe whiȝt of an ey.

Anoþ*er*: Tak of sarcocolle, *dragme* iij; of amyde, gu*m*y arabik, drag*e*, *dragme* ij; of cathmie argent*e*, of ceruse, *dragme* j *and* s*emis*; of ence*n*se, of opiu*m*, *dragme* j. Te*m*pre he*m* w*it*h þe wat*er* of roses oþ*er* w*it*h þe iuys of plau*n*teyn.

Anoþ*er*: Tak of dragag*e*, *dragme* j; of citre, *dragme* ij; of sarcocolle, *dragme* iiij; of m[e]myth, *dragme* viij. Te*m*pre he*m* w*it*h wat*er* of roses oþ*er* of reyn.

A collirie in þe wexyng of þe sicnesse to do a-wey þe
f. 35v ache: Tac of ceruse, *dragme* ij; | of cathmye, tuchie, gu*m*i arab*e*, dragag*e*, amyde, of eu*e*rich*e*, *dragme* j; of acacie, of opiu*m*, *dragme* s*emis*. Te*m*pr*e* he*m* w*it*h reyn-wat*er*.

Anoþ*er* collirie: Tac rosees, cathmye, gu*m*i arab*e*, dragag*e*, amyde, iiij *dragme*; ceruse, cost, ij *dragme*; of opiu*m*, *dragme* s*emis*. Te*m*pre he*m* w*it*h reyn-wat*er*. But aft*ur* cessyng of þe ache, ȝif þere leue eny web eþ*er* wem w*it*h-owty*n*, ony oþ*er* humo*ur* þ*er* hardyd, oþ*er* þe obtalmye w*it*h-owty*n* þe eiȝen, þ*o*u moost vse colliries þ*a*t bie*n* corrosyf *and* fretyng. But furst, ley þ*er*-to mollyficatifs to make*n* þe mat*er* neisch*e*, as femygrek oþ*er* lynsed. And aft*ur*, ȝif þe soor is ȝonge *and* newe, ley þ*er* to esy corosyues.

Esy corrosyues bie*n* as rewe, eufrace, ce*n*tru*m* galli, filago, liciu*m*, þe driȝt of an grene ofete, mirre, encense, sarcocolle, hony, *and* ceruse, camphore, cathmia, emachites, spik, me-mythe, [a]mber, gyng*er*, þe knot of a vyne, acacia, lymaile of goold, musk, *and* sich*e* oþ*er*.

9 memyth] *corr. from* momyth **12 of**[2]] *prec. by heading* The eiȝen **13 arabe**] *corr. from* arabey (y *canc. twice*) **27 amber**] *corr. from* limber

Strong corrosyues bie þe galle of eu*er*ych*e* best *and* p*ri*ncypaly of a rauenyn*g* briddes *and* of a bole, þe fatnesse of a quaile, castore, antymonye, bras j-brent, sandeuer, cop*er*ose, calamyna, magnes, tuchia, baume, þe dri3t of eu*er*iche beest j-brent *and* na*m*ly of a ma*n*, eu*er*ich*e* kynde of saalt, *and* sal-nitr*e*, sal armoniac, v*er*tegr*e*ce, þe i*n*n[e]re skyn of an*n* he*n*n*us* mawhe, alym, lau*n*ceolu*m* þ*a*t groweþ in wat*ur*, lymaile of bras, comyn, *and* pep*er*, þe stoon þ*a*t is | j- f. 36r foundyn a-mong lyme, aloes, þe blood of a blak flye, spume of þe see, os sepie, þe seed of spurge, chikenweed, *and* psilotru*m* þ*a*t is j-maad to don a-wey herys. But a-mong all*e* þese corrosyuys, tuchia is on of þe best for þe ei3en. But þ*o*u moste heetyn hy*m* ix siþis in þe feyr *and* que*n*chy*n* hi*m* as often-siþes in þe iuys of sowr grapys, oþ*er* of eufrasie, oþ*er* fenel, oþ*er* whi3t wyn, oþ*er* sich*e* oþ*er* þi*n*g. But þ*er* bien iij kyndes of tuchie: whi3t, *and* reed, *and* blak. *And* eu*er*ich*e* on of he*m* is mitigatif, *and* rep*er*cussif, *and* corosif, but þe whi3te is more rep*er*cussif in þe heete *and* in þe rednesse of þe ei3e*n*. Þe blac is mytigatif. And þe reed is moost rep*er*cussif.

And many of þese gret corosyues mote*n* bie wasche*n* in diu*er*se þi*n*ges to a-bate*n* her*e* malice. Calamina xal bie xx siþes j-que*n*chid in þe iuys of fenel, oþ*er* in childes vrine, oþ*er* in woma*n*n*us* mylk, oþ*er* in wyn of pomgarnad. Cathmia xal bie ix siþes j-wasche*n* in got*us* mylk, oþ*er* asse mylke, oþ*er* woma*n*n*us* mylk. Aloes xal by as ofty*n*-siþes in þe iuys of fenel. And antymonie *and* bras j-brent in þe same

6 **sal armoniac]** *corr. from* salarmoniac **innere]** *corr. from* i*n*nore
8 j-foundyn] *prec. by heading* The ei3en **12 of]** *in r.-h. margin*

12 þe[1]**]** *in r.-h. margin:* no*ta*

manere xul bie j-qwe*n*chid *and* j-waische, for þei bie*n* moost viole*n*t corosifs. And aft*ur*, þei mou*n* bien j-pit in colliries.

Su*m*me þinges bie*n* j-waischen to haue more viole*n*ce þa*n* þei hadden, as ence*n*se j-waische in þe iuys of celedoyne, and many oþ*er* þinges þ*at* serue*n* for oþ*er* sicnesses bi waisching lieseþ mych*e* of her*e* viole*n*ce, as lapis laȝuli, and f. 36v lapis armenic*us*, | j-waischen in wat*er*, *and* spurge seed in oyle. And scamone in þe iuys of plaunteyn is nat so laxatif as it was, ne aloes, *and* it bie j-waschi*n*, is nat so sotyl and so p*er*syng as it was, ne lym j-waische*n* ne is so brennyng as it was.

And medicines bien oþ*er*while j-brent to enc*r*esce here violence, as atrament *and* calamina. Su*m*me bie*n* j-brent to bie þe more sotil, as wat*er* cankre þ*at* is j-ȝeuy*n* to me*n* þ*at* bien etik. Su*m*me þi*ng*us bie*n* j-brent for þei xuldy*n* bie þe bet*er*e j-poudred, as sendel; su*m*me to liesyn here venimysnesse, as a scorpio*n* wha*n* me*n* takeþ hy*m* for þe stoon. And grettyr medicines þ*at* bie*n* of gret mat*er*, þorow bre*n*ny*n*g, þei wex þe more violent. Suttyl medicines in brennyng, liesen here violence, and mene medicines þ*at* bien nat riȝt sotel ne riȝt grete. But in makyng colliries þ*at* bie*n* corrysifs, þ*o*u moost medle w*ith* corrosifs, mytigatifs, *and* confortatifs, as wha*n* þei bien j-poudred, te*m*pre he*m* w*ith* þe wat*er* of rosees, oþ*er* þe iuys of plau*n*teyne, oþ*er* of fenel, oþ*er* of eufrase, oþ*er* of rwe, oþ*er* þe blood of a lapwynke oþ*er* of a swalwe. And siþþe, driȝe he*m* in þe su*n*ne. And so doo iij or iiij siþes. And so poudre it smal and bulte it þorow a smal clooþ. And siþþe, medle it w*ith* þe iuys of oon of þe for-seyd herbys, oþ*er* w*ith* þe blood of a capou*n*, oþ*er* of an

7 j-waischen] *prec. by heading* Aposteem **spurge]** *interl.* r hare, oþ*er* of a ram, oþ*er* of a boor. *And* so do it in his eiȝe. But loke þ*a*t þ*in* colliries bie*n* nat to st*r*ong | *and* violent, for harmyng of þe eiȝe. f. 37r And ȝif ony sich*e* bie in hese eiȝe, cast in a-noon woma*nn us* mylk. *And* gadere it owt as clene as þ*o*u myȝt. And siþe, lei to þe eiȝe mytigatifs *and* co*n*fortatifs, as dragag*e* resolued in coold wat*er*; oþ*er* þ*er* mussilage of p*er*sillie þ*a*t is þus j-maad: Tac þe seed of p*er*sillie *and* cast it in a vessel of coold wat*er*. *And* þe wat*er* vol wexe þicke as gelee oþ*er* gleir*e* of eyren. Wryng þ*a*t clooþ *and* kep it, for it is j-clepid mussilage. And in þe same man*er* þ*o*u mytist make mussilage of ocul*us* x*risti*. *And* boþe bie*n* good mytigatifs.

A good colirie: Tac of sarcocolle, encense, gu*m*i arab*e*, *and* of amyde, *dragme* iij; of liciu*m*, mirre, *and* ceruse, *dragme* ij; of aloes, tuchie, roses, *and* of ca*m*phere, *dragme* j; of opiu*m*, *dragme* j. And wha*n* þ*o*u ȝeuyst a ma*n* coliries, boþe bi-fore and aft*ur*, a-noynte þe eiȝen w*ith* wat*er* þ*a*t rosees or plau*n*teyn bie*n* j-soden i*n*ne, in greuau*n*ce þ*a*t comeþ of hete; but ȝif it comeþ of coold, w*ith* wat*er* of eufrase or of fenel. Jn coold causes, vse medicynes as þ*a*t was j-teld in þe last chapitre, and þe colliries of þ*i*s chapitr*e*. But ar þan þ*o*u ȝyue hy*m* colliries, make he*m* a plastre of beene mele in a bagge j-soden in wyn, oþ*er* of gyng*er and* a lytyl hony, oþ*er* sich*e* oþ*ere* as it was teeld in þe oþ*ere* chapitre, and baþi*n*ge also *and* st*ri*ctories as it was told þer*e*.

2 and] *prec. by heading* of the eiȝe **7** is] *follow. by canc.* iuys **17 water**] *follow. by exp.* of þat] *interl.* **20 medicynes**] *interl.* first e **23 and**] *follow. by canc. twice* of

6 mussilage] *in r.-h. margin:* no*ta* b*e*n*e* | Muscilag[e]

f. 37v A collirie: | Tac aloes, *and* myrre, *and* encense, *and* calamina, ceruse, tuchia, of eu*er*ich*e*, j-lich*e* mych*e*; of amyde, su*m*what more; of opiu*m*, wel lasse. *And* mak þ*er*-of a collirie.

Oþere sicnesses þ*er* bie*n* of þe eiȝen. Oon is a web oþ*er* a wem þ*at* hideþ þe mydel of þe eiȝe. And þis is in to maneres: Oþ*er*while he is whiȝt *and* þi*n*ne, and oþ*er*whiles he is þicke, as wha*n*ne obtalmie is nat clene j-helyd vp but þe rote a-bideþ stylle. Oþ*er*whiles þe web is nat whiȝt, but reed oþ*er* blak. But wha*n*ne al þe eiȝe is keuerid, þa*n* it is j-clepid a clooþ. And wha*n*ne it keuereþ þe oon cornere of þe eiȝe, þa*n* it is j-clepid vngula. And þis g*r*euau*n*ce comeþ of corupt humo*urs* as obtalmie doiþ. And xal bie helyd by corrosyues, co*n*fortatyu*us*, rep*er*cussiu*us*, mitigatyues, *and* st*ri*ctories, *and* blood-lety*n*g*us*, as obtalmie is j-helyd. But ȝif it comeþ of obtalmye oþ*er* of eny hurtyng of þe eiȝe þ*at* is nat weel j-helyd, þ*o*u most vsen consolidatyues in þi colliries, as sarcocolle, oþere aloes, mirre, encense, emachites, sandragu*n*, w*it*h þe white of an ei, oþ*er* w*it*h þe iuys of plau*n*teyne, oþ*er* w*it*h þe iuys of auence. And in þe by-gy*n*ny*n*g, it is good to vse mollytiu*us* ȝif it be so þ*at* þe eiȝen bie*n* nat ful moist. And siþe, worche w*it*h corrosyu*us*, first w*it*h esy, *and* siþþe w*it*h streng*ur*e.

Ȝif it nedeþ good mollytiu*us*, bie*n* woma*n*n*us* mylk, *and* þe wat*er* þ*at* þe hocke *and* þe holy-hocke bien j-soden i*n*ne,
f. 38r lynseed, femygrek, w*it*h þe iuys of fenel, and þe wat*er* | þ*at* floweþ of a snail wha*n* his hows is ip*er*sed. And þe beste of

1 **Tac**] *prec. by heading* ffor þe eiȝen 5 **Oþere**] *2-line space left for initial* 19 **ei**] *corr. from* eiȝe (ȝe *canc. twice*) 25 **þe**^{2}] *follow. by* hocke (c *oblit.*) **hocke**] *in l.-h. margin* 26 **water**] *catchword* (*in bottom margin*): þat floweþ of **þat**] *prec. by heading* ffor þe eiȝen

all*e* is oyl of notes þ*a*t is þ*us* j-maad: Tac notes *and* seeþ hem in wat*er* al hool. *And* siþþe, breke hem *and* tak owte þe kerneles, *and* stamp he*m*. *And* siþþe, wrynge hem þorow a clooþ. *And* þ*a*t oile is a nobil mollityf. And ȝif þe greuau*n*ce bie of newe, tak þe iuys of chicke*n*mete oþ*er* of reed popi. *And* it wul suffisen. Oþ*er* mak a collirie of mirre, aloes, liciu*m*, w*it*h þe iuys of fenel. And ȝif þese fretyn a-wey, tak su*m*me streng*ur*e fret*er*es, as os sepie, spume of þe see, calamyna, *and* tuchie: Þ*a*t is þe beest of he*m* alle. Oþ*er* seþe salt in vinegre *and* poudre it. *And* cast in-to þe eiȝe, jt freteþ a-wey þe web. And so dooþ þe iuys of celidoine, of v*er*ueyne, ȝif þe sor*e* bie newe. Also tac a reed snail *and* salt hy*m* in a bacyn. *And* lat hi*m* ligge*n* a-iij daies. *And* aft*ur*, set þ*in* bacyn a-slont and þ*a*t wat*er* þ*a*t comeþ fro hym, do it in his eiȝe. Also tac calamyna *and* tempre it w*it*h þe iuys of fenel. *And* do it in his eiȝe *and* lat it bie þere iij days. *And* þa*n* do a-wey þe piece þ*a*t it haþ j-frete a-wey. And siþþe, do of þe oþ*er* lico*ur* in his eiȝe.

A good poudre to frete*n* a-wey eu*er*ich*e* kynde of web in a ma*nn**us* eiȝe, *and* þei it bie old so þ*a*t mollificatifs goon bie-fore: Tak of amide, of sarcocolle, *dragme* ij; of roses, *dragme* s*emis*; of tuchie, *dragme* s*emis*. Te*m*pre he*m* w*it*h þe iuys of eufrace oþ*er* fenel. And siþ, driȝe þat fele daies in þe su*n*ne, and þa*n* do þ*er*-of in his eiȝe. And ȝif he mowe not wel suffren it, medle it w*it*h þe blood of an he*n*ne, or w*it*h þe iuys of su*m*me herbe þ*a*t is good for þe eiȝe*n*, as eufrace,

8 freteres] *interl.* first e **25 henne]** *follow. by canc. twice* oþ

1 Tac] *in r.-h. margin:* no*ta* **2 hem]** *in r.-h. margin:* no*ta* ben*e* mod **3 wrynge]** *in r.-h. margin:* Oile **25 blood]** *in r.-h. margin:* Good h*er*b[e] | þe eiȝen

plau*n*teyn, egremonye, ve*r*ueyne, endyue, filago, celydoyne, oþ*er* sich*e* oþ*er*e: Þere is no bet*er* medicyne for þis greuau*n*ce.

f. 38v And | vnderstond þ*at* þe beste man*er* to make poud*er*es smale for þe eiȝen is to rubben hem w*ith* þe iuys of þe for-seyd herbis, or a barbours wheston, oþ*er* in a weel scoryd bacyn. Anoþ*er*: Tac of hony dispumed, *dragme* iij; of hare blood, *dragme* ij; of coperose, *dragme* j. A-noþ*er*: Tac hony, *and* þe mylk of a biche, *and* hare blood. A-noþ*er*: Tac whiȝt wyn *and* smal wormes leene of þe erþe, *and* powne he*m* to-gidere. Oþ*er*: Pyt a pep*er* corn in þe knotte of a whiȝt vine, *and* rubbe it w*ith* whiȝt wyn on a westo*n*, *and* do licour su*m*what white in his eiȝe*n*. Oþ*er*: Tak þe blood of blake flien þ*at* sittyn on hockys oþ*er* on co*n*firie þ*at* schiteþ reed drit, *and* medl[e] yt in þ*in* hond w*ith* spotel; w*ith*-i*n*ne iij daies, it brekeþ þe web. And þe blood of an eel *and* his galle, and þe samonus also heeliþ sich*e* sicnesse; and þe grece of a quayle and þe fatnesse of an hare, for it brekeþ þe stoon in a ma*n*n*us* bleddre; and a lapwyng *and* her*e* brayn j-dried, and hoot blood of a swalwe, and þe poudre of scho solus j-brent; and þe blood of a grene ofete wha*n* þe heed *and* þe tail bien j-kyt of, for þei bie venenouse, *and* his driȝt al-so. And þe iuys of þe iij-leuyd gras þ*at* haþ whiȝt speckys is good for whiȝte webbys, and of hym þ*at* haþ þe blake for blake webbys, and gold oþ*ur* latu*n* y-froted on a wheston w*ith* vynegre til þe vinegre bie þicke, *and* aft*ur*ward j-dried is

4 vnderstond] *prec. by heading* The eiȝen **15 medle yt**] *corr. from* medlyt **18 for**] *corr. from* ffor **22 for**] *corr. from* ffor

13 blood] *in l.-h. margin:* m*em*or*a*b*i*le **14 confirie**] *in l.-h. margin:* no*ta* m*em*or*a*b*i*le

good *and* drieþ myche þe eiȝe*n*. Oþ*er*: Take þe iuys of cap*ri*folie *and* medle it w*it*h þe poudre of leed. *And* siþ, cast þ*er*-to vinegre *and* þe | iij part oile, *and* seeþ hem to-geder*e*. f. 39r *And* siþþe clanse it *and* do it in hese eiȝe wha*n* he gooþ to bedde, ȝif þe web bie newe.

Þe poudre of leed xal þ*us* bie maad: Tac leed *and* melte it ou*er* þ*er* fier *and* stere it w*it*h a grene aselyn sticke. *And* it wole turne to blac poudre, and þ*a*t is good for þis g*re*uau*n*ce. A-noþ*er* good collirie: Tac þe galles þ*a*t leueþ by raueyne *and* te*m*pre þ*er*-w*it*h þe poudre of mirr*e*, aloes, sarcocolle, encense, perles, *and* whiȝt coral, of eu*er*ichon of hem, j-liche myche. But loke þ*a*t þ*o*u legge nat eu*er*mor*e* corosyues, but oþ*er*while mytigatifs, *and* co*n*fortatifs, *and* mollytifs; for ellys þ*o*u mytest, þorow viole*n*ce of corosyues, destrie þe eiȝe. And wha*n* þ*o*u co*n*fortest þe eiȝe, co*n*forte hy*m* boþe w*it*h-i*n*ne *and* w*it*h-owte. And confort þe stomac, for þ*a*t is p*ro*fitabil to þe eiȝen. And in driȝe eiȝen, vse moist corosyues; in oold greuau*n*ces, stronge corrosyues *and* i*n*ne newe greuau*n*ces esy corosyues aft*ur* þ*in* discrecyon.

Also a ma*n*n*us* eiȝen bien oþ*er*whiles reed oþer infect. Reednesse comeþ of blood; infeccion comeþ of oþ*er* humo*urs* *and* of oþ*er*e sicnesses, as of þe ȝelwe euele, oþ*er* stoppyng of þe splene, oþ*er* heetyng of þe leuere. And to hele sich*e* infeccions, me moste helen ferst þe sicnesses þ*a*t bien cause of hem, and siþþe vse colliries þ*a*t bien a lytil corrosyf *and* mu*n*dificatif to frete*n* a-wey *and* to clens[e]n þ*a*t infeccio*un*

3 **iij**] *prec. by heading* The eiȝen   9 **good**] *in l.-h. margin*   13 **for**] *corr. from* ffor   20 **Also**] *2-line space left for initial*   23 **leuere**] *corr. from* spleuere (sp *canc. twice and exp.*)   26 **clensen**] *corr. from* clenson

8 **to**] *in r.-h. margin:* No*ta* bene

f. 39v *and* purge*n* þe body of þ*a*t humo*ur* | þ*a*t is encheson of þ*a*t infeccion. Of blood comeþ rednesse, *and* nat þ*a*t aloonly, but oþ*er*whiles a gobet of flesch*e* growyng on þe eiȝe. Oþ*er*whiles, for gret plente of blood *and* feblenesse of þe eiȝe, þe blood liþ j-co*n*geled on þe eiȝe *and* makeþ þe eiȝe*n* reede. Oþ*er*while þei bie*n* reede for gret ple*n*te of blood þ*a*t is in þe veinys. And oþ*er*whiles þorow fallyng oþ*er* þorow smytynge, blood falleþ in-to þe eiȝe *and* makeþ hem reed.

Ȝif þer*e* grow a pece of fleisch*e* on þe eiȝe, let frete it a-wey w*ith* strong corrosyues. But late nat hy*m* touche þe eiȝe. And ȝif it wul nat bie frete*n* a-wey, kyt it a-wey *and* strawe strong corrosiues byneþe*n* þ*a*t it grow nat a-ȝe*n*. And w*ith* a strictorie *and* blood-letyng, mak þ*a*t þe blood bie j-lettyd of his cours to þe eiȝe. And aft*ur*ward, ȝif hi*m* colliries þ*a*t mowe*n* clanse *and* co*n*forte þe eiȝe, as we teylde*n* bie-fore. And ȝif þ*er* bie mych*e* blood in þe veynis of þe eiȝe*n*, let hy*m* blood in þe veyn of þe heed in þe arm, or in þe veyn of þe elbow, oþ*er* of þe womb. And ȝif þe eiȝe bie kyt in þe whiȝt of þe eiȝe, oþ*er* þe whiȝt bie j-broke, hele it vp here-w*ith*: Tak sarcocolle, mastik, ence*n*se, sandragou*n*, emathite. *And* te*m*pre he*m* w*ith* sanguinarie þ*a*t is j-clepid schep*er*dus-purs, oþ*er* plaunteyn. Oþ*er* tac aloes *and* amyde, f. 40r *and* te*m*pre hem w*ith* þe blood of a culuere oþ*er* of | an hen, and lei no corrosyues, but ȝif þei bie*n* feble *and* here violence bie do a-wey. But vse here co*n*solidatyues, þ*a*t is to say, siche þi*n*ges þ*a*t wole*n* souden a þi*n*g þ*a*t is j-kyt oþ*er* to-broke, as co*n*firie, *and* daisye, *and* þe mydle confirye, *and* centorie, *and* plau*n*teyn, *and* aua*n*ce, *and* siche oþ*er*e, *and* sa*n*dragou*n*, *and* emathite. But loke þ*a*t þe collirie ne make nat þe eiȝe to

1 **þat**[2]] *prec. by heading* The eiȝen **16** **þe**[1]] *follow. by canc.* eiȝe
23 **an**] *prec. by heading* The eiȝen

ychche ne smerte. And ȝif þe blood is co*n*gelyd, þ*at* is to seie, j-hardyd *and* maad þicke þorow coold, þ*ou* must co*n*sume it, *and* dissolue*n* it, *and* departe*n* it fra*m* þe place þ*at* it is i*n*ne, as w*ith* þe iuys of verueyne *and* of plau*n*teyn j-medlid to-gedere. And þ*ou* must cle*n*se þe eiȝe w*ith* mu*n*dificatyues, as w*ith* þe iuys of endyue, oþ*er* þe wat*er* of a vine, oþ*er* comyn *and* þe iuys of rewe *and* wyn j-soden to-gidere, oþ*er* þe crust of a loof j-rosted *and* j-powned w*ith* iuys of rewe *and* w*ith* þe for-seid wyn j-plastred on þe eiȝe, oþ*er* encense *and* mastik j-medlyd w*ith* þe iuys of march *and* þe gleyre of an ey, oþ*er* isope j-soden i*n* wat*er* *and* j-plastred a-boue*n*, oþ*er* verte-g*r*ese cast i*n* wyn, *and* siþþe þe wyn wha*n* it is cleer*e*, j-cast in-to þe ei3en.

For ichchyng of þe eiȝen: Dragagaunt is good in colliries oþ*er* hym-self in coold wat*er*, p*er*sillie *and* his mussilage, oile of roses, *and* þe whiȝte of eyre*n*. But algatis bie þei ware of clawynge.

Moistnesse of þe eiȝe*n* comeþ of þe heed þ*at* is replet | f. 40v
w*ith* humo*urs*, as blereschipe of þe eiȝen comeþ of cooldnesse *and* of moistnesse of þe brayn. And þ*er*-fore it by-houeþ to purgen þe heed *and* na*m*ly of male*n*colie, as it was teld in þe sicnesse of þe heed. And aft*ur*ward, lat baþi*n* hym in a baaþ of lorel leeues, *and* of rewe, eg*r*emoyne, *and* beteyne, fenel, *and* oþ*er* herbys þ*at* bie*n* co*n*fortabil for þe brayn. And siþþe waisch his heed w*ith* þe wat*er* while it is warm. And siþþe 3if hi*m* su*m*what in hese nose to make*n* hym fnese. And make hym to chewe poudre of piretre, s[t]aphie, *and* seneuey. And what humo*ur* þ*at* falleþ a-down fra*m* his brayn, let hit passyn owt at hise mowþ. And siþþe

14 For] *corr. from* ffor **19 with**] *prec. by heading* Wepy*n*g of the eiȝen
28 staphie] *corr. from* scaphie

leie hym a bedde *and* lat a woma*n*[es] mylke þ*a*t fedeþ a knaue child [a-noynte] his eiȝen. And i*n*ne þis manere blereid-eiȝe*n* and aky*n*ge bien j-helyd. Aft*ur* make hi*m* a collirie co*n*fortatyf of spik, *and* foliu*m*, *and* wat*er* of roses, *and* eufrace, *and* fenel, *and* sych*e* oþ*er* þinges.

Wepynge of þe eiȝen comeþ oþ*er*while of enchesou*n*s w*it*h-oute-forþ, as of smokes, oþ*er* of wynd, oþ*er* dust, oþ*er* sich*e* oþ*er* þing, oþ*er* of a strok. Oþ*er*whiles it comeþ of w*it*h-i*n*ne, as of ioye, oþ*er* of sorow, oþ*er* of angur, oþur of plente of humo*ur*s in þe heed, as of feblenesse of þe veynis f. 41r þ*a*t bien in þe eiȝen. And ȝif | plente of humo*ur*s bie*n* þe enchesou*n*, a p*ur*gaciou*n* is p*ro*fitabil. And ȝif he haue g*re*t ple*n*te of blood, let hy*m* blood in þe veinys þ*a*t cle*n*syn þe eiȝe*n* *and* þe heed, as þe heed veyn of þe arme, oþ*er* þe veyne þ*a*t is bie-twyne þe þombe *and* þe nexte fynger, oþ*er* þe veyne of þe elbow. And make an enplastre of encense, mastik, bole, sandragou*n*, þe whiȝte of an ey, *and* a lytil wyn *and* a lytil vinegre, *and* lej þ*a*t on his forheed. But loke þ*a*t in non sicnesse of þe eiȝen, bie it of coold oþ*er* of heete, þ*o*u legge non hoot plastre to þe eiȝen. And ȝif þ*o*u leist a coold plastre to þe eiȝen þ*a*t bien riȝt hoote, ne late þ*o*u not þe plastre ligge ful longe, lese it catche heete of þe eiȝen. And ȝif wepy*n*g come of feblenesse of þe brayn, co*n*fort þe brayn. *And* in þe be-gy*n*nyng, make a collirie of ceruse, dragag*e*, foliu*m*, roses, of eu*er*iche, j-lyche mych*e*. And smyþis wat*er* is p*ro*fitabil for þis greuau*n*ce, and for þe web, and for þe

1 **womanes ... eiȝen]** *corr. from* woma*n* mylke his eiȝen þ*a*t fedeþ a knaue child **6 Wepynge]** *2-line space left for initial* 11 **plente]** *prec. by heading* Cankyr of the eiȝe

19 heete] *in r.-h. margin:* Reg*u*la ge[neralis] (*underl.*)

bries þ*a*t bien j-t*ur*ned i*n*warde. Also tac of ceruse, gu*m*i arab*e*, *and* of ence*n*se, *dragme* ij; of dragag*e*, *dragme* j; of opiu*m*, *dragme* s*emis*. Anoþ*er*: Distille a wat*er* of eg*re*moyne, of fenel, *and* ve*r*ueyne, *and* roses i*n* þe g*re*ttest q*ua*ntite.

For þe canker of þe eiȝe: ȝif [it] is of colre, [it] makeþ þe eiȝe hard, *and* freteþ a-wey þe bries, *and* makeþ þe eiȝe ful hoot. And þa*n*ne he xal bien j-helyd w*it*h a plastre j-maad of | litarge *and* of solatre, oþ*er* w*it*h hempseed *and* ocul*us* x*risti* f. 41v j-powned to-gider*e* *and* j-plastred on his eiȝe. But ȝif it bie of male*n*colie, þe eiȝe is ful hard *and* ful heuy. *And* þa*n*ne make a plastre of beene mele *and* boles galles.

For hurtyng of þe horned clooþ of þe eiȝe, *and* closeþ þe appel of þe eiȝe *and* þe humo*ur*s þ*a*t bie*n* a-bowten hym, þu most vsen co*n*solidatifs in þ*in* colliries, *and* no siche þinges þ*a*t wole make þe eiȝe to smerte ne itche, but mytigatyues *and* co*n*fortatyues. Narþeles, woma*n*n*us* mylk is nat ful good here, for it is to moist, but þe blood of culuere oþ*er* of a chike is good here, and þe consolidatifs þ*a*t weru*n* j-teld in þe sicnesse of þe eiȝen. Also þe wat*er* þ*a*t whete was j-sode*n* i*n*ne w*it*h oþ*er* co*n*solidatyues *and* co*n*fortatyues, as roses, *and* eufrace, *and* siche oþ*er* is ful good. And aft*ur* þu most legge siche þing*us* to þe eiȝe þ*a*t þe wou*n*de bie nat a-sene, þ*a*t is, þe iuys of mad*ur*, *and* boras, and þe fatnesse of an he*n*ne *and* þe mary of here bonys, *and* sich*e* oþ*er* þinges. And ȝif þere wexiþ ony postem*us*, as bleynys on þis party of þe eiȝe, tac apostolico*n* *and* medle it ou*er* þe feir w*it*h oile

1 of] *interl.* **5 quantite]** *interl.* **6 For]** *2-line space left for initial; corr. from* ffor **it[1]]** *corr. from* he **it[2]]** *corr. from* he **9 litarge]** *prec. by heading* Hurty*n*g of the eiȝe **11 is]** *interl.* **13 For]** *2-line space left for initial; corr. from* ffor **27 þe[1]]** *follow. by canc.* eȝe *and* w*ith* boles talwe. *And* wet a lytil clowt i*n* wyn, *and* siþþe a-noy*n*te it w*ith* þis oyneme*nt*, *and* leiȝe to þe eiȝe. Oþ*er* tac þe poud*re* of gyng*er* *and* aloes cicatryn, *and* medle he*m* w*ith* f. 42r hony, *and* ley vp-on þe eiȝen. |

Feblenesse of siȝt comeþ in many man*er*es, as bi sicnesse of þe eiȝen, as we ha*n* j-teld bi-fore; oþ*er* of sicnesse of þe heed, *and* þa*n* it is j-holpe*n* bie helyng of þilke sicnesse; oþ*er* of g*re*uau*n*ce of þe stomac, and þei bien a-me*n*did þorow helynge of þe stomac. Oþ*er*-while þe feblenesse of þe eiȝe comeþ of feblenesse of here spiritis, and here þ*o*u xalt vnd*er*stonde þ*at* siche spiritis bien smale bodies þ*at* bien i*n*ne a ma*n*n*us* eiȝe. And þei bie*n* þe inst*r*ume*nt*es of þ*at* þe siȝte seeþ forþ w*ith*, for siche spritys receyue*n* þe lithnesse of þilke þi*n*gus þ*at* a ma*n* j-seeþ. And þ*er*-fore wha*n* þei bie*n* feble, nedlyche þe siȝt most bien feble.

And for þis sicnesse a piȝe is ful profytabil i*n* many maneris. On manere is to etyn here j-sode*n* oþ*er* j-rosted. Anoþ*er* man*er* is to pulle*n* here *and* to take*n* owt here guttys, *and* brenne þe re*m*nawnt in a newe erþen pot þ*at* bie wel j-stopped a-boue. And þe poudre is p*ro*fitabil in metes, *and* drynkys, and i*n*ne colliries. And þilke poudre is good al-so for þe cardiacle, and for male*n*colie, and oþ*er* coold sicnesses, *and* for þe cankre in a ma*n*n*us* ȝerde. Anoþ*er* manere of þe piȝe is þis: Pulle here *and* tac owt here guttys, *and* seeþ þe oþ*er* del in whiȝt wyn tyl þe wyn bie sodyn a-

5 Feblenesse] *2-line space left for initial; corr. from* ffeblenesse; *prec. by heading* ffebylnesse of syȝt **12 þat**] *follow. by canc. and exp.* ma*n*n*us* **þe**[2]] *interl.* **13 for**] *corr. from* ffor **25 oþer del**] *corr. from* oþ*er*del

16 for] *in r.-h. margin:* no*ta* **23 Anoþer**] *in r.-h. margin:* no*ta*

wey *and* þe fleisch departed fro þe bonys. And þa*n*ne powne it al to-geder*e* *and* pit it i*n* a vessel. *And* lat þe þynne re*n*ne fro þe þicke | iij daies. *And* tac þa*n*ne lynet of a smal clene (f. 42v) lynet clowt, *and* wete it in þe lycour, *and* do of þe lyco*ur* boþe w*ith*-i*n*ne þe eiȝe *and* w*ith*-owte, for it doeþ a-wey þe dercnesse *and* þe smerty*n*g of þe eiȝe, *and* þe reednesse, *and* þe ache, *and* conforteþ þe spirit*us*. And netle seed also is good in dercnesse of þe eiȝen, *and* þe wat*er* þ*at* þe seed is j-soden i*n*ne; also a got*us* lyuere j-rosted *and* j-spreynt w*ith* poudre of pep*er* *and* j-ete, *and* þe lyco*ur* þ*er*-of j-dropped in his eiȝe. Also seeþ þe lyu*er*e *and* þe splene of a goot, *and* þe skymmyng þ*er*-of do it in hese eiȝe*n*. Also kyt þe lyu*er*e of a goot, *and* salt it, *and* seeþ it in vinegre, *and* hange þe eiȝen ou*er* þe smoke. Also distille a wat*er* of eufrace, celedoyne, rwe, eg*r*emoyne, fenel, *and* of roses. Also tac þe galle of an hare *and* of an eel, *and* te*m*pre he*m* w*ith* þe for-seyd wat*ur* *and* hony, oþ*er* w*ith* þe for-seyd wat*ur* bie hym-self. Also tac an hoot barly loof *and* breke hy*m* a-two. *And* cast þe powd*re* of carewey þ*er*-on *and* hoold þi*n* eiȝe*n* ou*er* þe smoke. Also seeþ turme*n*tille in wyn *and* drynk þe wyn, *and* lei þe herbe on þi eiȝe. And it is good for hem þ*at* han feire eiȝen *and* j-seeþ noþi*n*g, for w*ith*-i*n*ne ix daies it makeþ he*m* seen. Also tac þe iuys of fenel *and* of heihoue, *and* set it i*n*ne þe su*n*ne iij daies in a brasen vessel. *And* siþþe do þ*er*-of i*n*ne þe eiȝe oþ*er* a-noon do it in his eiȝe. Oþ*er* medle þe iuys of heyhoue *and* hony to-gedere; oþ*er* mak a plastre of comy*n* j-poudryd *and* whiȝt wyn, *and* ley it on hese eiȝe, but ley a clooþ bi-

3 iij] *prec. by heading* ffebylnesse **5 for**] *corr. from* ffor **20 and**[1]] *follow. by canc.* seeþ **drynk**] *interl.* **22 for**] *corr. from* ffor

21 eiȝe] *in l.-h. margin:* no*ta*

f. 43r

twene. Oþ*er* tac þe iuys of wermot *and* of rwe, of boþe j-lyche meche, *and* cast i*n*ne to þe ei3e; oþ*er* tac þe | iuys of rwe *and* hony *and* medle hem to-gidere *and* cast it in-to his ei3e. *And* it makeþ þe flowyng of þe wat*er* to cessyn. Oþ*er* tac gyng*er*, *and* þe iuys of fenel, *and* whi3t wyn, *and* medle hem to-gidere. *And* dri3e he*m* in þe su*n*ne *and* do þ*er*-of in þ*in* ei3en. Also medle þe iuys of celydonie, *and* of rwe, *and* of morwetydes dew, *and* hony, of eiþur j-lyche mych*e*. *And* drie it i*n*ne þe su*n*ne *and* aft*ur*ward do þ*er*-of in hese ei3e. Also tac a 3ong swalwe *and* pit owt here ei3e w*ith* a nedele. *And* aft*ur* iij daies, come a-3een *and* þ*o*u xal fynde here seen. Pulle of here heed þa*n*ne *and* bren it i*n*ne an erþen vessele. *And* make þ*er*-of smal poudre *and* medle þ*er*-w*ith* þe galle of a sowkyng qwelpe þ*at* is xxx daies old. *And* cast þ*er*-to half so myche of opobal3amu*m* *and* as myche of castore, *and* do þ*er*-of in hese ei3e.

A good poudre þ*at* clereþ þe si3t, co*n*forteþ þe stomac, *and* co*n*sumeþ corupt wy*n*des in a ma*n*n*us* body, *and* vse þ*er*-of eu*ery* day a lytil porciou*n*: Tak of loueache, anyse, ameos, march, canel, cardamome, origane, anet, carewey, fenel, silere mou*n*tayn, comyn, sauge, mynte, calamynte, eufrace, thime, pep*er*, ysope, p*er*sile, of eu*er*iche oon, *dragme* j; of ging*er*, liquoris, piliole, notemuge, *ounce* ij; of clowes, *and* gali*n*gale, *and* citre, *ounce* s*emis*; *and* 3if þ*o*u wolt, take *a pound* of piliole *and* 3if þ*o*u wolt, cast *pound* j of sug*re*. Þ*o*u mytest make*n* it in forme of an electuarie.

2 iuys] *prec. by heading* of sygth **4 flowyng**] *corr. from* fflowyng

10 nedele] *in r.-h. margin:* no*ta*

Anoþ*er* poud*re*: Tak of notemuge, ligni | aloes, sylere f. 43v mou*n*tayne, citre, mastik, rubarb*e*, eufrace, carawey, anete, fenel, *and* of masys, *dragme* ij; of gyng*er*, *and* of long pep*er*, *dragme* s*emis*. Mak here-of poudr*e* *and* lat hym vsen þ*a*t in hese mete.

A p*ro*fitable collirie for feble si3t: Tak hou*n*destonge, gallit*ri*cu*m*, rwe, cellidonie, eufrace, memythe, egremoyne, of eu*er*ich*e* of þese herbis, m*anipulum* s*emis*. Take þe iuys of þese herbys *and* seeþ hem w*ith* wyn. And cast þ*er*-to þis poudre: Tak aloes *and* tuchie þ*a*t is j-qwe*n*chid as we teld bifore; *and* sarcocolle, *and* þe ryndes of mirabol*e*, of eu*er*ich*e*, *dragme* ij; of whi3t pep*er*, camphore, whi3t coral *and* reed, *dragme* s*emis* of eu*er*ich*e*; of citre, *dragme* s*emis*; of marg*er*i p*er*les, *dragme* s*emis*. Þis collirie cleriþ þe si3t, *and* freteþ awey þe web, *and* stau*n*cheþ þe wateryng of þe ei3en, *and* doiþ a-wey þe reednesse of þe ei3e*n*.

Jn a mann*us* eei3lidis *and* his bries þ*er* bien many greuau*n*ces, as pimples, icchinge, cleuy*n*ge to-gedere by su*m* viscouse mat*er*e, turnyng þe bri3es in-ward, wormes in þe ei3e-ledis, *and* lyis a-mong þe herys.

Pymples *and* postem*us* bien oþ*er*whiles of viscouse mat*er*e j-gaderid to-gidere in a lytil skyn, oþ*er*whiles in þe man*er*e of scabbys, oþ*er*whiles in þe manere of stones. 3if it bie in þe firste man*er*e, it may bie helyd w*ith* a plastre aft*ur* þe q*ua*ntite of þe pympil j-maad of swynes galle *and* bene mele j-medlid to-gidere þ*er*-too, oþ*er* w*ith* a plastre of lily rotis *and* of affodille j-stamped to-gidere. 3if it bie in þe secu*n*de manere, as a scabbe, | mak a plastre of þe lilie roote, f. 44r

1 aloes] *prec. by heading* Sekenesse **17 Jn**] *2-line space left for initial* **23 scabbys**] *corr. from* scanbbys (*n canc. twice*) **28 mak**] *prec. by heading* of the ei3e-lydys *and* bran, *and* scabiose, *and* langedebeef; oþ*er* make hym su*m* oþ*er* medicine þ*a*t is p*ro*fitable for scabbys. Ȝif it bie in þe iij manere, take þe galle of an ylspil *and* l[e]y þ*er*-to; oþ*er* tak þe iuys of mellilot *and* a lytil of þe poudre of an audemau*n*t stoon, *and* medle he*m* to-gydere ou*er* þe fier, *and* ley it on a pece of leiþer*e* aft*ur* þe q*u*antite of þe g*re*uau*n*ce.

For ichynge, tac þe poudre of a reed wheston, *and* þe iuys, *and* atrame*n*t, *and* medle he*m* to-gidere in a bacyn. *And* siþþe driȝe it i*n*ne þe su*n*ne *and* keep it. Oþ*er* tac vinegre *and* lat it stond iij daies in a brasen vessel. *And* þa*n* cast þ*er*-to a lytil hony *and* ij pep*er* cornes j-poudred. *And* let it stonde a while i*n*ne þe su*n*ne *and* þ*er*-wiþ a-noynte hese bries.

For viscouse mat*er*e þ*a*t makeþ þe bries to cleue to-gidere, waisch*e* þe eiȝen w*ith* childes vrine oþ*er* þe skym of whiȝte sope *and* wat*er*. And ca*m*phore in wat*er* is ful good. Ȝif þe heris g*ro*weþ i*n*ward to-ward þe eiȝe, pulle*n* owt *and* wete an nedles poynt in liȝe, *and* let a drope of þe liȝe fallen as þ*er* þe here stood. And siþþe, waisch*e* þe eiȝen w*ith* iuys of grapes þ*a*t bie*n* nat ripe. And ȝif þe eiȝeledys be so fleischly þ*a*t me may nat wel pulle*n* owt þe heeris, frote he*m* wel w*ith* p*er*it*er*ie leeuys þ*a*t þei bleden, *and* siþþe pulle owt þe heeris be þe roote. *And* þa*n* a-noynte it w*ith* þe gleire of f. 44v eyren. And ȝif it bie | wynt*er*, resolue furst þ*er*-i*n*ne a lytel safru*n*, and so miȝtest do as ofte as it nedeþ. And asse pisse wole make þ*a*t heeris xul nat growe in þe bries.

For wurmes, tac þe iuys of camedreos *and* a-noynte þe briȝes; oþ*er* plastre þe herbe on his eiȝe*n*; oþ*er* tac aloes *and*

3 ley] *corr. from* loy **7 For**] *corr. from* ffor **14 For**] *corr. from* ffor **18 an**] *follow. by canc.* on **24 wynter**] *prec. by heading* Sekenesse **27 For**] *corr. from* ffor

frete it w*ith* whiȝt wyn on a wheston *and* do þ*er*-of in þi eiȝe.

For luys, tac wat*er* þ*a*t lupynes bie*n* j-soden i*n*ne. Ȝif þei bien heuy *and* grete, ley a plastre of p*er*it*er*ie on he*m*, oþ*er* þe rote of march*e*, oþ*er* þe leeues a lytel j-soden.

For cleuy*n*g of þe skyn in þe corneris of þe bries: Tac sauge *and* bren it, *and* medle it w*ith* mastik *and* olibanu*m*, *and* springe it þ*er*on. Oþ*er* tac serepinu*m* *and* dissolue it in wyn, *and* it wole soude þe place.

For swellyng of þe bries, lei gootes blood on he*m*, oþ*er* hony *and* sal armoniac to-gidere. Oþ*er* ley þ*er*-to mollityues þ*a*t we spoky*n* of bie-fore.

Wormes þ*a*t bien j-gaderid to-gider*e* on a bowe bien good for grete bries in þis wyse: Wryng he*m* þorow a lyne*n*ne clooþ *and* do iuys on þe bries. *And* þis iuys is good for smartyng, *and* akyngge, *and* swelly*n*g, *and* for werid eiȝen.

Jn a ma*n*n*us* eeren þ*er* bie*n* many many g*r*euau*n*ces, as ache, posteme, | flowyng of blood, flowyng of q*ui*tere, f. 45r wormes, ryngynge in þe eeren, fallyng of su*m*-thyng in-to þe eeren, *and* deefnesse. Ache comeþ of many enchesou*n*s: of posteme, of smytyng, of wynd w*ith*-i*n*ne þe eeren, of gret heete oþ*ur* of gret coold, oþ*ur* of su*m*-þi*n*g þ*a*t is j-falle*n* into þe eeren, oþ*ur* of su*m* corupt humo*ur* þ*a*t is in þe eeren. And ȝif it comeþ of su*m* corupt humo*ur*, þa*n*ne þ*er* is myche

3 For] *corr. from* ffor **6 For**] *corr. from* ffor **7 and**[1]] *follow. by canc.* bryn **10 For**] *corr. from* ffor **13 to-gidere**] *corr. from* to-gider*eus* (*us canc. twice*) **16 werid eiȝen**] *interl.* **18 Jn**] *2-line space left for initial* **19 flowyng**[1]] *prec. by heading* of the eere

24 corupt] *in r.-h. margin:* corruptt hu | mor

heuynesse in þe eer*e*, *and* na*m*ly ȝif it bie of coold. Ȝif it come of corupt wynd, þ*er* is ryngyng þ*er*-i*n*ne w*it*h-owtyn gret heuynesse. Oþ*er*whiles it comeþ of þe brayn, *and* þa*n* it dureþ co*n*tinueli*c*h*e*. Oþ*er*while it comeþ of þe stomac, *and* þa*n*ne it dureþ nat co*n*tinueli*c*h*e*. Of clene moistnesse ne of clene driȝenesse, þ*er* comeþ no g*r*et ache. Wha*n* þe ache is of heete, þe eere is hoot *and* reed, *and* þe ache is scharp. And ȝif it bie of eny hoot corupt humo*ur*, it is w*it*h pricchyng, *and* w*it*h smoke, *and* w*it*h a swift pouse, *and* lytil sleep, *and* in his sleep, he xal mete of reed þi*n*ges. And ȝif þ*at* corupt humo*ur* is of þe brayn, his for-heed *and* his chekys wole bie*n* reed; *and* is þurstful; *and* his heed akeþ. *And* coolde þi*n*ges confortyn hym *and* hoote þi*n*ges enc*r*escyn his greuau*n*ce. Ȝif þe ache bie of coold, þe eere is pale *and* þe ach*e* is nat ful
f. 45v greet. And ȝif þ*at* coold bie | of a corupt humo*ur*, þe ache is w*it*h mych*e* heuynesse, *and* in coold wederes þe ache is greuous. And ȝif þe humo*ur* bie of þe brayn, þe for-heed is pale *and* heuy *and* akeþ a lytil. And ȝif it comeþ of þe stomac, þe stomac is j-greued bi su*m* coold *and* haþ no talent to mete. And comy*n*ly þe ache of eeryn ne comeþ nat of coold, but it bie w*it*h su*m*me posteme, ne of gret heete, but it bie w*it*h a feuere. And ȝif þ*er* is a posteme w*it*h-i*n*ne-forþ, þe ach*e* is greuous w*it*h-i*n*ne. And ȝif þe posteme is su*m*whaȝt owtward, þa*n* þe eere is to-swolle su*m*what w*it*h-outen. And ȝif þe eere akeþ *and* þese toknes ne folweþ nat, loke in his eere *and* þ*er* þu mitest seen ȝif eny-þi*n*g is fallyn þ*er*-i*n*ne þ*at* makeþ hy*m* aken.

For ache þ*at* comeþ of heete, ȝif a corupt humo*ur* bie þe enchesou*n* þ*er*-of, let p*ur*ge*n* hym w*it*h siche þinges þ*at*

7 eere] *corr. from* heere (h *canc. and exp.*; first e *interl.*) **15 of**] *prec. by heading* Of the eerys **28 For**] *corr. from* ffor

purge*n* colre *and* p*ur*ge*n* blood. And siþþe worche as þ*ou* scholdest ȝif þ*er* wore no corupt humo*ur*, þ*at* is to seie, styue his eeren ou*er* wat*er* þ*at* hockes bie*n* j-sode*n* i*nn*e, *and* violet, *and* plau*n*teyn, *and* roses, *and* wermot, v*er*ueyne, *and* smal chaf of barlich*e* oþ*er* of ooten. *And* siþþe bryng hym to bedde *and* pit in his eere þe iuys of an oyne*n* *and* woma*nnus* mylk, oþ*er* þe iuys of syng*r*ene w*ith* þe oile of roses, oþ*er* þe oile of violet w*ith* þe iuys of coliaundr*e*, oþ*er* | ellys aft*ur* his f. 46r styue, let hym haue a sleep *and* swete weel. *And* þ*at* wol[e] doon a-wey þe ache. And vnd*er*stond þ*at* alle þe medicines þ*at* schulli*n* bie do in þe eeres xul bie warm *and* nat coold, *and* smale j-ground *and* nat grete. And strong medicines xul nat longe a-byde i*n* þe eere*n*, last þei drawyn to myche matere to þe eeren, ne no-þi*n*g xal bie do in þe eere*n* but it bie w*ith* oile oþ*er* w*ith* su*m* oþ*er* fatnesse, þ*at* it mow liȝtly come owt a-ȝen ; ne no*n* medicine xal bie doon i*n* þe eeren but ȝif þe heed bie j-stufed *and* þe heed j-p*ur*ged bi-fore, and þis js vnd*er*sto*n*d þere-as þe sicnesse is eeld. And sich*e* stufes oþ*er* fumigacyou*n*s xulle*n* bie of swyche þi*n*ges þ*at* bie*n* co*n*trarie to þe sicnesse. And ȝif þe sicnesse is of coold, þei xulle*n* bie coold. And þe best man*er* for þe stufyng of þe eere*n* is þ*at* a man ligge in his beed *and* ley his eere ou*er* þe poot þ*at* þe herbis bien j-soden i*nn*e, *and* helde it so stille til þe herbis wexyn coold, and þa*n* ligge dou*n* in his bed *and* tak a good swot. And þis xal bie*n* don in postem*es* of þe eere*n*, and in oþ*er* sicnesses þ*at* a ma*n* haþ long j-haad. And aft*ur* þis disposiciou*n*, leie þi medicines i*n* þe eer*e*. And ȝif þe ache bie of heete as j-seid bifore, tac a drope or too of letuse *and*

8 oþer] *catchword* (*in bottom margin*): ellys aft*ur* his **ellys**] *prec. by heading* The eerys **9 wole**] *corr. from* wolo

f. 46v medle it w*it*h as | myche of oile of rosees oþ*er* of violet. Oþ*er* seeþ in oile of rosees, acacie, violet, liciu*m*, *and* ij greyn*n*is of mastik. And siþþe clense it *and* do a drope þ*er*-of in þe eere w*it*h cotu*n*, oþ*er* sich*e* oþ*er* þi*n*g. Oþ*er* tac þe iuys of syngrene, *and* of letuse, *and* woman*us* milk, *and* seeþ he*m* to-gidere. *And* cast þ*er*-to ca*m*phore, þe seed of plau*n*teyne, *and* a lytil safru*n*. *And* cle*n*se it *and* pyt þ*er*-of in þ*in* eere, *and* stoppe it. And ȝif þe ache bie strong *and* g*r*euouce, tac acacie, *and* þe seed of popye, *and* of plau*n*teyn, *and* medle he*m* w*it*h roses, *and* woma*n*n*us* mylk, *and* þe whiȝte of an ey, *and* a lytul opiu*m* dissolued in vinegre. *And* cle*n*se it *and* do þ*er*-of in þi*n* eere. Oþ*er* medle oile of roses *and* of violet to-gidere, *and* do þ*er*-of in þi*n* eere. *And* a-noynte þe eer*e* w*it*h-owtyn w*it*h þe iuys of coold herbis, as it was seid in þe heed-ache þ*at* comeþ of heete.

Dietyng of he*m* þ*at* han þis sicnesse xa[l] bien as of men þ*at* han þe feuere t*er*cia*n*, saue it xal bie mor*e* laxe. But ȝif þe ache come of coold, let hy*m* haue p*ur*gaciou*n*s as it falleþ for þe humo*ur* þ*at* is þe encheson of þe ach*e*. And afturward mak hy*m* a stufe of þese herb*e* j-sode*n* i*n* wat*ur*: fenel, verueyne, wermot, wyld sauge, mynte, bawme, sauge, *and* salt; *and* a lytyl of wy*n* þ*er*-to. *And* let hym vse þis stufe iij niȝt*es* co*n*tinueli*che*, and eu*er*mor*e* stoppe a ma*n*n*us* eerys aft*ur* his stuffy*n*g. And iij niȝtis aft*ur*ward, do in his eeres f. 47r oile of | lorer*e*, *and* woma*n*n*us* milk, *and* gleire of eyren y-medled to-gidere. And ȝif it comeþ of þe stomac, let hi*m* vsen sich*e* þi*n*ges þ*at* co*n*forteþ þe stomac. And þese þi*n*ges bien comy*n* *and* p*ro*fitable for alle g*r*euau*n*ce of þe eeryn þ*at*

1 **myche**] *prec. by heading* Of the eerys 13 **violet**] *follow. by canc. twice* d 21 **fenel**] *corr. from* ffenel 22 **a lytyl**] *corr. from* alytyl 25 **lorere**] *prec. by heading* Apostem of the eerys

comeþ of coold, oile of lorer*e*, *and* of bytter alemau*n*des, *and* of rwe. And þe best stuphe is of been scales oþ*er* of beene*n* of he*m*-selfen j-medlyd w*it*h comy*n*. And aft*ur* þe stuphe, do i*n* þe eere oyle j-maad of bittere alemau*n*des.

A special medicine: Tac rwe, *and* oynou*n*s, *and* a lytil oile, *and* medle hem to-gider*e*. *And* siþe roste it in a wort leef vnd*er* axen *and* plastre þ*a*t w*it*h-oute þe eere. Oþ*er* powne wermot oþ*er* mugwort w*it*h oile of rwe oþ*er* of piliole *and* wyn. *And* siþþe roste it in a cool leef vnd*er* axen *and* lei it to þe eere. And in coold causes, tak þe iuys of garlek, *and* leek, *and* fenel, rwe, beteyne, *and* netles, *and* of onyou*n*s, *and* of chise-bolles, *and* þe iuys of yuy, *and* mastik, *and* woma*nn* *us* milk, of yche-on, a-lyche mych*e*. *And* powne he*m* to-gidere *and* pit in a holwe onyou*n*, *and* rost it in axes. *And* siþþe tac it owt *and* wryng it þorow a clooþ *and* do þ*er*-of in þe eer*e*. *And* it heleþ þe ach*e* *and* þe re*nn*yng of þe eeren. Diety*n*g of þis sicnesse xal bie as in a feu*ere* cotidian.

For þe postem of þe eeris ȝif it bie of coold oþ*er* of heete, þ*o*u maist know it bi þe toknes of þe last chapitre. And in helyng þis postim þu | xal nat wurche w*it*h rep*er*cussyues, f. 47v but w*it*h mytigatifs ȝif it is of heete, *and* w*it*h maturatyfs to make it wexe ripe. And ȝif þe posteme is of heete, make a plastre of oile of roses, *and* of violet, *and* þe rote of hockes *and* beet*es* j-medlyd to-gyder*e*. Oþ*er* tac þe fatnesse of a calf, *and* þe grece of an hen *and* of a gandre, *and* medle þ*er*-w*it*h violet, *and* rosees, *and* wex. *And* make a[n] oyneme*n*t to a-noynte þe eere*n* w*it*h-owte*n*. Oþ*er* mak a plastre of botyr, *and* hockes, *and* oile of violet oþ*er* of roses. Oþ*er* mak an

1 **bytter]** *corr. from* by*n*tter **19** **For]** *2-line space left for initial*; *corr. from* ffor **21** **xal]** *prec. by heading* Aposteem **24** **þe]** *interl.*

oyneme*n*t of ga*n*deris grece *and* he*n*ne grec*es* *and* þe mary of an hert. And ȝif þe ache bie ful greuous, tak oile of roses, *and* wex, *and* opiu*m*, *and* medle to-gidere, *and* do þ*er*-of in his eere; oþ*er* þe iuys of solatre, *and* oile of rooses, *and* þe whiȝte of an ey j-medlyd to-gidere, *and* j-doon þ*er*-of in þe eere w*ith* a wyke. Oþ*er* tac þe grece of an heron, *and* of an eel, *and* þe talwe of a gret bucke, *and* pit he*m* in an holow onyou*n* vnd*er* hoot axen. *And* siþ wry*n*g it þorow a clooþ *and* do þ*er*-of a drope or to i*n* þe eeres. Jt is good for ache, *and* heete, *and* defaute of hery*n*g, *and* to turne þe posteme to q*ui*ture. But ȝif it come of coold, vse þe oyneme*n*t*es* þ*at* weru*n* j-toold in þe last chapitre. *And* a-noynte it w*ith*-owte*n*-forþ w*ith* botere oþ*er* w*ith* deute oþ*er* fatnesse of beestis. *And* ley þ*er*-too oþ*er*e maturatyues þ*at* makeþ postem*us* ripe for-to breke. Cru*m*mes of breed j-sode*n* i*n* f. 48r wyn *and* | j-plastred bien good. And ȝif egremonie is medled þ*er*-w*ith* it is þe bett*er*e.

A good maturatif: Take g*r*ece, *and* oile, *and* hockes, *and* beetis, *and* eg*r*emoyne, *and* mak of he*m* a plast*r*e *and* lei to þe eere. Also tac þe iuys of an herbe þ*at* hatte schep*er*des-ȝerde; it heleþ þe postem*us* of þe eeren. And þe iuys of syng*r*ene j-medlid w*ith* oile of roses cesseþ þe ache of þe eeren *and* helpeþ me*n* þ*at* bie*n* deef. But wha*n* þe posty*m* js j-broke *and* þe q*ui*ture floweþ owt at þe eere, þ*o*u most vse mu*n*dificatifs to clense þe eere of his q*ui*ture. But þ*o*u xalt vnd*er*stond þ*at* q*ui*tur*e* of þe eerys comeþ oþ*er*whiles of breky*n*g of a posteme, oþ*er*wiles it comeþ of su*m* festre of þe eer*e*, oþ*er*while it comeþ of su*m* oþ*er* sicnesse of þe heed. But where-of-so it comeþ, þ*o*u xalt vse mu*n*dificatifs to

16 j-plastred] *prec. by heading* Of the eerys

clense þe eeren. And ȝif it comeþ of þe heed, vse medicines to purge þe heed of siche corupt humo*ur*s.

Good mu*n*dificatifs bien mirre, nytre, *and* hony j-medlid to-gidere; oþ*er* alym, *and* myrre, *and* vinegre; oþ*er* olibanu*m* resolued in þe iuys of schep*er*dis-purse; oþ*er* salt j-medlyd w*ith* woma*nnus* mylk; oþ*er* nitre, alym, *and* hony; oþ*er* comyn, castore, coost, j-medlyd w*ith* vinegr*e*; oþ*er* eu*er*ich*e* of þese bie hi*m*-self. And ȝif þese þi*n*ges cle*n*se nat þe eere, it is semlych*e* þ*at* þe quitur*e* comeþ of su*m* festre. *And* þa*n* þe heed moost bie*n* ofte-tymes j-schaud and he most bie cuppyd in þe necke, oþ*er* j-soke w*ith* wat*er*lechis to driȝe þe place a-bowte þe eeren *and* to make þe fluxe cessen. And siþþe | f. 48v make a strong medicine to goo to þe roote of þe eere. And ȝif cesseþ nat, þa*n* it is good to leue werke, laste þorow violence of medicyns, þe eere oþ*er* þe heed falle in-to a gret*ere* greuau*n*ce. Þe roote of þe whiȝte vyne *and* of a blak wyld vyne is þe best medicyne to clense þe eere of q*ui*tur*e* *and* of sych*e* filþe, *and* it is p*ro*fitable medicine for deefnesse. And Auycen say þ*at* þe galle of a crowe *and* of a snail j-soden to-gidere *and* j-cast in-to þe eere w*ith* wo*m*man*us* mylk clanseþ þe eere of long q*ui*turyng þ*at* haþ ȝore bie j-flowed. And so doiþ þe iuys of leek, *and* of centorie, *and* of þe maw of an hare, nat þe skyn, but þ*at* þ*at* is w*ith*-i*n*ne-forþ, *and* vynegr*e* j-medlyd to-gidere. Oþ*er* oile of a ma*nnus* dryt j-bre*n*t, oþ*er* þe iuys of þe roote of radich, oþ*er* cardamomu*m*, nytre, *and* driȝe figes j-clensed *and* j-sode*n* in þe iuys of rwe oþ*er* of radich*e*, *and* j-doon iij daies in-to þe erþe, jt is a

13 **make]** *prec. by heading* fflux of blood **27** **þe]** *follow. by* eere **erþe]** *fin l.-h. margin*

18 for] *in l.-h. margin:* d*ic*tum auice*n*

p*ro*fitabil medicine to make þe eeris clene of sich*e* filþe. But vnd*er*stond þ*at* aft*ur* þ*o*u hast doon ony sich*e* þi*n*g in-to a ma*nnus* eere, aft*ur* þ*at* oon hour*e* is j-passed, make hi*m* fnese, þ*at* þe medicine come clene owt, for drede of moor*e* harm.

Flowyng of blood at a ma*nn*es eeris oþ*er*-while it comeþ of smytynge, oþ*er*while it comeþ fro w*ith*-inne forþ, *and* þ*at* f. 49r may bie in | two man*er*es, for oþ*er*while it haþ a certeyn tyme for his flowynge, as þe iij or þe iiij day, oþ*er* more or lasse. And þis flowynge is nat good to bien j-stau*n*chid, *and* na*m*ly ȝif it comeþ of an-oþ*er* sicnesse, *and* p*ri*ncipaly in þe day þ*at* it xuld flow. A-noþ*er* flowynge þ*er* is þ*at* ne is nat at certeyn cours of flowyng, but comeþ oþ*er*while raþere, *and* oþ*er*while lattere. And þ*at* comeþ oþ*er*while of plente of blood *and* brekynge of su*m* veynys, oþ*er* ellys of su*m* postym þ*at* is j-brokyn ar þ*at* he bie fullych*e* ripe. And wheþer it bie oon or oþ*er*, it mot bie heelyd by mu*n*dificatyfs þ*at* mowen cl[e]nsyn þe eeren of þe blood þ*at* is w*ith*-i*n*ne, and w*ith* co*n*solidatyues þ*at* mowen sowden þ*at* place þ*at* is to-broke. And it is good to me*n*ge w*ith* he*m* special medicines þ*at* seruen to lete blood. And bie war þ*at* he fnese nat myche, ne þat noon ful scharp medicine, ne bytynge entre in-to þe eere.

A medycine for-to cle*n*se þe eere: Tak þe iuys of leek *and* of vynegre *and* medle he*m* to-gidere, oþ*er* wyn þ*at* galles bie*n* j-soden i*n*ne, *and* þe iuys of radich to-geder*e*, oþ*er* galles *and* vynegre to-gidere. And siþþe, tac þe iuys of

4 fnese] *interl.* first e **6 Flowyng]** *2-line space left for initial*; *corr. from* fflowyng **8 two]** *prec. by heading* at the eerys **for]** *corr. from* ffor **12 nat]** *in r.-h. margin* **18 clensyn]** *corr. from* clonsyn **24 for-to]** *interl.* for

schep*er*dys-purs *and* ence*n*se *and* medle he*m* to-gider*e*, *and* piȝt in-to þe eere, oþ*er* þe iuys of netle*n* *and* samdragou*n* j-medlyd to-gider*e*, oþ*er* ince*n*se *and* woma*nn**us* mylk j-medlyd to-gider*e*. Co*n*solidatifs | xulle*n* boþe bie leid w*i*t*h*-i*n*ne *and* w*i*t*h*-owte, and mu*n*dificatyues w*i*t*h*-i*n*ne þ*a*t wolle*n* make noo*n* icchyng. And eu*er*mor*e* aft*ur* þe brekynge of a postym in þe eere, mak a collirie in þe iuys of leek *and* ence*n*se smal j-poudred *and* medle to-gidere, oþ*er* oile of roses *and* mastik. And ȝif it woolde make þe eere to hoote, medle þ*er*-w*i*t*h* woma*nn**us* milk, for þis wole clense a-wey þe q*ui*turi*n*g *and* kepe it fro festrynge. And vnd*er*stond þ*a*t þ*er* is no medicine so good to cle*n*se þe eeris as a stufe in þe manere þ*a*t we told bie-for*e*. f. 49v

Also wormes in a ma*nn**us* eeren comy*n* in two maneris: Oon is j-gendrid w*i*t*h*-i*n*ne-forþ of corupcio*n* of þe eeris, anoþ*er* fro w*i*t*h*-owte crepi*n*g in-to þe eeres. And wheþ*er* þei come*n* in oo man*er* or oþ*er*, þei bie j-distriȝed by medycines þa*n* bien byttere. And for sych*e* wormes, tak oile of lorer*e*, *and* do it in-to þe eere, *and* stoppet an houre. And ȝif þ*er* bie a worm þ*er*-i*n*ne, þ*o*u xalt j-sie hi*m* in þe eere þ*er*-as þe oile was. And tak þa*n*ne þe iuys of wermot, *and* of calamynte, *and* of bittere alemaundes, *and* cast all*e* þ*a*t in a coole leef vnd*er* axene. *And* siþþe wryng owt þe oile *and* do þ*er*-of in þe eere, oþ*er* seeþ mirre *and* aloes in wyn *and* siþþe cast a drope þ*er*-of in þe eer*e*, oþ*er* w*i*t*h* a pipe me*n* may souken owt þe worm. Oþ*er* þe iuys of radich*e* oþ*er* of neep bie j-cast in-to þe eer*e* for it sleeþ eu*er*y crepi*n*g worm þ*a*t is in þe eere. Also | þe iuys of wermot, of centorie, of horehoune [and] of eleborus nig*er* sleeþ wormes in þe eeren. f. 50r

4 **xullen**] *prec. by heading* Of wormes **14** **Also**] *2-line space left for initial* **28** **þe**] *prec. by heading* in the eere

A good medicyne: Tac a rype appel *and* a wel smelly*n*ge *and* warm it at þe fier, þ*a*t he bie smellyng. *And* lei hy*m* al ny3t to þe eere. *And* ley þe ers of þe appel toward þe eere as ney3 as þ*o*u my3t, *and* a-morwe þ*o*u xalt fynde þe worm in þe myddel of þe appel. Me*n* may j-knowe wheþ*er* a worm bie in þe eer*e* bi icchi*n*g, *and* tynchynge, *and* meuynge w*ith*-i*n*ne þe eer*e*. And a[n] attircoppe is j-slawe þ*a*t is i*n* þe eer*e* w*ith* oolde oile of notes, oþ*er* wiþ seneuey, oþ*er* piliole, oþ*er* eleborus nig*er*, oþ*er* euforbe, oþ*er* þe iuys of radich*e* j-medlid w*ith* oile. And þe iuys of casteyn sleeþ eu*er*y kynde of wormes in þe eere, and so dooþ þe mylk of a figge tree, þe iuys of ce*n*torie, þe iuys of lupynes, þe iuys of wyld gourdes. And aft*ur* þ*a*t a worm is j-slawe or j-tak owt of þe eere, me moste take mu*n*dificatifs to cle*n*se þe eere, and co*n*solidatifs to heele*n* vp þe eere w*ith*-i*n*ne-forþ. And 3if þ*er* bie a flee in þi*n* eere, pyt a lytil wolle in þi*n* eere *and* he wole come to þe wolle. But 3if a stoon oþ*er* eny sich*e* dri3e þi*n*g falle in-to þe eere, tak a round stikke *and* make it smal at þe oon ende. *And* pit a lytel turmentyne at þe smal ende *and* do it in-to hese eere softly, þ*a*t þe eere bie nat j-g*r*eued. *And* so tak it

f. 50v owt, but bi-fore a-noynte þe eeren w*ith*-oute*n* w*ith* hoote | oynementis, as deute, marciato*n*, *and* sich*e* oþ*er*, and make hy*m* to fnese wel. And 3if wat*er* oþ*er* eny sich*e* weet þi*n*g bie falle*n* in-to his eere, þrist þe eere to-gedere harde oþ*er* pit þ*er*-i*n*ne cotu*n* oþ*er* a sponge to drie it vp.

3 **ers**] *corr. from* aers (a *exp.*; e *interl.*) 4 **a-morwe**] *follow. by canc. twice* i 22 **oynementis**] *prec. by heading* Ryngynge

1 **wel**] *in r.-h. margin:* no*ta*

Ryngynge in a ma*n*n*us* eeren oþ*er* noise lich*e* blowyng of hornes comeþ in diu*er*se man*er*s: Oþ*er*while, of gret wyndy mat*er* þ*a*t is in þe eere *and* moueþ vp-on down *and* al a-bowte w*ith*-i*n*ne-forþ *and* may nat out for his boistirnesse, *and* þa*n* þ*er* is a co*n*tinuel ryngynge *and* noyse in þe eeres; oþ*er*whiles, it comeþ of a viscouse corupt humo*ur* þ*a*t stoppeþ þe eere w*ith*-i*n*ne-forþ, *and* þa*n* þ*er* is mych*e* heuynesse in þe eeren. And ȝif it comeþ of heete, it comeþ w*ith* bitternesse of þe mowth, *and* heuynesse of þe riȝt eere, *and* reednesse, *and* heete. And ȝif it comeþ of coold, it is w*ith* co*n*t*ra*rie signes *and* heuynesse of þe lifte eere. Oþ*er*whiles, it comeþ of feblenesse of þe eere, *and* þa*n* þe ry*n*gi*n*ge is w*ith*-outyn þese for-seid signes. Of ryngi*n*ge þ*a*t is of wyndi mat*er*e enclosid oþ*er* of stoppi*n*ge þorow a viscouse mat*er* or humo*ur*, þ*er*e is oon manere cure, saue ȝif it bie of a corupt humo*ur*: Ȝif hi*m* furst a p*ur*gaciou*n* þ*a*t a-cordeþ to þe humo*ur*. Ȝif it bie of heete, to p*ur*ge*n* þe colre; ȝif it is of coold, to p*ur*ge þe male*n*colie. And make he*m* to fnese, and siþþe mak hy*m* a stufe of beene scalees | w*ith* anyse or comyn j-seden w*ith* f. 51r
he*m*, oþ*er* of cleene beenys j-soden bie hem-self. And ȝif it bie of heete, seeþ wermot þ*er*-w*ith*, and a-noon aft*ur* his stufe, do a drope in his eere of oile þ*a*t is j-maad of bytt*er* alemau*n*des. And þ*a*t is j-maad in þis wyse: Tac bitt*er*e alemau*n*des *and* sta*m*pe he*m*, *and* pyt he*m* in a closed vessel vnd*er* hoote axen. *And* siþþe wryng owt oile of hem þorow a clooþ. Oþ*ur* make a stufe of þese sedis j-sode in wat*er*: seed of fenel, *and* of p*er*sily, of anyse, carawey, dawk. And ȝif þ*o*u wolt, cast þ*er*-to laue*n*dr*e* *and* tyme. But ȝif þe stoppynge bie of coold, mak a collirie of mirre *and* castore. Oþ*er* tac þe iuys

1 **Ryngynge**] *2-line space left for initial* 19 **with**[1]] *prec. by heading* in the eere

of radich, oþ*er* of leek w*ith* oile of rosees, oþ*er* wo*m*man*us* mylk. Oþ*er* tac su*m* of þe oiles þ*at* we spokyn of in þe aky*n*ge of þe eeres. And ȝif it bie of feblenesse of þe eeren, tac þe iuys of wermot, *and* medle it w*ith* warm vinegre, *and* do þ*er*-of in þe eere. A good oyneme*n*t for þe eeris in alle man*er* greuau*n*ces þ*at* comeþ of coold: Tak peletre of spayne, *and* of castore, *dragme* j; of mirre, nytr*e*, long pep*er*, rwe, *dragme* ij; euforbe, *dragme* j. Poudre þis *and* medle it w*ith* iiij *ounce* of þe iuys of radich oþ*er* of leek. And loke þ*at* in medicynes of þe eeres, þ*ou* do no-þi*n*g w*ith*-i*n*ne-forþe þ*at* is scharp *and* byti*n*ge, but his malice bie rep*re*ssid *and* a-batyd by su*m* oþ*er* þi*n*g þ*at* is a mytigaciou*n* (nat þe iuys of radych
f. 51v þ*at* is oon of þe best for g*re*uance of | a mannys eeren).

Defnesse comeþ in many man*er*es, boþe of þe enchesou*n*s w*ith*-owte-forþ, as of smyti*n*ge, oþ*er* of enchesou*n*s w*ith*-i*n*neforþ þ*at* may bie in two man*er*es: Oþ*er* bi su*m* oþ*er* sicnesse of þe heed, as litarge or frenesi, or by his owne g*re*uau*n*ce w*ith*-oute*n* eny oþ*er* greuau*n*ce w*ith*-i*n*ne-forþ, as we han j-teld of bi-for*e*; oþ*er* bi stoppyng w*ith*-owty*n*-forþ by su*m* werte oþ*er* su*m* fleisch*e* þ*at* groweþ i*n*ne þe hole of þe eere. Ȝif deefnesse comeþ of a sicnesse of þe heed, it is j-heelyd bie helyng of þe sicnesse. Ȝif it comeþ of eny of þe forseyd g*re*uau*n*cis, jt is j-helid as þei bien. Ȝif it comeþ of wrett*es* oþ*er* of fleisch*e* þ*at* growyth bi-fore þe hoole of þe eere, jt xal bie heelyd w*ith* corrosyues þ*at* xulle*n* frete he*m* a-wey. Ȝif it comeþ of euel disposiciou*n* of þe eere w*ith*-i*n*ne-forþ, jt hath*e* p*ro*pre medicynes. Narþelees þe medicynes of oþ*er* g*re*uau*n*cys of þe eeren helpeþ, ȝif it mow bie j-heelyd, for þ*ou* xalt vnd*er*stond þ*at* olde sicnesses of þe

13 a] *prec. by heading* Deefnesse **14** **Defnesse**] *2-line space left for initial* **29** **for**] *corr. from* ffor eere*n*, *and* na*m*ly deefnesse, bien vncurabil, but deefnesse þ*at* is newe *and* oþ*er*wiles grett*ere* þa*n* oþ*er*-while, may be j-holpe. Deefnesse þ*er* is also, þ*ere*-as a ma*nn*e*s* herynge is by-[n]o[m]e*n* hym, is incurable but ȝif it bie more nwe. And of what enchesou*n* deefnesse is, men may j-know by þ*at* þ*at* is j-seid bi-for*e*. And ȝif it bie of ony corupt humo*ur*, ȝeyf hi*m* purgacyou*n*s aft*ur* þe kynde of þ*at* humo*ur*. *And* make | hi*m* f. 52r fnese, and siþþe make hy*m* a stufe of beene scales *and* of anyse. *And* siþþe do in his eere þe iuys of radich*e*. Oþ*er* seeþ lorer*e* leeu*es* *and* spyknard i*n* wyn, *and* lat þe smoke þ*er*-of comy*n* in-to þe eere þorow a pipe. Oþ*er* do empte eyren in oile *and* let he*m* rote þ*er*-i*n*ne *and* þa*n* do-þ*er* of in þe eeren. And in þe same man*er* þ*ou* maist do w*ith* þe iuys of syng*re*ne *and* of onyou*n*s j-cast in oile of lorer*e*. Oþ*ur* tac grene aischen bowes *and* ley he*m* in þe feyr, *and* tac of þe wat*er* þ*at* comeþ owt at þe endys of hem þe q*ua*ntite of an he*n*-ey-schelle-full*e*. *And* cast þ*er*-to two sponefull*e* of oile oþ*er* of bot*ure*, *and* oon sponefull*e* of þe iuys of sy*n*grene, *and* ij spone-full*e* of hony, *and* oon sponefull*e* of wo*m*man*us* milk þ*at* norischeþ a knaue child; ȝif it bie for a woma*n*, a maide-child. And do of þis a drope oþ*er* two in his eere *and* stoppe þe eere. Oþ*er* tac þe iuys of sy*n*g*re*ne *and* þe fatnesse of an eel, of boþe, j-lich*e* mych*e*, *and* do þ*er*-of i*n*ne þ*in* eer*e*, oþ*er* þe clene g*re*ce þ*at* droppeþ fra*m* a rostid eel is ful good, oþ*er* a boles galle j-medlyd w*ith* gootes pisse, oþ*er* castore, gu*m*me of yuy *and* of mirre j-medlyd w*ith* þe iuys of

3 **by-nomen**] *corr. from* by monie*n* 7 **him**] *prec. by heading* of the eere 24 **eere**] *corr. from* heer*e* (h *canc.*)

17 **hen-ey-schelle-fulle**] *in r.-h. margin:* no*ta* 22 **syngrene**] *in r.-h. margin:* no*ta*

radich, of rwe, wermot, oþ*er* of yuy. And ȝif it comeþ of heete, aft*ur* p*ur*gaciou*n*s *and* stufes, do þe iuys of syng*r*ene in þe eere j-medlyd w*it*h þe fatnesse of an eel. And þe same doiþ þe iuys of hou*n*destonge. Oþ*er*e þere-as þe deefnesse is coold, tak syngrene *and* do it in an erþen vessel j-closed xij f. 52v monþes vnd*ur* þe erþe. | And at þe ȝeris ende, tak þe moistnesse þ*at* cleueþ bie þe pottys syde *and* do þ*er*-of in his eeris. Oþ*er* þi*n*ges also þ*at* were*n* j-teld in þe ach*e* of þe eeren bien good for deefnesse, and þe iuys of a gorst *and* of sauyne ben good, boþe for oyneme*nt*es *and* stufes of þe eere*n*, for þei oppy*n* wel þe poris þ*at* bie*n* in þe eeres, *and* j-stopped w*it*h corupt humo*ur*s.

Jn a ma*n*n*us* nose þ*er* bien many greuau*n*ces, as þe pose, stynch*e* of þe nose-þirles, and flowyng of blood at þe nose; and w*it*h-oute*n*, þ*er* is a g*r*euau*n*ce þ*at* is j-clepyd gutta rosacea. Oþ*er* greua*n*nces þ*er* bie*n* also of þe nose: cancr*e* *and* fleisch*e* þ*at* stoppeþ þe nestrilles as noli me ta*n*gere. Of an vnkyndly humo*ur* *and* corupt þ*at* is a-bowte þe brayn is þe pose enge*n*drid, for þ*at* humo*ur* stoppeþ þe ou*er*part of þe nose *and* letteþ a ma*n* of his smellyng. And as su*m*me me*n* seyn þe pose ne is nat but a stoppyng of þe nestrilles þorouȝ a rewme, for as þei seyn, þe rewme falleþ oþ*er*while dou*n* into þe nose *and* makeþ þe pose. Oþ*er*while it falliþ a-dou*n* into þe chekys *and* makeþ he*m* swelle *and* aken. Oþ*er*wile jt falleþ down to þe roote of þe teeþ, *and* þa*n* it makeþ he*m* ake *and* roote. Oþ*er*while it falleþ to þe roote of þe tu*n*ge, *and* makeþ her*e* swelle *and* bie laxe, *and* bryngeþ here in-to a palesie, *and* makeþ a ma*n* to lese hese speche. Oþ*er*while, it

6 **And**] *prec. by heading* Greuawn*n*ce 13 **Jn**] *2-line space left for initial* 17 **fleische**] *corr. from* ffleisch*e* 19 **for**] *corr. from* ffor 22 **for**] *corr. from* ffor 27 **bryngeþ**] *interl.* e

falleþ down to þe breest, *and* makeþ þe breste streyt. Oþ*er*while, it falleþ down to þe liȝt oþ*er* to þe stomac, | oþ*er* f. 53r to þe reynes, oþ*er* in-to a ma*n*n*es* guttes. And but þe me*m*bre bie þe more myty to pit it a-wey fro hi*m*, it wole make þ*er* a posteme. Oþ*er*while, it falleþ dou*n* a-mo*n*g þe veynes *and* guttes in diu*er*se places of þe body. And oþ*er*while, it roteþ *and* heeteþ þe veinys *and* makeþ a ma*n* to falle*n* in-to a feuere. Alle þese greuau*n*ces comeþ of þe rewme, and þ*er*fore it is ful needfulþi*n*g for a ma*n* to kepyn hy*m* fro þ*a*t greuau*n*ce, last he falle in-to a grett[e]re. Jn þe pose, a ma*n* haþ mych*e* g*r*euau*n*ce *and* ache in his forheed *and* in hese eiȝen, *and* fneseþ ofte, *and* smelleþ febelich*e*. And ȝif it comeþ of heete, a ma*n* xal fele scharpnesse *and* gret heete in his nostrilles. And ȝif it comeþ of coold, he xal fele þe co*n*t*ra*rie þi*n*ges. Narþelees, of salt humo*ur* þ*a*t floweþ þorouȝ þe nose, þ*er* comeþ smertynge *and* scharpnesse, and siþ þis g*r*euau*n*ce comeþ of þe heed. In þe bi-gynnyng, ȝif hi*m* a p*ur*gaciou*n*, ne lat nat hi*m*-self waischi*n* his heed ne his feet. *And* ȝif hy*m* no*n* medicines, and þis j seie wheþ*er* he bi w*ith* feuer*e* or w*ith*-owtyn. Ne lei no*n* dissolutyues þ*er*-to in þe be-gy*n*nyng, ne scharp þi*n*ges as strong wyn; ne sich*e* þi*n*ges þ*a*t dissoluen more þa*n* co*n*sume*n* *and* wasten, as þi*n*ges þ*a*t myche pep*er* is i*n*ne; ne soure þi*n*ges, for þei wolde*n* make mat*er*e falle down to þe breest *and* make hi*m* catche a kow. And alle man*er* met*es* *and* drynkys þ*a*t he haþ xulle*n* bie*n* hoote. | And bi war of mych*e* etyng *and* f. 53v drynkynge, *and* of late soperes, *and* late drynkynges, *and* of mych*e* sleep, for þ*er* is no-þing þ*a*t encresceþ ne norisceþ

2 oþer[2]] *prec. by heading* of the nose **10 grettere**] *corr. from* grettore **13 scharpnesse**] *interl.* r **26 hoote**] *follow. by* And bewar **And**] *prec. by heading* Sekenesse of the nose **28 for**] *corr. from* ffor more þe rewme. And bi war of myche liȝt *and* myche smoke. And let hym nat blood, laste þe mat*ere* of þ*at* rewme bie drawe in-to þe veynis *and* be encheso*n* of more. Ne ȝif hi*m* no laxatif to make hi*m* a flux, laste þe mat*er* falle down to þe breest oþ*er* to þe stomac *and* bie cause of su*m* posteme oþ*er* of su*m* oþ*er* sich*e* g*re*uau*n*ce. But ȝif þe pose comeþ of coold, *and* bie nat a full*e* greet coold, make hi*m* a fumigaciou*n* of lignu*m* aloes, *and* encense, *and* calam*us* aromatic*us*, *and* of lapdanu*m*. And siþþe, make hi*m* a stufe of lignu*m* aloes, *and* of storax, *and* of lapdanu*m*. And aft*ur* his stufe, let hi*m* drynke a lytul wy*n*, oþ*er* make a stufe of lorer*e* leeuys *and* of aue*n*ce oþ*er* roses. And siþþe, a-noynte hese heed w*ith* hote oyles, as of lorere oþ*er* rewe. Oþ*er* þ*o*u miȝtest make hi*m* a stufe of hoote herbis *and* weel-smellynge, as piliole, mynte, *and* ca*m*mamille, beteyne, origan, *and* sich*e* oþ*ere*. And mak hy*m* a fumigaciou*n* w*ith* hoote seedis, as fenel, anyse, carawey whete bran, *and* sich*e* oþ*ere*. And ȝif þ*o*u ne haast he*m* all*e*, tak su*m* of hem. But þe beest stufe of all*e* js j-maad of olibanu*m* j-sode*n* in wyn, w*ith* roses, aue*n*ce, *and* f. 54r fenel. | After, make a plastre of affodille rootis j-braied w*ith* wyn *and* oile to-gidere, and j-warmed, *and* j-leid to þe heed. Good pillules: Tak of mirre, *dragme* v; of olibanu*m* *and* of lapdanu*m*, *dragme* v; of opiu*m*, he*n*nebane, hou*n*destonge, *and* radich*e*, of euerich*e*, *dragme* iij. *And* te*m*pre he*m* w*ith* wat*er* of roses. *And* make pillules þ*er*-of in þe q*ua*ntite of a fech*e*. *And* wha*n* he gooþ to bedde, ȝif hi*m* v of hem at

9 lapdanum] *follow. by canc.* And aft*ur* his stufe, let hy*m* drinke a lytil wyn. Oþ*er* make a stufe of lorer*e* leeues *and* of aue*n*ce (va *and* cat *interl. at the beginning and end of the fragment respectively*) **20 fenel**] *catchword* (*in bottom margin*): after make a plast*re* **After**] *prec. by heading* Of the nose oones. Oþ*er* good pillules, wan þe mat*er* floweþ fra*m* þe heed to þe breest: Tak of storak, mirre, *and* of opiu*m*, of eu*er*ich*e*, j-lich*e* mych*e*, *and* te*m*pre he*m* w*it*h dispumed hony. *And* make pillules of þe q*ua*ntite of a pese *and* ȝif ij or iij þ*er*-of wha*n* he goþ to bedde. But ȝif it comeþ of heete, make hi*m* a stufe of wat*er* [þat] mirre, camomille, *and* vinegre bie*n* j-sode*n* i*n*ne. Make þ*in* stufe i*n*ne þis wyse: Do of þ*a*t wat*er* on an hoot glowynge stoon *and* let þe fume þ*er*-of go vp into his nose. Anoynte þe fore-heed w*it*h oile of violet *and* bot*er*e j-medlid to-gidere. And ȝif it bie newe, p*ur*ge þe heed of þe humo*ur* *and* lei plastres þ*er*-to þ*a*t opiu*m* js j-medlid wiþ, for it is good wheþ*er* it come of heete oþ*er* of coold. Rewme þ*a*t comeþ of heete þ*a*t haþ bie long in þe heed, jt is ful hard ȝif it bie j-helid. And it is p*ro*fitabel in boþe causes to heele*n* þe heed w*it*h herbis þ*a*t bie*n* p*ro*fitabil þ*er*-fore, *and* nat schaue þe heed, but dodden it. *And* þa*n*ne þe heeris *and* þe oyneme*nt*es þ*a*t comeþ a-mo*n*g he*m* wolle*n* ligge | to- f. 54v gidere in þe manere of an emplastre.

Stynckyngge of þe nosethrilles comeþ oþ*er*while of humo*ur*s þ*a*t falle*n* down fro*m* þe heed to þe pores of þe þirles *and* ligge*n* þ*er*e *and* stynkyn. Oþ*er*while it comeþ of streiȝtnesse of þe nosethrilles, for corupt humo*ur*s liggen w*it*h-i*n*ne-forþ *and* mou*n* nat come out for streiȝtnesse of þe nostrilles. Oþ*er*wile it comeþ of bleynes *and* bot[c]hys w*it*h-i*n*ne-forþ, *and* ben nat wel j-clansed. Ȝif it bie of streiȝtnesse of þe nose-þirles, it is incurable. Ȝif it comeþ of boche oþ*er* of a buyle w*it*h-i*n*ne-forþ, it xal bie heelid þorow heelyng of

6 j-soden] *follow. by exp.* to-gidere **12 for**] *corr. from* ffor **17 to-gidere**] *prec. by heading* Stynche of the nose **19 Stynckyngge**] *2-line space left for initial* **22 for**] *corr. from* ffor **23 for**] *follow. by* for **24 botchys**] corr. from botthys

a boche. But ȝif it bie of þe heed, *and* þe nose bie hool *and* sou*n*d, p*ur*ge furst þe heed. And ȝif he haue heete *and* p*ri*ckynge in his nose, cast þ*er*-i*n*ne oile of roses *and* of violet, oþ*er* oon of he*m* *and* make hi*m* to fnese. And ȝif he haue no pose, lat waische þe heed w*i*t*h* wat*er* þ*a*t roses *and* violet, *and* þe rynde of popy is j-sode*n* i*n*ne, *and* plastre he*m* on his heed. Ȝif it bie of þe pose, heele þe pose. And ȝif it is of coold, *and* w*i*t*h*-oute*n* akynge *and* p*ri*ckyng, *and* he haue no pose, make hi*m* to fnese w*i*t*h* a poudre of piretre, *and* of canel, of castore, *and* of seneuey, of eu*er*ich*e*, j-lich*e* mych*e*. And ȝif þe nose ne mow nat suffre*n* siche scharp poudres, þ*o*u most vse esy desiccatyfs to driȝe vp þe nose, as poud*re* of roses oþ*er* of benen, oþ*er* of canel. Mastyk j-chewyd it is ful good, also to bie*n* j-cupped oþ*er* j-horned in þe necke-piȝt. | f. 55r

Flowyng of blood at a ma*n*n*us* nose comeþ in many man*er*es *and* of diu*er*se enchesou*n*s. Oþ*er*while it comeþ for scharpnesse *and* keneschipe of þe blood þ*a*t p*er*seeþ þe veynis, oþ*er*while for sotylte of þe blood, and oþ*er*while for gret multitude of þe blood. Ȝif it bie on þe furst man*er*e, þese bien þe tokenes: Þe blood is hoot, *and* cleere, *and* reed, *and* bitiþ þe nose in his flowinge. Ȝif it bie of þe secu*n*de man*er*e, þ*a*t blood is þi*n*ne, *and* myche flowynge where-eu*er*e it stondeþ. And ȝif it bie on þe þridde man*er*e, þ*er* comeþ mich*e* blood out at þe nose, *and* þe veynes bie*n* ful neesche *and* ful of blood. But of which*e* man*er*e þ*a*t it bie, it mai bie in two man*er*es: jn sicnesse oþ*er* owt of sicnesse. And it may bie in sicnesse in two man*er*es: Oþ*er* hauy*n*ge a certeyn tyme for his flowynge, as þe secu*n*de day or þe þridde; oþ*er*

16 **Flowyng]** *2-line space left for initial; prec. by heading* fflux of the nose

comynge oncertenlych*e*, oþ*er*while raþere oþ*er*while lattere. And wheþ*er* it in oon man*ere* or in oþ*ere*, ȝif it liȝteþ a ma*n* of his oþ*er* sicnesse, it is nat good to stau*n*che*n* it. Ȝif a ma*n* is feblere aft*ur* his bledi*n*ge *and* he haue toknes of liyf, it is good to stau*n*che*n* it, but nat sode*n*ly, but ȝif a ma*n* bie myche j-feblid bi hese bledi*ng*. And ȝit whiche of alle þese man*er*es nose-bledi*ng* bie, hit mai bie of þe lyuere, oþ*er* of þe splene, oþ*er* of þe emeraudis, oþ*er* in wo*m*me*n* of wiþ-holdynge of her*e* p*ur*gaciou*n*s. And sich*e* bledi*n*ge is p*ro*fitable. But ȝif it come of þe lyuere, þese bien þe toknes: greuau*n*ce of þe riȝt syde, reednesse of his vrine, | and f. 55v
bledynge of þe riȝt nose-þrille. And ȝif it is of þe splene, þe splene swelleþ *and* þe riȝt side is j-greued. *And* þe liȝft nose-þrille bleediþ. And ȝif in þe nose-bledyng þe lyu*ere* oþ*er* þe liȝt swelliþ, oþ*er* aftur þe stau*n*chyng of þe blood þe body is infect w*it*h*o*wtyn w*it*h ȝelwe spottes, it is a tokne of deeþ. Ȝif it is of mych*e* blood, þ*o*u moost worche w*it*h two man*ere* medicynes: Su*m* to make þe bleed þicke, as coliys of an eld he*n*ne, *and* harde ȝelkes of eyren, and oþ*er* þi*n*ges þ*at* we wol speke of in þe flux of þe wombe. Jt bie-houeþ also to haue medicynes þ*at* bie*n* st*ri*ctorie to legge*n* to þe foreheed *and* also to þe nose, to stau*n*che þe blood. And ȝif þ*er* floweþ mych*e* blood, it xal nat bie sodenly j-stau*n*chid ne bie strong st*ri*ctories; do by esy as sugr*e* roset, *and* sirip of roses, *and* oþ*ere* esy st*ri*ctories j-leid to þe fore-heed *and* to þe nose. And ȝif a ma*n* blede mych*e* for gret plente of blood, *and* he ne haue no feuere t*er*cia*n*, ne noo sich*e* scharpe sicnesse, let him bledyn at þe heed veyne of þe arme on þe same syde þ*at*

11 and] *prec. by heading* fflux of blood

8 oþer[1]] *in r.-h. margin:* no*ta*

hese nose bledeþ. And lat hese dietyng bie w*ith* smal ale *and* sich*e* met*es* as makeþ litel blood, as herbis *and* fruytes. And lat leggen co*n*solidatyues wiþ-owtyn, for þe gret ple*n*te of blood brekeþ þe veynes. But ȝif it come of sotylnesse of þe blood, lat hi*m* ete sich*e* met*es* þat makeþ þe blood þicke, as riys *and* hard ȝelkes of eiren, and oþ*er* metys þ*at* we xul
f. 56r speky*n* of in þe flux | of þe wombe. Many þi*n*ges þ*er* bie*n* þ*at* stau*n*cheþ blood, as coral emathites, *and* sang*ui*narie þ*at* is schep*er*dis-purs. Also a plastre j-maad or barly meele, *and* sandragu*n*, encense, *and* þe whiȝte of an ey j-medlid to-gidere; oþ*er* a clooþ j-wet in coold wat*er* *and* j-leid to þe fore-heed oþ*er* to þe þrote; oþ*er* haare heeris j-brent *and* medlid w*ith* gu*m*me arabik in þe iuys of plau*n*teyn, *and* j-pit in þe nose-þrilles. Also smellyng of stynckynge þi*n*ges is good, as of swynes dryt, *and* of hornes j-brent, oþ*er* heeris. And ȝif it bie of þe lyuere, make a plastre on þe lyuere of þe rynde of elm j-poudrid, *and* of sa*n*cdragou*n*, *and* bole, *and* mastik j-medelid w*ith* þe iuys of syng*re*ne, oþ*er* of v*er*ueyne, oþ*er* of plau*n*teyne. *And* cast þ*er*-to spodie *and* roses. And ȝit it comeþ of þe splene, do þ*er*-to medicines þ*at* xul bie teeld in þe sicnesse of þe splene. *And* do his p*ri*ue me*m*bres i*n* a disch w*ith* vinegre. Oþ*er* tak reed netlen *and* salt j-stamped to-gidere *and* do i*n* his nose, oþ*er* þe poudre of netle*n* j-brent, oþ*er* þe poudre of ey-schell*e* j-brent. Oþ*er* sang*ui*narie j-powned *and* j-hoold i*n* a ma*n*n*us* hoond stau*n*cheþ blood. Oþ*er* take wormes of þe erþe *and* pownne he*m* w*ith* ence*n*se *and* w*ith* þe whiȝt of an ey, *and* pit þ*er*-of in hese nose. And ley su*m* þ*er*-of i*n* þe man*er*e of a plaistre to his forhed. Oþ*er* pit vnsleckyd lym *and* coperose oþ*er* atreme*n*t vp-on þe

7 of[2]] *prec. by heading* at the nose

veyne, *and* it wole stau*n*che þe blood. And so wole an hoot yren j-leyd þ*er*-to wher*e*-eu*ere* it bie. | And þei it bie so þ*at* f. 56v þis is good to staunche blood at þe noose, it is p*ro*fitabil oþ*er*while to make þe nooseblede as in þe frenesie *and* in þe heedache. And þ*at* þ*o*u miȝtest do to pyt a braunche of sauyne in þe nostrille oþ*er* þe leef of mille-foil. Oþ*er* w*it*h swynes brustles j-pit in a stickes ende *and* j-kyt at þe oon ende *and* j-pit in-to þe nose, þei wolle*n* wiþ here scharpnesse make þe noose to blede.

Gvtta rosacea is an infecciou*n* of þe nose w*it*h-oute*n*-forþ of myche reednesse. And oþ*er*while, it is a tokne þ*at* a ma*n* is disposed to bie mesel. And ȝif it come, oþ*er*while of blood and oþ*er*while of colre, *and* it is nat þe morfeu, but it is j-clepid a rosey goute. And ȝif it comeþ of blood, þese bie*n* þe toknes: jchi*n*ge of þe nose *and* likynge i*n* þe ichinge, *and* brekynge vp of pymples þ*at* sone turneþ to q*ui*ture. But ȝif it comeþ of colre, þ*er* is icchi*n*ge *and* p*ri*ckynge in þe noose *and* pymples þ*at* bie*n* þ*er*-oon ne q*ui*tereþ but lytel. And þe place of þe g*re*uau*n*ce is hard in þe handly*n*ge. And ȝif it is of blood oþ*er* in þe necke oþ*er* in þe coppe of þe nose, he xal bie late blood oþ*er* j-cupped v[n]d*er* þe chyn. Oþ*er* wheþ*er* it bie of blood or of colre, make hi*m* a p*ur*gaciou*n*. But furst, to defie þe mat*ere*, lat hi*m* drincke of þe sirrip of fumyt*re* *and* oximel y-medlid to-gydere, of boþe, j-lich*e* mych*e*. Siþþe, make hym a stufe of coold herbis, as of fumyt*re*, scabyouse, *and* sich*e* oþ*ere*. And aft*ur* his p*ur*gaciou*n*, let hi*m* blood to drawe þe blood a-wey fro þe visage. And siþþe,

2 yren] *corr. from* eyren (first e *canc. twice and exp.*) **And**] *prec. by heading* Redenesse of the nose **10 Gvtta**] *2-line space left for initial* **13 þe**] *follow. by canc.* gowte **morfeu**] *corr. from* morfeue (first e *interl.*; last e *canc. twice*)

f. 57r make | a stufe of wat*er* þ*a*t wermot, *and* hockes, *and* violet, *and* þe smal chaf of barlich*e* *and* oof oote*n* bie*n* j-sode*n* i*n*ne. And siþþe, a-noynte hi*m* w*it*h þis oyneme*n*t: Tak barly mele, *and* femygrek also, *and* as myche of mader, *and* of plaunteyn j-poudred, *and* medle he*m* w*it*h þe iuys of oyneu*n*s *and* hony despumed. And ȝif it is an oold, make an oyneme*n*t of berace *and* pep*er* j-medlid w*it*h þe iuys of onyou*n*s *and* hony despumyd. Anoþ*er*: Tak þe iuys of heihoue *and* of chasteyns, *and* þe pouder of ciceres, boþe of whiȝte *and* of reede, *and* seeþ he*m* to-gidere. And siþe do þ*er*-to a porciou*n* of ca*m*phore *and* of borace. And ȝif þ*o*u castist þ*er*-to þe iuys of co*n*fyri and of mynte*n*, it wol bie weel þe bet*er*e, *and* þe poud*re* of coral is good to cast þ*er*-to. Of þe ca*n*cre of þe nose, *and* of noli me tang*er*e, *and* of fleisch*e*, *and* of buyles þ*a*t bie*n* in þe noose, we wol speke w*it*h goddys grace wha*n*ne we spekyn of postem*us* *and* ca*n*cris.

Jn a ma*n*nes mouþ þ*er* bien many greua*n*ces, as cleuy*n*ge of lippes, stynckyncge of mouþ w*it*h-i*n*ne-forþ, ache, *and* oþ*er* g*re*uau*n*ce of þe teeþ, *and* sicnesse of þe tu*n*ge. Cleuy*n*ge of lyppes is in many man*er*es, as of pymples j-broke, oþ*er* of smytynge, oþ*er* of euel humo*ur* *and* a corupt þ*a*t cleueþ þe lippes, oþ*er* of coold, oþ*er* of wynd, oþ*er* of
f. 57v cancre. But ȝif it bie of smytynge, i[t] | xal bie helid as oþ*er* wou*n*des. And ȝif it bie of eny of þese oþ*er* man*er*es, it may bie heelid w*it*h an oynement j-maad of oile of violet oþ*er* of roses *and* wex j-medled to-gidere; oþ*er* w*it*h an oyneme*n*t j-maad w*it*h þe iuys of sorel *and* of oile *and* wex to-gidere; oþ*er* w*it*h wexe *and* he*n*nebane seed j-soden in oyle. Also þe

1 a] *prec. by heading* The mowth **6** **an oynement**] *corr. from* a noyneme*n*t **17** **Jn**] *2-line space left for initial* **23** **it**[2]] *corr. from* is **xal**] *prec. by heading* The mowth

poudre of portulake heeliþ *and* hideþ þe cleuy*ng* of meseles lippes, ȝif portulake bie j-brent. For cleuy*ng* of þe lippes oþ*er* of þe tu*n*ge *and* for bladdres w*ith*-i*n*ne þe mouþ, make a oynement of poudre of liciu*m*, *and* amyde, *and* penydes j-medlid w*ith* þe wat*er* of roses. *And* a-noynte þ*er*-w*ith* þe same g*r*euau*n*ces. Anoþ*er* for þe same g*r*euau*n*ce *and* for cleuy*ng* of þe roof of þe mouþ: Take dragagant, *and* resolue hit in coold wat*er*, *and* cle*n*se it, *and* medle þ*er*w*ith* þe poudre of amyde. *And* þ*er*-w*ith* a-noynte þe soore w*ith* a feþere. And ȝif þe g*r*euau*n*ce bie of moist pymples, a-noynte it w*ith* clene hony, oþ*er* w*ith* þe poudre of beenen j-brent *and* hony, oþ*er* w*ith* þe poudre of portulake *and* hony j-medled. Also þe iuys of ce*n*torie, of wermot, *and* of aristologie þe rou*n*de is good þ*er*-fore. Also for cleuy*n*ge of þe lippes *and* of tetes, melt wex *and* oile of violet oþ*er* de olyue to-gidr*e*. *And* cast þ*er*-too þe poudr*e* of mastik *and* of olibanum | to-gydre, *and* þ*er*w*ith* a-noynte þe soore. Oþ*er* f. 58r
take poudre of roses *and* medlid w*ith* gu*m*me resolued in wat*er*. Oþ*er* medle sau*n*dres *and* þe poudre of roses, *and* gu*m*me, *and* ceruse, w*ith* wat*er* of roses, *and* a-noynte þe soore. Also tac þe grece of an hen, *and* of gandre, *and* of a malard, *and* medle þ*er*-w*ith* þe poudre of ence*n*se of mastik, of canel, *and* ceruse, *and* þ*er*-w*ith* a-noynte þe lippes. For cleuy*ng* of þe lippes þorow coold oþ*er* þo-row, an-oynte he*m* w*ith* hony *and* siþþe straw þ*er*-vp-on þe poudr*e* of colofyne. And ȝif þe lippes swellyn, make an oyneme*n*t of þe iuys of pasnep leeues *and* þe poudre of litarge j-medlid to-gidere, *and* þere-wiþ a-noynte þe lippes.

2 For] *corr. from* ffor **4 a**] *follow. by canc.* poudre **15 de olyue**] *corr. from* deolyue **17 to-gydre**] *prec. by heading* Stynche of the mowth **23 For**] *corr. from* ffor **25 siþþe**] *follow. by canc.* in resure

Stynkyng of þe mouþ comeþ oþ*er*while of corupcion of þe gomys *and* of þe teeþ; oþ*er*while it comeþ of þe stomac; oþ*er*while it comeþ of þe liȝte. Ȝif it comeþ of þe teeþ *and* of þe gomes, frete þ*in* gomes w*ith* þ*in* fyng*re and* þ*in* mowþ wul sti*nke*n. Ȝif it comeþ of þe stomac, þe mouþ sti*n*ckeþ whil a ma*n* is fastyng. *And* me*n* xal smelle þe sti*n*cke whil his mouþ is open. Ȝif it comeþ of þe liȝt, me*n* xal smelle*n* þe sti*n*che þei þe mouþ bie closed. Ȝif it comeþ of þe teeþ *and* of þe gomes, ȝif þ*er* bie eny roted fleisch*e*, let fretyt a-wey *and* f. 58v siþþe hele it vp. Ȝif þ*er* bie no roted fleische, | let waische þe mouþ w*ith* wyn þ*at* birche oþ*er* my*n*nte*n* bie j-sode i*n*ne *and* let frete wel þe gomes w*ith* a scharp lyne*n* clooþ, þ*at* þei bleden. *And* lat hi*m* ete origane, mynte, *and* peletr*e*, *and* þ*er*w*ith* frote here teeþ *and* heere gomys. And þis is good also ȝif þe fleisch*e* of þe gomys bie roted. Oþ*er* late he*m* waisch*e* here mouþ in þ*at* hoot glowyng pomyis is que*n*ched i*n*ne. And late hi*m* dri*n*kyn eu*er*y eue*n*tyd wyn þ*at* ysope, or canel, oþ*er* spik, oþ*er* quybibes ben y-soden i*n*ne. And lat hi*m* absteyne hi*m* fro*m* grete metys *and* euel j-sauered, *and* fram moist metis as mylke *and* siche oþ*er*e. And aft*er* eu*er*y meel, lat he*m* waisch*e* wel here mouþ *and* frete wel here gomys *and* here teeþ þ*at* no corupt mat*er*e a-byde a-mong here teeþ. And make þis pouder: Tak of pep*er*, *ounce* j; *and* of mynte, as myche; *and* of salge*m*me, as myche. *And* let hi*m* chewe þis poudre a good while in his mouþ *and* siþe swolewen it a-down. But ȝif it comeþ of þe stomac, it comeþ of a corupt flewme þ*at* is in þe stomac. *And* þa*n* þe stomac

1 **Stynkyng**] *2-line space left for initial* 6 **whil**[1]] *interl.* h **xal**] *follow. by* men xal 10 **let**] *prec. by heading* Stynche 16 **hoot**] *corr. from* hoote (e *canc. twice and exp.*) **glowyng**] *corr. from* glowynge (e *canc.*) **pomyis**] *prec. by canc. twice and exp.* pomys

most bien j-p*ur*ged of flewme, as we xul telle in þe sicnesse of þe stomac. And þei most absteyne he*m* fra*m* al man*ere* fisch*e*, flesch, *and* herb*e* þ*a*t make*n* mych*e* flewme i*n* a ma*nnus* body. | And lat he*m* waische*n* ofte-siþes wel her*e* f. 59r mouþ *and* frote wel here teeþ w*ith* a scharp clooþ. *And* let hem chewyn swete-smellyng thynges. Narþeles, myche chewyng of spic*er*ies ofte-siþes a-peireþ þe sauour of þe mouþ, for þei dissoluen myche þe corupciou*n* of þe gomes *and* maken þe mouþ sti*n*ken more þa*n* he dide. And lat hi*m* vse þese pilulees þ*a*t bie*n* good for alle manere stynckynges of þe mouþ: Take of clowes, notemuges, canel, *and* of maces, *ounce* viij; of reed sau*n*dres, *dragme* x; of quybibes, vij *dragme*; of cardamomu*m*, *dragme* vj; of lignu*m* aloes, *ounce* j; of gallia muscata, *dragme* v. Te*m*pre he*m* w*ith* þe iuys of my*n*te *and* make pillules of þe q*ua*ntite of a fetche. *And* þ*er*-of late hi*m* haue two vnd*er* hese tu*n*ge at ones. Also, tak good aloes *and* poudre he*m* *and* te*m*pre he*m* w*ith* þe iuys of wermot. And ȝeue hi*m* iij sponeful a-morewe *and* as mych*e* at eue. And a-noon aft*ur*, late hi*m* take as many sponefull*e* of hony. *And* lat hi*m* doo so eu*er*y day. By þis doynge many me*n* han bie heelid. And ȝif it comeþ of roted teeþ, late hi*m* rubbe his teeþ w*ith* þe poud*re* of hert*es*-horn j-brent. And ȝif it comeþ of þe heed, it js holmsome to eete hoote spices and weel-smelly*n*g. And ȝif it | comeþ of þe liȝte, men moste f. 59v hele þe liȝte. And ȝif þe stenche ne is nat distreyed bi alle þese man*er*es of medicynes, me moste hiden it in þe beste

4 **And**] *prec. by heading* of the mowth 7 **chewyng**] *corr. from* chewynge (e *canc.*) 8 **for**] *corr. from* ffor 9 **And**] *corr. from* cAnd (c *canc.*) 12 **quybibes**] *corr. from* quy*m*bibes 16 **hese**] *follow. by canc.* ta 23 **heed**] *follow. by canc.* lat hi*m* rubbe*n* his teeþ 24 **comeþ**] *prec. by heading* Tooth

wyse þ*a*t me may w*ith* pillules j-holden in a ma*n*nes mouþ of swete-smelli*n*g spices.

Jn a ma*n*nes teeþ bie*n* diu*er*se g*re*uau*n*ces: ache, wermes, sty*n*ckynge, rote*n*nesse. Ache comeþ in diu*er*se man*er*es: Oþ*er*while, of þe heed *and* of þe humo*ur* of þe heed þ*a*t falleþ dou*n* in-to þe teeþ, and þa*n* comely þe ou*er*teeþ akeþ. Oþ*er*while, it comeþ of þe stomac, *and* þa*n* þe neþ*er* teeþ akeþ. Oþ*er*while, it comeþ of to hoot metys þ*a*t a ma*n* etiþ, oþ*er* of to coolde, oþ*er* of a sodeyn chau*n*gynge fra*m* hoote met*es* to coold, oþ*er* of ri3t soure met*es*, or ri3th kene, oþ*er* of corupt mete þ*a*t cleueþ bie-twyn þe teeþ, for þe teeþ bie nat thicke j-now j-set, but a-twynny. Oþ*er*while, þe ache comeþ of corupt humo*ur*s þ*a*t bie*n* at þe roote of þe teeþ. And 3if it comeþ of heete of þe heed, þe chekys bien to-swolle*n*, *and* reede, *and* hoote. Jn ache þ*at* comeþ of coold þ*at* is palenesse of þe chekys *and* coold of þe teeþ. And 3if it comeþ of moistnesse, þ*er* is swellynge *and* sooftnesse of þe chekys. f. 60r And 3if it comeþ of drienesse, | þ*er* is hardnesse *and* litil swellynge w*ith* þe ache. And so 3if þe cheke bie swart reed *and* þe ache is ful kene. And 3if it bie of flewme, þei bien ful whi3te *and* þe ache is w*ith* heuynesse. Of blood comeþ reednesse *and* swellyng of chekys. Of malencolie comeþ swart 3elewnesse of þe chekyn, w*ith* lytil swellyng, *and* greet heuynesse i*n* þe ache. And 3if it comeþ of þe heed, me*n* may know it bi þe g*re*uau*n*ce of þe heed. And 3if it comeþ of kene humo*ur* a-mong þe teeþ, it makeþ wermes in þe teeþ, oþ*er* it makeþ þe teeþ holewe. And 3if it comeþ of þe heed *and* þ*er*

3 **Jn]** *2-line space left for initial* **17** **and]** *follow. by exp.* moistnesse **sooftnesse]** *interl.* **18** **þer]** *prec. by heading* ache **19 cheke]** *corr. from* acheke (a *canc. twice and exp.*) **21 comeþ]** *follow. by canc.* heuynesse

bie no rewme, lete hi*m* blood on þe heed veyne of þe arme. *And* ȝif þe body by ful of blood, lat hi*m* blede at þe veyne þ*a*t is vnd*er* þe tu*n*ge, for þ*a*t is good for þis greuau*n*ce, *and* for þe breeste, *and* to make a ma*n* haue a clere vois. But ȝif it comeþ of coold, ne let hi*m* not blood at no veyne, but let hy*m* bie cuppid in þe necke-pyt. And ȝif it comeþ of rewme, make þ*a*t þe humours flowen nat to þe teeþ, and ȝif it comeþ of heete, w*ith* fumigaciou*n*s of roses j-soden in wat*er*, oþ*er* oþere coold herb*e* þ*a*t mowen lette*n* þe humo*ur* of here cours. And ȝif þe rewme is of coold, make a fumigaciou*n* of encense. And in boþe causes, a fumigaciou*n* of he*n*nebane *and* of leek seed is good. And ȝif it comeþ of þe stomac, let hy*m* chiewe*n* portulake | oþ*er* solatre w*ith* venegre, *and* f. 60v purgen þe stomac of corupcio*n*. A strictorie to leggen to þe te*m*ples to stau*n*chyn þe flowyng of þe humo*ur* þ*a*t comeþ fra*m* þe heed and xal bie maad of mastik, of bole, of sanedragu*n*, *and* þe whiȝte of an ey. And it is good to leggen coold plastres to þe chyne w*ith* a q*ua*ntite of mynte j-medlid þ*er*-wiþ. But ȝif þe ache bie ful gret, ley a plastre w*ith*-owtyn of he*n*bane oþ*er* of opiu*m*. And medle galbanu*m*, mirre, *and* opiu*m* to-gider*e*, *and* ley to þe teeþ oþ*er* in þe tooþ, oþ*er* mirre w*ith* vynegr*e*, oþ*er* he*n*nebane by he*m*-self. But ȝif it bye of þe rewme, ley þ*er*-to no*n* vynegr*e*, *and*

13] *paragraph marks are in red in folios 60v, 61r, 61v, and 62r; headings are underl. in red and some initial letters are decorated in the same colour* **oþer**] *prec. by heading* Tooth-ache (*underl. in red and red decoration in initial letter t*) **14** **A strictorie**] *corr. from* Astrictorie **21** **oþer**] *corr. from* ooþ*er* (first o *interl.*; last o *oblit.*) **22** **oþer[1]**] *red decoration in letter o* **23** **and**] *follow. by canc. twice* ma

2 **veyne**] *in r.-h. margin:* no*ta* ben*e*

namly ȝif þe ache bie on þe syde, but make a plastre of roses, *and* of wat*er*-lilyen, *and* he*n*nebane w*ith* p*er*it*er*ie oþ*er* comyn. And ȝif all*e* þis ne helpe nat, it is semelych*e* þ*at* þe ache comeþ of su*m* worm, oþ*er* þ*at* þe teeþ bie*n* j-p*er*ceed by su*m* corupt humo*ur*, or j-roted. And ȝif it bie w*ith* swellyng of þe cheke, it is a token of a postem a-mong þe teeþ. And þ*at* xal bie j-helyd as þe posteme of þe gomes. And ȝif þe ache bie ful greuouse w*ith*-owte*n* swellyng, jt is a tokene of a
f. 61r worme. |For in þe by-gy*n*nyng of wormes in þe teeþ, þe ache is ful kene, *and* þa*n* it may bie helid w*ith* þe smoke of he*n*nebane. But aft*ur*ward it is ful hard to distreiȝe þe worm, but me*n* distreiȝe þe tooþ *and* drawe hi*m* owt. And þ*er*e-as þe ache is oold, it is p*er*ilouse to drawe*n* owt a tooþ. Jn ache þ*at* comeþ of blood, it suffiseþ to late hi*m* blood. And ȝif it comeþ of colre, let purgen hym w*ith* a colagoge *and* haue fumigaciou*n*s of coold herb*e*, *and* na*m*lych*e* of he*n*nebane. And ȝif it comeþ of flewme þ*at* falleþ down*n* fro*m* þe heed, me*n* mot let hit of his cours by strictoryes. And ȝif it comeþ of þe stomac, let p*ur*ge*n* þe stomac. *And* siþþe make a lytille bagge of þe q*ua*ntite of þi lytil fyng*er*, *and* fill*e* hit w*ith* þis poudr*e*: Tak piretr*e*, pep*er*, castor*e*, staphi, euforbe, *and* powne he*m* to-gidere. *And* do he*m* in þe bagge *and* seþ þe bagge in vynegr*e*. *And* siþe ley þe bagge by-twene his teeþ *and* lat hi*m* gnawe fast þ*er*-oon. And ȝif þe humo*ur*s comeþ

1 **bie**] *follow. by canc.* of 5 **And**] *red decoration in letter a* 6 **And**] *red decoration in letter a* 9 **For**] *2-line initial f in red; prec. by heading* Wormes in the teeth (*underl. in red and red decoration in letter w*) **by-gynnyng**] *corr. from* by-gy*n*nynge (e *canc.*) 14 **And**] *red decoration in letter a* 18 **And**] *red decoration in letter a* 20 **þis**] *in l.-h. margin* 24 **And**] *red decoration in letter a*

13 **tooþ**] *in r.-h. margin:* in oold aches | draw no teth

fra*m* þe heed to þe teeþ, make hym a gargarysme to gnawyn oon of wyn þ*a*t ysope is j-soden i*n*ne, *and* piretr*e*, *and* euforbe, *and* pep*er*. And make a plastre of armoniac *and* of poudr*e* of brymston | f. 61v j-knede by þe feere, *and* all*e* warm j-leid to þe place þ*a*t akeþ. And ȝif it comeþ of þe rewme, make hi*m* a fumigaciou*n* of þe smoke of ence*n*se *and* of clowes. And a-mong all*e* herbis, origane *and* me*n*[t]astre bien þe beste for ache of þe teeþ þ*a*t comeþ of coold, for þe wyn þ*a*t þei bie*n* j-sode*n* i*n*ne is p*ro*fitable to bien j-holdyn in þe mowþ, *and* þe herb*e* to bie j-plastred w*ith*-owtyn; also a plastre j-maad of hony *and* of salt, oþ*er* of hony *and* of storax. A strictorie to lygge*n* on þe temples: Tak þe poudre of ence*n*se, of mastik, *and* of spik j-medlid, w*ith* þe whiȝt of an ey. Many oþ*er* speciall*e* medicynes þ*er* bien for þe tooþ-ache: Oon is, tak þe wat*er* þ*a*t is distilled of reed netles, *and* wet a clowt þ*er*-i*n*ne *and* leie to þe cheke. Oþ*er*, tak þe iuys of netlen *and* medle þ*er*w*ith* half so myche of reed wyn. *And* wet a clowt *and* lei it to þe cheke. Oþ*er*, tak piretre *and* seeþ in vinegre *and* chiewe it a good while in þ*in* mouþ. *And* siþþe spit it owt *and* let þ*in* mouþ bie opene þ*a*t þe fleume þ*a*t falleþ in-to þe mouþ mow passe forþ. And in þe same man*er* þ*ou* mytest chiewe iiij greynes or v of s[t]aphie, oþ*er* mastik, oþ*er* galbanu*m*. *And* siþþe speet it out *and* let þe

3 **And**] *red decoration in letter a* 4 **j-knede**] *prec. by heading* Tooth-ache (*underl. in red and red decoration in initial letter t*) 7 **And**] *red decoration in letter a* **mentastre**] *corr. from* me*n*castre 8 **for**[2]] *corr. from* ffor 12 **A**] *red decoration* 15 **Oon**] *red decoration in initial letter o* 18 **Oþer**] *red decoration in letter o* 21 **And**] *red decoration in letter a* 22 **staphie**] *corr. from* scaphie 23 **þe**] *follow. by canc.* mouþ bie opyne

7 **And**] *in l.-h. margin:* no*ta* ben*e*

flewme ren out. Anoþ*er*, stampe pollipodie *and* salt j-medlid f. 62r to-gidere, *and* mak þ*er*-of a plast*re* | and ley to þe cheke. Oþ*er* tak þe iuys þ*er*-of in-to nose-thrilles. Oþ*er* frete þe teeþ w*ith* poudre þ*at* is j-maad of gyng*er*, *and* pep*er*, *and* piretre, *and* coost. And wat*er* þat an aische*n* roote is j-soden i*n*ne *and* j-holde in a ma*nn es* mouþ is profitabil*e*. And so is þe iuys of garlek *and* poudre of pep*er* þ*er*w*ith* *and* j-cast in-to þe eere on þe co*n*trarie syde. Hare brayn a-noynted on ȝonge children chekys makeþ here teeþ to waxyn. And þe roote of hou*n*destonge j-stamped *and* siþe j-froted w*ith* a litel oyle oþ*er* w*ith* botere is good to liggen vp-on þe cheke, and alym, *and* salt, *and* colu*m*bine, *and* v*er*ueyne j-soden to-gidere, *and* þe poudre of hem j-leid to þe sore teeþ. And þe iuys of karsen j-doon in þe eeris cesseþ þe ache of þe teeþ. Also seeþ þe root*es* of tyntinalle in wyn, *and* w*ith* þ*at* wyn, let wasche þe teeþ. And þe same doiþ þe rootis of netlen j-soden in vinegre *and* root*es* j-plastred to þe cheke. And so doiþ þe roote of pentafilon *and* of camedreos. And ȝif þe ache ne cesseþ nat bi alle þese medicines, þ*o*u most worche w*ith* stupefactyues, as he*n*nebane *and* opiu*m*. And ȝif þ*at* makeþ nat þe ache to ceessen, þ*o*u most drawen owt þe tooþ.

Rotenesse of þe teeþ comeþ of þe same enche-sou*n*s þ*at* þe tooþ-ache comeþ. *And* þei j-sauyd fra*m* rotyng by þi*n*ges

2 plastre] *catchword* (*in bottom margin*): *and* lei to þe cheke **and**[2]] *prec. by heading* Corupcyou*n* of teeth (*underl. in red and red decoration in initial letter c*) **3 Oþer**[1]] *red decoration in letter o* **6 And**] *red decoration in letter a* **13 And**] *red decoration in letter a* **14 Also**] *red decoration in letter a* **17 cheke**] *corr. from* chekeys (last e *interl.*; ys *exp.*) **And**] *red decoration in letter a* **18 And**] *red decoration in letter a* **22 Rotenesse**] *2-line initial r in red*

þ*at* co*n*forte*n* þe teeþ, as to frete*n* he*m* w*ith* þe poudr*e* of canel *and* w*ith* mastik, oþ*er* w*ith* þe poudre | of origan, oþ*er* f. 62v of mynte, oþ*er* of nytre. But it is nat good to frete þe teeþ w*ith* ri3t hoote spicis, for þ*at* wole make hem to roote wel þe raþere. Also mirre, *and* egremoyne, *and* v*er*ueyne, *and* galles þ*at* me*n* maken of enke, *and* olibanu*m* kepeþ þe teeþ fra*m* rotyng, *and* co*n*forteþ he*m* myche. And to dri3e þe teeþ aft*ur* mete w*ith* a dri3e ly*n*ne*n* clooþ is p*ro*fitabyl, *and* clenseþ he*m*, þ*at* no mete cleue nat, ne non corupciou*n* a-monge þe teeþ to make hem roten.

A mannes tonge haþ two s*er*uices. Oon is to tast w*ith* a ma*n*nes metes *and* drynckes; anoþ*er* is to speke. An þorou3 diu*er*se g*re*uau*n*ces þ*at* comeþ of corupt humo*urs*, a ma*n*nes tonge is oþ*er*while indisposed, þ*at* a ma*n* may naþ*er* speke ne taste. Greuances of þe tonge bie*n* postemys, *and* bladdris, oþ*er* stoppyng of her*e* senewys þorow corupt humo*urs* þ*at* make*n* þe tonge laxe, *and* falle in-to a palesie. And 3if þ*er* bie a posteme oþ*er* a bleyne on þe tonge, 3if it bie of blood, þe tonge is swolle, *and* reed, *and* hoot, *and* neische, *and* akynge. And 3if it is of colre, þe tonge is ful hoot, *and* cyt*ri*ne, þ*at* is to sey, a derke reed; þe ache is more scharp þa*n* of þe blood, *and* þe swalm ne þe softnesse is nat so myche as of blood. | f. 63r But 3if it is of flewme, þe tonge is coold, *and* swellyng, *and* neische, *and* of whi3te colo*ur*. Of malencolie, comeþ cooldnesse, *and* swart 3elwe colo*ur*. *And* þe tonge ne swelleþ nat, but is su*m*what j-drawe to-gidere. And þese bien þe toknes bi whiche me*n* may j-knowe what humo*ur* is þe

1 as] *red decoration in letter a* **2 oþer[1]]** *red decoration in letter o* **of]** *prec. by heading* Greuau*n*ce; *follow. by exp.* mastik **4 for]** *corr. from* ffor **11 A]** *2-line space left for initial* **23 But]** *prec. by heading* of the tonge enchesou*n* of þe palesye of þe tonge. And ȝif þe bleynys of þe tonge bie blake oþ*er* grene, it is a tokene þ*at* þe tonge is j-cancrid. For postem*us and* bleynnys þ*at* comeþ of coold, lat hi*m* vse hoote gargarism*us* to chiew in his mouþ *and* to make hi*m* fn[e]se; *and* hoot fumigaciou*n*s for þe heed, as w*ith* anet, mellilot, cammamille, *and* sansuke j-soden. And late a-noynte þe heed w*ith* hoote oynementis *and* enplastris on his heed, as coold þinges, and purgen his heed, as we tolde*n* in sicnesse of þe heed. *And* let hi*m* blood in boþe veynis vnd*er* þe tonge, and siþe late hi*m* waisch*e* þe mouþ w*ith* coold þi*n*ges. And a-noynte þe tonge as it was j-teld in þe cleuyng*e* of þe lyppis how men xuld heele bleynis of þe mouþ. And ȝif þe co*m*plexiou*n* of þe tonge bie colde, vse sych*e* þi*n*ges as we xul telle in þe palesie of þe tonge. And ȝif þe postem*us* bie hard, make hi*m* a gargarisme of milke, *and* of wat*er* þ*at* driȝe figges *and* fenel bie*n* j-sode*n* i*n*ne. And ȝif it bie of coold, f. 63v waisch*e* it w*ith* wat*er* of | camomille, *and* make a gargarisme of seneuey *and* of hony. For þe pemples þ*at* bien of hete, let hi*m* þe iuys of sichomour oþ*er* of weybrode vndere his tonge, oþ*er* þe iuys of solatre, *and* medle þ*er*-w*ith* reed saundres *and* wat*er* [þat] sumac, oþ*er* balaustia, oþ*er* mirre, oþ*er* rooses, bien j-soden i*n*ne.

A goode poud*re* for sich*e* postem*us* of þe tonge: Tak of dispumed hony, *ounce* vj; of þe iuys of þe erþe appel *and* of þe milke of a fige tre, *ounce* ij. Siþe seeþ he*m* to-gidere on an esy fiere and siþe medle þ*er*w*ith* þis poudre: Tac tartaru*m* of whiȝt wyn, *and* seneuey, of eiþ*er*, *ounce* j; of whiȝt pep*er*,

3 For] *corr. from* ffor **15 of**[1]] *follow. by* mylk (lk *exp.*) **milke**] *in r.-h. margin* **16 fenel**] *corr. from* ffenel **17 camomille**] *prec. by heading* Greuawn*n*ce **18 For**] *corr. from* ffor **21 oþer**[2]] *follow. by canc.* nir **25 a**] *corr. from* an

and a lityl sugre, *ounce* s*emis*; of borac*e*, *ounce* ij; of olibanu*m*, *and* of os sepie, *dragme* ij. Poudre al þese *and* medle he*m* w*ith* þe oþ*er*e for-seid þi*n*ges, *and* þ*er*w*ith* a-noynte þe soore w*ith*-i*n*ne þe mouþe. A whiȝt oyneme*n*t þ*at* is good for þe same greuau*n*ce: Tak of mastic *and* of olibanu*m*, *ounce* s*emis*; of litarge *and* of brend leed, *ounce* j; of ceruse, *ounce* iij; *and* do al þese in a morter*e* *and* medle he*m* w*ith* a lytil vinegre. *And* seeþ he*m* w*ith* a lytil oyle *and* eft-sones w*ith* vinegre. *And* medle he*m* w*ith* oon aft*ur* a-noþ*er* til it bie naþ*er* to þicke ne to þi*n*ne. But ȝif þe tonge haue þe palesie þorow su*m* corupt humo*ur* þ*at* stoppeþ þe senewis, of what humo*ur* þ*at* it bie, þ*ou* maist knowe it bie þe tokenes þ*at* we tolden bi-fore. And ȝif it bie of blood, lat hym blood at þe veynys þ*at* bien vnder*e* | þe tonge. And f. 64r siþþe, lat hoolde castore vnd*er* his to*n*ge, oþ*er* þe iuys of a wyld caule. And vnd*er*stonde þ*at* caul seed conforteþ myche þe tonge *and* þe þrote *and* þe tokene þ*er*-of is, for þe nyȝtyngale aft*er* þ*at* he haþ j-ete syche seedis he syngeþ faste. After-ward, lat waisch*e* hese mowþ w*ith* oximel, *and* pep*er*, *and* seneuey, *and* ysope *and* origane. Also lat waischen hese mouþ w*ith* oximel þ*at* mayþen bie*n* j-medlid w*ith*, *and* lat hi*m* hooldyn hese mouþ opene, þ*at* þe humo*ur*s flowen owt at þe mouþ. And let hi*m* chiewe drye piretre, oþ*er* mastik, oþ*er* s[t]aphie *and* mastik to-gidere. And lete hi*m* frotyn hese tonge w*ith* þe poudre of piretre, of pep*er*, of s[t]aphie, of seneuey, of castore, of gyngere, of salge*m*me, oþ*er* of salnitr*e*, oþ*er* of sal armoniac. And su*m*me cast þ*er*-to clowes,

14 þe[2]] *prec. by heading* of the tonge **21 mayþen**] *corr. from* may*n*þen **24 staphie**] *corr. from* scaphie **25 staphie**] *corr. from* scaphie

16 vnderstonde] *in r.-h. margin:* no*ta* be*n*e

notemuge, gali*n*gale, cardomomu*m*, spik, *and* sich*e* oþ*er* þi*n*ges. A gargarisme mai be maad of þe same þi*n*ges. Oþ*er* þus: Tac origane, piretre, gynger*e*, pep*er* whiȝt *and* blac *and* long, canel, ysope, nygille, sansuke, cost, of eu*er*yche, j-lyche myche. Te*m*pre he*m* w*ith* oximel. And herewiþ þ*o*u myȝtest also frete þe gomes oon boþe sydys, *and* þe tonge a-boue *and* by-neþe.

A sirip þ*er*for*e*: Tac aue*n*ce, of þe floures of borage, anthos, driȝe sauge, calamynte, origane, baies of lorer*e*, pyonye, laue*n*dre, þe herbe of þe palesie, *and* of carses, *ounce* j; of quibibes, reed saundrees, rooses, mellise, a-mom*e*, f. 64v *ounce* s*emis*. Pownne hem and make vp þi sirrip w*ith* | ij *pound* pounde of sugre.

An oyneme*n*t: Tac of of þe iuys of sauge, *ounce* j; of þe iuys of wermot, of maiorane, *and* of march, *ounce* j; of þe baies of lorere, iunip*er*i, castore, *ounce* j; of marciaton, *and* of oile of lorer*e*, *ounce* ij; of reed wex, q*ua*r[t] j. *And* medle hem to-gidere *and* þ*er*w*ith* a-noynte þe tonge.

A stufe for he*m* xal bie maad of mugweed, mynte, horehowne, origane, calamynte, carses; *and* of þe herbe of þe palesie and ȝif þe palesie bie of coold oþ*er* of ple*n*te of humo*urs* a-boute þe tonge. And þoo þ*at* han þis sicnesse moten leeue alle manere fleu*ma*tik metys, *and* oþ*er*e metys þ*at* bien euel to defye. And late he*m* vse sauge in here met*es*, *and* leek, *and* oynou*n*s, *and* leeue þei strong wyn *and* drynk smal wyn. And ne baþe*n* he*m* nat myche *and* na*m*ly wha*n* þei bien repleet.

A good gargarisme: Tak origane, piretre, pep*er* blac *and* whiȝt *and* long, gyng*er*, canel, ysope, nygille, sansuke, coost,

11 a-mome] *corr. from* amom*er* **12 ij**] *prec. by heading* Squinacie **13 pound**] *interl.* **25 and**[2]] *follow. by canc.* onyou*n*s

of eu*er*iche, iliche myche. Poudre he*m* *and* te*m*pre he*m* w*it*h sape, þ*at* is, swete vinegre, *and* make vt þ*in* gargarisme w*it*h oximel.

Sq*ui*nacie is a posteme of þe þrote þ*at* letteþ a ma*n* boþe to speke *and* for-to chiew hese mete. *And* it wole strangle a ma*n* but ȝif it bie holpyn. And ȝif þis postym bie | of blood, f. 65r þese bien þe tokenes: fulnesse of þe veynys, reednesse of þe visage, *and* swelli*n*ge, *and* hete, a gret pouse, *and* a strong, *and* a swyft. Of colre, þe ache *and* þe angwisch*e* is greet, [þe] hete is gret, *and* þirst, *and* bytt*er*nesse of þe mouþ, miche fume *and* smoke in þe wesynge. Þe pouse is voyid, but he is stronge *and* swyft. Of viscouse flewme, þ*er* is no*n* so gret ache as þ*er* is oþ*er* humo*ur*s. But þ*er* is a swalm, *and* þe place of þe sore is neische, *and* þe mouþ is on-sauery. And ȝif it bie of salt flewme, þe mouþ is ful salt *and* ful bitt*er*. *And* þe place a-bout þe soor, su*m*what is reed *and* hoot. But of whiche of þese humo*ur*s þe sq*ui*nacy bie, let hi*m* blede furst su*m*what on þe heed veyne of þe arme, siþe of oon of þe tonge veynes, and siþe on þe gret too, to drawe a-weyward þe blood fra*m* þe postym. And ȝif it bie of fleu*ma*goge to p*ur*gen hym of flewme, ȝif he mowe receyue*n* hit for g*r*euau*n*ce. But algatis let hi*m* blood as his statte askeþ. And ȝif he bie strong of co*m*plexiou*n* *and* ȝong, lat hi*m* blede þe mor*e*.

Diameron þ*at* is good for þe sq*ui*nacie *and* for oþ*er* greuau*n*ces of þe mouþ. Take mores, *and* of sicamour, j

3 oximel] *interl.* **4 Squinacie]** *2-line space left for initial* **6 of]** *prec. by heading* Squinacie **7 fulnesse]** *corr. from* ffulnesse **19 tonge veynes]** *corr. from* veynes tonge

17 squinacy] *in r.-h. margin:* Reg*ula* g[eneralis] (*underl.*)

pound; of hony, *pound* s*emis*; of sape, *ounce* iij. Seþe he*m* f. 65v to-gid*ere* in a tynne*n* vessel til it bie þicke *and* cleuy*n*ge. | W*ith* þis *and* þe iuys of plau*n*teyn, make hy*m* a gargarisme. But loke þ*at* þ*ou* legge noon coolde plastres w*ith*-owten-forþ in þis sicnesse, leste þei lette*n* hi*m* of breþi*n*ge *and* swellynge. A-noynte his þrote w*ith* dewte, *and* lei þ*er*-on wolle þ*at* is j-[shoren] of a scheep vnwasche.

Deute is þ*us* j-maad: Tak of þe rootis of bismalue, þ*at* is, þe holy-hocke, ij *pound*; of lynseed, of femygrek, *pound* s*emis*; of sq*ui*le, *pound* s*emis*. Clense he*m* weel *and* stampe he*m* weel to-gidere. *And* siþe do he*m* in viij pou*n*d of wat*er* *and* lat he*m* liȝe so to-gidere iiij daies. *And* siþe set it ou*er* þe feir *and* seeþ it softly til it bie þicke. *And* þa*n*ne wrynge it *and* cast þ*er*-to a litil hoot wat*er*. *And* wryng it sadly þ*at* þe iuys come owt clene. And ȝif þ*ou* haast ij pou*n*d of iuys, cast þ*er*-to iiij pound of oile *and* let he*m* seþe to-gidere til þe iuys bie co*n*sumed. *And* siþe caste þ*er*-to j *pound* of wexe *and* let he*m* medle wel to-gidere. *And* siþe caste þ*er*-to of t*ur*me*n*tyne, of galbanu*m*, *and* of gu*m*me of yuy, *ounce* ij; *and* siþe *pound* s*emis* of rosyn, *and* as myche of colofyne. *And* siþe, do it fro þe feir *and* kepe it. And þis is good for þe breest, *and* for greuau*n*ce of þe brest þ*at* comeþ of coold, and for þe postym of þe liȝt, *and* for membris þ*at* bien j-cooldid f. 66r *and* j-dried, | and for-to make postemys *and* bochches ripe for-to breke. And vnd*er*stonde þilke þ*at* ha*n* g*re*uau*n*ce in

3 With] *prec. by heading* Squinacye **10 squile**] *corr. from* sq*ui*lle (first l *canc. twice*) **17 j**] *follow. by canc.* pou*n*de **pound**] *interl.* **19 yuy**] *corr. from* y*n*uy*n* **24 and**[2]] *prec. by heading* Squinacie **25 þilke**] *corr. from* þ*at*ilke (*at canc. twice*)

18 wel] *in l.-h. margin:* no*ta* bene

here þrote, oþ*er* in here brest, oþ*er* in here spiritual me*m*bris, þ*at* is to seie, in þilke me*m*bris þ*at* bie*n* a-boue*n* þe mydrif, as þe herte *and* þe li3te, schulle*n* bie ny3 a*n* hoot fier, þ*at* þe eir*e* þ*at* þei reseyuen in drawyng breeþ bie hoot, for alle coolde þi*n*ges bie*n* neyful for postemes.

A good plast*re* to legge*n* w*it*h-outy*n* to make þe posteme to ripe*n* *and* is good for eu*er*y postym boþe w*it*h-i*n*ne a ma*n*n*us* body *and* w*it*h-owtyn: Tac þe root*es* of malue, *and* bismalue, *and* lilies, *and* seeþ he*m* in wat*er*. *And* siþe sta*m*p he*m* w*it*h* freisch3 grece *and* bot*er*e, *and* cast þ*er*-to mele of lynseed *and* of femygrek, *and* snayles, *and* sta*m*pe alle to-gidere. And 3if hi*m* a gargarisme of vinegr*e* þ*at* barlych*e* haþ j-leyn i*n*ne, and wat*er* þ*at* balustia, oþ*er* sumac, oþ*er* rosees, oþ*er* galles, bien j-sode*n* i*n*ne; oþ*er* lentes, oþ*er* medle w*it*h vinegr*e* þe iuys of p*er*silie oþ*er* of solatre. Oþ*er* make a gargarisme of asse mylk oþ*er* gotys mylke j-medlyd w*it*h sugre *and* a lytul safru*n*. And 3if hi*m* tisane to dri*n*ke w*it*h þe wat*er* þ*at* þe seedis of four*e* coolde herb*e* haue bie*n* j-waschy*n* i*n*ne. But 3if þe posteme bie of flewme, aft*er* his blood-latyng *and* his p*ur*gaciou*n*s, make hi*m* a gargarisme of sap of an noote tree, *and* anet, *and* memyth, oþ*er* of þe wat*er* þ*at* þe rynde | of a note tree is j-sode*n* i*n*ne oþ*er* of f. 66v mylberie tree, oþ*er* þe iuys of solatre is j-sode i*n*ne, wiþ liciu*m* oþ*er* w*it*h aloes. And 3if his mouþ smerte oþ*er* bie ful hoot, make hi*m* a gargarisme of mylke þ*at* is warm as it comeþ fra*m* mylkynge. And aft*er*ward þu my3tist vse strengore gargarismes, as wiþ sap of an note tree, w*it*h

15 iuys] *follow. by exp.* of **22** of[1]] *prec. by heading* Squinacye
26 And] *follow. by* aft

6 plastre] *in r.-h. margin:* no*ta* be*n*e

piretre, oþ*er* oximel, or þe mylk of a goot *and* whiȝt hou*n*dys drit j-poudrid *and* j-medlid to-gidere. Oþ*er* a-noynte his mouþ w*ith*-i*n*ne w*ith* a feþere. Oþ*er* poudre hou*n*dys driȝt smalle *and* medle it w*ith* bolys galle, *and* do it in his mouþ, *and* let it passe to þe soore. *And* a-noynte þe mouþ w*ith*-i*n*ne w*ith* hony, for boles galle *and* schepys galle ben good for þe sq*ui*nacie, and so ga*n*dris driȝt to bie*n* j-plastred w*ith*-oute*n*-forþ on þe þrote. And it wole drawen owt of a wou*n*de boþen yren *and* thornes. Oþ*er* make a plastre of galbanu*m* *and* of pich*e*. Oþ*er* heete galbanu*m* bi hi*m*-self *and* ley w*ith*-owte*n* to þe soor*e*, *and* it wole breke þe postym. And so wole a plast*re* j-maad of whete oþ*er* of sourdouȝ j-medlid w*ith* þe iuys of oy*n*nou*n*s, oþ*er* of whete *and* of wormes of þe erþe j-medlid. Anoþ*er*: Wha*n* þe mat*ere* of þe postym is defiȝed, þe ripe of þe postym is j-know bi þe neischenesse þ*er*-of, *and* a-batyng of þe heete *and* also of þe ache. Tak of dragagant,
f. 67r *dragme* v; of oile of alemau*n*des *and* of violet, | *quantum* s*ufficit*; of wat*er* [þat] barlich*e* haþ j-leyn i*n*ne a while, of lycorys, of hockys, of þe iuys of gourdys, *and* of plau*n*teyne, of eu*er*iche, j-liche myche. And of wat*er* þ*at* cassia fistula haþ bie*n* j-soden i*n*ne. And medele þese to-gidere *and* lat hi*m* vsyn it in þe man*ere* of a gargarisme. And ȝif þ*o*u wult raþer*e* haue it open, tak wat*er* þ*at* figges bien j-sode*n* i*n*ne *and* medle it w*ith* asse mykil oþ*er* houndys drit j-poudrid. And þis same dooþ gootis mylk oþ*er* asse mylk w*ith* p*er*silie, oþ*er* w*ith* þe seed of yreos þ*at* hatte flourdeliȝ *and* oile of

6 for[1]] *corr. from* ffor **9 yren**] *corr. from* ynren **17 quantum**] *prec. by heading* Squinacye **18 þat**] *corr. from* of **24 oþer**] *follow. by canc.* hoþ*er*

6 for[2]] *in l.-h. margin:* no*ta* m*emorab*ile

violet, oþ*er* botere j-medlid w*it*h whete mele. And ȝif al þis ne helpeþ nat *and* þe postym bie ripe, brise it w*it*h þi*n* hond oþ*er* w*it*h a staf, þ*at* it breke. And wha*n* it is j-broke, ȝif hi*m* þe ȝelkys of eyren y-soden w*it*h amide, *and* dragaga[n]t*e*, *and* oile of violet; oþ*er* w*it*h þe iuys of plau*n*teyn, *and* wat*er* þ*at* barliche *and* lycorys bien j-soden i*n*ne; oþ*er* figges *and* cassia fistula doon þ*er*-too *and* y-medlyd w*it*h oile of violet. And an oyneme*n*t to opene a postym of þe wesynge: Take of whiȝt wex *and* of oile of violet, xij *ounce*; of bot*er*e, viij *ounce*. Stampe he*m* to-gidere *and* so make þe oyneme*n*t. And late he*m* þ*at* ha*n* þis sicnesse bien j-norisched w*it*h bren j-clensed w*it*h wat*er*, *and* w*it*h oile of alemau*n*des, *and* oile of violet, w*it*h penydes, hockes, *and* arage, *and* b[e]etis, *and* gourdes. And let a-noynte þe wesyng w*it*h oile of violet, dragag*e*, *and* w*it*h gleire of eyren. | f. 67v

Horsnesse comeþ in two maneres: Oon is of humours þ*at* bien in þe vesselles þ*at* bie*n* enchesou*n*s of þe vois, þ*at* is to seie, in þe liȝte, oþ*er* in þe breste, oþ*er* þe þrote-bolle. Oþ*er*whiles, it comeþ of sicnesse of þe heed, as apoplexie, *and* epile*n*cie, oþ*er* falli*n*g down of þe pose in-to þe spiritual me*m*bris. Oþ*er*while it comeþ of febilnesse, *and* namlych*e* of sich*e* men þ*at* drynkyn mych*e* wat*er*, and þe cooldnesse of þe wat*er* streyneþ here breest, *and* hirteþ þe liȝte *and* þe þrote, þ*at* bie*n* þe instrume*n*t*es* of þe vois. And ȝif it comeþ of blood, þese bien þe tokenes: a moist couȝ, *and* reednesse of visage, swellyng *and* fulnesse of veynes, sweetnesse of þe mouþ, and wiþholdyng of blood þ*at* was to blede*n* at þe nose oþ*er* at su*m* oþ*er* place, oþ*er* defaute of blood-leti*n*ge i*n* sich*e* men þ*at* bien j-wont for-to blede. Of habu*n*dau*n*ce *and*

13 beetis] *corr. from* boetis **16 Horsnesse**] *2-line space left for initial; prec. by heading* Hoorsnesse plente of flewme þ*at* is a-boute þe li3te *and* þe brest, þese bien þe tokenes: a moist cou3, *and* an vnsauernesse of þe mouþ, *and* coold, *and* mych*e* spittynge, pale coloure, *and* myche greuau*n*ce a-ny3t, *and* myche sleuþe. Of febilnesse, þese bien þe tokenes: feblenesse of all*e* þe body, *and* leneschipe þ*at* comeþ of myche fastyng bi-foren, oþ*er* flux, oþ*er* oþ*er* þi*n*ges þ*at* makeþ a ma*n*nys body leene.

Horsnesse þ*at* comeþ of drynesse of þe breest, comeþ on two man*er*es: as of dust, oþ*er* smoke, oþ*er* su*m* sych*e* oþere þing þ*at* comeþ fram w*ith*-owtyn-forþ in-to þe breest; | oþ*er* of drynesse of þe places þ*at* a ma*n*nys breeþ passeþ þorou3, *and* þ*at* d*ri*nesse comeþ of wynd, oþ*er* of vse of salt metis *and* soure. *And* þe tokenes here-of bien a dri3e cou3e, *and* a drinesse of þe mouþ, *and* p*ri*ckynge w*ith*-i*n*ne-forþ. 3if þe hoorsnesse bie of blood, let hi*m* bledi*n* at þe heed veyne of þe arme aft*er* þ*at* his a-staat axeþ, and let purgen hym w*ith* a calogoge. And lat hi*m* vsen an electuarie j-maad of diapenidion *and* diarris, but þe ij partys xul bien of diapenidion *and* þe iij parte of diarris. And let hi*m* vse þese pillules: Tak of þe seed of melou*n*, of gourdis, of portulake, citon*e*, þe iuys of lycorys, of amyde, gu*m*me arab*e*, dragagant*e*, penydes, of euerich*e*-one, j-liche mych*e*. Te*m*pre he*m* wiþ þe sirryp of violet, oþ*er* w*ith* þe mussilage of p*er*silie, *and* þe iuys of hockes, *and* lei he*m* vnd*er* his tonge. But 3if it bie of fleume, let purgen hi*m* w*ith* a fleu*ma*goge. And siþe gyf hi*m* a gargorisme of oximel, and þe clansy*n*ge of piretre j-soden in meeþ. And let stufen hi*m* in wat*er* þ*at* yreos, *and* ysope, *and* sau*er*ey, *and* sauge, *and* fenel, *and* horsheel, *and* spik, *and* femigrek, *and* lynseed j-rostyd, *and*

f. 68r

10 fram] *in l.-h. margin* **oþer]** *prec. by heading* Hoorsnesse

calamynte, *and* pynes, [ben j-soden in]. *And* let hi*m* vse þe forseyd pillules. A-noþ*er*e good gargarisme is j-maad of piret*r*e, pep*er*, calamynte, puliole, origane, gy*n*ger*e*. And ȝif a ma*n* haþ nat j-haad þe grevaunce | f. 68v but litil while, let stufen his heed ouer warme wat*er* þ*a*t puliole *and* roses bie*n* j-soden i*n*ne. And let keuere weel his heed for catchi*n*ge of coold. *And* let hi*m* ete*n* dyapenydio*n* w*ith* tysane (tysane is wat*er* þ*a*t barliche is j-soden i*n*ne). And late hi*m* ete*n* in þe eue-tyd an ey *and* orpeme*n*t þ*er*-i*n*ne. An late a-noynte here breest, *and* þe nolle of here heed, *and* þe þrote-bolle w*ith* deute, oþ*er* marciaton, oþ*er* su*m* oþ*er* sich*e* oyneme*n*t. And let seþen driȝe figges *and* pyretre in swet wyn *and* ȝif hi*m* þ*a*t wyn for a gargarisme. Oþ*er* tac reed netlen croppes *and* sta*m*pe hem w*ith* þe ȝelkys of eyren j-broken on an hoot glowyng tilstoon. *And* let keueryn hese breeste w*ith* a warme lyne*n* clooþ. And lat hi*m* vsen þis electuarie: comyn j-rostyd, *ounce* j; of seneuey, *ounce* ij; of pep*er*, *ounce* ij; of canel, calamynte, piretre, *ounce* ij. But ȝif þe horsnesse come of drinesse, þ*o*u myȝtest j-knowe it bi þe for-seid tokenes, and by myche wakynge *and* lityl spyttynge oþ*er* noon, *and* þ*a*t is bitt*er* oþ*er* salt. *And* he haþ an hoot cowȝe, *and* a driȝe, *and* a greuouse, *and* his þrote-bolle is sore. And in þis greuance, þ*o*u xalt ȝeue hym no purgacion, but þ*o*u xalt vse mollityues to make þ*a*t neisch*e* þ*a*t is hardid, and lenytyues to make þ*a*t smoþe þ*a*t was rowȝ, *and* scharp, | f. 69r *and* hard, þorow drinesse. And so hi*m* is good to take þe coold dragagantu*m*, *and* diapapauar, w*ith* sugere of violet oþ*er* w*ith* diapenidion. And lat hi*m* holdyn vnd*er* his tonge þe seed of citonyes, *and* of p*er*silie, *and* dragagant*e*. And ȝif hi*m*

4 **grevaunce**] *f. 68v* | vaunce **but**] *prec. by heading* Hoorsnesse
25 þat[1]] *follow. by canc.* neisch **and**[2]] *prec. by heading* Hoorsnesse

a sirip of violet y-medlid w*ith* wat*er* of gourdys, nat of þe seed þ*at* is in þe greet gourdys, but of þe herbe þ*at* we clepen gourde in al þis tretys. And late hi*m* drynke wat*er* þ*at* dragagau*n*t*e*, *and* gu*m*me arabik, *and* þe seed of citonye, *and* hockes [ben jsoden in]. *And* sta*m*pe he*m* to-gid*ere* *and* medle he*m* w*ith* tysane þ*at* is j-maad of dragag*e* infuse. *And* let make pillules here-of *and* holde he*m* vnd*er* his to*n*ge. Dragagant*e* is a gu*m*me, but dragag*e* infuse is wha*n*ne þe dragag*e* is resolued in wat*er*, oþ*er* in tysane, oþ*er* eny sych*e* oþ*ere*. So gu*m*me arabik te*m*preþ enkes. A-noynte his breste *and* his þrote-bolle w*ith* bot*ere* þ*at* ne is nat j-salted. And ley a plastre on his breste of hockys j-sode*n* in bot*ere* oþ*ere* in oyle. A good electuarie: Tac of dragag*e*, gu*m*me arab*e*, amyde, of þe seed of citonyes, of gourdis, of melou*n*, of portulake, *ounce* iiij; of saffren, *ounce* j; of penydes, *ounce* vj. A-noþ*ere*: Tak of dragag*e*, *dragme* v; of gu*m*me arab*e*, amyde, swete alemau*n*dys, *and* of gourde seed, *dragme* ij; of penydes, xxx *dragme*, m*anipulum quantum* s*ufficit.* Anoþ*er*:
f. 69v Take of ceterak, maidenher*e*, | ysope, sauge, barlyche j-clensyd, liquorys, *and* þe iuys þ*er*-of as myche as þe likeþ. *And* seþe hem in wat*er* oþ*er* wyn *and* ȝyue he*m* to drynken. Þe dietyng xal bie cold *and* moist, cla*n*synge of bryn, *and* gootys mylk, oþ*er* schepis, þe colyis of an hen oþ*er* of a chike. And late hi*m* vsen penydes, *and* amyde, *and* applen j-rosted, *and* bot*ere* w*ith* alle man*ere* mete. And leue þei salt metys, *and* kene, *and* rostid, *and* fried, *and* fastynge, *and* anger, *and* cryi*n*ge, *and* excesse of etynge *and* of drynkynge, *and* wakynge, *and* alle manere coold.

19 ysope] *prec. by heading* Streytenesse

1 of[3]] *in r.-h. margin:* no*ta* ben*e*

Streytnesse of a ma*n*nes brest comeþ oþ*er*while of drynesse. *And* þe tokenes þ*er*-of bien leneschipe, pale colour, þirst *and* hoot couȝe *and* a driȝe, *and* myche wakynge. Þis nedeþ no purgaciou*n*, but þei xul bie helyd as þi[l]ke þ*a*t ha*n* horsnesse of drinesse of þe breste. Su*m*me ha*n* streitnesse of þe brest of humo*ur*s þ*a*t stoppe*n* here breste. And þ*a*t me knowe by myche spyttynge, *and* couȝe, *and* siche oþ*er*e þi*n*ges *and* tokenes. And xal bie j-heelyd as horsnesse þ*a*t comeþ of humo*ur*s of þe breste. And late hi*m* vsen diarres, diaprassiu*m*, diacalame*n*tu*m*, *and* diatrio*n*[piperion]. And late a-noynte her*e* brest w*i*t*h* marciaton | *and* oile of lorere. f. 70r And oþ*er*while lat hi*m* haue a fumigacio*n* of orpeme*n*t. And late stufe hi*m* w*i*t*h* horsel. And late vse to drynke wyn þ*a*t calamynte is j-soden i*n*ne.

Diapenydion is good for eu*ery* g*r*euau*n*ce of þe liȝte, *and* for þe couȝ, *and* for horsnesse, *and* streitnesse of þe breste þ*a*t comeþ of drynesse, *and* for tysik; *and* is j-maad þus: Take of penydes, *ounce* ij *and* s*emis*; of blau*n*chid alemau*n*dis *and* of whiȝt popi seed, *dragme* ij *and dragme* j; of canel, clowes, gyng*er*, þe iuys of licorys, dragagant*e*, gu*m* arabik, amyde, seed of gourdes, melone j-clensed, *dragme* j; of camphore, þe þridde part of *dragme* j; of þe siryp of þe violet, *quantum* s*ufficit*. Mak it in þis maner*e*: Tac *dragme* iij of violet *and* seeþ he*m* in a pou*n*d of wat*er* til þe v*er*tu of þe herbys bie in þe wat*er*. *And* tak þe wat*er and* cast to þe for-seid seedis j-stamped *and* þ*in* penydes. And ȝif þ*er* houeþ eny-þi*n*g of þ*in* seed*es* a-boue þe wat*er*, stamp it in a morter*e and* cast it to þe toþ*er*e. *And* þa*n* medle he*m* wel to-

1 **Streytnesse**] *2-line space left for initial* 4 **þilke**] *corr. from* þicke 11 **marciaton**] *f. 70r* | ciaton; *catchword* (*in bottom margin*): ciaton *and* oile **and**] *prec. by heading* of the breest 13 **horsel**] *interl.* r

gidere. And aft*er*ward, cast in þi pouderis *and* stere it wel til it bie wel j-medled. And late hi*m* vsen wel þis on eue *and* on morowe w*ith* tisane ȝif he haþ myche heete, and w*ith* wyn ȝif he haþ coold.

Diadragantu*m* þ*at* is coold is good for þe brest *and* for þe mouþ i*n* coold. But wha*n* a ma*n* vseþ it, he xal hoolden it in his mouþ tyl it bie dissolued. And is þus j-maad: Tak of dragagant*e*, *ounce* ij; of gu*m* arab*e*, *ounce* j *and ounce* ij; of amyde, *ounce* j *and* s*emis*; of lyquorys, *dragme* ij; of penydes, f. 70v | *ounce* iij; of þe seed of gourdes *and* of meloun, *dragme* ij; of camphore, *dragme* s*emis*; of þe sirip of violet, *quantum* s*ufficit*.

Diadragant*e* þ*at* is hoot is good for coolde couȝes þ*at* comeþ of flewme, *and* þ*at* mowe nat spitte, *and* for men þ*at* mow nat breþe*n*, *and* for þe postym of þe liȝt *and* of þe syde. And it is good for þe stomac *and* makeþ good digestiou*n*. And it is þus j-maad: Tak of dragagant þ*at* haþ bie iij daies infuse in clene wat*er*, *ounce* iij; of ysope, *ounce* j *and dragme* ij; of canel, *ounce* j; of gyng*er*, *ounce* ij; of liquorys *and* of his iuys, *dragme* j *and* xv grei*n*s. *And* make it in þis wyse: Clense þe dragagant *and* w*ith* sufficient hony seeþ it ou*er* þe fier til it bie þicke. And siþe do it fra*m* þe fier. And wha*n* it keleþ, cast i*n*ne þ*in* poudres *and* medle it al to-gidere. Anoþ*er* hoot dragagant: Tak of hony, viij *pound*; of dragagant, *dragme* iiij; of gu*m* arabik, *ounce* iij; of liquorys

8 **arabe**] *corr. from* arabeik (ik *canc. twice and exp.*) 10 **ounce**] *prec. by heading* Sekenesse 17 **dragagant**] *corr. from* dragagan*n*t (*n canc. twice*)

15 **þe**[2]] *in l.-h. margin:* no*ta* ben*e*

oþ*er* of his iuys, *ounce* ij; of spik, *dragme* j; of clowes, *ounce* j. And make þis as þe toþere.

Anoþ*er* sicnesse þ*er* is in a ma*n*nys brest þ*at* is þe couȝe. *And* þe mat*er*e of þ*at* sicnesse is þe wynd þ*at* a ma*n* breþeþ to delyuere hi*m* of su*m* corupcio*n* þ*at* is w*ith*-i*n*ne hi*m*. Oþ*er*while it is a sicnesse bie hi*m*-selfen; oþ*er*while it foloweþ a-noþ*er* sicnesse. And ȝif it is a sicnesse bie hi*m*-self, it comeþ of humo*ur*s þ*at* falleþ dou*n* fro þe heed in-to þe brest *and* in-to þe liȝte, oþ*er* of fumes, oþ*er* of humo*ur*s | þ*at* f. 71r comeþ in-to þe breste fra*m* þe stomac, oþ*er* þe lyuere, oþ*er* su*m* oþ*er*e place þ*at* is bi-neþe þe mydrif. Oþ*er* it comeþ of su*m* corupt humo*ur*s þ*at* bie*n* j-t*ur*ned in-to postemys in þe brest oþ*er*e in þe liȝte. And þese couȝes þ*at* comeþ of humo*ur*s, oþ*er* þei comeþ of hote humo*ur*s, as colre oþ*er* blood, oþ*er* þei come of coold humo*ur*s, as of þi*n*ne flewme oþ*er* of viscouse flewme þ*at* is þicke as byrdlym. And þere is a-noþ*er*e manere couȝe þ*at* is driȝe, *and* may come for thre enchesou*n*s, as for rowȝnesse of þe þrote, oþ*er* of þe brest, *and* þe liȝte, *and* þe þrote, oþ*er* of viscouse matere þ*at* is in þe liȝte, *and* þe liȝte wolde delyuery*n* hi*m* of þ*at* mat*er* *and* may nat. But þe mat*er* þ*er*-of is þi*n*ne *and* is meuyd vp by þe couȝe, and is j-sparplid a-brood, *and* wexþ driȝe or it comeþ to þe mouþ, *and* þ*at* makeþ it driȝe. Þe couȝe þ*at* comeþ of d*ri*nesse *and* scharpnesse of þe þrote is j-helyd as horsnesse þ*at* comeþ of rownesse of þe þrote. And þe couȝe þ*at* comeþ of d*ri*nesse of þe co*m*plexiou*n* of þe þrote is j-helyd w*ith* moist medicynes þ*at* bie*n* mollytif *and* lenytif, of þe whiche medicines it was j-spoken of in þe chapetre of horsnesse. And ȝif þe couȝe come of an-oþere sicnesse, it is j-helyd ȝif

3 Anoþer] *2-line space left for initial* **9 þat**] *prec. by heading* of the couȝe **20 him**] *interl.*

f. 71v he hele þe sicnesse of couȝe | þ*at* comeþ of heete, *and* of rowȝnesse, *and* greuau*n*ce of þe þrote, *and* myche þirst, *and* gret lykynge to drawe breeþ of coold eyr. And ȝif his visage bie reed, *and* his veynis ful of blood, *and* is mouþ swete, hit is a tokene þ*at* þe couȝe comeþ of blood. But ȝif þe mouþ bie bitt*er*e, *and* þe visage derk reed, and his breþing ful hoote *and* ful driȝe, it is a tokene of colre. Ȝif it bie of blood, let hi*m* blede at þe veyne of þe arme þ*at* is j-clepid basilica, oþ*er*e at þe veyne þ*at* is vnd*er* þe tonge. And ȝif he haue mych*e* blood, lat garsen hi*m* a-bowte*n* þe schuldr*is*. And wheþ*er* it bie of blood oþ*er* of colre, let p*ur*ge*n* hi*m* wiþ su*m* [c]alogoge, for þe same þ*at* p*ur*geþ colre purgeþ blood. And siþe, ȝeue hi*m* symple medicines in dietyng to a-batyn hese heete, oþ*er* his dr*i*nesse, oþ*er* boþe ȝif it nedeþ. And lat hi*m* vsen þe coolde diapapauer*e* þ*at* is þ*us* j-maad: Tak þe iuys of licorys, of dragag*e*, of gu*m* arabik, *dragme* x; of amyde, of þe seed of cytonie, *and* of portulake, *dragme* v; of þe seed of gourdes, of melou*n*, of letuse, *and* of hockys, *dragme* iiij. Tempre hem w*ith* þe syrip of violet oþ*er*e sape, þ*at* is, swete vinegre of swete wyn. And late hi*m* vsen electuaries w*ith* þe sirip of violet oþ*er* w*ith* þe wat*er* þ*at* wat*er*lilies oþ*er* here leeues bie*n* j-soden i*n*ne, *and* dragag*e*, *and* gu*m*i arabik, *and*
f. 72r lyc*o*rys, *and* þe seed of cytonies. |

A good sirip for hem: Tak innibes, *and* plu*m*mes, *and* þe violet, *and* þe iuys of gourdis, portulake, *and* þe seed of scariole, *and* gu*m* arabik, *and* dragag*e*, *and* sugr*e*. *And* seþe he*m* in wat*er* *and* siþe clense it. *And* cast þ*er*-to þe mussilage of p*er*silie *and* þe seed of cytonies. Anoþ*er*: Take violet,

1 **þat**] *prec. by heading* The couȝe 3 **breeþ**] *interl.* last e 12 **calogoge**] *corr. from* galogoge **for**] *corr. from* ffor 24 **A**] *prec. by heading* The couȝe **innibes**] *corr. from* inimbes

licoryis, þe seed of hockys *and* here floures, *and* seeþ he*m* in wat*er*; cast gu*m* arabik, *and* dragag*e*, *and* swete plo*m*mes, *and* penydes, *and* sugre, *and* make vp þi sirip. And þus þe [best is] to done in alle manere siripes þ*at* gu*m*me arabik *and* dragag*e* bien j-soden i*n*ne to resolue*n* hem wha*n* þe sirip is coold, for þei wolen myche raþere *and* betere bien dissolued in a coold lico*ur* þa*n* in an hoot. A-noþ*er* sirip of ysope þ*at* is good for þe couȝe *and* for þe stiche *and* ache in þe syde, and is þus j-maad: Tak of þe rote of fenel, of march, *and* of licoryis, *dragme* x; of maidenhere, þe seed of ci[t]onyes, of dragag*e*, *and* of hockys, *ounce* iiij; of clene barly, *dragme* v; xxx inimbes; of resynes j-maad cleene, *dragme* j; of figes, j *pound*. *And* seþe al þis in *pound* iiij of wat*er* til it come to *pound* j, *and* siþe cast þ*er*-to *pound* of penydes. Anoþ*ere* sirip of inimbes: Take inimbes, *and* of lycoris, xx *dragme*; of maidenher*e*, of violet, *and* of þe seed of hockes, *dragme* x; of þe seed of cy[t]onyes, of melou*n*, of letuse, of popi, of dragag*e*, barlich*e* j-clensed, *dragme* vj; of wat*er*, *pound* x; of penides, oþ*er* of sug*re*, | oþ*ere* of sape, f. 72v *pound* iiij. *And* make vp þi sirip.

Good pillules: Tak dragagant, gu*m* arabik, seed of portulake, of ci[t]onyes, *and* of melou*n*, of gourdis, of eu*e*rich*e*, *dragme* v; of blau*n*ched alemandis, *dragme* vj; of þe seed of letuse, of whiȝ popi seed, of amyde, *dragme* iiij, of penydes. Te*m*pre þis w*ith* þe iuys of hockys *and* make pillules þ*er*-of. Anoþ*er* for-to make pillules: Tak þe seed of

4 best is] *corr. from* is best **6 for**] *corr. from* ffor **11 citonyes**] *corr. from* ciconyes **14 to**] *follow. by canc. twice pound* **17 cytonyes**] *corr. from* cyconyes **19 water**] *follow. by canc.* til it come to *pound* j *and* siþe cast þ*er*-to *pound* of penydes. A-noþ*er* sirip **oþere**] *prec. by heading* The couȝe **22 citonyes**] *corr. from* ciconyes cy[t]onyes, of gourdes, of swete alemau*n*des, *and* of beenes j-blau*n*ched, *and* of hockes seed, *dragme* vij; of gu*m*me arabik, of dragag*e*, *dragme* iiij. Te*m*pre þis w*ith* þi mussilage of p*er*silie *and* make pillules of þe q*ua*ntite of a beene. Oþ*er*e good pillules: Tak of mirre, *dragme* vij; of encense, *dragme* v; of march, of he*n*nebane, *dragme* iiij; of þe rote of hou*n*destonge, *dragme* iij. Make vp þi pillules w*ith* wat*er* of roses of þe q*ua*ntite of a fetche *and* ȝif hi*m* twyes a wyke oon of þese w*ith* wat*er* of roses. *And* lat hi*m* holde*n* he*m* vnd*er* his tonge til it bie dissolued.

An oyneme*n*t for-to a-noynte þe breste: Medle whiȝt wex, *and* oile of violet, *and* bot*er*e to-gidere. Anoþ*er*e: Tak þe iuys of coold herbys, *and* of þe leues of þe wat*er*-lilie, *and* medle he*m* w*ith* wex, *and* oile, *and* bot*er*e. Anoþ*er*e is j-maad of wat*er*-lilie leues, *and* þe whiȝt of an ey, *and* woma*n*nes mylk, *and* oile of violet, *and* bot*er*e, *and* wex.
f. 73r Anoþ*er*: Tak oile of violet, popilion, | deute, þe mussilage of p*er*silie, *and* þe iuys of letuse, of eu*er*ich*e*, j-liche myche. *And* medle hem to-gidere, *and* þerewiþ a-noynte an oold lambes skyn on þ*at* syde þ*at* was next þe fleisch*e*, *and* on þ*at* same syde lat leggen it to þe breste. And it is good for alle greuau*n*ces of þe brest þ*at* comeþ of heete. And jt be-houeþ þ*at* þe hoote humo*ur*s þ*at* comeþ fra*m* þe heed bien defied, laste þei falle*n* dou*n* to þe lu*n*ge *and* lette*n* a ma*n* of his breþi*n*ge. Also it bihoueþ to loke wheþ*er* þe mat*er* bi þicke, oþ*er* þi*n*ne, oþ*er* viscouse. And ȝif þe brest bie hoot, *and* feele

1 cytonyes] *corr. from* cyconyes **17 popilion**] *f. 73r* | lion **deute**] *prec. by heading* The couȝe **18 persilie**] *corr. from* p*er*siliel (e *interl.*; last l *canc. twice*)

20 on[2]] *in r.-h. margin:* no*ta* b*e*n*e*

a scharp smoke come þorow his brest *and* his þrote, *and* he bie þirstfull*e* also, *and* spete lityl, *and* his colo*ur* bie swart *and* ȝelew, oþ*er* citrine þ*at* is swart reed, *and* his mouþ salt, þa*n* it is a tokene þ*at* it is a þi*n*ne humo*ur* þ*at* is enchesou*n* of his sicnesse. And he may bie maad þicke w*ith* þe sirip of inimbes.

A coold couȝe comeþ of a coold humo*ur*, as of flewme. *And* þe tokenes þ*er*-of bie*n* lytil þirst, co*n*fort of hoote þi*n*ges, lityl g*re*uau*n*ce. Malencolies *and* fleu*ma*tike metis doon hi*m* harme *and* greuau*n*ce; and ȝif he speteþ myche, he feleþ myche coold w*ith*-i*n*ne-forþ; *and* haþ ne þirst ne fume comyng vp þorouȝ his breste *and* his þrote. Þe flewme þ*at* is encheson | of his couȝe is gret *and* viscouse, and it be-houeþ f. 73v to maken it more sotyl þ*at* it mow come a-way more esyly w*ith* couȝyng*e*, oþ*er* in su*m*me oþ*er*e wyse, as we xul telle here-aft*er*. For þis coold couȝe, furst defie þe mat*er* w*ith* oximel squillytik. But adde þ*er*-to fenel seed, *and* march seed, *and* horehowne, *and* thyime, *and* epithime. And aft*er* xiiij daies, purge hym w*ith* a flewmagoge oþ*er* a malagoge. And siþe, make hym a stufe of hoot þi*n*ges *and* wel smellyng. And siþe, lat wassche his breest w*ith* wat*er* þ*at* sauge is j-soden i*n*ne. And oones in þe weke let hi*m* vsen þese pillules: Take ysope, mirre, *and* driȝe figges, in euene porcion, *and* medle hem w*ith* hony, *and* make pillules. A-noynte his breest w*ith* oyle of violet *and* of piliole j-medlyd to-gider*e*.

2 spete lityl] *corr. from* spetelityl **7 a**] *interl.* **11 myche**] *follow. by* he feleþ mych*e* **13 encheson**] *f. 73v* | cheson **of**] *prec. by heading* The couȝe **16 For**] *corr. from* ffor **18 after**] *follow. by* xij **19 xiiij**] *in l.-h. margin*

7 humour] *in r.-h. margin:* A cold cough

And lat hym vsyn diapenidion *and* diadragant*e* j-medlyd to-gider*e*. His dietyng xal bie moist *and* hoot, of gyng*er*, of safrou*n*, galyngale, comyn, ysope, saueray, *and* mynte, *and* good wyn j-warmed.

Þes medicines *and* dieti*n*ges is of þe cou3e þ*at* comeþ of
f. 74r malencolie, and þ*at* þu | my3test know by swart 3elow colo*ur* of þe ma*n*, and 3if his spittyng is lytyl *and* þicke, *and* 3if his cou3e greueþ hy*m* more wha*n* þe northe*n*wynd blowith þa*n* in oþ*er* wyndes, and in heruest more þa*n* in oþ*er* tymes of þe 3ere. But 3if it comeþ of flewme, þe tokenes wul be open þ*at* we ofte*n*-tymes haue spoke*n* of, and his cou3e is ful greuows on ny3t and in wynt*er*. And þe mat*er* of here cou3e moost bie defied w*ith* oxymel of radich *and* oximel duretik j-medlid to-gider*e*. And siþe, late stufe hym w*ith* hoote herbis *and* wel smellyng. And syþe, late hym vsen hote electuaries, as diacymynu*m*, diapigamu*m*, diacalamentu*m*, diapiretron, *and* siche oþ*er*e. And lat hym vsen þe salt þ*at* was spoken of in þe siknesse of þe heed. And make hi*m* a sirip of ysope, of horehowne, of calamynt, *and* of hony. And make hym a fumigaciou*n* of calam*us* aromatic*us*, terbentyne, orpeme*n*t, þe kydeneyren *and* þe fat-nesse of a goot j-cast vp-on colys. *And* lat hym hange*n* his mouþ ou*er* þe smoke. Fyges *and* ysope j-soden to-ged*er* co*n*forteþ myche þe li3te, and mirr*e*
f. 74v *and* lynseed w*ith* puryd hony. A good oximel is j-|maad of ysope, sauerey, whi3t horehowne, origan, p*er*silie, fenel, liquoryis, pynes, dri3e figges. Seþ al þese in vinegre tyl þei go

6 my3test] *prec. by heading* The cou3e **22 Fyges**] *corr. from* ffyges **24 maad**] *prec. by heading* The cou3e **25 fenel**] *corr. from* ffenel

12 ny3t] *in r.-h. margin:* no*ta* **23 to-geder**] *in r.-h. margin:* no*ta* p*er* splene

down to þe botme. *And* siþe clense þe vineg*re* *and* pyt þ*er*-to þi*n* hony. Also orpeme*n*t j-sta*m*ped smal *and* j-etyn wiþ a-monge is p*ro*fitable. And siþe late him vsen su*m* lenetif, as dragag*e*. Also xv ȝelkes of eyren, *and ounce* iij orpeme*n*t, *and* of terebentyne *ounce* j, *and* let leie þis þi*n*ne vp-on lynne*n* cloutys to drye. And siþe lei hem on colees *and* let hy*m* resceyue þe smoke in-to his mouþe. Aft*ur*ward, lat wetyn a fair lynne*n* clooth*e* in þe gleyre of eyren *and* þ*er*-on strawe orpeme*n*t smal poudred *and* lei it in þe su*n*ne tyl it bie drye. And of þe poudre let medle w*it*h pynes and lat hy*m* eten a lytyl þ*er*-of. *And* lat hi*m* vsen bot*er* to his mete. And ȝif þe couȝe bie of viscouse flewme, ȝyf hym a sirrip j-maad w*it*h horehowne, *and* þe rote of fenel, of radich, of march, *and* anyse. Also sych*e* viscouse flewme js dissoluyd in a ma*n*nes brest w*it*h calam*us* aromatic*us*, | oþ*er* w*it*h f. 75r
orpement *and* terbentyne, as it was told by-fore.

Alectuarie: Tak lynseed j-rosted, swete alemau*n*des, pynees, of eu*er*ych*e*, *dragme* x; of licorys, *dragme* x; of fenel, ysope, gyng*er*, *dragme* iiij; of pep*er*, *dragme* ij; of hony, *quantum* s*ufficit*. Anoþ*er*e: Take of spodie, *dragme* vij; of bole, j exag*e*; of notemuge, as mych*e*; of long pep*er*, *dragme* iij; of sugr*e*, xxx *dragme*; of hony *and* of bot*er*e, *quantum* s*ufficit*. Oon sponeful here-of is ful good for a driȝe couȝe. To me*n* þ*at* bie*n* ful lene *and* myche j-febelyd by þe couȝe, þou xalt nat make a fumigaciou*n* of orpeme*n*t, but to cesse þe flux of humo*ur*s þ*at* fallen down in-to his brest, þu xalt

7 **resceyue**] *interl.* y 12 **viscouse**] *interl.* first s 15 **oþer**] *prec. by heading* The couȝe 25 **to**] *follow. by canc. twice* se

23 **here-of**] *in r.-h. margin:* no*ta* p*er* c[ouȝe]

make hym a fumygacion of encense. Also tak a pyn-appel þ*at* haþ myche gu*m*me *and* siþe hym in wat*er*. *And* siþe clense þe wat*er* *and* cast þ*er*-to a lytil hony. *And* lat hym vse to drynk þ*er*-of a-morwetyd *and* an eue, þe q*ua*ntite of an henschel-ful w*it*h warm wat*er*, so þ*at* þe iij p*ar*ties bie of wat*er*, *and* þe iiij p*ar*t of þis drynk.

Diapiretru*m* is good for þis cou3e *and* for alle greuau*n*ces of þe breest þ*at* comeþ of coold. *And* it is good for þe splene, for þe veynes, *and* for þe stoon, *and* for f. 75v strangure, | *and* for womanes syknesse. And it þus j-maad: Take of newe piretre þ*at* js j-maad clene, xxv *dragme*; of canel, of spik, of anyse, of fenel, of sq*ui*nant*e*, vj *dragme*, m*anipulum quantum* s*ufficit*. Let hem vsen þ*er*-of a-morwetyd *and* on euyntid, *dragme* iiij.

Jn a ma*n*nes li3te þ*er* bien many g*re*ua*n*ces, as postemys, *and* gaderyng to-gidere of corupt humo*ur*s þei þ*er* bie no postym. Þe postteme of þe li3t is j-clepyd p*er*ipleumonye, but þ*er* is an-oþ*er* postym of þe mydryf *and* of þe sydes vnd*er* þe rybbys þ*at* is j-clepid pleuresye. *And* þese postemys a-cordyn mych*e* to-gid*er*e boþe in tokenes *and* eke in enchesouns þ*at* þei come*n* of. And by oon man*er* medicines þei bien j-heelyd. And þe tokene of boþe þese g*re*uau*n*ces bie*n* greuau*n*ces of þe brest, *and* of þe syde, cou3e, *and* a scharp feuere. And oþ*er*-while þ*er* foloweþ þese sicnesses, as spittyng of blood, *and* spetyng of glat, *and* of quit*ur*e. And aft*ur* þ*at* comeþ tysik *and* oþ*er* sicnesses þ*at* comeþ of plente

1 a pyn-appel] *corr. from* apyn appel **6 þis**] *follow. by* of þis **9 for**[2]] *corr. from* ffor **10 and**] *prec. by heading* Grevawn*n*ce **15 Jn**] *2-line space left for initial*

8 comeþ] *in r.-h. margin:* no*ta* p*er* splen[e] (*underl.*)

of humo*urs* in þe li3te oþ*er* a-bowte, as hardnesse to draw breþ *and* to breþen also. Jn þe holownesse of þe li3t þ*er* mown bie iij humo*urs* þ*a*t make*n* here | syik *and* letten f. 76r here-of here kyndely worchynge. And þilk humo*urs* bien flewme, colre, *and* male*n*colie. Of flewme, þese bien þe tokenes: hardnesse *and* greuau*n*ce to breþin, *and* oþ*er*whiles a cou3e *and* hoorsnesse, *and* þe g*r*euau*n*ce is more a-ni3t þa*n* aday, *and* in wynt*er* þa*n* in som*er*, *and* myche greuau*n*ce aft*ur* þ*a*t a man haþ j-etyn, *and* myche spetyng *and* diu*er*se, aft*ur* þe diu*er*site of flewmes; for of þe kyndelych*e* flewme, þe spetyng is watt*er*y *and* whi3t, þi*n*ne *and* vnsauery, *and* li3tly comeþ vp by a rechynge [and] spetynge. Of glasi flewme comeþ spetyng of gret gobettes *and* hard j-gaderyd, *and* pale *and* vnsau*er*y. *And* is g*r*euouse in þe spytyng, in-so-mych*e* þ*a*t it makeþ a noyse w*i*t*h*-i*n*ne-forþ *and* semeþ as þei it cleuyde w*i*t*h*-i*n*ne to þe breste oþ*er* to su*m* oþ*er* þing. Of flewme þ*a*t is j-clepid salt, þe spittyng is whi3t, *and* þicke, *and* salt, *and* esy for-to spitte. Of kene flewme *and* egre, comeþ þi*n*ne spittyng *and* vndefied, *and* moist *and* sowr. Of colre, þe tokynnes bien hardnesse of breþi*n*g, horsnesse, a dry3e cou3e, þirst, bitt*er*nesse of þe mouþ, drinesse of þe tonge, an hoot breþi*n*g, and here þirst is mor*e* j-kelyd bie coold or þan bie any drynke. Þe breste is hoot *and* j-feleþ | f. 76v hete comyn vp fra*m* þe depnesse of þe breste. And þei haue more greuau*n*ce a-day þa*n* a-ny3th, *and* in som*er* þa*n* in wynt*er*. And 3if it is of colre þ*a*t is citrine, þe spittyng is citrine *and* thicke, *and* comeþ out gobetmele. Of reed colre

3 syik] *prec. by heading* of the syde **5 flewme[1]]** *corr. from* fflewme **10 for]** *corr. from* ffor **12 glasi flewme]** *corr. from* glasiflewme **13 j-gaderyd]** *follow. by canc.* to-gedere **pale and]** *corr. from* pale*and* **23 j-feleþ]** *f. 76v* | feleþ **24 hete]** *prec. by heading* Grevau*n*ce þ*at* is reed oþ*er* of þe colour þ*at* ȝelkes of eyren bie*n*, þe spitty*ng* is citrine oþ*er* grene, *and* defied grene wha*n* it be-gynnyth*e* to bien j-bred. *And* it is esy in spetyng*e*. Of malencolie, þe tokenes bien þese: greuau*n*ce in breþing, couȝe, *and* gret greuau*n*ce in speti*ng*, *and* lytil þei spetyn, *and* þ*at* is ȝelwe *and* sour*e*, oþ*er* blac *and* sour*e*, *and* here greuau*n*ce is grett*er* in heruest þa*n* in wynt*er*. And in me*n* þ*at* bien oolde þ*er* is myche cold a-boutyn here breste þ*at* comeþ as hem semeþ fra*m* þe depnesse of here breste. *And* his brest is cold *and* þe colo*ur* of hese breste is ȝelwe oþ*er* blac. Oþ*er*whiles, þe veynes þ*at* bien a-boute þe liȝte bie*n* ful humo*urs*, *and* þirst þe liȝte to-gidere, *and* makeþ a ma*n* narwe j-brethid. And ȝif þ*at* repleciou*n* bie of ony oþ*er* humo*ur* þa*n* of blood, þu maist knowe it bi þese forseyd tokenes. And ȝif it bie of blood, þese bien þe tokenes: redynesse of þe visage, fulnesse of þe veynes, *and* swetnesse of þe mouþ, *and* oþ*er* tokenes of blood þ*at* han oftyn-seþes

f. 77r bie spoke of. And þe sekerest tokyn to knowe wheþ*er* | þe liȝte bie ful of humo*urs* is spyttyng, nat eu*ery* spetyng, but spetyng þ*at* comeþ w*ith* cowȝyng, for owt of þe heed þ*er* comeþ humo*urs* þorowȝ to holys in-to þe mouþ wha*n* a ma*n* draweþ breþ, *and* enforceþ hy*m* to spete. Anoþ*er* spetyng comeþ fra*m* a ma*nn*es chekys *and* his þrote, w*ith* a-forsyng to spete w*ith*-owtyn drawyng breþ. Also fra*m* þe breste þ*er* comeþ a spetyng*e*, w*ith* a rechyng *and* breþi*ng*. Owt of þe liȝte þ*er* comeþ spetyng w*ith* cowȝy*ng*. And fra*m* þe mydrif

8 cold] *follow. by exp.* in **a-boutyn]** *in l.-h. margin* **16 visage]** *interl.* i **18 þe^2]** *prec. by heading* of the syde **20 for]** *corr. from* ffor

21 holys] *in r.-h. margin:* no*ta*

and þe sydes it comyth w*ith* a stronge couȝe. Fra*m* þe stomac comeþ spetyng by his owne a-cord. And ȝif þese humo*urs* ligge*n* longe in þe liȝte, þei maken þ*er* a postym þ*at* is j-clepid p*er*ipleumonye. And of which*e* humo*ur* þ*at* he comeþ, þu maist knowe bie þe forseid tokenes. And oþ*er* special*e* toknes þ*er* bien of p*er*ipleumonie, as a co*n*tinuel feuer*e*, *and* a couȝe, *and* a gret g*r*euau*n*ce in þe breste, and namely in þe lift syde vnd*er* þe lift pappe, *and* vnd*er* þe xuld*er*-blad boþe be-hynde *and* by-fore up to schuld*er*, and heuynesse of þe eiȝen, *and* swellyng of þe veynes, *and* reednesse in þe mydly*n* of þe cheken. And þe same bie*n* þe tokenes of pleuresie, saue þ*at* in þe pleuresie is mych*e* ach*e* *and* greuau*n*ces a-bowte þe sydys *and* a-bowte þe ribbys. *And* þe couȝe comeþ fra*m* þe syde. But þ*er* bie*n* two | manerys of pleuresie, verri *and* not verri. f. 77v

Verri pleuresie is in þe mydrif, *and* he mai bie in ij manerys: oþ*er* a-boue, oþ*er* bie-neþe. Nat verri is in oon of þe sydis oþ*er* vnd*er* þe rybbys. And þese too han oon man*er* tokenes, saue þ*at* þei bie*n* more greuouse in verri pleuresie þa*n* in þe toþ*er*. And also in pleuresie of þe sydis, me*n* may fele oþ*er*while w*ith*-outyn-forþ þe posty*m* *and* þe boche, but of þe mydrif, me*n* xal nat so. And wha*n* þ*er* is but an esy couȝe, *and* wiþ oon couȝwi*n*ge or too, a ma*n* delyuerith*e* hym of glet, it is a good tokene. But wha*n*ne þe couȝe is t*ra*ueliows *and* litel deliuerau*n*ce of corupt mat*er*e, it is a tokene þ*at* þe mat*er*e of þe g*r*euau*n*ce is euel to defie *and* to delyueryn owt fro w*ith*-i*n*ne þorowȝ couȝwy*n*ge ne þorow spetyng*e*. A good exp*er*ience to white wheþ*er* þ*er* bie a

1 **Fram**] *corr. from* ffra*m* 13 **couȝe**] *follow. by canc. twice* s
14 **manerys**] *prec. by heading* Pleurisye

postym in þe li3te: Let hy*m* spetyn on colys. *And* 3if it stynkyth, þ*er* is a postym in þe li3te. A-noþ*er*: Let hym spetyn on wat*er*, *and* 3if it houeþ a-boue al to-gidere, þa*n* þe li3te is hool. But 3if su*m* þ*er*-of houe a-boue *and* su*m* þ*er*-of gooþ to þe ground, it is a tokene þ*at* þ*er* is a posteme in þe li3te. But in caas þe corupt speti*ng*e is holdyn up by þ*at*, þ*at* is good, þ*at* it may nat go to þe grou*n*de.

f. 78r Pleuresie þ*at* is in þe neþ*er* parte | of þe mydrif ne is nat so p*er*ilouse as a-bouen, ne in þe lift syde as in þe ri3t syde. But 3if þe li3te haue replecion of humo*ur*s *and* no posty*m*, 3if it bie of blood *and* 3if it be of eny oþ*er*, let hi*m* haue a p*ur*gaciou*n* a-cordyng*e* to þe humo*ur*. And vse medicines as it haþ bie told in horsnesse *and* streitnesse of þe breste *and* i*n* þe cou3e, for alle þese siknesses a-corden ful myche, boþe in medicynes *and* in dietyng*es*, *and* in tokenes, *and* enchesou*n*s þ*at* þei come*n* of. But 3if þ*er* bie a postym, wheþ*er* it bie in þe li3t, in þe mydryf, oþ*er* in þe sidis, ne whiþ-drawe þou nat his mete, but fede hym w*ith* co*n*fortabyl metys, as chekenes, *and* colyis, *and* alemau*n*de mylk, *and* tysane þ*at* dri3e figes, *and* dragag*e*, *and* lycoryis, *and* resynes bien j-soden i*n*ne. But 3if here greuau*n*ce bie of flewme, ne ete þei no figes. *And* 3if þei bie*n* costyf, ne 3yue hem no tisane, but 3if he*m* cru*m*mys of bred *and* þe clansyng of bryn j-soden w*ith* allemau*n*d mylk, and perees j-rosted, *and* chasteynes, *and* penydes, *and* blak plu*m*bes. But be þei ware of soure metys. Electuaries þ*at* bien goode for þese postemys bien diapenidion, *and*

8 **parte**] *catchword* (*in bottom margin*): of þe mydrif **of**] *prec. by heading* Pleuresye **14 for**] *corr. from* ffor **19 colyis**] *corr. from* coly*n*is **20 and**[3]] *follow. by canc. twice* s

1 postym] *in l.-h. margin:* no*ta*

diadragant, *and* sugre of violet, *and* sugre of rosees. Good siripis bie*n* þe sirip of i*n*nibes, oþ*er* of rosees, oþ*er* of violet. | f. 78v Oþ*er* siche oon: Take of barliche j-clensyd, of reisynes, of violet, innibes, þe seed of melou*n*, of gourdys, of amyde, dragag*e*, horshel, liquorys, reed citeres, blake plu*m*mes, þe seed of citonyes, þe rote of fenel, of p*er*sily, of march*e*, anet, ameos, caraway, anyse, dauk, pastinake, pynes, penydes, of eu*er*ych*e* of þese, vj *dragme*. *And* make here-of a sirip, þ*at* is to sey, seþe all*e* þese in wat*er* tyl þow suppose þ*at* þe v*er*tu of hem bie in þe wat*er*. And þa*n*ne cast þ*er*-to a q*ua*ntite of sugre to maken it swete. Anoþ*er*: Tak of barlych*e* j-clensyd, of resynes, of driȝe figes, of sugre, of þe roote *and* of þe iuys of liquorys, of damascenes, of violet, of þe seed of iiij coold herbis, of ysope, of þe rote of fenel, *and* of p*er*sile, of eu*er*ich*e* of þese, iij *dragme*. *And* w*it*h a pound of sugre, mak of hem a sirip for pluresie, *and* heete of þe breste, *and* for driȝe cowys, *and* for þe tysik in þe be-gynnyng*e*. Tak of violet, dragag*e*, þe seed citonyes, barlych*e* j-clensid, of þe seed of hockys *and* of gourdys, of eu*er*ych*e*, *dragme* vj; of i*n*nibes, xx. Seþe hem in iiij pound of wat*er*. *And* wha*n* it is j-soden, cast þ*er*-to *pound* j of sugre. A plastre: Tak þe rote of hooly-hocke, *and* þe leues of hockes, *and* þe rote of fenel, *and* lynseed, *and* driȝe figes, *and* oile, of eu*er*ych*e*, j-lyche myche, a q*ua*rt*er* of a powund. Seeþ hem | f. 79r to-gidere *and* stampe hem. *And* ley to his side, but a-noynte it bi-fore w*it*h dewte, oþ*er* popilion *and* oile of violet j-medlid to-gidere. *And* ofte-syþes renew þi plastre. A-noþ*er*: Tak þe rote of bismalue, *and* þe leues of malues, *and* lynsed, *and* femygrek, *and* driȝe figes, of eu*er*ych*e*, *dragme* j. *And* stampe he*m* to-

3 Oþer] *prec. by heading* Pleuresye **24 to-gidere**] *prec. by heading* Pleuresie

gidere *and* siþe cast þ*er*-to oile of rosees oþ*er* of violet, oþ*er* comy*n* ooile þ*at* is ooile de olyue, *and* mete oile *and* ley þis plastre to his syde. But furst a-noynte þe place as j-seid byfore. And s*um* me*n* cast þ*er*-to datys *and* reysynes, *and* barly mele. *And* it is þe best plast*re*, for it is mytigatif *and* maturatif. A-noþ*er*: Tak þe iuys of berule *and* of wat*er*cressu*m*, of boþe, j-lych*e* mych*e*, *and* medle he*m* w*ith* as mych*e* of oold swynes grece þat is j-mouled. *And* siþe cast þ*er*-to þe iij part of dispumyd hony. *And* siþe cast þ*er*-to þe poud*re* of lynseed *and* of femygrek, *and* whete mele, *and* medle he*m* wel to-gidere. And in þe verry pleuresy, cast þ*er*-to þe ooile of violet. And in boþe þese greua*n*nces, ȝif þei come of coold, lat a-noynte þe breste *and* þe syde w*ith* dewte; and ȝif it kome of hete, medle w*ith* þe dewte oyle of rooses oþ*er* ooile of violet, and siþe ley þ*er*-on wolle þ*at* is j-schore of oon-waschen schepe, so þ*at* all*e* þe wolle may catch*e* moistnesse, and all*e* warm ley it to | þe breste. And whan þe postym is to-brokyn and þe quiture bi-gynnyth to goon his wey, let hym vsyn sirripis þ*a*t bien mu*n*dificatif, *and* electuaries also, as þe sirip of i*n*nibes, *and* diapenidion, *and* diadrag*e*, *and* diacodion þ*a*t is diapapau*er*. But lat hym nat vsyn diacodion but þe botche hele nat as fast as he schuld. And þa*n*ne in pleuresie, lat hym vsen diadrag*e* wiþ a q*ua*ntite of mirre *and* of sau*n*dragu*n* j-do þ*er*-to in þe makyng*e*. Jn p*er*ipleumonie, let him vsyn dyapenidion w*ith* mirr*e* *and* sau*n*dragu*n*. And in all*e* þi medicines, þ*o*u moost take kepe to his hete *and* þe keneschipe of his feu*ere*. And þ*er*-aft*er*, þu moost ordeyne þi medicynes in heete *and* in coold. And ȝif he haue a kene feu*ere*, late his dietyng bie sotyl, *and* lityl,

f. 79v

15 ooile] *interl.* i **17 þe**[1]] *prec. by heading* Pleuresye **25 vsyn**] *corr. from* vsyni (i *canc. twice and exp.*)

and of soupyng þi*n*ges as broþes. 3if þe feu*ere* bie esy, he may vse grett*ere* metis. And ȝif he bie feble *and* þe mat*ere* bie of coold *and* þe feu*ere* is esy, he may vsen a colyis of an henne oþ*er* of a capou*n* w*ith* þe clensyng*e* of bren. And let hym kepe wel here hoondis, *and* her*e* armes, *and* her*e* feet fra*m* coold. Naþeles, ȝif þei catche a couȝe, ȝyue hem tysane of wheete. Clansynge of bren is whan men casten bryn in-to clene wat*er and* cla*n*siþ it þorow a clooth*e*. Þis clensynge of bryn is a good mu*n*dificatyf, *and* so it is good for postemys þ*at* bien w*ith*-i*n*ne a ma*n*. And for | as mych*e* as it is nat generatyf of mych*e* blood, it is good for men þ*at* han þe feueres. f. 80r

Spetyng of blood, ȝif it comeþ w*ith* cowȝwi*n*ge, it comeþ fra*m* þe liȝte oþ*er* fra*m* þe mydrif. 3if it comeþ w*ith*-owten couȝwe, it comeþ fra*m* as many places as oþ*ere* spetyng doiþ. Also it comeþ fra*m* oþ*er* parteys of a ma*n*nys body, of brysynge of veynes, as fra*m* þe stomac. *And* þ*at* greueþ a ma*n* by-neþi*n* his mydrif, *and* makeþ wlaten his meete, *and* makeþ hy*m* to haue euyl digestiou*n*, oþ*er* it comeþ fra*m* þe leuere *and* þa*n* þe greuau*n*ce is in þe riȝt syde. And ȝif it comeþ of þe splene, þa*n* it is in þe lyft syde. And ȝif it comeþ of þe heed, [it] is heuy and all*e* a ma*n*nys wyttes bien j-feblyd þ*er*-bie. And ȝif it comeþ of þe veynes of þe brayn *and* by nyȝte, here g*r*euau*n*ce is more þa*n* on þe day. And it comeþ wha*n* a ma*n* draweþ breeþ *and* arecheþ stro*n*glyche to spete. Fram þe liȝte it comyth w*ith* cowȝwy*n*ge and fra*m* þe

6 ȝyue] *corr. from* ȝy*n*ue **10 as**[1]**]** *prec. by heading* Spittyng of blood **13 Spetyng]** *2-line space left for initial* **20 greuaunce]** *corr. from* greuau*n*cee (last e *canc.*) **26 Fram]** *corr. from* ffram

8 water] *in l.-h. margin:* no*ta*

mydryf w*ith* a st*ro*ng couȝwe *and* is su*m*what fomy. But wha*n* it comeþ fra*m* þe breste, it is nat fomy. Oþ*er*whiles it comeþ of stoppyng of blood in syche places þ*at* it xuld flowe, as in women þ*at* haue nat here p*ur*gaciou*n*s and in hem þ*at* han þe emerawdes.

Bledy*ng* þ*at* comeþ of briche of veynes, comeþ in two
f. 80v man*er*es: as fra*m* w*ith*-i*n*ne-forþ, oþ*er* fra*m* su*m* enchesou*n* | w*ith*-outyn-forþ. Fra*m* w*ith*-i*n*ne, as for greet plente of blood þ*at* brekeþ þe veynes, oþ*er* of sotylte, oþ*er* of scharpnesse *and* keneschipe of þe blood þ*at* makeþ hy*m* to brekyn also. Fra*m* w*ith*-outy*n*-forþ, veynes byn j-brokyn þorow smytyng, or lepyng*e*, oþ*er* fallyng*e*, oþ*er* þorow mych*e* cryyng *and* sich*e* oþ*er* thi*n*ges. Spetyng of blood þ*at* comeþ in a greuouse sicnesse *and* liȝtteþ a ma*n* of his sicnesse, *and* is tokene of his heele; oþ*er* ellys heuyeþ a ma*n* ful mych*e* *and* is to-kene þ*at* he xal sone deiȝe, ne xal nat bie staunchid. But ȝif a ma*n* haue no sich*e* greuouse sicnesse, it is good to staunchyt, but dis[c]retely, as it was j-seyd in þe nose-bledyng. And ȝif it come of stoppyng of su*m* oþ*er* places, lat hi*m* vse medicynes to make þilke places flowe. And ȝif it comeþ of a strook, let helyn it by surgery. But bie þei ware fro wraþþe *and* cu*m*penyi*n*ge w*ith* wome*n*, *and* waky*ng*, *and* fastyng, *and* fra*m* soure met*es*, *and* salte, *and* kene, and namly fra*m* comyn, *and* fra*m* cachi*n*ge gret heete, fra*m* baþi*n*ge, mych*e* trauayle, mych*e* þouȝt, *and* mych*e* bysynesse, for þese þi*n*ges hety*n* þe spirytys, *and* make*n* hem drawyn owtward w*ith* þe blood, *and* brekeþ þe veynes of þe

8 **with-outyn-forþ]** *prec. by heading* Spyttyng **Fram]** *corr. from* ffra*m* **11** **Fram]** *corr. from* ffra*m* **12** **lepynge]** *follow. by canc.* g **18 discretely]** *corr. from* distretely **26 for]** *corr. from* ffor

which*e* brych*e* | comeþ spetyng of blood. And ȝif þe spetyng f. 81r of blood comeþ of gret mych*e* plente of blood, dyete þe pacient w*ith* sich*e* met*es* þ*at* genderiþ lytyl blood, as herbys *and* fruytis. And ȝif it come of keneschip of þe blood, ȝif hy*m* alteratyfs *and* siripys *and* electuaries, þ*at* is to sey, sich*e* þi*n*ges þ*at* mou*n* a-bate þe keneschipe of þe blood *and* turne it in-to a-noþ*er* kynde. And ȝif it come of sotylte of þe blood, ȝif hi*m* syche met*es and* drynkes þ*at* wole*n* make þicke blood, as we teldyn in bledyng of þe nose and we telle more in þe chapitr*e* of þe flux.

A good sirip for spetyng of blood where-of-eu*er* it come: Take ipoqwyssides, chimole, boole arm[oniac], acacie, coral whyȝt *and* reed, þe poudre of onyfacie, mu*m*mye, mynte, psidie, gallos, balaustia, gu*m* arabik, dragg*e*, symphite, corigiole, þe seed of plau*n*teyn, roris ciriacy, sumac, pentafilon, radich, sandragou*n*, of eu*er*ich*e* of þese, *ounce* j. Seeþ he*m* in reyn-wat*er* tyl þe iij part of þe wat*er* bie sodyn a-wey. And wha*n*ne it is j-clansyd, cast þ*er*-to iij *pound* of sugre. And ȝif þ*at* sirip to þe pacient w*ith* þe iuys of plau*n*teyne. And þe sirrip þ*at* is j-maad of plau*n*teyne is ful good also.

A confeccion þ*at* soud[i]þ *and* a-swageþ þe bledyng: Tak jpoq*ui*sides, acacie, | balaustia, of eu*er*ych*e*, *dragme* ij; of f. 81v galles, as mych*e*; of opiu*m and* of citre, *dragme* vj. Tempre hem w*ith* reynwat*er and* ȝyue hym to drynk w*ith* reynwat*er*. Also tak of spodie, *dragme* iiij; of þe seed of gourdis *and* of portulake, bole, carabie, of eu*er*ych*e*, *dragme* iij. Tempre hem w*ith* þe wat*er* of þe scheppard*es*-ȝerde.

1 **comeþ**] *prec. by heading* of blood **2 gret**] *interl.* **12 armoniac**] *corr. from* arm*er* **22 soudiþ**] *corr. from* soudrþ **23 balaustia**] *prec. by heading* Spyttyng of blood

An electuarie þ*a*t clansiþ þe breste w*it*h-i*n*ne forþ of blood: Tak of amyde, *dragme* v; of beene mele, of þe seed of melou*n* *and* of hockys, *dragme* vj; of barlych*e* j-clensyd, x *dragme*; of gu*m* arabik *and* of dragag*e*, *dragme* iij; of bole, of þe seed of ci[t]onyes, *and* of borage, *dragme* v. Poudre hem *and* do þ*er*-to m*anipulum* *quantum* s*ufficit*.

Also for blood þ*a*t is co*n*gelyd *and* liþ cooldyd in a ma*n*nys brest: Take tansey, *and* sta*m*pe it w*it*h vinegre, *and* wryng it. *And* ȝif hym to drynke oþ*er* let hym drynke þe iuys of tansey *and* vinegre to-gidere. Also for-to stau*n*che þe spety*n*g of blood: Tak of wermot, of anyse, of dauk, *dragme* iiij; of storac*e*, of opiu*m*, of mirr*e*, of citre, of anet, *dragme* iij; of canel, of castore, *dragme* ij; hony, *quantum* s*ufficit*. Ȝif hi*m* here-of a-morewetyd *and* on euene þe q*ua*ntite of a note wiþ wat*er* þ*a*t plau*n*teyn is j-sodyn i*n*ne, þ*a*t xal bie warm *and* nat coold. Dietyng of hem xal bie rostyd fleisch*e* þ*a*t is comynly vsyd, saue swynes fleschȝ, *and* wheete, *and* beenen
f. 82r j-broke *and* j-fryid w*it*h schepis talwe | *and* gootys talwe, also riȝs, *and* harde eyren, *and* crabbes of þe see þ*a*t bien medicinable *and* is good mete for þis sicnesse, and chesteynes j-sodyn *and* j-fryid w*it*h ȝelkys of eiren, *and* whete mele j-sodyn w*it*h mylk. Oþ*er*while spetyng of blood comeþ of wat*er*-lechis þ*a*t a ma*n* swelwiþ in w*it*h wat*er*. *And* þei biten his þrote *and* maken it to blede. And for-to sie hem, take a glasse*n* vessel *and* set it bi-twyne þe su*n*ne *and* his þrote. *And* þu xalt j-sien hem. Tak hem owt þa*n*ne w*it*h a peyre of scherys and siþe ȝif hi*m* a gargarisme of vinegre *and* salt

4 iij] *follow. by canc. twice and* **5** **citonyes**] *corr. from* ciconyes
18 **and**[2]] *prec. by heading* Spyttyng of glat **24** **it to**] *corr. from* itto
25 glassen] *corr. from* glasse*n*a (last a *canc. twice and exp.*)

oþ*er* garlek, but late he nat þe vinegre go dou*n* in his þrote. *And* siþe late hym vse þe for-seyd co*n*structyues.

Spetynge of glat *and* of quytere comeþ of infecciou*n* of þe li3te, as wha*n*ne corupt blood haaþ j-loyn in þe li3te *and* is j-rotyd, oþur corupt humo*ur*s ha*n* j-falle*n* down fra*m* þe heed *and* bien j-t*ur*ned to siche glat. Oþ*er*while siche spetyng comeþ of infecciou*n* of þe mydryf, oþ*er*while of a postym of þe lyuer*e* *and* corupt humo*ur*s in hym. Oþ*er*while it comeþ w*it*h a feuere, oþ*er*while w*it*h-outy*n* a fyuere. Tokenes here-of bien: spetyng þ*a*t is corupt, as quiture, leneschipe of þe body, smalschipe of þe necke, greuau*n*ce in breþing, swelli*n*g | f. 82v of þe ei3en. 3if þei haue a feu*er*e, let hem bie dietid as þilke þ*a*t haue þe pleuresie oþ*er* p*er*ipleumuonie. And 3if it comeþ of heete, 3eue hy*m* diapenydion, *and* þe coold diag*ra*gantu*m*, *and* diapapauer*e*, and þe sirip þ*a*t was j-told in þe coold cou3e, *and* a-noyntynges. And 3if þe spety*n*g styncke þ, *and* þe heeris of his heed falleþ a-way, and þe nayles of his fyng*re*s schrynkeþ *and* wexeþ narwe at þe endys, it is a tokene of deeþ. And 3if þis greuau*n*ce comeþ of coold, þe spetyng is corupt, as q*ui*t*ur*e, as whi3t or swart 3elwe. And þe cure here is as of þe coold cou3e. And 3if hy*m* medycines to restreyne þe humo*ur*s *and* to clense þe breest as it haþ bie told bi-fore.

A good plastre for hem to leggen on here breste by-neþen: Tak spica celtica, *and* apiu*m* rana*rum*, *and* anet, *and* seeþ hem in wyn *and* in oyle. Also centorie j-soden in oile of car[s]es *and* plast*ri*d a-boue is good. And 3if þei han no

3 **Spetynge**] *2-line space left for initial* 12 **of**] *prec. by heading* Spittyng **22 restreyne**] *interl.* second e **24 A good**] *corr. from* Agood **25 spica celtica**] *corr. from* spicaceltica **27 carses**] *corr. from* cartes

feu*er*es, gotis mylk is good þ*at* stoones of þe ryu*er*e bien j-quen*n*chyd i*n*ne.

A good ellectuarie for an oold couȝe *and* for spety*n*g glat: Tak piretre, bit*er*e alemau*n*des, laureole, and radiche, of f. 83r euerich, j-lyche mych*e*; hony, *quantum* s*ufficit*. | Te*m*pre hem to-gidere *and* ȝif hi*m* on morwe *and* on euene, þe qua*n*tite of a walsch*e*-note. A-noþ*er*: Tak of eu*er*ych*e*, j-lych*e* mych*e*, of femy-grek, *and* lynseed j-rostyd, *and* caraway; of hony, *quantum* s*ufficit*. Anoþ*er*: Take horehowne *and* orobȝ, of eiþ*er*, *dragme* iij; of citre, mirr*e*, gyng*er*, ysope, long pep*er*, anyse, of eu*er*ych*e*, exag*e* j; of hony, *quantum* s*ufficit*. A-noþ*er*: Tak of calamynt þ*at* groweþ in ȝerdys, also in feldis, of p*er*silie, of syleos, *dragme* vj; of march seed *and* of ameos, *dragme* j; of ysope, *dragme* viij; of pep*er*, *dragme* iij; of hony, *quantum* s*ufficit*. Also horshel j-poudred *and* j-medlyd w*it*h hony is good þ*er*-fore. Ȝif hi*m* þ*er*-of on eue *and* on morwe þe q*ua*ntite of a walsch*e*-note. Aristologia rotu*n*da j-sode*n* in wat*er* is good also. *And* for þe couȝe, let hi*m* dri*n*ke þ*er*-of on eue *and* on morwe.

Goode pillules for hem þ*at* han þis greuau*n*ce of rewme fallyng a-down to þe brest: Tak of galbanu*m*, myrr*e*, storac*e*, olibanu*m* dragg*e*, ylyche mych*e*. Medle he*m* to-gidere w*it*h an hoot pestel *and* make þe pillules of þe q*ua*ntite of a vech*e*. *And* ȝif hi*m* þ*er*-of v or vj at onys. Euerich*e* manere crabbe of þe see is good for þis sicnesse. And ȝif þei ha*n*ne þe f. 83v feu*er*es, ȝif it he*m* w*it*h tisane. | Ȝif þei haue no feu*er*es, ȝif it he*m* w*it*h wyn. And vnd*er*stonde þ*at* ȝif þilke þ*at* han p*er*ipleumonie ne bien nat clene j-purged w*it*h-i*n*ne xiiij daies oþ*er* xx aft*er* þe brekyng of þe postym, þei xul falle in-

5 **Tempre**] *prec. by heading* of glat 25 **hanne**] *interl.* 26 **if**] *prec. by heading* Tysyk

to þis greuau*n*ce. And þa*n*ne but þei bien holpyn *and* j-heelyd w*it**h*-i*n*ne xl daies oþ*er* j-p*ur*geid, þei fallyn in-to a tysik.

Tjsyk is a destruccio*n* of þe kyndlych*e* moistnesse of a ma*n*nes body. But þ*er* bien two man*er*es of tisyk: Oon is a verri tysik *and* þe oþ*er* is nat a verri tysik. Verri tisyk is a destreyng of þe kyndlyche moistnesse of a ma*n*nes body þorow sicnesse *and* corupciou*n* of þe liȝte. But þe tisyk þ*a*t is nat verri comeþ nat of þe liȝte, but of su*m* oþ*er*e enchesou*n*. Verri tysik comeþ in iij man*er*es. Oon is of a posty*m* of þe liȝte þ*a*t was nat wele j-heelyd. Anoþ*er*e is of humo*ur*s þ*a*t bien kene, as salt flewme *and* colre, *and* falleþ a-dou*n* fro þe heed in-to þe liȝte *and* apeiriþ here. But þe iij man*er*e is of humo*ur*s þ*a*t come*n* fra*m* oþ*er* places *and* apeiriþ þe liȝt, as of squina*n*cie, oþ*er* of pleuresie, oþ*er* of greuau*n*ce of þe lyuere, oþ*er* of þe splene, oþ*er* of su*m* oþ*er* place. Tisik also þ*a*t is nat verri is in iij man*er*es. Þe first is w*it**h* gret heete w*it**h*-outyn-forþ on a ma*n*nys body. *And* þ*a*t is j-heelyd | as f. 84r þe feuere etik. Þe toþ*er* is of gret drynesse *and* cold. *And* þ*a*t is j-heelyd as spetyng of glat þ*a*t comeþ of drinesse *and* of coold. Þe iij man*er* comeþ of mych*e* flewme þ*a*t is in a ma*n*nes body, *and* þ*a*t is j-helyd as þe flux of a ma*n*nys wombe. Of verri tysik þ*a*t we wole spekyn of now, þe tokenes bien co*n*tinuel heete, *and* su*m* more, as in hem þ*a*t a feu*er*e þ*er*-wiþ, jn su*m*me lasse, as in hem þ*a*t ha*n* no feu*er*e; þirst, *and* drynesse of þe tu*n*ge, smalnesse of þe neck, *and* leneschipe of all*e* þe body, costifnesse of þe wombe, corupciou*n* of þe nailes, holwnesse of þe eiȝen, and ache of þe left schuld*er*-blad vp-to þe schulderyn. And comynlych*e*,

3 Tjsyk] *2-line space left for initial* **17 as]** *prec. by heading* Tisyk siche me*n* bie*n* disposyd to þis sicnesse þ*a*t bien lene of body, *and* bien streite a-bowte þe breste, *and* han hiȝe schuldrys. Tokenes of deeþ in þis sicnesse bien: fallyng of heer*es*, feuerys, streynyng to-gidere *and* corupcion of þe endys of here naylys, fallyng down of his browys, a sy*m*ple flux of his wo*m*be. Syche men xul speke deyi*n*ge, *and* diȝe spekyng*e*. Also lat hym spetyn in a basyn *and* on morwe cast þ*er*-to hoot wat*er and* stere it, *and* ȝif þ*er*e goiþ bi þe ground þicke drosse, he is incurabile. Oþ*er* ȝif his breþ styncke in his sicnesse, *and* was bie-fore wel smellyng, þ*er* now he is incurable. Also a verry tysyk haþ þis tokene: a co*n*tinuel couȝe. And ȝif it come of heete, his spetyng is citrine, oþ*er* f. 84v ȝelwe as safru*n*, oþ*er* grene. *And* þe body febeliþ mych*e* | eu*er*y day *and* openly. It xal bie heelyd as þe couȝe þ*a*t comeþ of heete. But ȝif it comeþ of coold, þe spetyng is whiȝt oþ*er* ȝelwe, *and* it xal bie heelyd as þe coold couȝe. But wha*n*ne tisyk comeþ of a wound of þe liȝt, þ*o*u moost ȝif hi*m* mu*n*dificatifs *and* co*n*solidatyfs. *And* þ*o*u moost bie ware leste þe q*ui*ture a-byde stille in þe breste. And ȝif þ*a*t happeneþ, *and* he mow nat spete wel *and* delyu*er*e hym of þ*a*t corupciou*n*, ȝyue hi*m* hony þ*a*t jsope *and* violet bie*n* j-sodyn i*n*ne. A good electuarie for þis greua*n*nce: Tak of resynes þ*a*t bien clene, *dragme* xx; of hockes seed, *dragme* iij; of crabbes of þe see, xxx *dragme*; of þe leuys of wat*er*lilies, of schep*er*des-ȝerde, of plau*n*teyne, *dragme* v; of liquorys, *ounce* j. Seþ al þese in iij pound of wat*er* in-to ij pownd *and* cast þ*er*-to a pound of sape oþ*er* ij pound of sugr*e*, *and* make

4 **feuerys**] *corr. from* ffeuerys 5 **fallyng**] *corr. from* ffallyng 14 **euery**] *prec. by heading* Tysyk 17 **of**[1]] *follow. by* of

1 **disposyd**] *in r.-h. margin:* Caue Sp*er*haw[ke]

þ*er*-of a sirip. Aft*er*ward, take of gu*m* arabik, of dragagau*n*t, of þe seed of citonyes, *dragme* viij; of amyde, of þe seed of portulake, *dragme* vij; of popy seed, *dragme* v. Poudre al þis *and* medle he*m* w*it*h þe forseyd sirip *and* 3if it in þe man*ere* of an electuarie. Hit is good for p*er*ipleumonys, *and* pleuresie, *and* for a feble stomac. And aft*ur* þ*at* þe postem*us* bien to-broken *and* bie nat wel j-clensyd, þis sirip *and* þis electuarie bie*n* goode. And wha*n*ne þe mat*er* wexeþ hard, it is good | to 3euyn hym hoote medicines þ*at* mowen hete hi*m* f. 85r w*it*h-inne-forþ, *and* clense hi*m* *and* make hym to haue a cou3e. And siche bien þe seed of orobus, *and* of aristologia rotu*n*da *and* longa, *and* of long pep*er*, canel, anyse, *and* [ci]cori, coost, cassia fistula, spik, *and* sich*e* oþ*ere*. But þ*o*u xalt nat vse þese 3if he haue a strong feuere, but wha*n* þe mat*er* is fleu*ma*tik. And 3if he bie costyf, p*ur*ge hym w*it*h esy clist*ere*s þ*at* bie*n* j-maad of molitifs, for a strong flux is p*er*ilouse in þis sicnesse. And 3if he haue oon, staunche it as soone as þu my3t, but do it disc*re*tely, for drede of more p*er*ile. And 3if þ*at* þe wound of þe li3t dri3e to slowly, wheþ*er* þe wou*n*d bie of an hertyng*e* oþ*er* of a boche, þu moost 3euy*n* hym subtiliatyfs to maken þe mat*ere* sotyl, þ*at* it may þe raþer*e* comyn owt *and* þe wou*n*d þe raþ*er* bien dri3e. And 3if it bie w*it*h a rewme, 3if hym bole armoniac w*it*h þe iuys of plaunteyn, oþ*er* w*it*h dragagau*n*t oþ*er* licoryis, for it drieþ *and* regendrieþ þe flesch*e*.

A good medycyne to sowde veynes þ*at* bien tobroke in þe li3te oþ*er* in þe breste: Take of bole, of amyde, *dragme* iiij; of carabe, of þe seed of myrte, of coral, of spodie, of

7 **to-broken]** *follow. by canc.* *and* **9** **to]** *prec. by heading* Tysyk **13** **cicori]** *corr. from* acori **16** **for]** *corr. from* ffor **26** **sowde veynes]** *corr. from* sowdeveynes

emachites, *dragme* v; of gu*m* arabik, of þe iuys of lycorys, *dragme* vij; of crabbes of þe see j-brend, of þe seed of f. 85v pursylane, *dragme* x. Poudre al þese *and* medle it | w*ith* þe iuys of plau*n*teyn, *and* make rounde balles þ*er*-of. *And* ȝif hym at ones þe q*ua*ntite of j exag*e* w*ith* þe iuys of purselane oþ*er* of gourdys. Anoþ*er* þ*a*t is good for bleynes, *and* wou*n*dys of þe liȝte, *and* cle*n*-seþ hi*m* *and* soudeþ hem a-ȝen: Tak of balaustia *and* of rosees, *dragme* iij; of sau*n*dragu*n*, of amyde, of ence*n*se, *dragme* j; of carabe, of saffren, *dragme* s*emis*. Te*m*pre he*m* w*ith* þe iuys of citonyes, *and* make þ*er*-of round balles. *And* ȝif hi*m* here-of j exag*e* w*ith* coold wat*er*. Naþeles, tak kepe þ*a*t he xal nat vsen þese driȝe medicynes but þe mat*er*e bie j-clensyd. *And* þ*a*t þ*o*u miȝt j-knowe ȝif he ne spete no glat ne gobetis of þe liȝte, for þ*er* may no wound bie j-helyd *and* driȝed but ȝif it bie j-clensyd. And þa*n*ne he may vsyn in his medicines rosees, *and* bala[u]stia, dragg*e*, mastik, carabe, bole, sau*n*dragou*n*, mirre, emachites, þe seed of plau*n*teyn, *and* sich*e* oþ*er* thynges.

A good electuarie for he*m* þ*a*t han þis sicnesse w*ith* a feuere: Tak of þe seed of gourdys *and* of melou*n*, *ounce* j; of letuse, violet, lycoryis *and* his iuys, of þe seed of popi, of amyde, of dragg*e*, *ounce* ij. Medle he*m* w*ith* wat*er* þ*a*t lycorys haþ j-soden i*n*ne *and* dragg*e* haþ bie resoluyd i*n*ne. Ȝeue hi*m* of þis electuarie a-morwetyde *and* on euene, for it f. 86r restorith*e* his kyndlych*e* moistnesse | *and* saueþ it þ*a*t it is nat

3 with] *prec. by heading* Tysyk **6 gourdys**] *interl.* r **9 carabe**] *corr. from* carabre (r *canc. twice and exp.*) **14 for**] *corr. from* ffor **17 balaustia**] *corr. from* bala*n*stia **25 moistnesse**] *catchword* (*in bottom margin*): *and* saueþ it þ*a*t it **and**] *prec. by heading* Tysyk

24 eue] *in l.-h. margin:* no*ta*

destrei3ed þorou3 vnkynde heete of þe feu*er*e. Take of rosees, *dragme* j; of spodye *and* of þe iuys of liquoryis, *dragme* v; of amide, of portulake, of endyue, *dragme* iij; of gou[r]de seed, of meloun, of sau*n*dres, *dragme* ij. Te*m*pre it w*ith* þe iuys of p*er*silye *and* w*ith* sirip of violet. And vnd*er*stonde þ*at* siripes *and* electuaries for me*n* þ*at* ha*n* þe tysik ne xul nat bie j-maad ou*er* þe feyr as oþ*er* electuaryes bien, but þei xul bie maad in tynne vessel þ*at* xal bie set in a caudrou*n* of seþi*n*g wat*er* ou*er* þe fyer*e*, for 3if it were j-maad ou*er* þe fyer*e*, þe spises xulde lesyn myche of here kynde and þe smoke of þe feyr wolde medle w*ith* þe medycines þ*at* xulde aft*er*warde noy3e þe breste ful mych*e*.

P*ro*fitabyl þi*n*ges þ*at* clensyn þe breste bien gargarismis j-maad of wheey of got*us* mylk, *and* wat*er* þ*at* lycorys *and* barlych*e* is j-soden i*n*ne, oþ*er* barlych*e* j-soden w*ith* lycorys *and* w*ith* radych*e*. Also seeþ crabbes of þe see tyl þe fisch3 dep*ar*te fra*m* þe boones, *and* siþe tak þe colyis of þ*at* [f]isch3 *and* medle it w*ith* barlich*e* *and* make hi*m* a gargarisme þ*er*-of. *And* let hi*m* swolwe su*m*what þ*er*-of i*n*ne to his stomac, for it restoreþ þe kyndlych*e* moistnesse of a ma*n*nes body. Snayles j-sooden w*ith* spices as it is j-telde in þe feuere etik, and as touchi*n*g þis poynt of tysik, medycines of etik bie*n* p*ro*fitabyl *and* good. And wha*n*ne tysik haaþ a feuere | w*ith* f. 86v hym, þu moost loke wheþ*er*e it comeþ of heete oþ*er* of coold. *And* þ*er*aft*er* þu moost ordyne þ*in* medicines as it was j-teeld

4 **Tempre**] *follow. by exp.* he*m* it] *interl.* 9 **þe**[1]] *follow. by canc. twice* feir*e* *and canc.* foyr*e* **for**] *corr. from* ffor **17 fisch3**] *corr. from* sisch3 **23 with**] *prec. by heading* Tysyk **24 of heete**] *corr. from* ofheete **25 ordyne**] *corr. from* ordyyne (first y *canc.*)

13 Profitabyl] *in r.-h. margin:* no*ta*

in þe chapitr*e* of hoorsnesse *and* of þe couȝe. And medycynes þ*at* were j-telde þ*er*e bien good here, for all*e* sicnesses of þe breest acorden in medicynes *and* in enchesou*n*s. And ȝif þe pacie*n*t bie febyl *and* þe feu*er*e violent, tak of cassia fistula, *dragme* v; of driȝe violet floures, *dragme* vij; of reysyns clensyd, *dragme* xx; i*n*nibes, xx; sebestem, xxx. Seeþ all*e* þese in iiij *pound* of wat*er* til it come to half a pound. *And* siþe cast þ*er*-to xx *dragme* of hempseed. *And* let clensyn it *and* ȝif hi*m* þ*er*-of to drynke. Dietyng of hy*m* þat haaþ þe tisyk of wound of þe liȝte xal bie of coold þi*n*ges, *and* moost, *and* co*n*glutynatif, as of þe þiees *and* þe feet of pigges, *and* he*n*nes, *and* chikenes, *and* lambren, *and* kydis, *and* good breed of whete, *and* wyn ȝif he haue no feuere, and ellis meeþ þ*at* lycorys haþ bien j-soden i*n*ne *and* dragg*e* resoluyd. But ȝif tisyk come of humo*urs*, here dietyng xal bie of pork, *and* fischȝ of freischȝ wat*er*, *and* na*m*ly scalyd fischȝ, as pyke, perche, roche *and* brem, *and* fruyt, *and* driȝe siripis. And ȝif it come of þe rewme, me*n* most a-bate þe humorys bi su*m*
f. 87r st*ri*ctoryes of here cours, | as it haaþ bien j-teld sufficiently here-bi-fore. But all*e* fisycyens a-corden nat here-i*n*ne þ*at* woundes of þe liȝte bie*n* incurable, for þei mow nat bie*n* j-heelyd w*ith*-owtyn clensyng, *and* þei mow nat bie*n* j-clensyd w*ith*-owtyn cowȝyng, *and* þe couȝe wole drawe hy*m* a-brood *and* make hy*m* feblere þ*a*t he was, *and* fullere of corupt humo*urs* þa*n* he was, *and* so þ*at* he xulde helpe doiþ harm. *And* þ*er*-fore þei mote*n* nedys bien incurable.

Diaradon abbatis is good for tysik, *and* for etik, *and* for þe cardiacle, *and* for ȝelwe euele, *and* many oþ*er* sicnesses

5 violet] *interl.* i **19 as**] *prec. by heading* Tysyk

3 And] *in l.-h. margin:* no*ta*

and is þus j-maad: Take whiȝte sau*n*dris *and* reede, *dragme* ij *and* s*emis*; of gu*m* arabik, dragg*e*, spodie, *dragme* ij; of asaru*m*, spik, mastik, cardomom*um*, citr*e*, ȝilobalsamu*m*, clowes, gallie muscat*e*, anise, fenel seed, canel, þe iuys of liquorys, reubarb*e*, þe seed of basilicon, berbere, scariole, porcelane, gourde, melou*n*, of eu*ery*choone, *dragme* j; margarit*es*, þe boon þat is in an hert*es* herte, *dragme* s*emis*; of gyng*er*, of rosees, *ounce* j *and dragme* iij; of camphore, vij greyns; of musk, iij greyns *and* s*emis*. *And* medle he*m* togidere *and* lat hi*m* drynke on morwetyd *and* on euene wiþ þe sirip of rosees. But medle þ*er*wiþ rose wat*er* oþ*er* coold wat*er*.

A sirip for p*er*ipleumonie, *and* pleuresie, *and* tisik, *and* etik: Tak iiij *pound* of wat*er and* do þ*er*-i*n*ne *ounce* s*emis* of violet; of licoryis, | of whiȝt popy, *dragme* s*emis*; of þe seed f. 87v
of citonyes *and* of hock*es* j-clensid, *and* of coton, *and* of melou*n*, *and* of gourdis, *and* of purselane, gu*m* arab*e*, dragg*e*, of eu*ery*ch*e* of þese, *dragme* iij. Sta*m*pe all*e* þese *and* do in þe forseid wat*er* in a bagge. *And* siþe clense þe wat*er and* cast þ*er*-to ij pound of sugre *and* make vp þ*in* sirip.

Triasandry is good also for þe tysik, *and* for þe stomac, *and* for þe ȝelwe e[uel], *and* is þus j-maad: Tac of sau*n*dris, boþe of reed *and* of whiȝt, *and* citryn roses, *and* sugre, ij *pound*; reubarb*e*, spodie, þe iuys of licoryis, þe seed of purselane, þe wheiȝte of xviij *half a pound*; amyde, gu*m* arab*e*, dragg*e*, þe seed of go*ur*d*es*, of melou*n*, *and* of scariole, sol*e* j; camphore, j *dragme*. And su*m* me*n* q*ua*draplieþ þe rosees of þe sirip of þe rosees, *quantum* s*ufficit*. Let hi*m*

15 of[2]] *prec. by heading* Defaute **20 pound**] *follow. by interl. pound*
22 euel] *corr. from* elue

vsen here-of a-morwetyd *and* at mydday þe q*ua*ntite of a chasteyn wiþ coold wat*er*.

A man haaþ defaute in breþi*n*ge, su*m*me in drawyng breþ, su*m*me in letyng owt here breþ, su*m* in boþe, su*m*me in breþi*n*ge to fast. And þis greuau*n*ce comeþ of þe same enchesou*n*s þ*at* streytnesse of þe breest *and* þe couȝe comeþ, *and* þe same man*er* þei bien j-heelyd as þei bien. Naþeles, þ*er* bien oþ*er* special medicines for þis sicnesse, as ȝif it bie of gret humo*ur*s þ*at* stoppen þe brest, ȝif hym subtilyatyfs *and* dissolutyues, as oximel squillityk oþ*er* sympel, oþ*er* ysope j-f. 88r soden | in hony. Oþ*er* make hym a sirip of þese þinges: Take of horehowne, *dragme* xx; of licorys, x *dragme*; of march, of radich, of fenel seed, of anyse, calamynte, ysope, *and* of maydynhere, *dragme* v; of femig*r*ek, *and* lynseed, *dragme* iij; of clene reysyns, c*ent dragme*; figes, xx; of penydes, vj *ounce*, m*anipulum quantum* s*ufficit*. Make here-of a sirip *and* late hi*m* vsen smal wyn *and* cleer*e*. *And* late make hym rounde balles of anyse, *and* suphur-vise, of castore, of armoniak, *and* melanopip*er*, of eu*er*ych*e* of þese, j-lych*e* mych*e*. Stampe hem *and* medle he*m* w*it*h wat*er and* w*it*h hony, *and* make rou*n*d balles.

A good emplastre to ligge*n* on here breste: Tak lilie rot*es*, *and* malues, *and* bismalues, *and* beet*es*, *and* driȝe figes, *and* reysyns, *and* alemau*n*dys, *and* pynes j-clensyd. Sta*m*pe hem wiþ wyn *and* siþe do þ*er*-to mele *and* grece.

Good pillules also here-fore: Tak of myrr*e*, storac*e*, cal*e*, galbanu*m*, castore, *and* of pep*er*, vj *dragme*; of opiu*m*, *dragme* iiij. Te*m*pre he*m* vp wiþ tisane þ*at* dragg*e* is resoluyd i*n*ne. *And* ȝif hi*m* þ*er*-of x oþ*er* xj. Bawme is good for þis

3 A] *2-line space left for initial* **10 j-soden]** *f. 88r* | soden **11 in]** *prec. by heading* in brethyng **17 hym]** *follow. by canc.* l greuau*n*ce, *and dragme* j of ge*n*ciane j-poudryd *and* j-etyn w*ith* an ey *and* wiþ wyn is p*ro*fitable. And so is *dragme* j of orpime*n*t j-etyn w*ith* an ey. And oþ*er* þi*n*ges þat were j-seed in þe couȝe bien good here. And þe diu*er*site of þe enchesouns of þe sicnesse, let ordeyne þi medycynes as it was bie-fore-seid | in oþ*er*e greuaunces of þe breste. f. 88v

A mannes herte þ*a*t is þe p*ri*ncipal membre of a mannes body haþ a sicnesse þ*a*t is j-clepid þe cardiacle. And þ*a*t may bie on two man*er*es: Oon is of humo*ur*s þ*a*t bie*n* enclosyd w*ith*-i*n*ne þe vttere skynnes of þe herte, *and* þilke make þe herte to tre*m*ble *and* to quake. Anoþ*er* cardiacle þ*er* is þ*a*t is of þe spirytis þ*a*t bie*n* w*ith*-i*n*ne þe herte, *and* þ*a*t is j-clepid syncopis. But þe furst manere cardiacle comeþ oþ*er*while of siche humo*ur*s *and* makeþ a ma*n* to haue a feuere. *And* oþ*er*while he comeþ w*ith*-outyn a feuere, *and* oþ*er*whilee þe feu*er*e is scharp, *and* oþ*er*while esy. But what man*er*e feu*er*e it bie, it makeþ a ma*n* to haue an hoot swet, *and* his kyndly hete draweþ outeward fra*m* þe hert *and* fra*m* w*ith*-i*n*ne-forþ, *and* brekeþ owt at þe porys þ*a*t bien w*ith*-owtyn-forþ in þe skyn. Oþ*er*while, þis g*r*euau*n*ce comeþ of corupt wynd þ*a*t is e*n*closid in þe herte, and þa*n* it is j-clepid lepyng of þe herte. Oþ*er*while, it comeþ of corupt humour*er*es *and* kene þ*a*t bien in þe mouþ of þe stomac *and* goiþ vp to þe hert by smale veines *and* g*r*euyth þe hert. Oþ*er*while, it comeþ fra*m* sich*e* humo*ur*s þ*a*t come*n* fra*m* þe lyuer*e* to þe herte. | Oþ*er*while, f. 89r it comeþ of wormes þ*a*t bie*n* i*n* þe stomac oþ*er* in þe guttes, *and* prickeþ he*m*, *and* þe herte haþ co*m*passiou*n* of here

4 **And]** *follow. by* di **þe[2]]** *in r.-h. margin* **6 bie-fore-seid]** *follow. by* in **in]** *prec. by heading* Cardyacle **7 A]** *2-line space left for initial* **10 þilke]** *follow. by and* þilke **22 of]** *follow. by canc. and exp.* a **25 Oþerwhile]** *prec. by heading* Cardiacle

greuau*n*ce *and* is j-greuyd also. And þis greuau*n*ce of þe herte oþ*er* it comeþ of blood þ*a*t haþ mych*e* colre, oþ*er* of blood þ*a*t haþ myche male*n*colie. And þe tokenes of þis sicnesse bie*n* tre*m*blyng *and* lepyng of þe hert *and* of oþ*er* me*m*brys, hot swete w*ith*-outyn-forþ, *and* myche passyng a-wey of heete by pores, feblenesse of senewys, pale coloure, leene *and* j-wastyd a-wey as me*n* þ*a*t ha*n* þe tysik or þe etik, w*ith* mych*e* ach*e* *and* greuau*n*ce a-boute þe herte. And þei mowe slepe but lityl, and ofte-siþes þei bie*n* costyf, and here pouse is swyft, and here vrine is reed, and þei trembelyn as men don for g*r*et coold. And wha*n*ne it is of colre, þe herte tre*m*beleþ, *and* þei ha*n* mych*e* heete, myche þirst, *and* deep breþinge. And wha*n*ne it comeþ of male*n*colie, þe hert tre*m*bleþ, *and* þe ma*n* haþ mych*e* sorwe, *and* sleuþe, *and* ne is nat þirstful. And wha*n* þis sicnesse comeþ of eny oþ*er* sicnesse of eny oþ*er* me*m*bre, let ȝyue þe pacie*n*t sich*e* þi*n*ges þ*a*t co*n*forteþ þe herte while þe oþ*er* me*m*bre is on helyng. f. 89v But ȝif þe greuau*n*ce is p*r*incipaly of þe herte *and* it bie | of colre, let hym blede at þe arme veyne þ*a*t is j-clepid basilica ȝif þu seest þ*a*t it is neede, as ȝif þe ma*n* bie repleet of blood *and* ȝong. Ellys lat garsyn hym in places þ*a*t bien couenable þ*er*-to *and* neiȝe þe herte. And siþe ȝif hy*m* a sirip of borage, and siþe ȝif hym a calogoge to purge hym of colre. And siþe ȝif hym þe iuys of borage, *and* of scariole, *and* of pomegarnade. And in þe same man*er* do in a feuere wha*n* þ*er* is mat*er* j-last þ*a*t he ne is j-purgyd of. Aft*er*ward, a-noynte all*e* his body w*ith* muscilage of p*er*silie, *and* w*ith* þe whiȝte of an ey, *and* a lytyl popilion; oþ*er* w*ith* þe wat*er* þ*a*t dragg*e* haþ bie resoluyd i*n*ne j-medlyd w*ith* þe muscilage of p*er*sillie.

3 sicnesse] *corr. from* sicnesses (last s *exp.*) **18 of**[2]] *prec. by heading* Cardiakyl **28 lytyl popilion**] *corr. from* lytylpopilion

Aft*er*ward while þe body is moist, lat strawe þ*er*-on poudre of roses, of galles, of bole, of acasie, of ypo-quyscidos, *and* of sich*e* oþ*er* st*ri*ctoryes. And let hym vsen coold electuaries, as t*ri*asendi, rosa[t]a nouella, diarodon, diacameron, dyanthos muscat*e*, diamargariton, pocio muscata, diacitoniton, muscat*e*, *and* medle w*it*h he*m* oþ*er*e hoot electuaries. But lete þe coold haue þe maistre. Also, sugre roset, *and* sugre of violet, *and* diapapau*er* bie*n* good for hem. And þe piȝe is good as it was j-telde in þe sicnesse of þe eiȝe. And ȝif it bie a riche ma*n* *and* a worþi, ȝyue hy*m* dyarodou*n*, | julij. A special sirip for þis sicnesse: Tak borage, *and* mace, *and* spodie, *and* horsel, *and* þe seed of citonyes, *and* lignu*m* aloes, galyngale, amoni*e*, canel, þe rynde of pome citryne, whiȝt coral, *and* make vp þi sirip w*it*h sufficient sugre. Here dietyng xal bie of siche metis þ*at* bien esy to defiȝe. And late hym vse oftyn-siþes þe for-seid a-noyntyng of here body. And late hy*m* smelle ofte-siþes to colde þy*n*ges þ*at* bien aromatik, as roses *and* floures of violet, of borage, of basilico*n*, of bawme, *and* þe rynd of a reed appel. *And* make poudre of þe same þi*n*ges, *and* do it in a bagge, *and* lei it on þe stomac. And lat strewyn in þe hows þ*at* he lieþ i*n*ne salyen leuys, *and* vyne leeuys, *and* roses, *and* leeuys of violet, *and* wat*er*-lilien, *and* of sich*e* oþ*er* coold herb*e*. And ȝif it comeþ of coold, ȝif hym poudr*e* of canel, spik, cardamom*e*, *and* ȝedwarie, of eu*er*ich*e*, j-lich*e* mych*e*. And ȝif it comeþ of male*n*colie, p*ur*ge he*m* w*it*h myrabolan*e* ind*e*, *and* epithime, *and* sene, w*it*h gootis mylk, *and* sych*e* oþ*er* þi*n*ges. And ȝif þe cardiacle comeþ of male*n*colye *and* of colre to-gidere, lat his p*ur*gaciou*n* *and* his oþ*er* medicyns bie j-maad of þilke þi*n*ges þ*at* p*ur*ge*n* colre *and* malencolie, as

f. 90r

4 **rosata**] *corr. from* rosaca 10 **julij**] *interl.* (julij *oblit.*); *prec. by heading* Cardiacle

iora fortissima galieni, *and* þe grett*ere* stomaticon. And siþe f. 90v lete ȝif hym confortabyl electuaries *and* wel smellynge. | *And* medle w*ith* hem þe lymaile of goold *and* þe poudre of þe bon þ*at* is in an hert*es* hert. *And* let a-noynte here breste w*ith* hoote oynement*es and* aromatyk, *and* oþ*ere* hoote oiles þ*at* bie*n* myche bet*ere*. And late hym vsen good met*es and* good drynkys þ*at* gendreþ good blood, and smale briddes j-soden w*ith* spices, *and* herbis. *And* late hi*m* vsen ofte-tymes in his metys lymaile of goolde *and* þe poudre of margeri perles (þei bien goode for þe cardiacle þ*at* is w*ith* a feuere also). And in þ*at* cardiacle þ*at* is w*ith* g*re*t heete, lat froten þe sooles of þe ma*n*nes fete *and* þe pawme of his hondys w*ith* coold oiles. And wete [a] ly*n*nen cloþ in wat*er* of roses *and* lei it to his nostrilles. And late hi*m* ligge*n* in a coold place þ*at* is ful of coold floures *and* coold leeues *and* j-spreynt w*ith* coold wat*er*. And a-noynte hi*m* a-bowte þe te*m*ples w*ith* iuys of solatre, *and* of syngrene, *and* of sich*e* oþ*er* coold herb*e*. And a-noynte hese necke *and* his chyne w*ith* oile of myrtys *and* of saleyne. *And* siþe cast þ*er*-up-on poudre of roses *and* of saundres.

Oile of myrtes is j-maad of þe leues of myrtes j-soden f. 91r in comyn oile xxx daies i*n* þe | su*n*ne. Comyn oile is oile de oliue þ*at* is mete oile. And riȝt as oile of myrtes is j-maad, so is maad al man*er* oiles þ*at* bie*n* j-mad of leues oþ*er* of floures, as oile of rosees, oþ*ere* oile of violet, *and* siche oþ*ere*.

2 **And**] *prec. by heading* Cardiacle **9** **margeri**] *follow. by* pe*ri*les **perles**] *in r.-h. margin* **13** **wete**] *follow. by and* **15** **leeues**] *corr. from* leeoues (second e *interl.*; o *exp.*) **22** **sunne**] *prec. by heading* Cardiacle

24 **j-mad**] *in r.-h. margin:* no*ta*

Also a-noynte his breste w*ith* þe whiȝt of an ey *and* w*ith* þe iuys of citonyes j-medlid to-gidere. Oþ*er* make a plastre of iij kyndes of sau*n*dres, *and* rosees, *and* þe schauy*n*ge of þe yuer j-medlid to-gidere w*ith* oile of violet *and* w*ith* wat*er* of rosees. And ȝif þe cardiacle comeþ of þe stomac, make hym caste, oþ*er* ȝif hy*m* a p*ur*gaciou*n* of myrabolan*e* citryne, cassia fistula, manna *and* plu*m*mes. *And* make hi*m* a plastre w*ith*-outyn of saundrys, *and* barly mele, *and* smyþes axen, *and* siche oþ*er* þi*n*ges, oþ*er* þe forseyd plastres. And ȝeue hi*m* coold electuaries as it was told bie-fore, and ȝif it comeþ of þe lyu*er*e, as it xal bie teld in his sicnesse. And ȝif it comeþ of myche wakyng oþ*er* of mych*e* fastyng, ȝeue hi*m* dyanysu*m*, dyacitonycon oþ*er* diasp*er*mat[ic]on. And ȝif þu haue nat þese, take anyse *and* seeþ it in wat*er*. *And* in þ*a*t wat*er* wete wolle þ*a*t is j-schoore of an on-wasche scheyp, *and* ley þ*a*t vp-on þe hert. And ley oþ*er* medicynes in diu*er*se places | f. 91v þ*a*t bien dissolutyfs *and* mown dissolue corupt humo*urs* þ*a*t bien boþe in þe stomac *and* in þe herte, a*n*d for þis sicnesse ȝit þe pye is p*ro*fitable.

And ȝif þis sicnesse come of fleu*ma*tyk mat*er* oþ*er* of colrik þ*a*t is a-boute þe liȝte, it is j-clepyd a tre*m*belyng cardiacle, for wha*n*ne a ma*n* leiþ his hand on þe herte, he trembleþ. *And* ne haþ nat hese kyndly meuyng as he xuld haue. And to þis cardiacle it is p*ro*fitable to make a gargarisme of loueach*e*, ysope, *and* sauerey, *and* þe iuys of licoryis, *and* radich*e*, *and* yreos, *and* origane, *and* calamy*n*te, *and* horehowne j-soden jn meeþ. And late hi*m* vsen þis gargarisme a-morwe *and* on euene, and let hi*m* swelwyn down of þe same decocciou*n*. And siþe let p*ur*gen hym w*ith*

17 þat] *prec. by heading* Cardiacle **22 for]** *corr. from* ffor **27 meeþ]** *interl.* last e

iera j-medlid w*ith* þe poudre of radich*e* *and* of lycorys, *and* w*ith* þe iuys of radich*e* *and* of yrees. *And* siþe lat a-noynte hi*m* w*ith* mel roset despumed.

Symple medicynes *and* na*m*lych*e* for þe cardiacle bien coral, margarites, goold, *and* þe boon þ*at* is in an hertys herte, ca[r]pobalȝamu*m*, clowes *and* a p*re*ciouse stoon þ*at* hite jaci*nctus*. And to he*m* þ*at* han þe cardiacle of coold *and* of male*n*colie, it is a p*ro*fitable medicine [t]o drynk good wyn. And to hem þ*at* haan a cardiacle of corupt humo*urs* f. 92r *and* of þe stomac *and* na*m*ly of gret heete, me*n* xal | nat ȝyue hem hoote metis þ*at* wolen sone bie defied, but oþ*ere* metis þ*at* wolen longe bie indefiȝi*n*ge, as he*n*nes, *and* oold caponys, *and* swynes feet, *and* barlyche, *and* whete, *and* siche oþere þinges.

Syncopis is a greua*n*ce of þe herte *and* may bie clepid a cardiacle, for as myche as it is a sicnesse of þe hert. But it comeþ nat of humo*urs* as þe oþ*ere* cardiacle doiþ, but of þe greuau*n*ce of þe spiritys of þe herte, and þ*at* is in two man*eres*. Oon is wha*n* þei ben j-gaderid to-gidere in þe hert *and* þe herte haþ mo þa*n* he xuld haue, as it hapneþ wha*n* a ma*n* falleþ fra*m* a sodeyn gladnesse in-to a soden sorwe, oþ*er* falleþ fram a greet heete in-to a gret colde. But þe toþ*er* man*er* is wha*n* a ma*n*nes spirites goon sodenly out of his herte *and* bien j-sparlied a-brood in al þe body, as it hapneþ wha*n* a ma*n* falleþ in-to a soden ioy aft*er* his sorwe, oþ*er* in-to a gret heete aft*er* a gret coold. And of bothe þese man*eres* a man may liȝtly deiȝe but ȝif he bie þe raþ*er* j-holpe. Þis sicnesse comeþ also of to gret plente of humo*urs* in a ma*n*nes

8 to] *corr. from* do **drynk**] *interl.* r **10 nat**] *prec. by heading* Or Syncopis **15 Syncopis**] *2-line space left for initial* **19 þe hert**] *corr. from* þehert **25 ioy**] *corr. from* iooy (first o *exp. and oblit.*; last o *interl.*)

body þ*a*t þirsteþ þe herte to-gidere; oþ*er*whiles of a-ventysyng of a ma*n*nes body *and* to gret feblenesse, as it hapneþ by siche me*n* þ*a*t han j-had a long duryng flux, oþ*er* su*m* oþ*er* man*er* leesyng of blood, oþ*er* þorow myche stondyng in þe su*n*ne þ*a*t j-haþ draw out a ma*n*nes kyndlych*e* heete *and* his spiritys. Oþ*er*-while it comeþ of plente of humo*urs* þ*a*t bie*n* in þe stomac, *and* þanne | a man schal f. 92v wlate myche, *and* caste ofte-siþes, and þe hyndrere parte of heed wole ake, *and* namly bie-fore mete. And whiȝle he haþ his accesse, he semeþ þ*a*t he seeþ myche þi*n*g bi-fore hese eiȝe*n* þ*a*t is nat þere. And þis cardiacle þ*a*t comeþ of þe stomac ne lasteþ nat longe. Oþ*er*while it is of plente of humo*urs* þ*a*t bie*n* in þe guttes. And ȝif it bie of male*n*col*e*, þ*er* is heuynesse *and* g*r*euau*n*ce in þe wo*m*be [and] swellyng. Of colre comeþ ache *and* p*ri*ckyng. Of flewme comeþ heuynesse *and* swollyng, *and* oþ*er* siche tokenys aft*er* þe kynde of þe humo*ur*. Oþ*er*while it comeþ to women þorow beryng of a deid child, for þe veynes brekyn *and* blood floweþ owt more þa*n* it schulde. Oþ*er*while it comeþ of to myche strechyng of þe mod*er* as wha*n*ne it is to myche j-streiȝt in-to þe riȝt syde, oþ*er* in-to þe lift syde, oþ*er* upward, oþ*er* downward. Oþ*er*while it comeþ of begy*n*ny*n*g of co*n*ceyuy*n*g, for wi[t]h-holdyng of blood þ*a*t scholde kyndly flowe ne were here co*n*ceyuy*n*g. Oþ*er*whyle it comeþ in þe iiij monþe, for þe soule of þe child bi-gynnyth þa*n*ne to worche in his body. Oþ*er*while it comeþ in þe ix monþe wha*n* þe child is a-boute to passyn owt fra*m* his mod*er*is wo*m*be. And

4 sum oþer] *corr. from* su*m*oþer **7 a**] *prec. by heading* Sincopis
14 þe] *follow. by canc.* guttes **17 humour**] *corr. from* humours (s *exp.*)
18 of] *follow. by canc.* chyldren **22 of**[1]] *follow. by canc.* breþi*n*g
23 for] *corr. from* ffor **24 þe**] *follow. by canc.* by-gy*n*ny*n*g

oþ*er*while þe sicnesse comeþ of suffocacyou*n* of þe mod*er*. f. 93r *And* oþ*er*wyle þat | dureþ ij daies *and* ij nytes. And so þis sicnesse is oþ*er*while a sicnesse bie hy*m*-self, oþ*er*while it comeþ of a-noþ*er* sicnesse. But how-eu*er*e it bie, þu xalt hie to hele þis sicnesse, ȝhe wel raþ*er* þan þe sicnesse þat it comeþ of. And ȝif it bie of to gret plente of spirit*es* þ*a*t bien enclosyd in þe hert *and* bien j-ru*n*ne fra*m* w*i*t*h*-outen in-to þe herte, wheþ*er* it bie a sicnesse bie hi*m*-self, oþ*er* come of a-noþ*er* sicnesse, le[t] byndyn his fyngris w*i*t*h* þwonges *and* his toon also, þ*a*t þe spiritys *and* þe blood mown drawyn outward fra*m* þe hert. *And* closen þe nostrilles *and* oppyn his mouþ þ*a*t þe fume may come owt of his mouþ. *And* let wry*n*gyn hi*m* weel by þe noose, *and* pulle*n* hy*m* by þe heerys of his beerd *and* also of his heed. *And* let hym bye kyssid of su*m* frend þ*a*t loueþ hym weel. *And* let fretyn wel his hondys *and* þis wole make hi*m* aryssen vp of his accesse. And ȝif it comeþ of a-ventesyng *and* of feblenesse of his body, ȝyue hym in tyme of his accesse wyn þ*a*t clowes *and* sauge bien j-soden i*n*ne, oþ*er* þe broþ of an henne, oþ*er* of a capou*n*. And ȝif it bie of myche plente of blood oþ*er* of other*e* humo*urs*, let a-batyn hi*m* bie blood-letyng*e* oþ*er* by su*m* oþ*er*e p*ur*gaciou*n* aft*er* þe kynde of þe humo*ur*. And ȝif f. 93v it bie of gret plente of humo*urs* of þe | stomac, let hym caste. And ȝif it bie of hoot humo*urs*, ȝyue hym coolde medicynes. *And* ȝif it bie of coold humo*urs*, ȝif hym hoote medicynes, as we schul seyn in þe siknesse of þe stomac. And ȝif it bie of

2 dureþ] *prec. by heading* Syncopis **4 how-euere it**] *corr. from* eu*er*eit **10 blood**] *follow. by canc. and exp.* u **23 stomac**] *prec. by heading* Cardiacle

12 fume] *in r.-h. margin:* no*ta*

fulnesse of þe guttes, p*ur*ge hym w*ith* a clist*er*e oþ*er* a suppositorie. And ȝif it bie of þe ouere gutte, purge hy*m* w*ith* a-noþer p*ur*gaciou*n*, as we wollen tellen in þe sicnesse of þe guttes. And ȝif it comeþ of heete of þe su*n*ne oþ*er* of eny sych*e* oþ*er* heete, let spryngyn his visage w*ith* wat*er* of rosees, *and* leie on his visage *and* a-boute*n* hy*m* saleyn leeues. And ȝif it comeþ of þe mod*er* þ*at* is streiȝt vpward, oþer*e* downward, oþ*er* on syde for þ*er* þa*n* it schulde, let þe woma*n* walke on here bare feet til it bie as it schuld bie. And late seþe fenel seed, *and* p*er*seile seed, *and* siche oþ*er*e þi*n*ges þ*at* bien good for þe mod*er* in wat*er*. *And* let weten felt oþ*er* a-noþ*er* wolle*n* clooþ in þe wat*er* *and* leggen it on þe mod*er*. And ȝif it bie of beryng childryn, ȝeue here sugre roset, oþ*er* þe sirip of rosees, oþ*er* diapapau*er*, oþ*er* dyacitonyton. And lat here liggen vpriȝt *and* here feet heiȝere þa*n* here heed. *And* let cuppe*n* here at þe rote of here pappes. And ȝif sche haue no feu*er*e, lat here haue a baaþ of st*ri*cto-ries. *And* ellys late wetyn a clooþ in water*e* þat | strictories bien j- f. 94r
soden i*n*ne *and* leie þ*at* clooþ on þe mod*er*. And ȝif it comeþ of women þ*at* han late co*n*ceyuyd, lat here vsen confortabil electuaries *and* wel smellyng. *And* let sp*ri*ngyn here foreheed w*ith* wat*er* of roses. And ȝif þe mod*er* bie fallen down *and* bie lowere, þa*n* it xuld bie be a-boute to heuyn here vp bi strencþe of medicynes. *And* let here smellyn to hert*es*-horn j-brent *and* haue þe fume þ*er*-of in here nose *and* þe fume of storat. And ȝif it comeþ of gret flewme þ*at* is in a ma*n*nes

3 sicnesse of] *corr. from* sicnesseof **9 on here]** *corr. from* onhere **10 fenel seed]** *corr. from* fenelseed **16 rote]** *corr. from* þrote (þ *canc. twice*) **18 þat]** *catchword* (*in bottom margin*): st*ri*ctories bien **strictories]** *prec. by heading* Tysyk guttes, *and* ȝif he haue þe feueres, let heetyn a tyil-stoon *and* do hym i*n* vinegre. *And* þa*n* wrap hym in a clene lynen clooþ *and* leie to his herte. And ȝif he haþ nat þe feueres, ȝif hym t*ri*acle diatesseron w*it*h wyn þ*at* aue*n*ce *and* rwe bien j-soden i*n*ne. And in þe same man*er* do in þe suffocaciou*n* of þe mod*er*.

Triacle dyatessero*n* is þus j-maad: Tak of myrre, of aristologie rou*n*de, of ge*n*cian, of baies of lorere j-maad clene, *ounce* j *and ounce* ij; of ditan*n*dre, pigamy, camedreos, *dragme* j *and ounce* ij; *and* viij grei*n*s of gu*m*me of yuy; of calcance j-brent, *dragme* j; of hony, *quantum* s*ufficit*. Oþ*er* men doon here-to femygrek, nigelle, *and* ȝedwarie, of eu*er*ych*e*-oon, *ounce* j, *dragme* ij; *and* of aspalte, as mych*e* as. All*e* þese schullen bien j-pouderid *and* j-medlid w*it*h þe forseid hony. Þis t*ri*acle is good for men þ*at* bie*n* j-poysend oþ*er* j-byte of eny venymouse beste oþ*er* of a wood hound. And it xal bie dru*n*ke*n* w*it*h þe iuys of myntyn. And it is
f. 94v good to legge*n* | on venemouse postemys in þe man*er*e of an oynnement. And it is good for þe feu*er*e q*ua*rteyn *and* for þe cotidyan feuere to drynkyn wyþ þe iuys of pygamy oþ*er* of genciane. And it is good for hem þat bien greuyd in here stomac, oþ*er* in here lyuere, oþ*er* in þe splene. And ȝif syncopis come of bledyng at þe nose, ȝif it bie at þe liȝft nostrylle, let cuppen hym a-boute þe splene on þe liȝft syde, wiþoute*n* gar-synge to drawyn þe blood downward fra*m* þe nose. Ȝif þe nose blede on þe riȝt nostrelle, do so oon þe riȝt

1 **he**] *corr. from* hae (a *canc.*; e *interl.*) 13 **eueryche-oon**] *corr. from* eu*er*ych*e*on (cn *canc. and exp.*) 18 **on**] *prec. by heading* Tysyk 26 **riȝt nostrelle**] *corr. from* riȝtnostrelle

7 **þus**] *in r.-h. margin:* no*ta* b*e*n*e* te*riaca*

syde. And ȝif it comeþ of ventesyng of þe body, oþ*er* of mych*e* bledyng, let hi*m* drynken good wyn j-medlyd w*ith* coold wat*er*. Ȝif he haue no feu*ere* lat hym smelle swete-smellynges as roses, *and* siche oþ*er* þinges. And it is p*ro*fitabyl to hetyn a pece of goold oþ*er* of syluere in þe fyer *and* que*n*che it ofte-siþes in þe wyn þ*at* he schal drynke. And siche xal nat baþe hem, ne bie j-lete blood, for þ*at* wole drawen þe spiritys of here herte owtward. And þ*er*fore it bihoueþ to lyggyn hi*m* in a coold place *and* maken it coold w*ith* coold leeues, as it was j-told in þe cardiacle. And ȝif þis greua*n*ce come of myche beyng*e* in þe su*n*ne, oþ*er* of longe dwellynge in a baaþ, ne cast ne cold wat*er* in his visage but it bie medlyd w*ith* wyn. But set hym in þe wynde, oþ*er* w*ith* craft blowe | wynd on hym. And þe smel of gourdes is ful (f. 95r) profitabil for hem. And ȝif it comeþ of gret coold, let hi*m* vsen hoot electuaries. *And* late hym drynke good wyn *and* smelle to wel sauerid þi*n*ges.

A mannes stomac haþ many g*re*uau*n*ces. Þe furst is greuau*n*ce in swolewynge of mete *and* drynk. Anoþ*er* is on-resonabyl appetit to mete *and* to drynke. Anoþ*er* is þurst; anoþ*er* is defaute of þurst. Oþ*er* greuau*n*ces þ*er* bie*n*, as bolkyng, ȝyxynge, abho*mi*n*a*ciou*n* to mete *and* drynke, and wille for-to castyn, turnyng vp-so-dou*n* a ma*n*nes stomac, gret hete of þe stomac, and aposty*m* of þe stomac.

Greua*n*ce of swolewynge comeþ in iij man*er*es *and* of iij enchesou*n*s: of gret heete, *and* of gret coold, of þe wesyng. But þa*n* wha*n* he swolewiþ, it is greuouse; but so he may swolewe a lytil *and* a lytil. *And* he is þirstful ȝif it comeþ of

2 drynken] *interl.* r **7 for]** *corr. from* ffor **11 greuance]** *follow. by exp.* bie **come]** *interl.* **14 wynd]** *prec. by heading* Stomak **18 A]** *2-line space left for initial*

heete, *and* haaþ mych*e* heete *and* row3nesse in his wesyng. *And* to helyn hym of þis g*r*euau*n*ce, 3yue hym cassia fistula, *and* plu*m*bes, *and* i*n*nibes. And 3if hym nedeþ, let hym blood *and* ellys p*ur*ge hym. And siþe 3if hym coold siripis to akelyn hym wiþ, as violet, *and* of plu*m*bes w*ith* þe iuys of gourdys. And late hym etyn coolde herbys, as purselane, gourdys, violet, arage, letuse, *and* sich*e* oþ*er*e. And a-noynte hym w*ith* oyneme*nt*es *and* ley coold plastres also þ*er*-to to a-bate*n* þe heete. And 3if it comeþ of coold, lat hy*m* vsyn f. 95v alectuarie | þ*at* is j-maad of hony roset, *and* scariole, *and* þe iuys of march j-medlyd to-gidere.

Hony roset is j-maad of hony *and* of roses j-hacked smalle *and* j-soden i*n*ne hony ou*er* þe feer. Jn-to a pownd of rooses þu xalt haue ij *pound* of hony. Also let hi*m* vsen hoot electuaries þ*at* weryn teld in þe cou3e. Jn a-noþ*er*e man*er* þis greuau*n*ce comeþ of a postym þ*at* is in þe wesy*n*g. *And* þa*n* he haþ gret greuau*n*ce þ*er*-i*n*ne, *and* na*m*ly while he swoleweþ. And 3if þe postym is hoot, þu mytest j-knowe by þe for-seid tokenes. And 3if it comeþ of coold, þ*er* is heuynesse in þe wesynge wiþouten þilke tokenes. And 3if it is an hoot postym, do as it was j-seid raþ*er*e. Wha*n*ne it comeþ of hete w*ith*-outyn postym, leie coold plastres w*ith*-outyn-forþ *and* coold pillules vnd*er* þe tonge, and norisch*e* hym w*ith* alemau*n*d mylk, *and* w*ith* gourdys, *and* tysane, *and* sich*e* oþ*er*e þi*n*ges. And 3if it bie a coold postym, 3yue hym ysope j-soden in hony, *and* þe sirip of horehoune þ*at* was j-spoke in þe cow3e. And 3if it bie w*ith* a feuere, 3if hym tisane w*ith* alemau*n*d mylk *and* w*ith* sugre. And 3if þe

10 þat] *prec. by heading* Stomak

11 march] *in l.-h. margin:* no*ta* honyroset (honyroset *underl.*)

postym breke, cle*n*se hym w*it*h tisane, *and* alemaunt mylk, *and* calamynte j-medlyd to-gidere. And ȝif he bie riȝth feble, ȝyf hym gotys mylk to drynke þ*at* a reed glowȝyng stoon haþ bien ofte-siþes j-que*n*chid i*n*ne. And ȝif it bie an hoot postym, let þe plastre þ*at* schal make hym ripe bie j-maad of p*er*silie | f. 96r *and* of lynseed j-tempryd w*it*h mylk. And ȝif it bie of coold, let maken þe plastre of femygrek *and* þe seed of cotou*n* j-meynd w*it*h bot*er*e. Jn þe iij man*er*e, þis greuau*n*ce comeþ of a wound of þe wesyng. *And* þa*n*ne he feleþ þ*er*-i*n*ne boþe ache *and* prechyng *and* namlye wha*n* he eteþ soure metis oþ*er* salt. And þese wou*n*dys xulle bien j-helyd wiþ þe iuys of plau*n*teyn, bole, *and* t*ur*mentyn, *and* hony j-medlyd to-gidere. Þis medycine is p*ro*fitabil þei þe wound bie oold. And ȝif þe wound bie w*it*h-owtyn, þe for-seid medicyne xal bie leid þ*er*-to in þe man*er*e of an oynneme*n*t. And ȝif it bie w*it*h-i*n*ne-forþ, late hi*m* swolwe is medicine. And ȝif it bie w*it*h a feuere, ȝif hym his medicine w*it*h a tysane. Ȝif he haþ no feu*er*e, ȝeue hi*m* w*it*h mellicrate. Mellicrate is maad of wyn *and* hony j-soden to-gidere, but þe ij parties bien wyn *and* þe iij part is hony. And oþ*er* þi*n*ges bie*n* p*ro*fitable þ*at* weryn told in wou*n*dys of þe liȝte. And siche medicynes þ*at* schullen bien swolewyd ne xul nat bie sodenlyche swolewyd a-down, but all*e* by ese. *And* þa*n*ne þei schulle stonde to profiȝt.

Defaute *and* lesyng of a ma*n*nes appetit is in two man*er*es, oþ*er* þorouȝ coolde humo*ur*s þ*at* bien in þe stomac

3 haþ] *follow. by* haþ **5 hym**] *follow. by exp.* riche **6 and**] *prec. by heading* Stomak **25 Defaute**] *2-line space left for initial*

1 hym] *in l.-h. margin:* look **19 hony**] *in r.-h. margin:* Mellicrate no*ta* (Mellicrate *underl.*)

þ*a*t bie rawe *and* vndefiȝed, *and* þa*n* is sowr*e* bolkyng, *and* he ne is nat þirstful, *and* þe stomac defeeþ febely *and* swelleþ. Jt comeþ also of colric humo*urs* þ*a*t bien in þe stomac. *And* þe tokenes of hem bien an hoot bolkyng, bitt*er*nesse of þe f. 96v mouþ, *and* greet þurst, *and* swyftly he defieþ | gret mete as beef *and* sich*e* oþ*er*e mete. Jn þe secu*n*de man*er*e, it comeþ wha*n* a ma*n* haþ lost his desyre *and* his wille to mete. *And* is in two man*er*is. Oon is þorow corupcion of þe stomac. *And* þe tokene þ*er*-of is þ*a*t a man haaþ abho*mi*n*a*ciou*n* to þ*a*t mete þ*a*t he louyd by-fore. And þis is a p*er*ilouse greuau*n*ce in longe sicnesses *and* na*m*lych*e* in þe blody fluxe. Þe toþ*er* man*er* comeþ þorouȝ corupciou*n* of a mannes wit, as in men þ*a*t bien frentik oþ*er* wode, *and* han j-lost here wit, *and* so þei leesyn appetit to mete *and* to drynke. An vnresonabil appetit is wha*n*ne a ma*n* haþ wille to ete aft*ur* þ*a*t he haþ j-ete riȝt j-now. And þ*er* bien two kyndes of þis appetit. Þe ton is clepid an houndys appetit. *And* þ*a*t is wha*n* a ma*n* eteþ mych*e* mor*e* þa*n* hy*m* nedeþ *and* so[n]e aft*ur* castiþ it vp as an hound. Þe secu*n*de man*er*e is wha*n*ne a ma*n* defieþ his mete þou he ete mych*e* mor*e* þa*n* hi*m* nedeþ; oþ*er* þei he defyed nat, he casteþ it nat, but late it passe forþ þorow his guttes. And þis vnresonabyl appetit comeþ of þe stomakes coldnesse *and* of malencolie þ*a*t is in þe mouþ of þe stomac. For þu xalt vnd*er*stonde þ*a*t þe stomac desiriþ mete boþe for sustenau*n*ce of hi*m*-self *and* for all*e* þe body. And in þe ou*er* part of þe stomac is feeli*n*ge. And wha*n*ne þ*a*t þe humo*ur* of male*n*colie

5 **gret**] *prec. by heading* Stomak 10 **he louyd**] *corr. from* helouyd 11 **þe blody**] *corr. from* þeblody 13 **bien frentik**] *corr. from* bienfrentik (frentik: n *interl.*) 15 **riȝt**] *interl.* 17 **man**] *follow. by canc. twice* t 18 **sone**] *corr. from* soþe 23 **For**] *corr. from* ffor 25 **of**[2]] *follow. by canc. twice* his *and exp.* body (bo *canc. twice*) **þe**[3]] *interl.*

droppeþ on þ*at* ou*er* party of þe stomac, þe stomac j-feeliþ þe keneschipe of þis | malencolie *and* wylneþ *and* desireþ more f. 97r mete kyndly. But wha*n*ne þ*er* is to myche of þis malencolie in þe mouþ of þe stomac, it makeþ þe appetit vnresonabil, *and* wylneþ more þa*n* he may defiȝe *and* makeþ hi*m* casten it vp. For me*n* þ*at* ha*n* þis greua*n*ce, it is p*ro*fitabil to dri*n*ck good reed wyn, *and* myche fastyng, *and* na*m*ly sich*e* wyn þat is þicke in þe mouþ *and* swete. And lete hym vsen hoot electuaries þ*at* bie*n* su*m*what bitt*er*e, as dia[tri]onpip*er*ion, diacalamentu*m*, diapigamu*m*, diacene, diaprassion, dyacymynu*m*, *and* siche oþ*er*e. And late a-noynte here stomak*es* w*it*h hoote oyneme*ntes* *and* leggen hoot plastres þ*er*-on. And lat he*m* nat ete soure þi*n*ges. But ȝif þei desire vnctuose þi*n*ges, ȝif hem in godd*es* name, boþe in þe begynnyng of here appetit, *and* þe mydle, *and* i*n* þe ende.

Diatrionpip*er*ion is good to dissolue*n* corupt wyndys *and* humo*ur*s of þe stomac, *and* co*n*forteþ þe stomac *and* þe guttes boþe, *and* is þus j-maad: Tak of pep*er* boþe whiȝt *and* blac *and* long, of canel, of gyng*er*, of fenel seed, of anyse, of mastyk, of aȝaru*m*, *ounce* j; of xilobalsamu*m*, of cassie, of spik, of amoni*e*, *ounce* s*emis*; of cardamomu*m*, of march, ameos, citre, clowes, coost, *and* of maces, *ounce* iiij; hony, *quantum* s*ufficit*. Also let hym vse*n* dyaȝinȝiber, dialange, *and* siche oþ*er*e electuaries þ*at* clenseþ þe stomak of corrupt humo*ur*s. And ȝif þe | stomac bie feble þat he may nat f. 97v hoolde þe metys þ*at* he resceyueþ, þa*n*ne vn*n*ctuose met*es*

1 of þe] *corr. from* ofþe **2 malencolie**] *prec. by heading* Stomak
6 For] *corr. from* ffor **9 diatrionpiperion**] *corr. from* diaconp*er*ip*er*ion
25 stomac] *prec. by heading* Stomak **bie**] *interl.*

16 good] *in r.-h. margin:* no*ta* ben*e*

bien neyful. Vnctuose met*es* bien fate met*es* *and* alle manere fatnesse *and* oiles. But ȝif hym smellyng electuaryes *and* bit*ere* also, *and* sauery soure met*es* also. And ȝif it comeþ of hete þat ane*n*teseþ þe stomac *and* makeþ hym feble, let hym vse reste, *and* sleep, *and* coold eir*e*, and anoynte here stomac w*ith* oile of rosees *and* of violet. And ȝif hym coold sirypis to dryncke, as of violet *and* of rosees. And in siche vnresonabyl appetitys þ*at* comeþ of corupt humo*urs* of þe stomac, it is p*ro*fitable to make*n* hem casten, *and* purgen hem of þilke humo*urs*. And þ*o*u myȝt doon by anete *and* hony. *And* schal maken hem castyn wiþ-outyn gret trauaile. But furst late hem ete freischȝ fischȝ [and] rootys of herbys wiþ oximel. *And* siþe late hy*m* dryncke good wyn, *and* þa*n*ne þei xullyn esyli casten. And aft*er*ward, late dietyn hem w*ith* dei*n*teys, boþe of fleischȝ *and* of fyschȝ. And make a plastre w*ith*-outyn-forþ on þe stomac of mastik, of spik, rooses, wermot, *and* oþ*ere* syche þi*n*ges. And for wome*n* þ*at* bien w*ith* childe, make a sirip of clowys, canel, notemuge, maces, q*ui*bibes, calamynte, origan, mynte, sene, saundrys whiȝt *and*
f. 98r reed, *and* cardamom*e*. *And* cast þ*er*-to a sponefull*e* | of vynegre. *And* siþe make vp þi sirip w*ith* sufficyent sugre. Þe sirip doiþ a-wey an vnresonabyl appetyt *and* makeþ a good appetyt, *and* letteþ a man of castyng. But oþ*er*while þis vnresonabyl appetyt comeþ of humo*urs* þ*at* bie*n* rawe *and* vndefiȝed. *And* þa*n*ne it is p*ro*fitabil to make hy*m* to castyn *and* to p*ur*gyn hym by su*m* p*ur*gaciou*n* by-neþeforþ. And siþe ȝif hym good met*es* *and* good drynkys to make good

9 **to]** *follow. by canc.* ma **20** **and]** *follow. by* cardamonu*m* (u*m* *canc.)* **cardamome]** *in l.-h. margin* **of]** *prec. by heading* Thurst

9 maken] *in l.-h. margin:* No*ta*

humo*urs*. And ȝif hy*m* good *and* co*n*fortabyl electuaries, *and* sirypis, *and* swetesmellyng *and* emplastres. And a-mong all*e* herbys, þe moost p*ro*fitabyl bien mynte, *and* wermot, *and* rewe. And ȝif þe humo*urs* bie*n* colric, lat p*ur*gyn hym also. *And* siþe ȝif hym soure met*es* *and* coolde. And eu*er*ych*e* defaute of appetyt þ*at* comeþ of euel co*m*plexiou*n* of þe stomac, as of to greet heete oþ*er* of to gret coold, schal bie heelid bie þe contrarie, as ȝif it is of heet it moyst bie heelyd by colde medicynes.

Defaute of þurst comeþ in four*e* man*er*es, oþ*er* of euel humo*urs* þ*at* bie*n* in þe stomac þ*at* bie*n* coold *and* moiste. And þ*at* is j-heelyd ȝif þe stomac is j-purged of þilke humo*urs* *and* siþe is j-feed wiþ good driȝe met*es* *and* leueþ moist met*es*. And let hy*m* vse*n* hoot electuaries *and* driȝe, as diat*ri*onpip*er*on. And late hy*m* vsyn hoote sauces in his mete | *and* no vinegre. Also it comeþ of gret coold of þe stomac, f. 98v
and þ*at* is j-helyd by hote medicyines. And þis defaute of þurst comeþ of feblenesse of þe stomac *and* of corupciou*n* of þe felyng of þe stomac, *and* þis is in-curable *and* tokene of deeþ. And it comeþ of lesyng of a ma*n*nes wit that makeþ hym lesyn boþe appetit to mete *and* to drynk. And þis may bien holpyn ȝif þe man is brouȝt in-to his wit a-ȝeen.

Mjche þurst comeþ in many manerys, oþ*er*while of gret hete of þe breest, oþ*er*while of þe metys þ*at* a ma*n* eteþ, oþ*er*while of hete of þe eir, oþ*er* of mych*e* trauayle. Þurst þ*at* comeþ of þe stomac is in two man*er*es: Oþ*er* for to hoote metis *and* to-kene þ*at* a ma*n* haþ j-etyn; oþ*er* for corupt humo*urs* þ*at* bien in þe stomac as colre, oþ*er* salt flewme.

10 **Defaute**] *2-line space left for initial* 16 **and**] *prec. by heading* Thurst 19 **þe**[1]] *interl.* 22 **a-ȝeen**] *follow. by* h*abet* ille (*added in a different hand*) 23 **Mjche**] *2-line space left for initial*

And ȝif þis þurst come of colre, þe mouþ is hoot *and* bitt*ere*, *and* na*m*ly aft*er* þ*at* a ma*n* haþ j-dru*n*kyn coold wat*er*. And he may j-felyn how þe smoke comeþ vp in-to his þrote. And ȝif it is of salt flewme, he xal j-fele saltnesse in his mouþ. *And* his þurst is j-kelyd þorowe drynckynge of warm wat*er*. And ȝif it comeþ of heete, coold wat*er* wole stau*n*che*n* it. Þurst þ*at* comeþ of hete of þe breest is raþ*er* j-stau*n*chyd þorow drawyng breþ of coold eire þa*n* þorow eny drynck. f. 99r Naþeles, ȝif sich*e* gret þurst come | of corupt humo*urs*, oþ*er* in þe stomac, oþ*er* byneþe in þe guttes, oþ*er* in þe breste a-boue, let p*ur*ge*n* hi*m* wiþ a medicyne þ*at* is a-cordyng to þe humo*ur*. And ȝif it comeþ of mych*e* blood, let hy*m* bledyn. And siþe ȝif hym coold siripis, as of gourdys oþ*er* of violet w*ith* sugre, oþ*ere* þe muscilage of p*er*silie wiþ þe sirip of violet. And norysche hym w*ith* tysane, *and* purselane, letuse, vinegre, *and* blites. And late hym bie in reste, boþe of body *and* of spekyng. *And* late make þe eir*e* coold w*ith* coold þi*n*ges, as it was j-seid in þe cardiacle. And late make hym a plastre of gourdys, portulake, *and* of sych*e* oþ*ere* coold þi*n*ges.

Good pillules to hoolde vnd*er* a ma*n*nes tu*n*ge þ*at* haþ gret þurst for hete, *and* þei bie*n* goode for men þ*at* goon ouere contrey *and* han no wat*er* to dryncke, *and* þei bien good for me*n* þ*at* han þe feuerys, *and* þei bien þ*us* j-maad: Tak of dragg*e* *and* of þe seed of purselane, *dragme* iij; of þe seed of gourdys, of melou*n*, *and* of letuse, *dragme* ij; of sau*n*drys *and* of gu*m* arab*e*, *dragme* ij. Poudre al þese *and*

9 come] *f. 99r* | me of] *prec. by heading* Thurst **18 it**] *follow. by canc.* w **27 arabe**] *corr. from* arabeik (ik *exp.*)

21 hoolde] *in r.-h. margin:* no*ta* opti*me* Sp (*underl.*)

te*m*pre it w*it*h wat*er* of rosees. *And* make balles oþ*er*e pillules þ*er*-of as gret as a bene. *And* lat hem ligge*n* vnd*er* his tou*n*ge tyl þei bien molten. And ȝif þe þurst come of colre þ*at* is in þe stomac, let purge*n* hy*m* [wiþ sum] cologoge *and* make hym casten. And siþe ȝyf hy*m* þe sirip of violet, oþ*er*e þe muscilage of p*er*sillie, | oþ*er*e þe seed of citonyes. f. 99v

A good sirip þ*at* stauncheþ a ma*n*nys þirst, *and* makeþ hym moist, *and* co*n*forteþ þe stomac to defiȝen his mete: Take of violet, xx *dragme*; of plu*m*bes, of i*n*nibes, of oxifistula, *dragme* c*ent*; of spodie, *dragme* ij. Seeþ al þis in viij pound of wat*er* til it come to iij pownd. *And* þa*n*ne cle*n*se it *and* cast þ*er*-to a powund of þe iuys of swete pomegarnadis. Anoþ*er* good dryncke for þe same: Tak of driȝe rosees, *dragme* v; of oxifistula, *dragme* v; of cassia fistula, *dragme* ij; of þe seed of citonyes, of dragg*e*, *dragme* ij; of fenel seed, *dragme* j. Do al þis in ij *pound* of hoot scaldyng wat*er* al a-niȝth, *and* on þe morwe ȝif hy*m* to dryncke þ*er*-of fastyng *pound* s*emis*. But ȝif þe þurst come of salt flewme, ȝif hi*m* a p*ur*ga-ciou*n* *and* siþe late hym dri*n*cke þe wat*er* þ*at* fenel seed *and* march seed bien j-soden i*n*ne. And ȝeue hym to dryncke mellicrate j-medlyd w*it*h warm wat*er* oþ*er* good smal whiȝt wyn. Dietyng of hym xal bie good met*es* þ*at* bien nat salt. And ȝif a ma*n* is a-þurst a-niȝth, late hi*m* slepe *and* þ*at* wole kele his þurst, or ellys ȝif hym dryncke.

Bolkyng: Su*m* is smoky *and* hoot, *and* su*m* is sowr*e*. Þe furst comeþ of hete *and* of hote humo*ur*s þ*at* bien in þe stomac. Þe secu*n*de is of coolde hum*ur*os oþ*er* of feble heete

6 oþere[2]] *prec. by heading* Bolkyng **14 cassia fistula**] *corr. from* cassiafistula **24 hym**] *follow. by canc. and oblit.* di **25 Bolkyng**] *2-line space left for initial* **and**[1]] *follow. by canc. and exp.* su*m*

of þe stomac. For bolkyng þat comeþ of heete *and* of colric humo*urs* in þe stomac, let p*ur*gyn hym, and siþe late hym vsen coolde þi*n*ges boþe in medicines *and* also in hese dieti*n*ge. And let hym vsyn coold electuaries, as þe coold f. 100r dyacitonyto*n*, | triasendri, diarodon abbatis, sugre roset, *and* sug*re* violet, *and* þe sirip of roses *and* þe sirip of violet j-maad vp w*ith* vinegre. And here dietyng xal bie of met*es* *and* dryncky s þ*a*t bien nat ful hoot, as chyken, *and* partriches, *and* smale birdys, *and* scalyd fischȝ, *and* wyn j-medlyd w*ith* wat*er*, *and* coold frytis, *and* coold a-noynti*n*ges a-boute þe stomac, *and* coolde plastres j-leid þ*er*-to, *and* a te*mp*e*r*at baaþ naþ*er* to hoot ne to coold. But ȝif þe bolkyng comeþ of cold of þe stomac, it may bie in two man*ere*s: Oþ*er* of coold humo*urs* þ*a*t bien in þe stomac *and* makeþ þe stomac swelle, *and* heuy, *and* makeþ a ma*n* delyuere wynd by-neþe-forþe, or ellys it comeþ of cooldnesse of þe stomac wiþ-owtyn sich*e* humo*urs*. And þ*a*t greuau*n*ce is j-holpy*n* by hoote medicynes *and* w*ith* hoote oyneme*nt*es *and* em-plaistris. And ȝif þ*er* wex mych*e* wynd boþe a-bove *and* be-neþen, make hym a poudre of mastik, comyn, louage, anyse, gyng*er*, carawey, long pep*er*, *and* sich*e* oþ*ere* þi*n*ges.

A good medicine for bolkynge *and* to destriȝe corupte wyndes of þe stomac: Tak of mastik, comyn, louage, anise, fenel seed, squinant, gyng*er*, carawey, ameos, amoni*e*, sileris mo*n*tane, long pep*er*, ȝedware, galyngale, oȝymi, calame

1 For] *corr. from* ffor **2 siþe late**] *corr. from* siþelate **5 dyacitonyton**] *interl.* nyto*n* **triasendri**] *prec. by heading* Bolkyng **8 hoot**] *follow. by canc.* as ciky **24 seed**] *follow. by canc.* s

22 bolkynge] *in r.-h. margin:* C | no*ta* bene

aromatik, cassia lignea, maces, maiorane, of eu*ery*ch*e*, j-lyche myche. Poudre he*m* *and* medle he*m* w*ith* | hony roset. f. 100v

A good electuarie foor cooldnesse of þe stomac, *and* for wyndes, *and* for soure bolkynges, *and* for vnresonabil appetit, *and* makeþ a ma*n*nes mouþ j-wel j-saueryd, *and* is þus j-maad: Tak of canel, *and* of long pep*er* *and* of blak, of clowes, lignu*m* aloes, cassie, citre, spik, asa*rum*, sq*ui*nant*e*, gali*n*gale, calam*us* aromatic*us*, carpobalȝamu*m*, ȝilobalȝamu*m*, ameos, *and* of gyng*er*, *dragme* iij; of sugre, *dragme* iiij; of mastik, *dragme* j; of aristol[ogie] þe rou*n*de, of polie, of lycoryis, *dragme* iiij *and* s*emis*; hony, *quantum* s*ufficit*.

A good poudere for me*n* þ*at* bie*n* discoleryd *and* han feble siȝt *and* digestiou*n*: Tak canel, gynger, cardamom*e*, pep*er*, sauereie, maiorane, anyse, fenel, carawey, netle seed, gali*n*gale, eufrace, of eu*ery*ch*e*, *dragme* s*emis*; of note-muge, sq*ui*nant*e*, folie, *dragme* ij; of citre, *dragme* j *and* s*emis*; of yren clene j-waisch*e* *and* j-dried, *dragme* ij. Let hy*m* vsen þe poudre þ*at* is j-maad of alle þese j-medlyd to-gidere in hys metys *and* drynkys.

A good sirip *and* an hoot, for coldnesse of þe stomac, *and* for sowre bolkyngys of þe stomac, *and* for wy*n*dys of þe stomac: Tak xx *pound* of wat*er* *and* do he*m* in a *pound* of reysyns, of calamynte, mynte, *and* nepte, of eu*ery*che of he*m*, *ounce* iij. *And* lat alle þese bie*n* a day *and* a nyȝth in þ*at* wat*er*. Aft*er*ward, clense þat wat*er* *and* do þ*er*-to x *pound* of

2 hony] *prec. by heading* Bolkyng **10 aristologie**] *corr. from* aristol*e* **15 netle**] *interl.* t **16 eueryche**] *follow. by exp.* j-lich*e* mych*e* **21 of þe**] *corr. from* ofþe

21 A] *in l.-h. margin:* no*ta*

f. 101r hony. And seeþ þ*at* wel | ou*er* an esy fyer. Aftyr-ward, cast þi poudre þ*er*-to. Tak of mastik, cardamom*e*, blac pep*er and* long, of eu*er*ych*e*, *dragme* iij *and* s*emis*. *And* poudre hem *and* medle þis poudere w*i*t*h* þe wat*er*. *And* do hony þ*er*-to *and* kep it.

Diasp*er*mat[ic]on is good for heuynesse of þe heed, *and* turnyng of þe brayn, *and* for aky*n*g *and* sqwellyng of his chekys, *and* for siky*n*ge, *and* strei3tnesse of breþi*n*ge, *and* narweschipe of þe breste, *and* for me*n* þ*at* han j-lost here speche, *and* for ache of þe stomac *and* hardnesse, *and* sowre bolkynges, *and* for a feble stomac þ*at* may nat holden his mete but casteþ it up oþ*er* lat it passe down vndefi3eid, *and* is good also for þe splene, *and* for greuau*n*ce of þe mod*er*, *and* is þus j-maad: Tak of long pep*er*, *dragme* ix; of gyng*er*, *dragme* viij; of carawey, of louage, *dragme* vj; of p*er*sily, macedo, ameos, femygrek, dauk, siler*e* montayne, amoni*e*, comyn, march seed, fenel seed, anyse, *dragme* ij; hony, *quantum* s*ufficit*. Anoþ*er*e diasp*er*mat[ic]o*n* þ*at* is good for swellyng of þe wo*m*be *and* for he*m* þ*at* mow nat wel defi3en here mete: Tac carawey, anyse, cardamom*e*, canel, ameos, march*e*, *dragme* iij; of pep*er*, *dragme* iij; of sugre oþ*er* of hony, *quantum* s*ufficit*.

3ixi*n*ge comeþ in many man*er*ys, oþ*er*while of excesse of etyng oþ*er* of drynckynge þ*at* makeþ þe stomac to ful. *And* þ*at* may bie in two man*er*es, for all*e* þe stomac may bie
f. 101v to ful of mete, oþ*er* þe mouþ of þe stomac mai bie to | full

1 ouer] *prec. by heading* 3ixyng **3 of**] *follow. by* of **4 And**] *follow. by canc.* cast þ*er* do **5 kep it**] *corr. from* kepit **11 holden**] *interl.* l **23 ixinge**] *2-line space left for initial* **26 full**] *prec. by heading* 3yxyng

12 mete] *in r.-h. margin:* no*ta*

and syche ȝixynges comyn aft*ur* mete. *And* me*n* stau*n*chyn it in makyng a ma*n* a-gast, oþ*er* a-schamyd, oþ*er* riȝt glaad, oþ*ere* ȝif he piȝt his fyng*er* depe in his mouþ *and* holdiþ hym þere a whyle. Oþ*er*while ȝixi*n*ge comeþ of corupt humo*urs* þ*at* bie*n* in þe stomac *and* makeþ þe stomac feble. *And* þis ȝixi*n*ge comeþ raþere by-fore mete þa*n* aft*er*. *And* it is j-holpen ȝif þe stomac bie j-p*ur*gyd of þilk humo*urs* bi castynge, oþ*er* a-noþ*er* purgaciou*n* þ*at* is a-cordy*n*g to þe humo*ur* þ*at* is enchesou*n* of þe ȝixi*n*ge, and siþe in noryschynge þe ma*n* w*ith* goode met*es* *and* wiþ goode drynckys *and* leuyng surfetes. Oþ*er*while it comeþ of cooldnesse þ*at* is in þe ou*er* part of þe stomac þ*at* makeþ þ*at* party han a cra*m*pe, *and* is vnmyȝtty to delyueryn hym of þe corupt humo*urs* þ*at* bien in þe stomac. Oþ*er*while it comeþ of a-ventesyng *and* of feblenesse of þe stomac. *And* þat may bie in two manerys: Oþ*er* of colric humours þ*at* han longe j-leyn in þe stomac *and* j-maad þe stomac feble, oþ*er* of su*m* oþ*er* sicnesse þ*at* haþ j-feblyd þe stomac, as of flux oþ*er* of a feu*ere*. And wha*n*ne it is of a feuere, it is p*er*ilouse. But ȝif þe stomac is j-feblyd *and* ȝixiþ of a long flux þ*at* a ma*n* haþ j-haad, þ*o*u xalt diete*n* þ*at* ma*n* w*ith* co*n*fortabyl þi*n*ges, as w*ith* þe brooþ of an hoot henne or a capou*n*. And ȝyue hym electuaries þ*at* wole*n* make hy*m* moist w*ith*-i*n*ne-forþ, as dyapenydyon *and* diadragantou*n*. *And* ȝyue hym | f. 102r tysane to drynck, *and* þe sirip of violet wiþ þe muscilage of p*er*silye, *and* þe seed of citonyes. And make a plastre to liggen on his stomac of lynseed [and] of femygrek j-soden in oile. And anoynte þe stomac w*ith* þe oile of violet *and* of roses, *and* w*ith* þe muscilage of p*er*silye, *and* þe iuys of citonyes. And

1 **aftur**] *follow. by canc. twice and exp.* w **24** **hym**] *catchword* (*in bottom margin*): tysane to drynck **tysane**] *prec. by heading* ȝyxyng

ȝif þe ȝixi*n*ge come of kene metys, þe same þi*n*ges bien profitable. And late hem þ*a*t han ȝixi*n*ge of a-ventisynge of þe stomac vsen sugre roset *and* coold herbys *and* moiste, as purselane, *and* letuse, *and* cheries, *and* soure plu*m*bes, *and* sich*e* oþ*er*e. And weet a clooþ in warm wat*er* þ*a*t violet *and* hockes bien j-soden i*n*ne, *and* leie þ*a*t cloþ fro*m* þe mouþ of his stomac dou*n* to his me*m*bris *and* to his sydis. And make hy*m* a plastre of lynseed j-soden in wat*er*. *And* siþe cast þ*er*-to oile of violet, *and* woma*n*n*es* mylk, *and* sych*e* oþ*er* þi*n*ges, as þe rote of hocke *and* þe holy-hocke, *and* ley þ*a*t plastre on his stomac. And ȝif it comeþ of humo*ur*s þ*a*t filleþ þe stomac *and* þe humo*ur*s bien hoote, make hi*m* þis sirrip: Tak þe rot*es* of fenel, *and* of p*er*sili, *and* of wermot, hertistonge, endyue, comyn, raw silk, spicnard. Stampe hem to-gidere *and* seeþ hem in wat*er*. *And* make vp þi sirip *and* ȝif it hym to dryncke. Aft*er*ward purge hym w*it*h su*m* sirip þ*a*t is laxatif or w*it*h su*m* oþ*er* p*ur*gaciou*n*. And siþe ȝif hym coolde þi*n*ges boþe in medicines *and* oþ*er*wyse. But ȝif it be of coold humo*ur*s, ȝif hi*m* oximel componed. And siþe ȝif hy*m* a p*ur*gaciou*n*. And ȝif hym þe iuys of wermot w*it*h sugre *and* hony, oþ*er* aloes, oþ*er* castore w*it*h þe iuys of mynte, oþ*er* pyt þ*er*-to mastik, oþere þe watere þat carawei is
f. 102v j-sode*n* i*n*ne w*it*h | rwe, oþ*er* rwe w*it*h hony, nat raw, but soden w*it*h hony, and siþe ȝif hym hoot electuaries And make a stufe for þe stomac of wyn þ*a*t þese þi*n*ges bie*n* j-soden i*n*ne: origane, souþ*er*newode, calamy*n*te, samsuke, rwe, mynte, *and* sich*e* oþ*er*e. And of þe herbis make a plastre *and* lei on þe stomac. Anoi*n*te also þe stomac w*it*h oile of lorere, oþ*er* w*it*h su*m* oþ*er* sich*e* hoot oile. And ȝif he bie repleet of

23 rwe[1]] *prec. by heading* ȝyxyng

blood, lat hi*m* bleede. *And* ȝif hym cassia fistula w*ith* warm wat*er*, oþ*er* w*ith* þe iuys of a po*m*me-garnade. And ȝif þe stomac bie hard, tak dates, *and* cast a-wey þe stones, *and* powne þe re*m*nawnt w*ith* freisch grece. *And* make a plastre þ*er*-of *and* lei vp-on his stomac. Jt is good also for ȝixi*n*ge þ*at* comeþ of heete oþ*er* of coold, and siþe co*n*forte þe stomac as it was j-teeld bi-fore. *And* make hym to smelle wele to a brent clooþ. And make hi*m* ete wel *and* dri*n*ke also. And ȝif ȝixi*n*ge comeþ of coold of þe stomac w*ith*-owtyn sich*e* humo*urs*, it wole bie liȝtlych*e* j-holpe as þorow drynckyng of warm wyn *and* a-noyntynge of hoote oynement*es* w*ith*-owte-forþ. *And* lat all*e* here met*es and* here dryncky s bie warm. Fnesi*n*ge also stau*n*chiþ þis ȝixi*n*ge, *and* oksynge also þ*at* comeþ of to myche etynge *and* dryncky nge. And pillules þ*at* bien j-maad of aloes, *and* mastik, *and* þe iuys of wermot bien gode here also. Oþ*er* ȝif hi*m* to dri*n*ke wyn þ*at* rwe is j-soden i*n*ne j-medlyd w*ith* hony, oþ*er* þe seed of march, oþ*er* of caraway, oþ*er* anyse, oþ*er* calamynte, oþ*er* souþ*er*wode, oþ*er* reubarbe, oþ*er* gyng*er*, oþ*er* eny hoot electuarie þ*at* we han spoke of bifore. And | lat a-noi*n*t hym w*ith* hote oiles, f. 103r
as of lorer*e and* siche oþ*er*e. And ȝif ȝixi*n*ge come of kene met*es* þ*at* a ma*n* haþ j-etyn, let hym dry*n*ke coold wat*er*, oþ*er* þe sirip of violet, oþ*er* of plu*m*mes. And þu mytest stau*n*che euery man*er* ȝixi*n*ge ȝif þ*o*u makest a ma*n* wel a-ferd, and þorow fnesynge, *and* ȝif men byndeþ fast his hondys *and* his feet. Also ȝif a ma*n* holdeþ his breeþ, his ȝixi*n*ge wole cesse. A good poudre for corupt wyndys of þe stomac: Tac of fenel seed, *pound* j; of ameos, anet, carawei, *pound*

13 Fnesinge] *corr. from* ffnesi*n*ge **20 lat**] *prec. by heading* Castyng

27 for] *in r.-h. margin:* no*ta* C

s*emis*; of ysope, piliole, origa*n*, calami*n*te, *ounce* j; of cardamom*e*, of canel, *ounce* s*emis*; of folie, of gyng*er*, *dragme* ij. Mak poudre of al þis *and* ȝif hy*m* w*it*h oþ*er*e met*es* *and* bi hym-selfyn also.

Castyng *and* spewynge *and* wille for-to caste comeþ of corupt hum*ur*es þ*at* bie*n* in þe stomac. *And* of sich*e* corupt hum*ur*es þ*at* bie*n* in þe stomac comeþ a-noþ*er*e g*r*euau*n*ce þ*at* is abho*mi*n*a*cio*u*n *and* wlati*n*ge of mete *and* of dry*n*ke, for siche corupt hum*ur*es, ȝif þei bie*n* in þe mouþ of þe stomac, þei destryen a ma*n*nes appetit. And ȝif þei bien w*it*h-i*n*neforþ in þe stomac, þei ma-ken þe stomac feble þ*at* he may nat defieȝe*n* þe mete þ*at* he reseiueþ. *And* þese ij enchesouns maken a ma*n* to wlatyn hese mete *and* haue wil for-to caste. And ȝif þese hum*ur*es bien in þe mouþ of þe stomac, þa*n* a ma*n* xal caste liȝtlych*e* *and* delyuere hy*m* of þilke hum*ur*es. And ȝif þei bien by-neþeforþe, he xal caste w*it*h more greuau*n*ce. But ȝif þei bien in þe porys of þe stomac, a ma*n* xal wha*n*ne he haþ g*r*et wyl to caste, caste but f. 103v a lytil, *and* þ*at* xal bie w*it*h gret | greua*n*ce. And ȝif þei bien w*it*h-i*n*ne or betwynne þe ij skynnes of þe stomac, a man xal haue g*r*et wille to caste, but he xal cast no-þing. *And* þis is clepid nausea. Þese bien þe gret greuau*n*ces of þe stomac þ*at* comeþ of corupt humo*ur*s. But ȝif colrick me*n* han abho*mi*n*a*cio*u*n to mete þorouȝ sich*e* corupt humo*ur*s, vnneþe þei mou*n* bie heelid, but fleu*ma*tik men mou*n* lytly. And þei han wille to caste *and* mown cast wele, þat is a good tokene, for þa*n*ne þe corupt humo*ur*s bie*n* in þe stomac, *and* mou*n* liȝtlych*e* bie j-browȝt owt. But ȝif a ma*n* wlateþ his mete

5 Castyng] *2-line space left for initial* **8 for**] *corr. from* ffor **10 a mannes**] *corr. from* ama*n*nes **19 greuance**] *prec. by heading* Castyng **20 man**] *follow. by canc.* x **27 for**] *corr. from* ffor *and* haþ wille to caste *and* mai nat, þ*at* is a feble tokene, for þa*n*ne þe humo*urs* bien in þe porys of þe stomac, oþ*er* by-twene þe ij skynnes of þe stomac. And oþ*er*while þese g*r*euau*n*ces come*n* of distemperyng of þe stomac w*ith*-owte sich*e* corupt hum*ur*os. And oþ*er*while þei come*n* of hoote humo*urs* *and* oþ*er*whiles of coold. 3if þe greuau*n*ce comeþ of hoote humo*urs* þ*at* bien in þe stomac, þe mouþ of þe stomac is heuy *and* hoot, *and* þ*er* is p*r*ickyng a-boute þe mouþ of þe stomac, *and* þe mouþ is bitt*er*, *and* þei han an hoot bolkyng. But ȝif þe stomac is distemperid w*ith* heete *and* haaþ noon siche hum*ur*es, a ma*n* xal haue alle þe forseid signes *and* heyuynesse of þe stomac. And ȝif þese greuau*n*ces bie*n* of coold hum*ur*es, þe stomac is heuy *and* coold, *and* þe mouþ is vnsauery, *and* his bolkyng is soure. But ȝif þe stomac is but distemperyd w*ith* coold *and* ne haþ noon corupt hum*ur*es in hym, þa*n*ne he xal haue alle þe forseid signes, saue heuynesse of þe stomac. | f. 104r

And of þis sicnesse comeþ akyng of þe heed, scotomye, *and* turnyng of þe brayn, leesyng of appetite, feblenesse of all*e* þe body; and wha*n* þei han j-ete, þan þei bien ful feble. And oþ*er* þei han a flux, oþ*er* a gret wille to caste. And ȝif siche corupt hum*ur*es bien be-twine þe ij skynes of þe stomac, wheþ*er* þei bien hoote oþ*er* coold, þei han þe for-seid signes, saue ȝif þe hum*ur*es bien coolde *and* bien a-boute þe mouþ of þe stomac, þei make*n* a ma*n* to haue appetit to mete. But wha*n*ne he haþ j-ete, it makeþ hym to haue wille for-to caste. Castynge comeþ oþ*er*while of feblenesse of þe stomac, *and* comynly þa*n*ne a man haþ more wille to casten aft*er* mete þa*n* bi-fore. And þis feblenesse may be in ij man*er*es,

1 for] *corr. from* ffor **18 And**] *prec. by heading* Castyng

oþ*er* of þe ouer*e* party of þe stomac, oþ*er* of þe neþere party. And ʒif þe feblenesse bie of þe ou*er* party of þe stomac, a ma*n* xal cast liʒtly þe mete þ*at* he haþ last j-ete. But ʒif it bie of [þe] neþere party, he xal cast w*ith* gret greuau*n*ce þ*at* mete þ*at* he haþ furst j-ete. And in all*e* þese sicnesses þ*at* comeþ of corupt hum*ur*es, it is p*ro*fitabil to caste *and* to p*ur*ge þe stomac of corupt hum*ur*es. And ʒif þe hum*ur*es bien colric, make hym caste by-fore mete, *and* na*m*ly ʒif þe hum*ur*es byn nat in þe porys ne by-twene þe ij skynnes. And þu myʒtest make hym caste w*ith* esy medycines, as w*ith* tisane, mellicrate, oþ*er* w*ith* warm wat*er*; oþ*er* sta*m*pe þe seed of arage, *and* radich, *and* rapes to-gidere, *and* seþe hem to-gidere in wat*er*. *And* late hym dryncke þat. Oþ*er*: Tac þe iuys of lilye rotys, *and* salge*m*me, *and* mete oile, of eu*er*ych*e*, j-
f. 104v lyche myche, *and* lat hym dryncke | þ*er*-of fasti*n*ge. But ʒif þe humo*ur*s bien in þe medle of þe stomac, oþ*er* in þe grownd, oþ*er* in [þe] porys, oþ*er*e ʒif þe humo*ur*s bien viscouse, it is bet*er*e to cast aft*er* mete þa*n* bie-fore. And ʒif þese greuau*n*ces comen of an hoote distemp*er*aunce of þe stomac w*ith*-owtyn humo*ur*s, it suffisiþ too coold wat*er*. But ar þan þu ʒyue a ma*n* þese medicines for-to caste, late furst defie þe humo*ur*s þ*at* bie*n* in þe stomac, ʒif þei bien colric, w*ith* þe sirip of violet or w*ith* sirip of vinegre, *and* w*ith* herbis, as hockys, *and* blites, *and* arage, *and* siche oþ*er*e. And ʒif þ*er* bie mych*e* mat*er*e þ*at* heueþ þe stomac mych*e*, make a plastre w*ith*-owtyn of hockys, *and* of radich, *and* of þe holy-hocke, *and* of beetis, *and* of lynseed. *And* lei þe plastre bi-

3 liʒtly] *follow. by* and **8 namly**] *follow. by canc.* by **15 þer-of**] *prec. by heading* Castyng **17 grownd**] *follow. by exp.* of þe **oþer in**] *in r.-h. margin* **24 blites**] *corr. from* blitess (first s *interl.*; last s *oblit.*) **25 make**] *follow. by canc. and exp.* þa

fore on þe stomac, *and* by-hynde on þe rugh, of hockys j-stamped *and* j-friȝed in grece. And a-noynte his breste w*ith* dewte *and* w*ith* bot*er*e ij daies, or iij, or more, ȝif it nedeþ er þu make hym to caste. And wha*n*ne þ*o*u wult make a ma*n* cast aft*er* mete, late hym eete rootes *and* fruyt aft*er* his oþ*er* mete. And siþe w*ith*-i*n*ne ij houres aft*er* mete, make hym caste. But ȝif þese g*re*uau*n*ces come*n* of coold hum*ur*s, furst to defie þilke hum*ur*s ȝif hym oximel squillitik oþ*er* oximel of radich iij daies to-gidere. And siþe make hym cast wiþ þe iuys of radich, oþ*er* of walwort, oþ*er* of serpe*n*tarie þ*at* wole slee an addre in a ma*n*nes wombe, oþ*er* þe iuys of spurge. Oþ*er* ȝif hym nedeþ stre*n*gere medicinys, ȝyue hym þe iuys of gourdys, oþ*er* þe iuys of lesse centorie. But for su*m*folk ne | mow nat receyue*n* sych*e* strong medicines to make hem f. 105r casten, it is nedeful to telle of su*m* þi*n*ges þ*at* wole make a ma*n* to caste*n* ȝif þei bien anoi*n*ted on his bodi w*ith*-owtyn. And oon siche medicine is: Tac þe galle of what beest þ*at* þe likeþ *and* a-noi*n*te a ma*n*nes body fro þe nauele upward: He xal haue delyuerau*n*ce by-neþe. And þe same kynde haþ ierarufa. And ȝif þu a-noi*n*tist þe ou*er* lacertys of a ma*n*nes arme w*ith* þe drastys of oile, he xal caste. And ȝif þu a-noi*n*test þe neþ*er* lacert*es*, he xal go to pryuei.

An oyneme*n*t laxatif w*ith* who*m*, ȝif þ*o*u a-noyntest a ma*n*nes stomac, he xal caste, *and* ȝif þu a-noyntest his nauele, he xal go to pryuei, and ȝif þu a-noi*n*test þ*er*-wiþ his reynes bi-hynde, it wole make hy*m* costyf: Tac þe rote of electarie,

14 mow] *prec. by heading* Castyng 23 **An oynement**] *corr. from* Anoyneme*n*t

10 þat] *in l.-h. margin:* no*ta* **18 þe**] *in r.-h. margin:* no*ta* **20 And**] *in r.-h. margin:* no*ta*

dragme vij; of coconydie, of scamonye, *dragme* ij; of þe iuys [of] titymalle, *dragme* v; of turmentyne, *dragme* iiij; of ciclame*n*, *dragme* iiij; of elebor*us* nig*er*, *dragme* vj; of hony, *quantum* s*ufficit*.

A-noþ*er* oyneme*n*t w*ith* whom ȝif þu a-noi*n*tist a ma*n*nes hondys it wole make hym caste*n*, *and* ȝif þu a-noi*n*test his feet, it wole make hym to haue sege, and ȝif it delyuereþ of to mych*e* mat*ere*, a-no*n*cte his fete *and* his hoondys w*ith* popilion: Take peletre of spayne, *and* elebor*us* nig*er*, hermodactiles, henbane, accoru*n*, þe iuys of syngrene, *and* of brionye, of þese, j-lych*e* mych*e*, *and* medle he*m* w*ith*
f. 105v swyn*es* grece. | And ȝif þu maist nat make a ma*n* to cast for no-þing, make hym a p*ur*gaciou*n* to delyuere hym by-neþeforþ aft*er* þe kynde of þe humo*ur* þ*at* neyeþ þe stomac. As ȝif it bie of colre, ȝif hym a cologoge of mirab*e* ci[tri], oþ*er* reub*e* w*ith* þe iuys of plaunteyne. Ȝif it bie of flewme, ȝyue hi*m* a fleu*ma*goge of mirab*e* ke[be] oþ*er* yerapigra w*ith* þe iuys of calamynte. Ȝif it bie of male*n*colie, ȝif hi*m* a malagoge of mirab*e* ind[i], oþ*er* diacene, oþ*er* su*m* sych*e* oþ*ere*. And aft*ur* his p*ur*gaciou*n*, wheþ*er* it bie a-bouyn or by-neþen, conforte þe stomac w*ith* co*n*fortabyl metis, *and* drynckys, *and* electuaries, *and* siripis, *and* poudrys, *and* a-noi*n*tyngys w*ith*-owtyn-forþ, w*ith* hoote oyneme*ntes* oþ*er* coold, aft*er* þe kynde of þe humo*ur* þ*at* greueþ þe stomac.

A ful good oyneme*n*t boþe for þe stomac, *and* for stoppyng of þe lyuere, *and* also of þe splene: Tak þe fatnesse þ*at* hangeþ w*ith*-owtyn-forþ vp-on scheepis legg*es* *and* drie it in þe caniculere daies in þe su*n*ne. *And* siþe medle it w*ith*

3 iiij] *follow. by dragme* iiij **9 peletre**] *corr. from* pieletre (i *exp.*; first e *interl.*) **10 syngrene**] *corr. from* syngrenee (first e *oblit.*; last e *interl.*) **12 And**] *prec. by heading* Stawnch*e* **nat**] *follow. by exp.* cast for oile *and* þ*er*-wiþ a-noynte þe stomac. Oþ*er* seeþ þ*a*t fatnesse w*it*h schepis wolle þ*a*t is j-schore vnwasche *and* plastre þ*a*t wolle bi-fore þe stomac. And a ful good sirip for þis g*r*euau*n*ce of þe stomac is j-maad of þe iuys of mynten j-clarefied *and* siþe j-cast þ*er*-to sugre aft*er* þe q*ua*ntite of þe lico*ur*.

A good emplastre is for þe stomac of mastic, *and* rooses, *and* myntes j-stampid to-gidere, oþ*er* þe iuys of myntes, and vi*n*eg*r*e, *and* sowr breed.

To lette a man to caste but oþ*er*whiles it is needful | to f. 106r
lette a ma*n* to caste, for so longe a ma*n* miȝt vsen it, þ*a*t it xuld bie ful hard to destrie it. And þ*er*for*e* it is profitabyl to telle medicines to stau*n*chyn castynge. Fyrst, lat p*ur*gen þe stomac of þe humours þ*a*t make hym cast. And ȝif he is costyf, make hym neische j-wombyd. And ȝif his on þe flux, stoppe hym w*it*h su*m* st*ri*ctories. And diete hy*m* w*it*h met*es* þ*a*t wole make a ma*n* costif, as w*it*h barlich*e* breed, *and* rosteed met*es*, *and* chekens, *and* partriches, *and* sich*e* oþ*er*e. *And* late hym vse vinegre for sause and siþe ȝif hym a sirip const*ri*ctif. And make hym a plastre strictorie of mynt*es*, *and* of co*n*firie, *and* mastik, *and* vinegre, *and* cytonies, *and* sowr bred, *and* reyn-wat*er* þ*a*t goold is ofte siþes j-que*n*chyd i*n*ne ceessiþ casti*n*g. And ȝif þe stomac bie feble *and* þe sekenesse oold, make hym a sirip of clowes, *and* notemuge, *and* canel, *and* lignu*m* aloes, *and* mastik, *and* mynte, *and* spodie, *and* accacie, *and* sich*e* oþ*er* þi*n*ges. Oþ*er* ȝif þe greuau*n*ce bie of hoot humo*ur*s, tak mastik *and* lei it on an hoot tyyl, *and* siþe

8 of… breed] *interl.* **9 breed**] *interl.* last e **10 To**] *2-line space left for initial* **to**[2]] *prec. by heading* of castyng **11 to**] *interl.* **for**] *corr. from* ffor **13 Fyrst**] *corr. from* ffyrst **22 j-quenchyd**] j *follow. by exp.* soden; que*n*chyd *in l.-h. margin*

lei it on his stomac al warm. And seeþe galles, rooses, *and* myntes, *and* þe rynde of an ook in vi*n*egre. *And* þ*er*-i*n*ne wete a spou*n*ge of þe see *and* lei it al warm to his stomac. Oþ*er* make a plastre of bole, *and* mastik, *and* sau*n*dragou*n* diste*m*perid w*it*h þe whi3t of an ey. Oþ*er* late hym dry*n*ke wat*er* of roses þ*at* poudre of mastik is j-sode*n* i*n*ne. Oþ*er* make a plastre of meele, *and* of þe iuys of mynten, *and* of rooses, *and* of plau*n*teyne, *and* vi*n*egre. And 3if it bie of coold, mak hym a poudre of comyn, *and* of baies of lorere,
f. 106v *and* mastik, *and* olibanu*m*. | And a-noynte hys stomac w*it*h oile of lorere, oþ*er* comyn oile, þ*at* piliole haþ bie j-soden i*n*ne. And þe forseid sirip of myntis is good for all*e* þese g*r*euau*n*ces. And 3if castyng comeþ of feblenesse of þe stomac, let hym vsen confortabil þi*n*ges. And 3if it comeþ of to myche etyng, late hy*m* vse abstine*n*ce þ*at* is þe moost sou*er*eyn medicyne. *And* late hym caste aft*er* þ*at* he haþ mych*e* j-ete. And 3if he casteþ blood, it be-tokeneþ breche of su*m* veyne of þe stomac oþ*er* of su*m* oþ*er* place. And þa*n*ne 3if a ma*n* bie ful of blood, let hym blood. Oþ*er* ellys let cuppen hym on his þi3es oþ*er* on his leggis. And siþe late 3yue hym calamynte to dryncke j-soden w*it*h gotis mylk and oþ*er* medicynes þat were j-teld in spetyng of blood bien good here. 3if a ma*n*nes stomac bie myche j-feblid bie longe abstine*n*ce *and* fasti*n*ge, let diete*n* hym w*it*h co*n*fortabil metis, *and* dryncKes, *and* electuaries. *And* make hym leuyn all*e* þe ocupaciowns of his sowle, but it bie myrthe or gladnesse. And late hy*m* vsen a plastre on his stomac of mynten, aloes, mastik, *and* wermot, of eu*er*yche, j-lyche myche. *And* stampe hem *and* medle hem w*it*h oile of rosees,

9 **lorere**] *corr. from* lorerer (last r *canc. twice*) **10** **And**] *prec. by heading* Stoppyng of vomyte

and leie to þe stomac. And ofte-siþes ano*n*cte his stomac w*ith* oile of rooses. *And* let hym vsen a powdre j-maad of clowes, *and* galynggale, canel, gyng*er*, maces, quybibes, *and* lignu*m* aloes, amonye, calam*us* aromatic*us*, storac*e*, cara[b]e, *and* anet, of sugre, as myche as of all*e* þe oþere. *And* let hym vsen | at his mete þe wheiȝte of a *dragme* of þe poudre. f. 107r

The mouþ of þe stomac is oþ*er*whiles j-turned vp-so-down *and* makeþ a ma*n* to haue a co*n*tinuel wille to caste. And þis comeþ of an awhood colrik humo*ur* þ*a*t is in þe stomac, *and* wha*n*ne he meueþ vpward, he draweþ oþ*er* humo*urs* w*ith* hym. Oþ*er*while it comeþ for þe mouþ of þe stomac is feble, *and* þe botme is strong to pyt owt þe hum*ur*os þ*a*t bie*n* in hi*m*. Ȝif it comeþ in þe furst manere, þ*o*u most ȝyue hy*m* coold þi*n*ges in medicines to destrie þilke hoote colric humo*urs*. And ȝif it comeþ in þe secu*n*de man*ere*, it is p*ro*fitabil aft*ur* his oþ*er* metis þ*a*t he vse fruytis þ*a*t wole make hym coostif. *And* let hym ete lytil, *and* dri*n*ke lityl, *and* traueile litil. And let make*n* hym a plastre on his stomac of mastic *and* of mynte. *And* let hym eten þe lymail of goold w*ith* an ey, oþ*er* late hy*m* drync wat*er* oþ*er* wyn þ*a*t goold haaþ ofte siþes bie*n* j-que*n*chid i*n*ne. Oþ*er* mak hy*m* þis plastre: Tak galbanu*m*, *and* oppoponak, *and* serapinu*m*, *and* ammoniak, *and* lei hem in vi*n*egre al nyȝth. *And* aft*er*ward seeþ hem ou*er* þe feer. *And* þa*n*ne cast þ*er*-to mastik, olibanu*m*, coost, mirre, sandragou*n*, notemuge *and* put þis in a clooþ, *and* leie on his stomac. Oþ*ere* medicines þ*a*t were*n* j-told for castyng bie*n* good for þis sicnesse.

4 carabe] *corr. from* caralke **5 as**[1]] *in l.-h. margin* **myche**] *prec. by* as (s *oblit.*) **6 at**] *prec. by heading* Stomak **7 The**] *2-line space left for initial*

Oþ*er*while þe neþ*er*er parte of þe stomac is febler*e* þa*n* þe
f. 107v ou*er* part *and* for feblenesse is t*ur*ned vp-so-down. | And þis comen of two enchesou*ns*, as of gret abstinence oþ*er* of gret surfet. Ȝif it bie of gret abstinence, he most bie co*n*forted bie co*n*fortabil metis *and* drynckys *and* medicines. Ȝif it bie of surfeet, he most cast, þ*at* he bie delyu*er*ed of þe corupt humo*ur*s þ*at* bien in his stomac. Siþe he mote bie rewlid w*it*h abstine*n*ce *and* w*it*h reste. And siþe ȝyue hym electuaries *and* oþ*er* medicines to co*n*forte wel þe stomac, þ*at* he mow wel defiȝen his mete. And make a plastre of galles *and* of plau*n*teyne. And late hym vsen metis *and* electuaries þ*at* bie*n* of kynde to make a ma*n* coostif, as it xal bie toold whan we spekyn of þe flux.

Ache of þe stomac comeþ oþ*er*whiles of hete, oþ*er*while of coold. *And* þ*at* is in ij man*er*es: Oþ*er* of corupt hum*ur*os þ*at* bien in þe stomac, oþ*er* of a distemperyng of an heete oþ*er* of coold w*it*h-owte*n* sich*e* hum*ur*os. Tokenes of heete bien a smart ache, þurst, fulnesse, hoot bolkyng þ*at* brenneþ þe roof of þe mouþ, and hoote met*es* *and* drynk*es* encresceþ þe ac[h]e. His vrine is of an heiȝ coloure. And ȝif þ*er* bie hoot corupt hum*urus* in þe stomac, his mouþ is bitt*er* *and* he haþ wille for-to caste. And þ*at* þ*at* passeþ fra*m* hym at his fou*n*dement is forbrent. And þese han oon man*er*e cure, saue ȝif þat þ*er* bie corupt hum*urus* in þe stomac, þe stomac mote furst bie p*ur*ged of he*m*, *and* siþe haue oþ*er* medicines to a-
f. 108r bate*n* þe heete.| But ȝif þe ache comeþ of coold, he bolkeþ

1 **þe**[1]] *corr. from* þere (er *canc. twice*) **feblere**] *follow. by canc. twice* þat **þan þe**] *in r.-h. margin* **2 And**] *prec. by heading* Ache **5 confortabil metis**] *corr. from* co*n*fortabilmetis **14 Ache**] *2-line space left for initial* **18 fulnesse**] *corr. from* ffulnesse **26 But**] *prec. by heading* of the stomak

ofte, *and* hoote metis co*n*forten hym, *and* coold met*es* greuyn hym. And ȝif þ*er* bie*n* coold hum*ur*os in þe stomac, his bolkyng is sowr*e*, *and* þ*a*t he casteþ is fleu*ma*tik *and* so his dirt is also. And oþ*er*-while, wha*n* þe ache comeþ of coold w*it*h-owte*n* sich*e* corupt hum*ur*os, a ma*n* is costif. But þese hum*ur*os mown bien oþ*er*while bitwixe þe to skynnes of þe stomac, oþ*er*whiles in þe porys of þe stomac, oþ*er*whiles in þe stomac, as jt was j-teld bi-fore. Oþ*er*while ache of þe stomac *and* of þe guttes comeþ also comyn of corupt wyndys þ*a*t bien in he*m*, *and* is j-knowe bie noise *and* hurlyng in þe wombe. And wha*n* þei bien delyuered of sich*e* wynd*es*, þei bien mych*e* j-liȝtid. *And* þei bolken mych*e*, but þei bien nat delyuered of noon corupt hum*ur*os. And in þis same man*er*e comeþ ache in a ma*nn**es* guttes. And riȝth as þe stomac may bie j-greuyd w*it*h thre man*er*e hum*ur*os, þ*a*t is to seie, w*it*h colre, flewme, *and* male*n*colie, riȝt so þe guttes mown. But wha*n* þe stomac is j-greuyd bie ony of þese hum*ur*os, me*n* may j-know bi what humo*ur* it is bi þ*a*t þat j-haþ bie told bi-fore. And ȝif þe guttes bie*n* j-greuyd be ony of þese hum*ur*es, men xal j-knowe of what humo*ur* it is bie a ma*nn**es* drit; for of kyndlych*e* flewme comeþ whiȝt drit *and* þi*n*ne; of glasi flewme comeþ whiȝt drit *and* þicke, w*it*h mych*e* flewme j-medlid þ*er*-wiþ. And but ȝif a ma*n* bie þe raþer j-holpen, he xal | fallen in-to a flux oþ*er* in-to a-noþ*er* f. 108v greuau*n*ce of þe guttes þ*a*t is j-clepid colica passio. Of salt flewme comeþ pale drit *and* þi*n*ne. Of swete flewme comeþ drit þ*a*t is naþ*er* riȝt þicke ne riȝt þi*n*ne, *and* þei feelen heete in here guttes. Of sowre flewme comeþ driȝt þ*a*t haþ mych*e*

1 **ofte and**] *corr. from* ofte*and* 11 **wyndes**] *follow. by exp.* hum*ur*os
18 **it**] *follow. by exp.* is 19 **bien j-greuyd**] *corr. from* bie*n*j-greuyd
21 **for**] *corr. from* ffor 24 **fallen**] *prec. by heading* Ache

fome *and* many belles, *and* þei bie*n* blake oþ*er*whiles *and* oþ*er*whiles swart ȝelwe, *and* þei feelyn coold in here guttes. Of colre þ*a*t is in þe guttes þe tokenys bien: Þe dryȝt is citryne oþ*er* grene, *and* þei felyn hete, *and* smertyng, *and* biti*n*g in here gutt*es*, *and* þei bie*n* þirstful, *and* here mouþ is driȝe. And but þei bie*n* þe raþ*er* j-holpe*n*, þei xul fallen in-to a blodi flux. Of malencolie, þe toknes bie*n* swart ȝelwe driȝt oþ*er* blak, myche noyse *and* [h]urlyng of wy*n*d*es* in þe gutt*es*, *and* coold. Oþ*er*while þis ache comeþ of apostym in þe stomac þ*a*t is nat wel j-heelid. Oþ*er*while it comeþ of etyng of su*m* sory metys. Oþ*er*while þe stomac akeþ *and* swelleþ, for þe driȝt is j-hardid in a ma*nn*es wombe. Oþ*er*while ache *and* swellyng comeþ of þe dropesy. Ȝif it comeþ of hoot corupt hum*ur*os, let p*ur*ge þe stomac of þilke corupt hum*ur*os as it haþ be teld her*e* bie-fore w*it*h myrabol*e* oþ*er* reub*e*. Aft*er*ward, boile hockes in oile of violet *and* lei it

f. 109r to þe stomac. Oþ*er* tac þe iuys of si*n*grene *and* of penywort, | *and* a-noynte a clooþ þ*er*-wiþ, *and* lei it to þe stomac. Oþ*er* make a plastre of whiȝt sau*n*drys *and* of reed, *and* of oile of rooses, *and* vi*n*egre j-medlid to-gidere, *and* of spodie, *and* of barlych*e* mele, *and* ca[m]phore, *and* þe iuys of sy*n*grene. Oþ*er* a-noynte þe stomac w*it*h oile of rooses *and* oile of violet. And of electuaries, let hym vsen t*ri*asendri, *and* oximel sympel, *and* stomaticon þat is coold. *And* let hym vsen coold siripis, as of violet *and* wat*er* also þ*a*t þe sedis of coold herbis bien j-soden i*n*ne. Also seeþ þe iuys of plau*n*teyn tyl þe halfendel bie j-sode*n* a-wey. *And* make it vp in þe

4 **and biting**] *in l.-h. margin* 8 **hurlyng**] *corr. from* burlyng 17 **penywort**] *f. 109r* | nywort 18 **and**[1]] *prec. by heading* of the stomak 19 **reed**] *follow. by canc.* and 20 **to-gidere**] *follow. by* oþ*er* of whiȝt sau*n*dris *and* of reed **spodie**] *follow. by canc. and*

man*er* of a sirip, *and* pit þ*er*-to a lityl reubarbe *and* let hym dryncke þ*er*-of. And it is good to dryncke a good q*ua*ntite of cold wat*er and* siþe make hym caste. And a-noynte þe pawmes of here hondis *and* þe sooles of here feet w*ith* oile of violet, oþ*er* of rosees, oþ*er* popilion, oþ*er* w*ith* vynegre j-spreynt on hem. And let vse to etyn purselane *and* oþ*er* coold herb*e*. But ȝif þis comeþ of coold hum*ur*os, let a-noynte þe stomac w*ith* hoote oyneme*nt*es. And let seeþe p*er*it*er*ie in whiȝt wynne *and* leggen it al warm to þe stomac, *and* ofte-siþes renewe it. And ȝif þ*er* is eny wyndy mat*er* in her*e* stomac, it is p*ro*fitabil to setten an horn oþ*er* a cuppe on þe stomac wiþ-owtyn garsynge. And ȝif he bie a riche ma*n*, let | hym dryncke bawme, oþ*er* let hym dryncyn of þe f. 109v gu*m*me of an yuy tre þe q*ua*ntite of þre peses at onys. And make hym a plastre of mastik, *and* of olybanu*m*, *and* of þe baies of lorere, *and* of oile j-medlid to-gidere. Calamynte is also ful p*ro*fitabil for he*m*, *and* a plastre j-maad þ*er*-of; *and* of rewe *and* of hony j-soden to-gidere is ful good al-so. And so is a plastre of rewe *and* of origane j-soden i*n* hony. And let hem vsyn diasp*er*mat[ic]on, *and* dyacymynu*m*, *and* diamargariton. And let seeþe aue*n*ce w*ith* his rotes *and* sauge in whiȝt wyn *and* þ*er*-w*ith* let stufen hys wombe. *And* let hym drynckyn of þ*a*t wyn. And þis is good ȝif a ma*n*nes stomac akeþ for dri*n*ckyng of coold wat*er*. And let hi*m* vsen a powdre j-maad of comyn, *and* canel, *and* coliau*n*dre seed. And let hy*m* drynckyn wyn medlyd w*ith* wat*er*. Oft vse þei hit þ*a*t fenel seed, *and* p*er*sely seed, *and* mastik, *and* olibanu*m* han bien j-soden i*m*me. And þe same medicynes þ*a*t

2 good[2]] *in r.-h. margin* **3 cold**] *corr. from* coldd (last d *interl.*) **6 on**] *interl. and follow. by exp.* of **let**] *follow. by canc. twice* h **13 hym**[1]] *prec. by heading* The stomak **23 þat**] *corr. from* þate (e *canc. and exp.*)

destriȝen þese wyndes destreiȝen sowre balkynges. And for swellyng of þe stomac, tak þe seed of rewe, *and* þe baies of a lorere tree, *and* þe seed of p*er*silie, *and* of march, *and* of caraway, of dauk, hemlok, *and* of p*er*itorie. *And* stampe all*e* þese *and* seþe he*m* in a lytil wyn tyl þe wyn bie co*n*sumid. And siþe cast þ*er*-to a lytil oile of lorere, oþ*er* of rewe, oþ*er* of anet, oþ*er* of pilyole. *And* make þ*er*-of a plastre *and* lei on his stomac. And let hy*m* vsen electuaries as dyacyminu*m*, dyasp*er*mat[ic]on, *and* siche oþere.

f. 110r A good dryncke also for swellinge | of þe stomac *and* for-to destreiȝen sich*e* corupt wyndis: Tak of fenel seed, comyn, anyse, *dragme* vj; þe longe astrolog*e*, squynant, carpobalsame, *dragme* iij; of calami*n*te, spik, ameos, spodie, *dragme* ij; of maces, gyng*er*, clowes, *dragme* j. Stampe alle þese togydere *and* seeþ hem in iij *pound* of þe iuys of fenel. *And* siþe cast þ*er*-to a q*ua*ntite of sugre. And of þis dry*n*c late hym drync þe weiȝte of *dragme* iij at oones.

Diacalamentu*m* is good also for coold of þe stomac, *and* for wynd*es*, *and* for eu*er*y g*r*euau*n*ce of þe breste þat comeþ of coold, *and* na*m*ly for olde men, *and* for he*m* þ*a*t han þe coold couȝe. And it is þus j-maad: Tac of calamynte, of piliole, of melanopip*er*, si-sileos, of p*er*sili, *dragme* iij *and dragme* ij; of louage, *dragme* j *and dragme* j; of ameos,

1 **balkynges**] *interl.* l 7 **make þer-of**] *corr. from* makeþ*er*-of 10 **swellinge**] *f. 110r* | linge; *catchword* (*in bottom margin*): lyng of þe stomac **of**] *prec. by heading* The stomak 17 **þe**] *follow. by canc. twice* q*ua*

1 **balkynges**] *in l.-h. margin:* for the swell | ing of the stomack (ck *interl.*) **18 stomac**] *in r.-h. margin:* no*ta*

thyme, anet, canel, gyng*er*, *dragme* j; of hony, *quantum* s*ufficit*.

Diacitonyton hoot þ*a*t is good for castynge, *and* for corupt wynd*es* þ*a*t bien in a ma*n*nes body, *and* co*n*forteþ a ma*n*nes kyndly heete of his body. *And* is good for men þ*a*t han a neische wombe. *And* is þus j-maad: Take citonyes *and* seeþ he*m* wel in wat*er*. *And* siþe pile of þe rynde *and* make hym clene w*ith*-i*n*ne-forþ also. And to iiij *pound* of hem cast iiij *pound* of despumed hony i*n* a morter *and* stampe hem wel to-gidere. Siþe boyle it ou*er* þe feir til it wex þicke *and* stere it eu*er*-more til it bie wel j-soden. Þe tokene þ*er*of is so þicke þat it wole nat goo þorouȝ a st*re*yno*ur* ne þorow ne clooþ. But lat it nat bie ropi in þe mouþ as glew is, but schort in þe mouþ. | And wha*n*ne it is so, set it dou*n* of þe f. 110v fier*e* *and* medle þ*er*wiþ þese powdres w*ith* a sklice: Tak of canel, *dragme* j *and* s*emis*; of gyng*er*, *dragme* j; of pep*er*, of gali*n*gale, *ounce* s*emis*; of clowes, of notemuges, *dragme* iij; of spik, of lignu*m* aloes, of maces, of cardamomu*m*, *dragme* ij; of ȝedeware, *dragme* s*emis*, *and* tempre it w*ith* a lityl musk. And ȝif þu wylt make*n* it laxatif to eu*er*ich*e* powdre þ*er*-of, put *dragme* s*emis* of scamone, *and* wha*n*ne it is coold, medle he*m* wel to-gidere. *And* lat he*m* vse*n* here-of aft*er* mete *and* aft*er* sopere.

Diacitonyto*n* þ*a*t is coold is þus j-maad: Tak of citonyes þ*a*t bien j-maad clene as j-seid raþ*er*e *pound* j *and* s*emis*; of rooses, of sau*n*drys, *dragme* iij; of reubarb, of lycorys, of þe seed of purselane, of letuse, *dragme* j; of clowes, of canel, *dragme* s*emis*; of anyse, of gyng*er*, of þe sirip of rosees,

14 **And**] *prec. by heading* Aposteem **19** **lityl musk**] *corr. from* litylmusk

quantum sufficit. Make þis as þe oþ*er* was j-maad *and* at þe laste pit þ*er*-to a pounde of sugre.

Apostym is oþ*er*while in a ma*n*n*es* stomac *and* þ*a*t may bie in diu*er*se wysis, for oþ*er*whiles he is w*i*t*h*-i*n*ne þe stomac, oþ*er*whiles w*i*t*h*-outyn, oþ*er*whiles bitwyne þe to skynnes of þe stomac. Ʒif it bie w*i*t*h*-i*n*ne þe stomac, ar þa*n* þe postym bie rotyd, su*m* of þe mat*er* comeþ owte bie casti*n*ge. *And* wha*n* þe postym haþ j-cauȝt is roote, he is myche j-heuyed aft*er* mete. Ʒif þe postym bie w*i*t*h*-owtyn, þe swellyng is a-seene w*i*t*h*-owtyn. *And* þei he casteþ, þ*er*
f. 111r comeþ no-þi*n*g fra*m* þe stomac | þ*a*t bie-tokeneþ þe postym. Wha*n* he is bie-twyn þe to skynn*es*, he feleþ heuynesse *and* g*r*euau*n*ce in þe stomac w*i*t*h*-outen þese oþ*er* signes. And þese postem*us* come oþ*er*while of hoot corupt hum*ur*os, oþ*er*while of coold. Ʒif þe postym bie of hoot corupt hum*ur*os, oþ*er* it is of colre, oþ*er* of blood. Ʒif it is of colre, he feleþ gret heete *and* bre*n*ny*n*g, *and* mych*e* leepi*n*g, *and* heuynesse in his stomac, *and* his mouþ is driȝe *and* bitt*er*, *and* his herte foileþ hym ofte-siþes, in-so-mych*e* þ*a*t he falleþ a-down as þei he were j-swou*n*nyd. *And* þei ha*n* mych*e* greuau*n*ce boþe to swelewe *and* to drawe breeþ, *and* comynly þei han a feu*er* tercian þ*er*-wiþ. Ʒif it is of blood, it haþ þe same tokenys but þei bien nat so violent. But ȝif þe postym come of coold hum*ur*os, oþ*er* it is of flewme, oþ*er* of male*n*colie. Ʒif it bie of flewme, þe postym swelleþ mych*e* *and* is neisch*e*, *and* he feleþ mych*e* heuynesse in his stomac, but is ache is nat ful gret *and* he haþ lytyl þirst or noon. *And* þei spottyn mych*e* *and* all*e* here body is heuy *and* slow, *and* alle here wytt*es* bien stoneied *and* j-dulled as þ*a*t þei

3 Apostym] *2-line space left for initial* **4 for]** *corr. from* ffor **11 þat]** *prec. by heading* in the stomak

hadde litargie, *and* þei han an esy feu*er*e. But ȝif þe postym bie of male*n*colie, he feleþ mych*e* hardnesse in his stomac. *And* þe mat*er* of þe postym is gaderid to-gidere *and* mych*e* heuynesch*e* þei feelyn also. *And* þei han a sowr bolkyng *and* þei feelyn mych*e* greuau*n*ce in here | stomac. Þei mown [f. 111v] slepyn but a lytyl for a gret corupt wynd þ*a*t smyteþ vp in-to here heed. And wha*n* þe postym*us* bien in þe botme of þe stomac, þei febelyn þe stomac ful myche, so þ*a*t oþ*er*while þe stomac may nat hoolde þe mete þ*a*t haþ receyued, *and* þa*n* þilke me*n* han a co*n*tinuel flux. Oþ*er*whiles þe stomac is so feble þ*a*t he may nat wel delyuere hym of þ*a*t mete þ*a*t is in hym, *and* þa*n* a ma*n* is co*n*tinuellych*e* costyf.

Ȝif þis postym come of heete, let hym blede at his arme, ȝif he haue grete plente of blode. And siþe let dieten hym w*it*h couenabyl met*es*, as w*it*h letuse, purselane, *and* gourdys, endyue, blet*es*, *and* þe clensyng of breen, almau*n*d mylk, *and* w*it*h þe iuys of ciceres, *and* þe colyis of a chekyn *and* of partriches *and* oþ*er* smale briddes. And late he*m* etyn walsche-nootys *and* make hym grewel w*it*h goot*es* whey. And lat hym etyn perys, *and* applys j-soden, *and* chasteyns nat hard, but neische. And ȝif hym þe sirip of rooses, oþ*er* of violet, oþ*er* of þe iuys of solatre *and* of scariole, w*it*h cassia fistula *and* wiþ manna. And wha*n* þei bien wel j-soden, cast þ*er*-to su*m* sugr*e*. And lei coold rep*er*cussyues wiþoute*n*-forþ in-to þe vij dai. And anoi*n*te hi*m* w*it*h oile of rooses, oþ*er* of violet, oþ*er* of myrtes, oþ*er* of wat*er*-lilies, *and* w*it*h þe wat*er* of rooses, *and* w*it*h þe iuys of plau*n*teyn, *and* of letuse, *and* of purselane, *and* of pymp*er*enelle, | *and* of turmentille, *and* [f. 112r]

5 stomac] *prec. by heading* Aposteem **16** of] *follow. by* bryn breen] *in l.-h. margin* **28** and[2]] *prec. by heading* in the stomak

violet, *and* solatre, *and* of saffren, of eu*er*ich*e* of þese, take j-lych*e* mych*e*. *And* medle he*m* wel to-gider*e* *and* þ*er*-wiþ a-noi*n*te þe stomac. And weet cotou*n* oþ*er* a lyne*n* clooþ þ*er*-i*n*ne *and* lei it on þe stomac. And twies renew it in þe wyntris day *and* þries in þe som*er* dai. Anoþ*er* ful p*ro*fitable: Tak of saffren, of me-my[t]he, acacie, alfice, þe iuys of mynte, spodie bole, *dragme* v; of oile of roses, *quantum* s*ufficit*. Tempr*e* he*m* to-gider*e*. Also in þe bi-gy*n*ny*n*g of sich*e* apostym, make a plastre of sau*n*dris, rooses, vi*n*egre, *and* of oile. Ley þat on þe stomak. But ȝif þe mat*er*e mowe nat bie re[m]ewid from her*e* place bie þese coold plastres, þu most make plastres to make þe postym rype, as it was j-teld in þe chapitre of þe sq*ui*nance. Oþ*er* make a plastre of barly mele *and* of ȝelkys of eyren. Oþ*er* make a plastre of hockys *and* grou*n*deswily, *and* hoolyhockys, *and* swynes grece. But ȝif þe postym bie of coold, let diete*n* hym w*ith* temp*er*at hoot metis. *And* make hy*m* potage of þe clansyng o[f] breen *and* of almau*n*d mylk, oþ*er* mylk of noot*es*. Oþ*er* make hym a colyis of chekenys, oþ*er* furme*n*te, oþ*er* riȝs j-maad w*ith* almau*n*d mylk. And rooste he*m* good applen *and* fille he*m* w*ith* sugre. And make he*m* þis sirip: Tak a lityl spik *and* as mych*e* of asaru*m*, anise, anet, oȝimu*m*, yreos, femygrek, horsel, caperus, calam*us* aromatic*us*, cassia lignea, mastik,
f. 112v mynte, | wermot, *and* fenel seed, of eu*er*ich*e* of þese, ix

1 **of**[1]] *follow. by* safren **saffren**] *interl.* 6 **me-mythe**] *corr. from* me-myche 11 **remewid**] *corr. from* renewid 17 **of**[2]] *corr. from* ob 21 **as myche**] *corr. from* asmych*e* 24 **wermot**] *prec. by heading* Aposteem **fenel**] *corr. from* ffenel **þese**] *follow. by exp.* j-liche mych*e*

16 **postym**] *in r.-h. margin:* no*ta*

dragme. Seþe all*e* þese in wat*er and* cast þ*er*-to *pound* j of sugre. *And* lat hym vse þis sirip boþe in forme of medicine *and* of drynk. And let hym no blood but ȝif he haue riȝt grette plente of blood. But tac merch seed, dauk, comyn, anyse, fenel seed, spik, sq*ui*nant, baume, maiorane, lynseed, femygrek, mastik, cardomomu*m*, q*ui*bibes, aloes, cassia lignea, camomylle, þe fleisch*e* of dates, of ou*er*ich*e* of þese, j-lych*e* mych*e*. And wiþ þis wat*er*, waisch*e* þe wombe bi-fore þe stomak, and weet wolle in þ*at* wat*er*, *and* lei on his stomac. And pit all*e* þese herbis þ*at* bien j-soden in a ly*n*nen bagge *and* lei to þe stomac. Oþ*er* tak myrre, *and* bedelliu*m*, *and* alloes aroma[ti]c, hoolihocke, wermot, drie figges, femigrek, *and* grece, of eu*er*ich*e*, j-lych*e* mych*e*. *And* medle hem w*ith* þe iuys of march, *and* a lytil iuys of cool, *and* w*ith* bot*er*e. Also tak satureie *and* ambrose *and* stamp hem to-gidere w*ith*-outen eny oþ*er*e liquor*e*. *And* lei þ*er*-of a plastre on þe stomac *and* ofte-siþes renewe it. Oþ*er* tac lilie rot*es* *and* beet*es* *and* medle hem wiþ wyn *and* wiþ oile in a mortere. *And* siþe warm it *and* plastre þ*at* on hys stomac. Oþ*er* tak beenes *and* do a-wey þe hoole. *And* seeþ þe re*m*nau*n*t in wyn *and* oile *and* leie to his stomac. And wha*n*ne þe postym | is to-broke, þu muste vse f. 113r
mu*n*dificatyues to clense þe stomac of quiture. Tokene of þ*at* brekyng is þ*at* quiture brekeþ a-wey fro*m* þe stomac. And wha*n* þe postym is wiþ-i*n*ne þe stomac, þe q*ui*ture passeþ a-wei by-neþe, oþ*er* a-boue þorou þe mouþ. And ȝif it is wiþ-owtyn, it passeþ forþ by-neþe also. And ȝif he is by-twynne

5 fenel] *corr. from* ffenel **15 satureie**] *interl.* first e **19 on**] *follow. by exp.* þe **hys**] *interl.* **22 is**] *prec. by heading* in the stomak **25 is**] *follow. by* wiþ þe (wiþ: þ *oblit.*; þe: *canc. twice*) **wiþ-inne**] *in r.-h. margin:* wiþ w*ith*-i*n*ne þe skynnes of þe stomac, þa*n* þe q*ui*ture passeþ a-wey w*ith* þe vrine. And for-to clense þe stomac of þis quiture, seeþ barlich*e* in goot*es* mylk. *And* siþe clense it *and* seþe þ*er*-i*n*ne dragagant, *and* gu*m* arab*e*, licoryis, penides, horsel, orobus, reisenes, yreos, xilobalȝamu*m*, *and* sugre. And ȝif þe q*ui*ture greueþ hy*m* sore wha*n* it passeþ a-wei fra*m* hym, ȝif hym triacle wiþ wat*er* þ*at* is j-sod*en* i*n*ne, a-iij daies or iiij. Also to make hy*m* clene, ȝif hy*m* meeþ by hy*m*-seelf, oþ*er* j-meedlyd w*ith* wyn, oþ*er* w*ith* salt *and* þe poudre of nytre. And ȝif he bie j-purgid bie his vrine, ȝif hym of þe medicines þ*at* bien j-teeld in stranguria. And siþe, ȝeue hym co*n*solidatyues to souden þat place þ*at* is j-broken, and reyn-wat*er* þ*at* myr[t]ell*e* *and* galles bien j-soden i*n*ne j-medlyd w*ith* sugre. And wiþ-oute, lei plastr[e]s þ*at* bie*n* st*ri*ctories, as it xal bie told in þe flux.

Stomaticon þ*at* is coold is good for all*e* vnkynde heet*es*
f. 113v of a ma*n*nes stomac | *and* que*n*cheþ a ma*n*nes thurst. *And* is þus j-maad: Tac of sugre, *pound* j; of sau*n*dris whiȝt *and* of reed, *dragme* j *and* *semis*; of spodie, of þe seed of purselane, of scariole, of þe seed of melou*n*, of þe iuys of licorys, of rooses, of violet, of wat*er*-lilies, *dragme* j. Take þe forseid sugr*e* *and* put it in a ti*n*nen vessel ou*er* þe fier*e* w*ith* a pou*n*d of roose wat*er*, *and* let it seþe tyl þe wat*er* bie wasted a-wei. And siþe cast in þe powdre of all*e* þese oþ*er* þi*n*ges *and* stire it wel wiþ a sklice. *And* tak a lityl þ*er*-of *and* leie on a boord oþ*er* on a ston. And ȝif it bie so hard þ*at* þu mai kyt it esily

3 barliche] *follow. by exp.* of **in**] *interl.* **10 of**[1]] *follow. by canc. twice and exp.* þe **13 myrtelle**] *corr. from* myrcell*e* **14 plastres**] *corr. from* plastros **17 and**] *prec. by heading* Stomak **23 water bie**] *corr. from* wat*er*bie

w*ith* a knyf, þanne it is j-soden j-now. Let hym vse þ*er*-of þe morwetyd *and* at mydday w*ith* coold welle wat*er*.

Stomaticon þat is hoot is co*n*fortabil for þe stomac *and* helpeþ to defyen a ma*n*nes mete. *And* is profitable for þe greuau*n*ce þ*a*t is i*n*ne þe ou*er* guttes of a ma*n*n*es* wo*m*be. *And* is þus j-maad: Take of sugre, *pound* j, *and* of wat*er* as myche; of canel, of gyng*er*, *dragme* ij; of clowes, of gali*n*gale, *dragme* j; of notemuge, of spik, of lignu*m* aloes, of cardamom*e*, of maces, *dragme* s*emis*. Make it as þe oþ*er* was j-maad. And ȝif þu wolt haue it laxatif, cast þ*er*-to *ounce* j of scamone w*ith* þe oþ*er* poud*res*. Anoþ*er* stomaticon þ*a*t is laxatif: Tak of clowes, *dragme* iiij; of cardamome, of gyng*er*, of notemuge, of gali*n*gale, *ounce* j; of sugre, j *pound*; of scamone, *ounce* ij. Make it as þe oþ*ere* was maad.

Colides is a greuau*n*ce of þe stomac oþ*er* of þe guttes þ*a*t makeþ a man | haue so gret wyl to schite þ*a*t hym schal f. 114r
seme þat he xuld schite owt hese guttes. And ȝif it bie in þe stomac, it makeþ a ma*n* boþe caste *and* schite. And þis greuau*n*ce comeþ oþ*er*whiles of corupt humo*urs* þ*a*t bien in þe stomac oþ*er* in þe guttys, and þ*a*t may bie of colre oþ*er* of flewme. Ȝif it is of colre, it is ful violent *and* ful p*er*ilouse *and* w*ith* greet hete. Ȝif it is flewme, it is nat so p*er*ilouse. Oþ*er*whiles it comeþ of to myche etyng *and* drynck*y*ng; oþ*er*whiles for a ma*n*nys wombe haþ j-leyn on-hillid, *and* cauȝt coold in his sleep; oþ*er*while it comeþ of etyng of kene met*es*. But where-of-eu*er* þis sicnesse comeþ, þ*o*u xalt nat

5 a] *follow. by canc.* v **14 oþere…maad**] *interl.* **15 Colides**] *2-line space left for initial* **16 haue**] *prec. by heading* Or guttys **22 flewme**] *corr. from* fflewme

13 ounce] *in l.-h. margin:* S

encrescyn his fluxe ne his casti*n*ge, for þ*a*t xuld make hym more feble. But þ*o*u xalt ȝiue hy*m* co*n*fortabil met*es and* medicines þ*a*t bien st*ri*ctories. But þ*o*u xalt nat bie*n* a-bowtyn to stau*n*chy*n* hym sodenly, ne no man*er* of flux, but esily, for drede of more perel. And þ*er*fore let hy*m* vsen sugre roset, *and* diarodon abbat*es*, *and* rosata nouella. And [if] colric hum*ur*os bien enchesou*n* of þis sicnesse, let a-noynte hy*m* w*it*h coold þi*n*ges. *And* let bathy*n* hy*m* in a baþ to cessen his flux, as it xal bie teld in þe chapitre of þe flux. But ȝif it comeþ of coold, let hym vsen an electuarie þ*a*t is j-clepid dianthos, oþ*er* ȝinȝiber*e* alexand*ri*nu*m*. *And* ȝif hym þe sirip of mynte *and* make hy*m* a baaþ of myntes *and* of oþ*er* herbys þ*a*t bien hoote *and* st*ri*ctories. And ȝif it comeþ of heete, lete hy*m* dry*n*cke þe sirip of rooses. And ȝif þe ma*n* f. 114v is stro*n*g | of co*m*plexiou*n* þ*a*t haþ þis sicnesse, wheþ*er* it bie of hete oþ*er* of coold, þu muste ȝyue hym esy medicines to make hym caste, as meeþ j-medlid w*it*h a lityl warm salt-wat*er and* a litil oile. And late a-noi*n*te hy*m* w*it*h oile of rosees ȝif it comeþ of heete; ȝif it comeþ of coold, w*it*h su*m* hoot oynement*es*. Mynte is ful p*ro*fitabil for þis sicnesse ȝif it comeþ of coold, and for alle coold greua*n*nces of þe stomac: Medle þe iuys þ*er*-of w*it*h warm wat*er* ȝif it comeþ of heete; w*it*h wyn ȝif it comeþ of coold. And lat he*m* þ*a*t han þis sicnesse dryncke no coold wat*er* but ȝif þei han a ful gret lust *and* desire þ*er*-to, *and* ȝit ȝif hym but a lityl þ*er*-of. But ȝif þe flux bie of an hoot colric humo*ur*, þ*o*u myȝtest sauely let hym dryncke coold wat*er*. And so þ*o*u myȝtest ȝif a ma*n*n*es* lyuere is diste*m*p*er*ed w*it*h hete and in dissent*er*ie

15 of] *prec. by heading* Stomak

also. And ȝif alle þese helpeþ hy*m* nat, ȝif hy*m* good t*ri*acle, for þ*at* stau*n*cheþ eu*er*y flux.

A good plastre ȝif þ*at* sicnesse comeþ of heete: Take spodie *and* barly mele, *and* te*m*pr*e* hem w*ith* þe whiȝte of an ey *and* w*ith* þe iuys of plau*n*teyn *and* of mynten. *And* leie þ*at* plastre fra*m* þe mouþ of þe stomac down to hys preuy membrys. *And* on þe same man*er* lei it be-hynde on hys bakke. But ȝif it comeþ of coold, make a plastre of spodie *and* whete mele j-te*m*perid w*ith* þe iuys of mynte. *And* plastre it fra*m* þe mouþ of þe stomac downward boþe by-hynde *and* by-fore. And fore þis sicnesse is violent *and* draweþ þe mari owt of a manys bonys *and* wasteþ hys kyndly moostnesse, | it be-houeþ to stau*n*che þe flux as sone as men f. 115r
mai in feire manere, as it xal bie teld in þe chapitre of þe flux. And it is nedful to ȝyue*n* hym co*n*fortabil metys *and* medicines to restoryn hym hys kyndly moistnesse as it is j-teeld in þe feu*er* etik, for mych*e* of his moistnesse is j-wasted þorow violence of þe for-seid flux.

Jn a ma*n*nes guttes *and* of a ma*nn*es gutt*es* þ*er* bie*n* many sicnessis: Þe flux *and* a[n]-oþ*ere* g*r*euau*n*ce þ*at* is j-clepid colica passio, *and* wormes bie*n* j-gendryd also in a ma*nn*es gutt*es* þ*at* greueþ a ma*n* ful mych*e*. Anoþ*er* greuau*n*ce is wha*n* a ma*n* may nat schyte *and* ȝit he haþ gret wil þ*er*-to. Anoþ*er* g*r*euau*n*ce is wha*n* þe gutte þ*at* gooþ to a ma*nn*es fu*n*deme*n*t falleþ owt þ*er*-ate. Fluxes, þ*er* bie*n* foure man*ere* of kyndes. Oon is j-clepid dissent*er*ie, *and* þ*at* is

13 it] *prec. by heading* Or guttys **16 j-teeld**] *corr. from* j-teeldin (in *canc. and exp.*) **17 myche of**] *in l.-h. margin* **19 Jn**] *2-line space left for initial* **25 Fluxes**] *corr. from* ffluxes

1 helpeþ] *in l.-h. margin:* no*ta* b*e*n*e*

wha*n* a ma*n* schiteþ blood j-medlid w*ith* þe schauy*n*ge of his gutt*es*. Anoþ*er* flux is wha*n* þe blood passeþ fra*m* a ma*n* w*ith*-owtyn sich*e* medlyng, *and* þat is clepid þe blodi flux. Anoþ*er* þ*er* is þat is j-clepid a sympil flux, *and* þat is wha*n* a man is delyuerid of þat þat is in his wombe sone aft*er* þat þat it is defied, but it passeþ a-wey fra*m* hy*m* al neisch*e*. But þe iiij man*er* of flux is wha*n* a ma*n* is delyueryd of his mete as hool as he etiþ it, *and* þat is j-clepid lienterie.

Dissent*er*ie comeþ of diu*er*se enchesou*n*s, oþ*er*whiles fra*m* w*ith*-outyn, oþ*er*whiles fra*m* w*ith*-i*n*ne. Fra*m* w*ith*-outyn, it comeþ as of ful kene | f. 115v medicynes, oþ*er* of metys oþ*er* of dryncky*s* þat bien full*e* laxatif, oþ*er* of fallyng down*e* fra*m* an heiȝ place, oþ*er* of a strok of a ma*n*nys rugge, oþ*er* of a coold þat a man haþ j-cauȝt on his wombe oþ*er* in his feet. Fram w*ith*-i*n*ne-forþ, þis sicnesse comeþ of corupt hum*ur*os þat bien i*n*ne þe guttes, as of colre, oþ*er*e of sory blood, oþ*er* of salt flewme, oþ*er* malencolie. Oþ*er* it is of a febil rotentif, oþ*er* of a strong*e* expulsiue, þat is to say, oþ*er* þe guttes bien feble to hoolden þe mete w*ith*-i*n*ne, oþ*er* ful strong to put out þat þat is in hem.

Of dissenterie þ*er* bie*n* iij man*er*es: Oon is in þe ou*er*moost gutt*es*, anoþ*er* is in þe mydle gutt*es*, and þe iij in þe neþ*er*most gutt*es*. And in oon manere of dissenterie, þat þat passeþ fra*m* a ma*n* is as þei it were waschyng of fleisch*e*, *and* þat flux mai liȝtly bie j-helid. Jn a-noþ*er*e dissenterie, þ*er* passeþ fra*m* a man as þei were schauyng of parchemyn. But in þe thred man*er* of dissent*er*ie, þ*er* passeþ fra*m* a ma*n* hool gobet*es* of his gutt*es*, *and* þat is incurable. Wha*n* þis

5 man] *interl.* **his**] *follow. by exp.* body **10 Fram**] *corr. from* fFra*m* **11 ful kene**] *corr. from* fulkene **medicynes**] *prec. by heading* Sekenesse **15 Fram**] *corr. from* fFram

sicnesse comeþ of þe ouer*e* gutt*es*, þei felyn greua*n*nce a-bowte*n* þe nauele. *And* þe mat*er* þ*at* passeþ fra*m* hem is lyk þe waschyng of fleisch*e* wiþ-oute sich*e* schauy*n*ge, for þei bie*n* so thy*n*ne þ*at* þ*er* comeþ no sich*e* schauynge fra*m* he*m*. But wha*n*ne þis sicnesse comeþ fra*m* þe neþ*er* gutt*es*, þa*n* þe greuau*n*ce is be-neþe þe nauele, *and* þei bien delyueryd of mat*er* lyk þe schauy*n*g of gutt*es* *and* of blood to-gider*e*. *And* þe blood ne is nat j-medlid w*it*h þe dryt, but lyiþ | gobet-mele bie hym-self. But wha*n* þe flux comeþ fra*m* þe ou*er* gutt*es*, þe blood is j-medlid w*it*h þe drit for-to goiþ a long wey, *and* men xal nat ri3t wel p*er*seyue þe blood. But wha*n* it comeþ of þe mydil gutt*es*, þa*n* þe greuau*n*ce is a-boute þe nauele, su*m*what a-boue *and* su*m*what by-neþe. And of what humo*ur* þis comeþ, þu maist j-knowe bi þat þ*at* was j-teld in þe ache of þe stomac. Naþeles, of colre, þe dri3t mai bie in two man*er*es j-colurd, oþ*er* 3elwe, oþ*er* grene *and* j-medlid w*it*h blood. Of malencolie, it is blac *and* j-medlid w*it*h blood. Of salt flewme, it is a derk pale colour*e* *and* medlid w*it*h blood. Of corupt blood, it is nei3 of blak colo*ur* *and* j-medlid w*it*h blood. Oþ*er*whiles dissent*er*ie comeþ in certeyn tymes *and* in certen cours, *and* a ma*n* is mych*e* j-li3ttyd aft*er* his flux. And sich*e* man*er* flux xal nat bie j-stau*n*chid til he wolle cessen hym-self. But þ*er* is a-noþ*er* dissent*er*ie þ*at* comeþ on-certeynlych*e*, *and* greueþ a ma*n* *and* febleþ hym ful mych*e*. *And* hy*m*, men xal bie a-bowte to stau*n*che w*it*h medycynes.

f. 116r

For dissent*er*ie þ*at* comeþ of heete *and* of hoote kene hum*ur*os þ*at* bie*n* in þe gutt*es*, make hym a p*ur*gacıou*n* of

8 gobet-mele] *prec. by heading* in the guttys **11 whan]** *follow. by canc. and exp.* þe **24 man]** *follow. by and* greueþ a ma*n* **27 For]** *corr. from* ffor

mirabol*e* cit*ri* *and* indj. And ʒif it is of oþ*er* hum*ur*os, p*ur*ge hym w*it*h medicynes þ*a*t ben approprid to þe hum*ur*os. Mirabolan*e* cit*ri* p*ur*geþ colre, and þ*a*t þ*a*t purgeþ colre p*ur*geþ blood. Kebul*e* indi purgeþ flewme. Bellerici emblici
f. 116v p*ur*geþ male*n*colie. But wha*n*ne þ*o*u xalt make | þi p*ur*gaciou*n*, ʒif it bie a strong boistrus man of complexiou*n*, poudre þi medicine *and* lat hym etyn þ*a*t poudre oþ*er* drynckyn it. But ʒif it bie an-oþ*er* feble ma*n* of co*m*plexiou*n*, oþ*er* a ma*n* þ*a*t haþ bie j-noryschid wiþ deynteis, tak of þi medicine *ounce* j oþ*er* *ounce* s*emis*, *and* do þe powdre here-of in reyn-wat*er*, oþ*er* in wat*er* of rosees, oþ*er* in gotys whey, oþ*er* in wat*er* þ*a*t mastik or plau*n*teyn haþ j-soden i*n*ne. And cle[n]se þ*a*t wat*er* *and* lat hym dryncke þ*er*-of. But wha*n*ne þu ʒyuest a ma*n* sych*e* clensyng*e*, do þ*er*-i*n*ne þe more of mirabolan*e*. And wha*n*ne þ*o*u seist bi a mannys driʒt þ*a*t he is wel j-p*ur*geid of þ*a*t humo*ur* þ*a*t is cause of his sicnesse, þa*n* þu xalt bie a-boute to stau*n*che is flux by medicines þ*a*t bien st*ri*ctoryes. And þan ʒif hym an electuarie j-maad of diaconidion, *and* myclete, *and* athanasia j-medlid to-gidere. And ʒif he is a delicat ma*n*, do þ*er*-to a lityl sugre, *and* a lytil of sandragou*n*, *and* of bole, *and* of mastik, *and* of a ston þ*a*t is j-clepid emachites, *and* ʒif hym þis w*it*h þe iuys of plau*n*teyn ar þan he ete or dryncke. And lat settyn hys feet in salt warm wat*er* þ*a*t restabouis is j-sode*n* i*n*ne, for þ*a*t is good for eu*er*ich*e* flux. Oþ*er*, aft*er* þe medicyne, make hy*m* a
f. 117r baþe | þ*a*t rooses, *and* plau*n*teyn, *and* symphite, *and* restabou*es*, *and* sang*ui*narie, *and* schep*er*dys-ʒard*ese*, *and*

4 blood] *follow. by canc. and exp.* be **5 þi]** *prec. by heading* Sekenesse **26 þat]** *prec. by heading* in the guttys

4 blood] *in r.-h. margin:* no*ta*

galles, *and* þe rynde of an openers tree *and* of a chyry tree *and* of [a] citonye tree bien j-sode*n* i*n*ne, *and* sich*e* oþ*er* stri-ctories. And wha*n*ne he comeþ out of þe baaþ, let hym haue rest. *And* ȝyf hym dia[c]odiou*n*, *and* athanasia, *and* myclete j-medlid to-gidere. Anoþ*er* good baaþ for þis sicnesse to stau*n*che þe flux: Tak rosees, plau*n*teyn, co*n*firie, daie-eiȝe, *and* þe rynd of a blak þorn, *and* þe rynde of an ook, *and* þe blostmes of an ook, *and* þe hooles of beenes, *and* akrene of ookys, *and* chasteynes. Seeþ all*e* þese in wat*er*, *and* wha*n* þei arn wele j-soden, cast þ*er*-to þe v part of vi*n*egre. *And* lat hym sittyn a good while in þ*at* baaþ. Anoþ*er* good baaþ: Tak of reyn-wat*er* as myche as of all*e* oþ*er* þi*n*ges þ*at* þu makyst of þi baaþ, *and* seeþ þer-i*n*ne of a blak þorn, *and* openers tree, *and* of chiry tree, *and* of chasteyn tree, *and* of ook, *and* of plau*n*teyn, *and* confirie, *and* dayes-eiȝe, mynte, sloon, bole, þe blosmes of okes, pentafilon, þe hooles of an akrene, *and* of beenys. *And* cast to þ*at* wat*er* þe v part or þe vj part of strong vi*n*egre *and* seeþ al þis a good while to-gidere til þe wat*er* wexe blac *and* þicke. *And* siþe lat wrappe þe sike-ma*n* | f. 117v
in a schete *and* lat hym sitte þ*er*-i*n*ne a good while. A good plastre for þis sicnesse: [Tak of acacie], *and* [of] ypoquyscidos, *and* of þe iuys of plau*n*teyn, of eu*er*ych*e*, j-lych*e* myche; of whete mele, *quantum* s*ufficit*. Medle hem to-gidere *and* make a plastre þ*er*-of fra*m* þe nauele to þe schaar. A good fumigaciou*n*: Take colofonye *and* þe poudre of oþ*er* thyng*es* þ*at* wole make a ma*n* costyf, *and* strawe he*m* in brennyng*e* coles. *And* lete þe smoke þ*er*-of smytyn vp in-to here fou*n*dement. Oþ*er* tak qwyck eelys *and* leie hem on

4 **diacodioun**] *corr. from* diagodiou*n* 16 **pentafilon**] *interl.* filon *and follow. by exp.* folium 19 **wrappe**] *follow. by canc. twice* þ 20 **in**] *prec. by heading* fflux callyd dissenterye

þe bre*nn*ynge coles. *And* lat þe smoke of hem smyte vp in-to a ma*n*nes fou*n*dement. This fumigaciou*n* is good for al man*er* flux. Oþ*er* tak a bre*nn*yng tyl-stoon *and* que*n*che hym in vi*n*egre. *And* let þe smoke þ*er*-of smyte vp in-to a ma*nn*es fou*n*dement.

Dietyng of hem þ*at* han þis sicnesse xal bie of rostyd met*es*, *and* noon broþþes but ȝif þei bien j-maad þicke w*ith* spic*erie* *and* w*ith* þe poudre of sych*e* thyng*es* þ*at* wole make a ma*n* costif. And make hym breed of millefoile *and* of plau*n*teyne. And lete hym etyn an hen oþ*er* a partrich*e* j-rosted *and* j-fassyd w*ith*-i*n*ne w*ith* wex *and* a-noynted w*ith*-oute w*ith* wex. Oþ*er* fasse an heen w*ith* þe powdre of bole, sandragou*n*, coral, emathites, canel, clowes, gu*m*me arabik, f. 118r *and* dragagant*e*. And ȝif | þu wolt, medle þ*er*-wiþ ȝelkys of eyren, *and* wex, *and* chese. Rooste þe heen *and* late hym ete*n* here. Oþ*er* tak an oold hen *and* seeþ heere in reyn-wat*er* oþ*er* in stondyng wat*er* of a sisterne til þe heen bie half j-soden j-now. Siþe do þ*er*-to agresta *and* sumac wel j-wasschyn, *and* let hem seþe to-gid*ere* til þe fleisch falle fra*m* þe bonys. Þa*n* tak þ*at* *and* stampe it wel in a mort*er*. *And* medle þe broþ þ*er*-wiþ, *and* stampe þ*er*-wiþ ȝelkys of eyren *and* cru*mmes* of bred, *and* make it in man*ere* of mortrewys. *And* ȝif hi*m* þ*er*-of to hys mete. And ȝif þu sp*ri*ngist þ*er*-upon þe poudre of canel, clowes, bole, sandragou*n*, dragagant, it wol be wele þe bet*ere*. Also late make hym riys oþ*er*

6 **of²**] *follow. by exp.* sto 11 **with-oute**] *corr. from* w*ith*-i*n*ne-oute (i*n*ne *exp.*) 12 **with²**] *follow. by canc.* bole 14 **ȝif**] *catchword* (*in bottom margin*): þu wolt (*underl.*) **þu**] *prec. by heading* Dissenterye **22 mortrewys**] *interl.* e

1 vp] *in l.-h. margin:* no*ta*

fur-mente wiþ almau*n*d mylk, oþ*er* note mylk, oþ*er* goot*es* mylk. But ȝif þu makest it w*it*h got*es* mylk, que*n*che þ*er*-i*n*ne stonys of a rennyng wat*er* þ*a*t bien glowyng hote, oftesiþes que*n*che siche stonys in þe mylk *and* þa*n*ne þe mylk xal bie ful medicinabyl for þe flux. Meele also þ*a*t xal bie doon in þe potage of men þ*a*t han þis sicnesse xal bie put in a pot of erþe, *and* j-stopped *and* j-baken i*n* a[n] ouene as longe as þe breed is. Here drynck xal be, ȝif þei han feuerys, wat*er* of rooses, oþ*er* reyn-wat*er* þ*a*t mastik is j-soden i*n*ne. Ȝif þei haue no feu*ere*, ȝyf hem good reed wyn j-medlyd wiþ a lytil | f. 118v wat*er*, oþ*er* breen vp-on a tyl-stoon, mastik, *and* gu*m*me arabik. *And* seeþe þe poudre þ*er*-of in wat*er* *and* late hym drycke þe wat*er*. Oþ*er* make hym grwel of femygrek oþ*er* of letuse, *and* let hym vsyn it vij daies ȝif is stomac is a-uentisid. And oold chese j-soden in hony is good for hem also.

A sirip for þis sicnesse: Tak of roses, *ounce* iij; of plau*n*teyn seed, *ounce* j; of myrtilles, of sumac, *ounce* ij; of planteyn, m*anipulum* j; of good sugre, *pound* j; of athanasie, of myclete, of dyacodion, *ounce* ij. Seþe þese spices in reyn-wat*er*. *And* siþe clense þ*a*t wat*er* *and* aft*er*ward þe sugre. *And* þa*n*ne clarifie it vp *and* kepe it.

Anoþ*ere* sirip: Tak of rooses, *ounce* ij; of þe seed of planteyn, *ounce* j; of myrtelles, of sumac, *ounce* ij; of planteyn, m*anipulum* j; of sugre, ij ij oz. Seþe þe spices in reyn-wat*er*, *and* siþe clense it, *and* cast in þi sugr*e*.

A good plastre for þis sicnesse: Tak of roose, *ounce* j; of sumac, *ounce* ij; of bedellie, of mastik, of encense, *ounce* ij;

11 water] *prec. by heading* Dissenterye **25 oz**] *interl.*

1 wiþ] *in r.-h. margin:* no*ta*

of spodie, of sandragou*n*, of bole armoniac, *ounce* ij; of galles, of psidie, of balaustia, *ounce* s*emis*; of wermot, *ounce* ij; of þe iuys of mynte, *ounce* s*emis*; of þe iuys of planteyn, *ounce* ij; of whete mele *and* of þe whiȝt of eyren, *quantum* s*ufficit*. Medle hem to-gidere. Vnd*er*stond þ*at* for myrte, þ*ou* myȝtest take louage; *and* for myr[t]illes, louage seed; for
f. 119r balaustia, þ*ou* myȝtest | take þe blosm*es* of ookes; for psidie, þe rynde*s* of ookys. Oþ*er* special medicines þ*er* bie*n* for þis sicnesse. Oon is: Tak a quyk turtyl *and* bren here in þe feyren in an ouene. *And* put þ*er*-to *ounce* ij of saundragou*n* *and* as myche of mu*m*mye. *And* wha*n* al þ*at* is wel j-brent, make poudre þ*er*-of *and* let hym vsyn þ*at* boþe in met*es* *and* in drynck*es*. Oþ*er*: Stampe þe seed of planteyne *and* medle it w*ith* þe whiȝt of eyren. *And* roost it on a tylston*e* *and* let hy*m* ete þ*at*. Oþ*er*: Tak mylk of a kow *and* þe iuys of mynte. *And* let hym dryncke þorow ij pypes, j-liche myche of eyþere.

A good powd*re* for þis sicnesse: Tak rooses, plau*n*teyn, camomille, encense, canel, mu*m*mye, mastik, turme*n*tille, bole, balaustie, psidie, sandragou*n*, galles, maces, of eu*er*ich*e* of þe*m* take j-lich*e* mych*e*, *and* put sugre þ*er*-to. *And* vse þis in medicinys *and* i*n* met*es* *and* i*n* dryncky*s*. Cowe mylk also is ful profitabyl for þis sicnesse, but araie it as j-seid bi-fore of got*es* mylk.

Athanasia is good for þis flux but þ*ou* xal dryncke it þa*n* w*ith* þe iuys of mynten. And for þe flowyng of blood þ*at*

6 myrtilles] *corr. from* myrcilles **for**[2]] *corr. from* ffor **7 take**] *prec. by heading* Dissenterye **for**] *corr. from* ffor **8 ryndes**] *interl.* e
23 ful profitabyl] *corr. from* fulprofitabyl

13 it] *in r.-h. margin:* no*ta*

wom*en* han, it is good j-dru*n*ck w*ith* þe iuys of plau*n*teyn. And it wole stau*n*che bledyng at þe nose ȝif it be cast þ*er*-i*n*ne w*ith* þe iuys of sang*ui*narie. *And* it is þus j-maad: Tak of canel *and* of | cassia fistula, *dragme* iij; of greynys, vij; of f. 119v saffru*n*, of sq*ui*nant*e*, of storac*e*, of cal*e*, of valerian, of henbane, of mark, of dauk, of silery mou*n*teyn, anyse, opiu*m*, *dragme* j *and* s*emis*; iij grei*n*s of spik; of castore, of þe leeuys of myrte, of emachites, of sandragou*n*, of coral, of cost, of bole, of simphite, of asaru*m*, of acorus, of þe rynde of pomegarnade, of þe leeuys of a lorere, of iuen, of macropip*er*, of lencropip*er*, *and* of p*er*sily, *dragme* j *quantum* s*ufficit*. And wha*n* þu ȝeuyst a ma*n* here-of, ȝif hym *dragme* iij w*ith* þe forseid iuys. Alle þese medicines bien for flux þ*at* comeþ of greua*n*nce of þe ou*er*e guttes *and* also of þe medil gutt*es*. But ȝif þe neþ*er* gutt*es* bien a-peirid, þe moost p*ro*fitabil worchyng is w*ith* suppositories *and* clisteries to make þe guttes clene. But wha*n* þu ȝeuist a clist*er*ie in þis sicnesse, þou xal nat put it ful depe in ne ful hastiliche. Þou xal nat dryue in þe mat*er*e in-to his wombe, but esily, for hirtynge of þe gutt*es*. And a-noi*n*t it w*ith* oyle oþ*er* su*m* oþ*er* sich*e* soft þi*n*ge þ*at* it mow go in esylich*e*. And wha*n* a ma*n* delyueriþ hy*m* of þe mat*er*e of his clist*er*ie, loke wheþ*er* he bie deliuerid of as mych*e* as he resceyuid, þa*n* it is wel. And þanne late hy*m* resceyue a-þre clist*er*ies or a-foure tyl þe mat*er*e come as clere owt, as it was j-þrowe in-to his wombe. And wha*n* it is soo, þe gutt*es* bien wel j-clensid. And but | þei bien wel j-clensid, þei mown neu*er* bien wel j- f. 120r heelid. And aft*er* þ*at* tyme þ*o*u hast ȝouyn hym a clist*er*ie

4 cassia] *prec. by heading* Dissenterye **7 iij**] *follow. by canc.* gei*n*s gre **9 bole**] *corr. from* bbole (last b *interl.*) **18 þou**] *interl.* o **27 þei**[1]] *prec. by heading* The blody flux mu*n*dificatif, þou must ȝeue hy*m* a clist*er*ie st*ri*ctorie to maken his flux cessyn. Oon good clist*er*ie is j-maad of got*es* talwe þ*at* is a-bowten his kydeneyren, but medle oile þ*er*-wiþ. Anoþ*er*e: Resolue dragagant in tisane *and* medle þ*er*-wiþ woma*nn*es mylk *and* þe ȝelk*es* of eyren. But ar þa*n* þ*o*u ȝif hy*m* þese clist*er*ies, ȝyue hym medicines to p*ur*gen hym as it was j-seid bie-fore. Oþ*er*: Seþe barlich*e* j-hool in got*es* talwe *and* cast þ*er*-to purid hony þ*at* wol clense þe gutt*es*, wheþ*er* it bie j-dru*n*k oþ*er* j-take w*it*h a clist*er*ie. Oþ*er*: Wat*er* þ*at* lentes *and* femygrek bien j-soden i*n*ne *and* siþe cast þ*er*-to a litil hony. A clist*er*ie st*ri*ctorie: Take t*ri*acle *and* resolue it in wat*er* of rooses, *and* cast þ*er*-to *ounce semis* of musk *and* of mu*m*mye. Oþ*er*: Tak whete *and* breke it *and* seeþ it in cow mylk in þe man*er*e of þi*n*ne grwel. *And* cast þ*er*-to mastik, *and* bole, *and* sandragou*n*, *and* galles, of eu*er*ich*e*, j-lich*e* mych*e*. And wha*n* þou ȝeuyst a ma*n* a clist*er*ie, þ*o*u maist ȝeue hy*m* þe q*ua*ntite of a *pound* at ones.

Blodi flux comeþ oþ*er*while of gret plente of blood þ*at* a ma*n* haaþ, *and* þa*n* a mann*es* veynis bien ful of blood. Oþ*er*whiles it comeþ of su*m* wou*n*de, *and* þ*at* a ma*n* may know bi his eiȝe. Oþ*er*while it comeþ þorow keneschip of þ*at* blood þ*at* persiþ *and* brekeþ þe veynes of þe gutt*es*. *And* þa*n* f. 120v a ma*n* xal j-fele smertyng *and* gret hete in his gutt*es*. | Oþ*er*while, it comeþ for febylnesse of þe lyuere, *and* þ*at* is j-knowe whan þese for-seid signes lackeþ.

Ȝyf it comeþ of gret plente of blood, let hym blede in þe arme at þe lyuere veyne. And diete hym w*it*h met*es and* drynkys þ*at* genderyth*e* but lytel blood, as herbys *and*

16 þou[1]] *interl.* o **18 Blodi**] *2-line space left for initial* **23 guttes**] *follow. by* o **24 Oþerwhile**] *prec. by heading* Blody flux **for**] *corr. from* ffor

fruȝth. And let hym absteyn hym fro bathyng*e* of fresch*e* wat*er* *and* fram mych*e* sleep*e* *and* mych*e* reeste.

Ȝyf it comeþ of keneschyp*e* of blood, late p*ur*ge hym as it was j-teeld in dissent*er*ie. *And* siþe staunche þe flux, as it was j-teld þere.

Ȝif it come of febilnesse of þe lyuere, þ*er* comeþ a gret q*ua*ntite of blood j-gloderyd to-gydere at onys, w*ith*-outyn eny oþ*er* þing*e* j-meynd þ*er*-wyth*e*. *And* they ben j-greuyd in þe riȝth syde. And þ*o*u must ȝeue hym co*n*fortabyl electuarys as sugr*e* rooset, *and* let þe iiij part þ*er*-of ben of diacodion. And ȝyf þ*er*-of boþe in þe moreȝtyde *and* at eue *and* at mydday. *And* ȝyf hy*m* t*r*iasendri, and syþe þe sirip*e* of rosys or ellys þis sirip*e*: Tac rooses, saundres, myrtelles, sumac, *and* mynten*e*. Seeþe hem in wat*er*, *and* clense it, *and* cast þ*er*-to sugre. And tac rooses, *and* sau*n*dres, *and* a lytil spodie, *and* poudre hem, *and* medle hem w*ith* as mych*e* of barly mele. *And* siþe tempre it vp w*ith* wat*er* of rooses *and* w*ith* þe juse of mynte, *and* make a plastre | f. 121r þ*er*-of. Also make coolde plastres of þe iuys of h*er*bys þ*at* bien st*r*ictories, *and* of wat*er* of rooses *and* vinegre, *and* of þe iij kyndes of saundrys. *And* put þ*er*-to cow mylk, as mych*e* as þ*o*u hast of all*e* þe oþ*er*. And anoi*n*te hy*m* be-fore þe lyuere w*ith* oile of rooses j-medelyd w*ith* camphore. Oþ*er*: Tac spodie, *and* rooses, *and* canel, *and* cow mylk, of eu*er*ych*e*, *ounce* s*emis*; of bole, of amyde, of carse seed, *dragme* iij; of sandragou*n*, *and* of blac popy, *dragme* j. Te*m*pre hem w*ith* þe juys of mynten*e* *and* of plaunten, *and* make round ball*e* þ*er*-of w*ith* wat*er* þ*at* rooses, mynten*e*, *and* plau*n*ten ben j-soden ine. And aft*er*ward make thys plaistere: Haue a good q*ua*ntite of

7 onys] *corr. from* atonys **10 sugre**] *follow. by canc. twice* s **18 þer-of**] *prec. by heading* Diarrya þe iuys of plantein *and* of mynten. *And* w*ith* oon þ*er*-of medele barly mele oþ*er* whete mele *and* plastr*e* þ*at* on a clooþ. *And* w*ith* þe oþ*er* party of þe iuys, anoi*n*te þe place bifore þe lyuere. And siþe straw þ*er*-on whi3t sau*n*drys *and* of reed j-poudred. And siþe lei þe clowte w*ith* þe plastre al a-boue. And late hym abstene hy*m* fra*m* moist met*es*. And 3if al þis ne helpeþ nat, 3if hym streng*er* medicines þ*at* wer*e* j-tel in dissent*er*ie.

Djarria is a flux of þe wombe w*ith*-outyn flowyng of blood *and* w*ith*-outyn schauyng*e* of hys guttys, *and* hys mete is su*m*what defied ar þan it passiþ fram hym. And þis
f. 121v sicnesse comeþ | of þe same enchesou*n* þ*at* dissenterie doiþ. But naþeles, 3if colrik humo*ur*s ben þe enchesou*n* of þis sicnesse, p*ur*ge hym w*ith* wat*er* þ*at* cassia fistula is j-soden i*n*ne, *and* tamarynd *and* mirabol*e* cit*ri* ben j-soden i*n*ne. 3if it be of flewme, p*ur*ge hym w*ith* þe wat*er* þ*at* *ounce* j of polipodie, *and ounce* vij of agaryk, *and* iij *ounce* of [k]ebul*e* ben j-soden i*n*ne. 3if it be of malencolie, purge he*m* w*ith* wat*er* þ*at* sene, *and* epithyme, *and* myrabolan*e* indj ben j-soden i*n*ne. And aft*er* hys p*ur*gaciou*n*, 3if hym medicines þ*at* ben co*n*fortabil, *and* st*ri*ctories, as it was j-teld in dissent*er*ie. 3if it come of a rewme þ*at* falleþ a-down fra*m* þe heed in-to þe gutt*es*, hys dry3t is whi3t *and* full*e* of spumes *and* of bolles. *And* þanne þ*o*u xalt hele þe rewme as it was j-teld before. And siþe purge þe gutt*es* of flewme *and* hele hy*m* as it was j-teeld in dissent*er*ie. Miclete is a good medicine for þese fluxes *and* for gnawi*n*ges *and* hurli*n*ges in a mann*es*

2 a clooþ] *corr. from* aclooþ **4 saundrys**] *interl.* r **9 Djarria**] *2-line space left for initial* **12 of**] *prec. by heading* Diarria **15 inne**[1]] *follow. by canc. and exp.* 3yf it be of ffle **16 flewme**] *corr. from* fflewme **17 kebule**] *corr. from* bebul*e*

wombe. *And* is þus j-maad: Tak of myrabol*e* cit*ri and* indj, kebul*e*, þ*at* ben j-maad clene *and* ben j-roostid, *dragme* j *and* s*emis*; of bell*e*, of emblic*e* j-rostid, *dragme* j *and* s*emis*; of comyn, of anyse, of fenel seed, of ameos, of careaway, *dragme* j *and* s*emis*. Poudre þilke thing*es* þ*at* ben j-rostyd *and* lei all*e* þem to-gidere a-nyȝt *and* a-day in vi*n*egre. *And* þan do þ*er*-to of bole, of balaustie, of sumac, of mastik, *and* of gu*m*me arab*e*, *dragme* j *and* xv | grei*n*s. Frie all*e* þese in f. 122r oile of rooses *and* siþe tempre it vp w*ith* þe sirip of myrtes. *And* ȝyf hym here-of w*ith* reyn-wat*er* erlich*e*, *and* at mydday, *and* at þe euyn-tyde.

Ljentirie is a flux whan a man is delyuerid of hys mete al hool as he etiþ it. And þis sicnesse comeþ of corupt humo*ur*s þ*at* ben in þe stomac oþ*er* in þe gutt*es*, oþ*er* of su*m* postym þ*at* is in hem, oþ*er* of febilnesse of hem, oþ*er* of to mych*e* etyng*e and* drynkyng*e* at oon mele. And wheþ*er*-of-eu*er* it be, þ*o*u maist j-knowe be þe tokenys þ*at* han be teld here-be-fore. And medicines þ*at* wull*e* heele dissent*er*ie wole heele þe flux. Naþeles, þ*er* be special p*ur*gaciou*n*s for þis flux, as ȝif it be of coold hum*ur*os: Tak þ*at* þ*at* is w*ith*-i*n*ne a goorde, *and* polipodie, *and* fenell*e* sede, *and* sq*ui*nant. *And* seþ hem in wat*er*, *and* do in þ*at ounce* j of kebull*e*, *and* lat it stonde soo al nyȝt. *And* on morwe, lat hym drynke of þ*at* wat*er*. Oþ*er* tac of polipodie, *dragme* iiij, *and* seeþ hem in wat*er*. *And* clense þ*at* wat*er and* resolue þ*er*-i*n*ne of agarik, of turbith*e*, of hermedactil*e*, *dragme* ij. *And* let it stonde so al nyȝt. *And* a-morwe, clense it *and* let hym drynke of þ*at* wat*er*. And þ*o*u muste late hym drynke wat*er* þ*at* fenel sede,

8 greins] *prec. by heading* Lientirie **12 Ljentirie**] *2-line space left for initial* **27 it**] *follow. by canc.* nawth *and* polipodie, *and* anyse, *and* a lytyl mastik ben j-soden i*n*ne. *And* cast þ*er*-to *dragme* ij of esula. Aft*er* hys p*ur*gaciou*n*, ȝif hym hoot electuaris *and* confortabil, as diacimin*um*, diat*ri*onpip*er*ion, *and* sich*e* oþ*er*. Also lete hym f. 122v ete kene met*es*, as oynouns, *and* leek*es*, *and* mustard, | *and* garlek, *and* carses, *and* oþ*er*e salt met*es*. And siþe ȝyf hym a lityl wat*er* to make hym caste. And aft*er* hys p*ur*gaciou*n*, late hym baþe hym in syche a baaþ as it was j-teeld in dissent*er*ie. And whane he comeþ owt of þe baaþ, ȝyf hym myclete *and* athanasia w*it*h þe iuys of mynt. And a-noynte hym boþe be-hynde *and* a-fore, fra*m* a-boue þe stomac dou*n* be-neþe þe schare wiþ dispumed hony. *And* spryng þ*er*-oon þe poudre of mastik, *and* of ence*n*se, *and* of seneuey, *and* of mynten. But ȝif þis flux come of hoote hum*ur*os, p*ur*ge hym w*it*h *ounce* s*emis* of þe coold dragag*e*. *And* medlee þ*er*-wiþ *ounce* ij of myrabol*e* cit*ri*. Aft*er*ward, make hy*m* a baaþ of rooses, of plauntei*n*, *and* of sich*e* oþ*er* coold st*ri*ctories. And aft*er*ward ȝyf hym myclete *and* late hym be in reeste. *And* a-noi*n*te hys wombe *and* hys rugge also wiþ þe gleire of eiren. *And* sp*ri*ng*e* it al thyk w*it*h þe flowre of beenen in þe man*er* of a plastere. And in boþen enchesou*n*s, triacle j-drunke*n* w*it*h þe iuys of mynten js p*ro*fitabil.

Colica passio is a greuua*n*ces of a gut þ*at* is j-clepid colon. And jlica passio is a g*r*euaunces of an-oþ*er* smal gutte þ*at* is j-clepid jlion. And þese greuuau*n*ces a-corden mych*e* boþe in enchesons, *and* in toknes *and* in cures; *and* su*m*what

1 **lytyl**] *follow. by canc. twice* hon 5 **and**[3]] *prec. by heading* Colica
16 ij] *corr. from* iij (first i *canc. twice and exp.*) **23 Colica**] *2-line space left for initial*

22 with] *in l.-h. margin:* no*ta* ben*e*

þei discorden, | [f. 123r] for colon lithe a-bowte þe naule and is toward þe schare a-long, oþ*er*whiles in þe ri3t syde, oþ*er*while in þe lyft syde. Oþ*er*while it gooþ j-wharte ou*er* þe wombe in þe man*er* of a g*er*dyl. Oþ*er*while it is be-fore, oþ*er*whiles it is be-hynde vp to þe reyns, and oþ*er*while in þe ri3t side, *and* oþ*er*while in þe li3ft syde. And it walkeþ fra*m* oon place to a-noþ*er*, *and* it a ful greuouse peyn as it were a woman þ*a*t traueileþ of a childe. And þe ache makeþ a man oþ*er*whiles to lese hys wi3t, *and* ofte-siþes makeþ a man to falle in-to þe feu*er*ys. And su*m*me clepe þe greuau*n*ce styches. And boþe þese greuaunces come*n* of diu*er*se enchesou*n*s. Oon is grete heete in þe guttes þ*a*t dryeþ þe dri3t, þ*a*t it may nat passe fram þe gutt*es*. Anoþ*er* is mete *and* drynk þ*a*t makeþ a ma*n* costif. Anoþ*er* is viscouse flewme þ*a*t wiþ-holdiþ þe dri3t þ*a*t it may nat passen a-way. Anoþ*er* is a gret corupt wynd þ*a*t is in þe gutte *and* letteþ þe dri3t of his issu. Anoþ*er*e is a postym þ*a*t is in þe gutt*es*. Anoþ*er* is g*r*et plente of worm*es* þ*a*t ben in þe gutt*es*. Anoþ*er* is febylnesse of þe gutt*es* þ*a*t mou*n* nat delyuere hem of þe dri3t *and* of oþ*er* corupciou*n*s þ*a*t is in hem.

3if it comeþ of hete of colre þ*a*t is in þe gutt*es*, he is costif *and* he w*ith*-holdyn his vrine. *And* þe ache is ful | [f. 123v] kene, *and* ful scharp*e*, *and* his face citrine, *and* he feliþ gret hete in his gutt*es*, *and* he is thrust-full*e*.

3if it come of costif met*es and* drynk*es*, þe pacient may know þ*a*t hym-self be þe met*es and* drynk*es* þ*a*t he haþ j-etyn. 3if it come of salt flewme, þe g*r*euaunce ne mevith nawt mych*e* a-bowte, but a-bideþ stille in oon place, *and* þe ache is

1 **for**] *prec. by heading* Passio; *corr. from* ffor 3 **þe**[2]] *follow. by exp.* bely 15 **corupt wynd**] *corr. from* coruptwynd 23 **kene**] *prec. by heading* Colica 24 **guttes**] *follow. by canc. twice* þat

ful kene *and* full*e* t*ra*ueilouse. Hys vrine is of febyl colo*ur*, *and* hys face pale, of þe colo*ur* of leed; *and* he is nawt thristfull*e* *and* hys greuaunce is moost on nyȝth. Þe dryȝth þ*a*t passeþ fra*m* hym is lytil, *and* þ*a*t is ful of spume *and* of bolles, *and* viscouse, as þe gleir*e* of an ey wha*n* it is well*e* j-sterid. *And* gret will*e* þei haue to go to p*re*uye, *and* mown no-þi*n*g do þ*er*e. Ȝyf it come of corupt wynd, þe wynd makeþ myche hurlyng*e* *and* myche noyse in his wombe, *and* walkeþ a-bowte fra*m* place to place to haue is issu out. And wha*n* he is deliu*er*id of þ*a*t wynd, oþ*er* a-boue oþ*er* by neþe, he is mych*e* j-esyd. And oþ*er*-while sich*e* a wynd wreestiþ a mann*es* gutt*es* a-bowte, as ho-so wole wynd a ȝerde. And ȝif me bloweþ þa*n*ne in hys fou*n*deme*n*t, he is mych*e* j-esyd *and* þe gut is browt in-to hys kynde. Ȝif it come of a postym
f. 124r þ*a*t is in þe gutt*es*, it is j-know | be þe gret greuaunce þ*a*t þe man haaþ eu*er*-more a-bidyng*e* stille in oon place. *And* þ*er*-wiþ he haþ a feu*er* *and* gret ach*e* in his gutt*es*, *and* gret hete, *and* mych*e* þirst, *and* lityl sleep, *and* he wlateþ his mete, and is j-helyd as a postym of þe stomac is. Ȝif it come of wormes þ*a*t xal j-know it be þe token*es* þ*a*t xul be toold in þe next chapit*re*. Ȝif it come of febylnesse of þe gutt*es* *and* of long wiþholdyng*e* of drit, þe pacient may j-know þ*a*t hym-self ȝif þ*er*e many daies ha*n* j-passid siþþe he was at sege.

For þis greuaunce ȝif it come of heete oþ*er* of hoote colric hum*ur*os: Seeþ coold herb*e* in wat*er* *and* to þ*a*t wat*er* cast a litel oile of rooses, oþ*er* of violet, oþ*er* of bot*er*. And wete in þ*a*t wat*er* wulle þ*a*t is schore on-wassche oþ*er* a

15 be] *prec. by heading* Passio **21 febylnesse**] *corr. from* ffebylnesse **24 For**] *corr. from* ffor

25 water^2] *in r.-h. margin:* no*ta*

lynne*n* clooþ. *And* þ*er*-wiþ waisch his wombe wele to abate þe ach*e*. Oþ*er* waisch*e* hym in þ*a*t wyse w*ith* wat*er* þ*a*t violet, *and* rooses, *and* wermot, *and* loueage ben j-soden i*n*ne. Oþ*er* take þe iuys of solatre, of hock*es*, *and* of loueage, *and* vinegre þ*a*t hock*es*, violet, *and* anyse ben j-soden i*n*ne *and* medle hem togidere. And knocke whete in a morter*e*, *and* medle þ*er*-wiþ, and seþe it tyl it be thicke, *and* þ*er*of make a plastre. *And* lei to hys wombe *and* it wull*e* sesse þe ache. Oþ*er* seþe þe rote of holy-hocke *and* make | f. 124v a plastre þ*er*-of. Oþ*er* make hym a suppositorie of lard wha*n* hys greuau*n*ce comeþ to hym [and] put it in þe fou*n*de-ment. Oþ*er* ȝyf hy*m* a clyst*er*e in þis wyse: Seeþ mynt, wermote, *and* beetes in wat*er*, *and* clense þe wat*er*. *And* w*ith* þ*a*t wat*er* medle whete bryn. *And* siþe clense it *and* cast þ*er*-to *dragme* iij of oile, *and dragme* j of salge*m*me, *and dragme* s*emis* of þe electuarie þ*a*t is j-maad of þe iuys of rooses. And of þis medicine late hym receyve at on*es* a *pound* þorow a clist*er*ie. And for-to make þe clist*er*ie goo esilich*e* i*n*, a-noynte hys fou*n*deme*n*t w*ith* þe iuys of syneg*re*ne oþ*er* of violet, and lat baþe hym in a baaþ of m*er*curie, *and* of hock*es*, groundyswily, *and* of purselane. And þis is good ȝif þe sicnesse comeþ of coold hum*ur*os. And lete make hym a sirip of violet, *and* of plu*m*bys, *and* of iiij coold sed*es*, *and* of manna, *and* of cassia fistula. *And* lat p*ur*gen hym w*ith* su*m* cologoge as it haaþ been j-teld here-be-fore. And rewle hym boþe in medicynes *and* in met*es*, as it haaþ ben j-teld in þe ache of þe stomak*e* þ*a*t comeþ of heete. But ȝif it be of coold

6 hem] *follow. by* to **9 rote**] *corr. from* reote a] *prec. by heading* Colica **24 cassia fistula**] *corr. from* cassiafistula

2 hym] *in r.-h. margin:* no*ta* bene

hum*ur*os, bie a-bowte to p*ur*ge hym softly of þilk hum*ur*os, as it was j-teeld in þe ache of þe stomac. And a-noi*n*te þe place þ*at* is j-greuyd w*ith* dewte, arrogon, *and* marciaton. f. 125r And siþe ȝif hym a clist*er*ie mollitif | to make þe mat*er*e neisch*e*, and siþe a biti*n*ge clist*er*ie to make hym bie diliu*er*id of þ*at* mat*er*ie.

A mollificatyf clyst*er*ie is j-maad of wat*er* þ*at* hock*es*, oþ*er* lynseed, oþ*er* oþere moist herb*e* ben j-soden i*n*ne, and bren, oþ*er* barlych*e* oþ*er* whete. *And* siþe cast þ*er*-to a lityl hony *and* oile. Oþ*er* seeþ þe roote of þe holyhocke in tysane *and* cast þ*er*-to a lytil hony *and* oile. A clist*er*ie is j-maad of wat*er* þ*at* þe for-seid herbis ben j-soden i*n*ne *and* m*er*curie w*ith* hem. *And* siþe do þ*er*to hony, *and* oile, *and* salt þ*at* is j-relentid in wat*er*, *and* þ*er*-to cast scamone, oþ*er* su*m* oþ*er* medicyne þ*at* is a-cordyng þ*er*-to. Oþ*er* seþe rew, *and* calamynt, *and* centorie, *and* wermot, *and* p*er*itorie. *And* cast þ*er*-to salt-ge*m*me, *and* hony, *and* oile, of þem þre, *ounce* s*emis*. *And* of þis clist*er*ie, lat hym reseyue a pou*n*d at oon*es*. But late hy*m* neu*er* take a bitynge clist*er*ie but ȝif he haue j-haad a mollificatif be-fore, for drede of more p*er*eel. Oþ*er* take a lytil bagge of comyn *and* of bryn to-ged*er* *and* seeþ it in iij p*ar*t*es* of oile *and* þe iiij parte of iuys of rewe tyl þe iuys be j-wastyd a-wey. *And* lat cast þ*at* oile in-to hys wombe þorowȝ a clist*er*ie. Oþ*er* late hym ete t*ri*acle diatesseron. Oþ*er* seeþ in salt-wat*er*: wermot, *and* comyn, *and* anyse, *and* bet*es*, *and* merch, *and* maiorane, *and* wat*er*-carsen, *and*

4 to] *prec. by heading* Passio 5 **bitinge clisterie**] *corr. from* biti*n*geclist*er*ie 11 **A clisterie**] *corr. from* Aclist*er*ie 19 **hym**] *follow. by canc.* l 24 **triacle**] *follow. by canc. twice* dat

7 mollificatyf] *in r.-h. margin:* no*ta*

ȝarde-crassen, *and* mynte, *and* origane, *and* souþ*er*newode, *and* bawme, *and* horehoune, of eu*er*ich*e* | of þese, *ounce* f. 125v s*emis*. *And* as þese herbys seþen, br[e]ke them. And in þ*at* wat*er*, wete wulle þ*at* is j-schore on-waysch*e*, *and* leie to þe wombe, *and* renewe it ofte-siþes, *and* all*e* warm lei it þ*er*-to. Oþ*er* take oolde oile, oþ*er* oold bot*er*e, *and* hony, *and* strong vinegre, *and* salt, of eu*er*ich*e*, j-lich*e* mych*e*. *And* medle it wel to-gidere ou*er* þe fere til it be þicke. *And* þ*er*-i*n*ne wete wooll*e* þ*at* is vn-waisschen*e*, oþ*er* a felte, *and* lei it to hys wombe, for it wull*e* helpyn a ma*n* þei þe sicnesse haue j-holdyn hym longe, but renew it ofte-siþes. Oþ*er* seþe oold oile, *and* strong vinegre, *and* swynes grece to-gidere tyl it be þicke *and* þ*er*-i*n*ne wete a felt oþ*er* on-waisch*e* wulle, *and* leie it to hys wombe. But ȝif hym no laxatif tyl he haue wille for-to go to seege. A good oyneme*n*t for þis greuaunce: Tak drie fig*es*, *and* reisen*es*, *and* beet*es*, *and* oynou*n*s. *And* stamp*e* he*m* w*it*h oile *and* w*it*h wyn drast*es* to-gid*er*e. *And* lat it stond so iij daies to-gid*er*e. *And* seeþe it well*e* *and* cle*n*se it. *And* þa*n* cast þ*er*-to þe poudre of spurge seed, *and* of grashopp*er*es, *and* of euforbe, *and* of castore, *and* quyk brymston, *and* wax, *and* þ*er*-wiþ a-noi*n*te hys wombe. Also tak a spo*n*full*e* of þe poudere of grashopperis *and* as mych*e* of þe poudre of spurge seed. *And* let hy*m* medle he*m* to-gid*er*e *and* dry*n*k half at oon tyme *and* half at an-oþ*er* tyme. Also good pillules ȝif it comeþ of flewmatik hum*ur*os: | Tak f. 126r of diagredie, of aloes, of spurge, of þat is w*it*h-i*n*ne a wild

2 of[2]] *prec. by heading* Colica **12 strong**] *follow. by canc. and exp.* oile **25 humuros**] *catchword* (*in bottom margin*): tak of diag*r*edie **Tak**] *prec. by heading* Passio

5 lei] *in l.-h. margin:* no*ta*

gourde, of euforbe, of turbith, of reubarb*e*, of mastik, j-lich*e* mych*e* of eu*er*ich*e* of hem. Poudre he*m* all*e* *and* medle w*ith* oximel o*þer* w*ith* a wyld cool. *And* mak pillules here-of of þe q*ua*ntite of a beene. And ȝif he*m* to hym as he is of powere to vnderfonge hem.

And ȝif þis sicnesse come of wynd, it is j-heelid in þe same man*er* as þei it come of coold hum*ur*os. Naþeles þ*er* ben special medicines þ*er*fore. Oon js: Make a plastere of comyn j-soden in wyn *and* lei to hys wombe. But furst make hy*m* a suppositorie. Also make hy*m* a fumigaciou*n* of p*er*itorie j-soden in wyn. *And* let hym drynkyn of þ*at* wyn *and* plastre þe herbe on hys wombe, for p*er*itorie is a special medicine for sich*e* wyndes boþe w*ith*-i*n*ne-forth*e* *and* w*ith*-outyn. Anoþ*er*: Tak þe erþe þ*at* liye be-fore þe oxe stalle oþ*er* an horsys mangeer þ*at* is j-trodyn *and* be-pyssed. Heete it wel a-ȝens þe feer *and* all*e* hoot lei it to hys wombe. Anoþ*er*: Tak hoot schepis dryt *and* medle þ*er*-wiþ gotys talow in a mortere. *And* do þ*er*-to a litil pich*e*. Heet it *and* make þ*er*-of a plastre on leþere *and* lei it on hys wombe. And let hym vsen diasp*er*mat[ic]on *and* oþ*er*e electuaries þ*at* destruen oþ*er* corupt wyndes. *And* make hym absteine fro wyndi met*es*, as fra*m* beene*n*, *and* peesen, *and* herbys, *and* frut*es*.
f. 126v Naþeles, | carsen ben goode boþe w*ith*-i*n*ne *and* w*ith*-owte. And late hym vsen suppositories, *and* clist*er*ies, *and* medicines þ*at* ben laxatif, and late hym vse no costyf met*es*. Ȝif þis sicnesse comeþ of a postym, hele it as þe postym of þe

12 **for**] *corr. from* ffor   23 **carsen**] *prec. by heading* Wormes   **and**] *interl.*

12 **plastre**] *in r.-h. margin:* no*ta* p*er*i | torye   14 **stalle**] *in r.-h. margin:* no*ta*

stomac. 3if it come of wormes, hele it as it xal be teld i*n*ne þe next chapitre. 3if it come of febylnesse of þe gutt*es*, let hym vsen confortabil electuaries, as dian[t]hes, *and* diamargariton, w*it*h wat*er* þ*at* baume, *and* mynte, *and* maiorane, *and* karses ben j-soden i*n*ne.

Wormes ben j-genderid in a man*es* gutt*es* of di-uerse schaap, boþe for diu*er*site of a ma*nn**es* gutt*es*, *and* for diu*er*site of þe mat*er*e þ*at* þei ben j-genderid of. Of salt flewme, þ*er* come longe wormes *and* smale, *and* þei ben in þe smale gutt*es*. Sexe gutt*es* a man haaþ in hys wombe, iij smale *and* iij grete. And in þe smale gutt*es* ben smale worm*es* engenderid, and grete wormes ben genderid in þe grete guttes. Of swete flewme ben j-genderid longe wormes *and* broode. Of sowre flewme ben j-genderid schort worm*es* *and* rounde. Of kyndelich*e* flewme be*n* j-gend*er*id schort worm*es* *and* brode, of þe schaap of a gourde. Of glasi flewme be non wormes engend*er*id, for cooldnesse of þe mat*er*e. And þe greuaunce of þe worm*es* is ful kene *and* makeþ men oþ*er*whiles as þei were frentyk*e*. Oþ*er*whiles, | men han loost f. 127r here wyt for sorow. Su*m* men þei make lese here speche, as þei hadden þe litarge. Su*m* me*n* fallen down to grounde, as þou3 þei hadden þe epilencie. Su*m* wome*n* swonden*n* as þei hadden þe suffocacion of þe mod*er*. Su*m* grinden w*it*h here teeþ as þei hadden goutes. Su*m* han ache in here wo*m*be as þe hadden collica passio. Tokenes of þese wormes ben: ychynge of þe nostrilles *and* of þe lippes, stinckyng of þe

2 come of] *corr. from* comeof **3 electuaries**] *follow. by canc. and* dragges **dianthes**] *corr. from* dianches **6 Wormes**] *2-line space left for initial* **19 men**] *prec. by heading* in the guttys **20 Sum men**] *corr. from* Su*m*men **22 Sum women**] *corr. from* Su*m*wome*n* **26 stinckyng**] *corr. from* stingyng (first g *canc. and exp.*; ck *interl.*)

mowþe, hurlyng of þe wombe, *and* meuyng*e* w*ith*-i*n*ne þe gutt*es* as þei it were a quwyk þing. *And* þei gon vp *and* down in a ma*nnes* wombe, *and* oþ*er*while crepyn owte at his noose *and* oþ*er*whiles at hys mouþ. *And* hys teeþ sti*n*ckiþ *and* greuueþ. *And* gryndeþ w*ith* hys teeþ *and* na*m*ly in hys sleep. *And* þ*er* falleþ a gret itchy*n*g ou*er*al hys body. Oþ*er*while þei maken a ma*n* rysyn vp of hys sleep as þei he were wood. *And* þei maken a ma*n* to haue a febyl coloure, *and* haue ache in hys stomac *and* also in hys gutt*es*, *and* a[k]i*n*ge *and* pric[k]i*n*ge in hem, *and* namly be-fore mete. And oþ*er*while þei wlaten here mete, and oþ*er*while þei haue an hound*es* appetit, and oþ*er*while þei haue wil to cast. And oþ*er*while þ*er* comeþ dropis of blood at a ma*nnes* foundeme*n*t as þe wormes biten þe gutt*es* w*ith*-i*n*ne-foorþ *and* þei make al a mann*es* body ful febyl. And þ*er* is a difference be-twyn men
f. 127v þ*at* han wormes *and* hem | þ*at* ben frentyk *and* woode, for woode men pleyne*n* he*m* on here heed, *and* þese on here wombe. Frentik me*n* han þe feu*er*es in here accesse *and* leesen here wyȝt for þe tyme; þese men doon nat soo. A man þ*at* haþ þe litargie haþ a feu*er*e comely þ*er*-wyth; þese ma*n* ha*n* nat soo. And þ*at* haþ þe epilencie vomeþ, and þ*at* haþ þe cathalemsie castiþ, but þese men doon nat soo. And þ*at* haþ appoplexie haþ ache in hys heede, but þese men han in here wombe.

Suffocaciou*n* of þe mod*er* comeþ of greuaunce of þe mod*er*, but þis is of þe wombe and suffocaciou*n*. Let here absteyne *and* hie xal haue þe more eese, but þese han more

9 akinge] *corr. from* ali*n*ge **10 prickinge**] *corr. from* pricli*n*ge **16 þat²**] *prec. by heading* Wormes **for**] *corr. from* ffor **18 Frentik**] *corr. from* ffrentik **feueres**] *corr. from* ffeu*er*es **20 haþ¹**] *follow. by canc. and exp.* nat **22 doon**] *follow. by canc.* at

eese fulle þa*n* fasti*n*ge. And þ*er*fore alle tho þ*a*t han wormes schulle dyne be-tymes, laste þe wormes for defaute of mete gnawe þe stomac *and* þe gutt*es*. And gen*er*aly bittere metis medicines, *and* wel smellyng*e*, *and* soure medicines sleen wormes. And swete met*es* þ*a*t engendryn wat*er*i blood, gendriþ wormes *and* noryschet hem, as herb*e* *and* fruȝt *and* na*m*lyche þe substaunce of þe herb*e* *and* þe pareles of þe fruȝt. And in slei*n*ge of wormes, it is profitabil a-iij daies to late a ma*n* ete swete mylk *and* lete þe wormes fillen hem well*e* þ*er*-wiþ. And aft*er*ward late hy*m* take su*m* bitt*er* medicine, *and* þ*a*t xal slee hem soone. Eu*er*e wha*n* þu ȝeuist a medicine, | medle bitt*er*e þi*n*ges *and* swete to-gidere, as f. 127rbis
wormosede w*it*h wort; þe iuys of wermot w*it*h mylk, oþ*er* w*it*h hony. Special medicines þ*a*t sleen wormes ben aloes, þe iuys of wermot, of centorie, of cookyl, þe poudre of h*er*t*es*-horn j-brent, þe poudre of bit*ur* lupines, þe leues of a beche tree, þe leuys of caperis. For childeren þ*a*t han wormes, late he*m* drynk þe iuys of p*er*sicarie w*it*h goot*es* mylk. Bu[t] ȝif þe chyldren ben riȝt ȝou*n*ge *and* mou*n* drynke no bittere medicines, make he*m* plasteris *and* lei on here wombe. Oon js: Take wermot, cockyl, *and* vi*n*egre, *and* stampe he*m* to-gidere *and* make þ*er*-of a plastre. Oþ*er*: Tak þe poudre of h*er*tys-horn j-brent *and* te*m*pre it w*it*h salt-wat*er*. *And* do a litil hony þ*er*-to *and* make þ*er*-of a plastre. Oþ*er*: Make smale cakes of centorie, *and* of ȝel[k]es of eiren, *and* of whete meele. *And* let hy*m* ete þ*er*-of twies a wyke. Oþ*er* a-noi*n*te hy*m* a-bowte þe stomac *and* aboute þe nauele w*it*h booles

12 medle] *prec. by heading* in the guttys **13 wormosede**] *corr. from* wormode (de *exp.*; sede *interl.*) **17 For**] *corr. from* ffor

19 moun] *in r.-h. margin:* no*ta*

galle *and* w*ith* iuys of centorie. *And* pyt þ*er*-to, ȝif þ*o*u wylt, þe iuys of walwort *and* of elerne. *And* a-noi*n*te al þe wombe þ*er*-w*ith* ou*er*al: Jt sleeþ þe wurm*es* *and* bryngeþ he*m* oute also. Oþ*er* make a plastre of wat*er*-crassys to-broke *and* yhat in a pa*n*ne. Oþ*er* late hym drynk þe iuys of coost, *and* of mynte*n*, *and* of origane, *and* calami*n*te. Oþ*er* tak þe poudre f. 127vbis of bytt*er* lupines *and* of þe poudr*e* | of hert*es*-horn j-brent, *ounce* j; of þe poudre of gras-hopp*er*es, *ounce* iij. Medle it w*ith* hony *and* let hym etyn it. Oþ*er* ȝif hym genciane to drynke, it wole slee wormes, *and* an addre, ȝif it be in a mann*es* wombe; and so wole þe roote of dragance j-dru*n*ke. A plastre for childeren: Tac centorie, cockyl, vi*n*egre, *and* þe iuys of wermot, *and* a litil salt, *and* oile oþ*er* bot*er*e, *and* medle hem to-gidere. A streng*er* plaistere for men: Tac wermot, þe iuys of plau*n*ten, of march*e*, of p*er*sicarie, of beche tre leeues, of þe lasse centorie, iuys of boles galle, of eu*er*ich*e* of þese, j-liche myche. *And* make þ*er*of a plaistere. Also ij dropes or iij of þe iuys of titymalle, oþ*er* of þe wylde goorde j-dru*n*ke, sleeþ þe wormes. But wha*n* þe wormes ben j-slaw, men [m]ust be a-bowt to brynge hem oute w*ith* su*m* medicine as w*ith* sich*e* thyngis þ*at* purgeþ flewme. Also þe iuys of sta*n*crop j-dru*n*ke oþ*er* of orpyn, *and* þe herbys ben j-plaistred on þe wombe, þ*at* dryueþ out wormes þ*at* ben j-slawe. Oþ*er* ȝif þe wormes ben in þe ou*er*er*e* gutt*es*, make hym a stronge clist*er*ie of þe iuys of wermot, of lupines, of scamone, of nytre, of salt, *and* of hony, oþ*er* of boles galle,

7 of[3]] *prec. by heading* Wormes in the guttys **13 oile**] *follow. by canc. and* a litel (litel *also exp.*) **oþer**] *in l.-h. margin* **20 must**] *corr. from* bust

2 of[2]] *in r.-h. margin:* no*ta* **10 and**] *in l.-h. margin:* no*ta* ben*e*

and of þe iuys of centorie *and* of sotherne-woode. But fyrst a-noi*n*te he hys | hers wi*th* oile, þ*a*t þe clist*er*ie mowe esile f. 128r goon i*n*ne. Oþ*er*e make hym a clist*er*ie of þe wat*er* þ*a*t þe kerneles of beches *and* of chiristones ben j-sode i*n*ne, oþ*er* of þe wat*er* þ*a*t þe rynde of a noote tre is j-soden i*n*ne, for þ*a*t sleeþ þe wormes *and* dryueþ hem owte. But wha*n* þilk schort wormes of þe schap of a gourde ben neiȝ a manes ers, men mot ȝeue hy*m* scharp*e* clisteries *and* kene, as jerapigra j-medlid wi*th* galle. But furst a-noi*n*te þe ers wi*th* oile. Wyn þ*a*t þe rootes of a pomegarnat tree *and* of an aisch*e* be*n* j-sode*n* i*n*ne is good to drynke to slee wormes.

T̀enasmon is wha*n* a man haþ gret wille to schiȝt *and* he is on-myti þ*er*-to. *And* it semeþ a ma*n* as þouȝ he schulde eu*er*more schite, *and* wha*n* he comeþ to p*ri*uei, he mai no-þi*n*g do þ*er*-to. And þis greuau*n*ce is of a mann*es* gutte þ*a*t is clepid longae *and* þ*a*t gut gooþ dou*n* to a ma*n*n*es* ers. And þis greuau*n*ce comeþ of a kene colric humo*ur* þ*a*t is in þ*a*t gutte, oþ*er* of a glasi flewme. Ȝif it comeþ of a colric humo*ur*, þ*er* is heete *and* p*ri*ckyng, *and* oþ*er*whiles ȝichi*n*ge, *and* oþ*er*whiles smertynge wi*th*-i*n*ne a ma*n*n*es* ers, for þe keneschip of colre fleeþ oþ*er*while þe gutte wi*th*-i*n*ne-foorþ, *and* makeþ it smerte. *And* oþ*er*whiles dropis of blood fallen out. Wha*n* it comeþ of salt flewme, þ*a*t þristeþ *and* p*er*sseþ þe gutte a-doun, *and* þei felyn coold wi*th*-i*n*ne-forþe. *And* þ*a*t mat*er* þat | passeþ fram them is whiȝt, oþ*er* pale wi*th* f. 128v muscilages. And oþ*er*whiles þ*er* comeþ þ*er*wiþ dropes of

2 hers] *prec. by heading* T̀enasmon **5 þe water**] *corr. from* þewat*er* **12 Tenasmon**] *2-line space left for initial* **a man**] *interl.* **20 for**] *corr. from* ffor **25 passeþ**] *prec. by heading* T̀enasmon

6 þat] *in r.-h. margin:* no*ta* b*e*n*e*

blood of so gret enforsynge þ*at* a man enforceþ hy*m*-self to schite. And wha*n*ne þis sicnesse comeþ of colre oþ*er* of flewme, it be-houeþ suppositories, *and* clist*er*ies, *and* p*ur*gaciou*n*s, as colica passio dooþ. Ȝif it comeþ of su*m* kene medicine þ*at* a ma*n* haaþ j-take, make hym a clist*er*ie of wat*er* þ*at* whete bryn haþ be j-sode*n* i*n*ne. And ȝif it be of colre, p*ur*ge hym w*it*h þe same, oþ*er* w*it*h su*m* oþ*er* p*ur*gaciou*n*, as it haiþ be teld her*e*-before. And sone ordeine þ*at* he be p*ur*geid, last þ*at* he falle in-to dissent*er*ie. Aft*er*-ward, late baþe hym in freisch*e* wat*er*, *and* siþe la[t] hym restyn. *And* þe next day, late hym blood vnd*er* þe ancle w*it*h-oute-forþ. And siþe seþe hock*es*, *and* violet, *and* holy-hock*es*, *and* bet*es*, oþ*er* barly meele, oþ*er* femygrek *and* lyn-seed in reyn-wat*er*. *And* þ*er*wiþ waisch*e* hese wombe *and* hys fondeme*n*t. And make hym a fumygaciou*n* of oold yren j-hat *and* vinegre j-sprent þ*er*-on. Oþ*er*, of a myll[n]e-stoon oþ*er* of a querne stoon j-hat, cast þe leeues of leek *and* make smoke þ*er*-of passen vp in-to hys fou*n*dement. Oþ*er* tac cootu*n* *and* weete it in oile of violet oþ*er* in schepis talwe, *and* put it in-to hys ers. Also tac an hool pyn-appel wha*n* þe
f. 129r kyrnelys be*n* oute | *and* liȝt hym in þe feir*e* til he be wel j-liȝtid. *And* siþe que*n*che þe liȝe þ*er*of *and* sp*r*ing þ*er*-on þe poudre of comyn, *and* of sauyne, *and* of colofonye. And late hym sittyn on a hooled stool, þ*at* þe smoke smyte to hys fou*n*deme*n*t. *And* lat hy*m* sitten so as long as he mai wel suffren it. And ofte-siþes late hys ers ȝokyn *and* be wasche w*it*h wat*er* þ*at* bren *and* hoolihockyn ben j-soden i*n*ne. And

4 **colica passio**] *corr. from* colicapassio 10 **lat**] *corr. from* lac 15 **yren**] *corr. from* eyren (first e *canc. twice*) 19 **of violet**] *corr. from* ofviolet 21 **kyrnelys ben**] *corr. from* kyrnelysbe*n* **and**] *prec. by heading* Tenasmon

late seþen a bagge w*ith* bren in wat*er* *and* late hy*m* ofte*n*-siþes sitten on þat bagge while it is hoot. But ȝif it be of glasi flewme, late purgen hy*m* w*ith* þe purgaciou*n* þat was j-teeld in lienterie, oþ*er* w*ith* su*m* oþere þat a-cordeþ to flewme as it haþ ben j-teld here-be-fore. And siþe make hy*m* a fumigaciou*n* of mynte, *and* of þe leeues of leek, *and* a litil castorie sode*n* i*n* wyn. And make hy*m* also a fumygaciou*n* *and* a waschi*ng* of ysope, piliole, origane *and* beet*es* j-soden in wat*er*. Also make poudre of ysope, of calamynte, *and* origane, oþ*er* of here flowres, *and* do þat poudre in hys ers. Oþ*er* ȝif þe gutte falle out wha*n* he gooþ to sege, spri*ng* þe poudre þ*er*-on. Also a-noi*n*te his lend*es* *and* his reynes w*ith* warm hony, *and* spri*ng* þ*er*-on poudre of colofonye, *and* of carses, *and* of piliole, *and* of origane. *And* siþe bynd it vp w*ith* a swaþeles. Oþ*er* heete a boord of a pyn-appel tree til þe gu*m*me swete owte þ*er*-of, *and* lete þe pacient sitte al bare on þat bord whil he is hoot. Also heete weel a tylestoon, *and* lei þ*er*-on peritorie oþ*er* wermot, *and* let hi*m* sitte þ*er*-on*n*. Oþ*er* on sich*e* | an hoot tylstoon, leie a baggeful of þe f. 129v poudre of bayes of a lore[re tre], and of carse seed, *and* of piliole, *and* of mastik, *and* of encense. And algate kepe þe pacient fra*m* coold. Also make hym ligge on hys wombe *and* a-no*n*cte hys leendis *and* his rugge vp-on to þe secu*n*de ioint of his chine w*ith* petroile. *And* siþe spri*ng* þer-on þe for-seid poudre of baies of lorere *and* of þe oþ*er* þi*n*ges, *and* siþe bynd it fast w*ith* a swaþel. A suppo-sitorie *and* þ*er* is no betyr for þis sicnesse: Tak of myrre, *dragme* iij; of olibanu*m*,

16 pacient] *follow. by canc. and exp.* sitte a **19 an**] *prec. by heading* Sekenesse **þe**] *interl.* **20 a**] *interl.*

1 seþen] *in r.-h. margin:* nota **18 lei**] *in r.-h. margin:* nota

dragme j; of ameos, *dragme* j; of opiu*m*, *dragme* s*emis*; of saffren, x grei*n*s. Medle he*m* w*it*h hony oþ*er* stamp hem wiþ an hoot pestel*e*.

Fallyng out of a mann*es* ers is fallyng out of þ*a*t gutte þ*a*t is j-clepid longao. *And* þis sicnesse comeþ of di-u*er*se enchesons, as of to gret a-forsyng þ*a*t a man a-forseþ hym to schi3t, as it is in dissent*er*ie *and* i*n* tenasmon. Oþ*er*while, it comeþ of an hoot heuy humo*ur* þ*a*t pitteþ *and* þristeþ out þe gutte at þe ers. 3if it come in þe first man*er*, it is j-knowe be dissent*er*ie oþ*er* tenasmon þ*a*t a ma*n* haþ j-haad. 3if it be in secu*n*de man*er*, it is j-know be heuynesse *and* coold þ*a*t a ma*n* feleþ be-neþe-forþ, and he haaþ [sete] oon a marbelstoon oþ*er* on su*m* oþ*er* coold stoones in coold tymes þ*a*t haþ maad hy*m* haue þis greuau*n*ce. 3if it be in þe iij man*er*e, he feleþ coold be-neþe-foorth*e*, *and* þe gut is neisch*e* *and* slideri, *and* þ*a*t þat passeþ fra*m* hym gooith*e* a- f. 130r 3ens his wille, | oþ*er* þ*a*t he wot nat þ*er*-of; *and* his colo*ur* is pale. For-to help*e* a man here-of, me moot 3eue a ma*n* an esy p*ur*gacion to p*ur*gen hym of flewme, *and* an esy clist*er*ie also, as it was j-teeld in colica passio. Oþ*er* make hy*m* an esy clist*er*ie of hony *and* of woma*n*n*es* mylk j-warmed. *And* þ*a*t purgeþ boþe flewme, colre *and* male*n*colie. And i*n* þe same man*er*e doiþ wat*er* þ*a*t lentes *and* wermot ben j-soden i*n*ne, *and* a lytyl hony cast þ*er*-to. A soueren remedi for þis greuaunce: Sta*m*pe garlec in clene wat*er*, *and* tac þ*a*t wat*er*,

1 **opium**] *follow. by canc. twice* s*emis* 2 **with**] *follow. by* hi*m*w*it*h 4 **Fallyng**] *2-line space left for initial* 5 **þis**] *interl.* 17 **oþer**] *prec. by heading* of the ers 18 **For-to**] *corr. from* ffor-to 20 **colica passio**] *corr. from* colicapassio 22 **flewme**] *corr. from* fflewme

22 **malencolie**] *in r.-h. margin:* no*ta* b*ene*

o*þer* þe wat*er* þ*a*t garlec haþ ben soden i*n*ne, *and* lat hys ers
ȝokyn wel þ*er*-i*n*ne. And aft*er*ward, take þe poudre of
hert*es*-horn j-bre*n*t, and of pyn-appel j-brent, *and* of
encense, *and* of mastik, and sp*ri*ng þ*er*-on. And þis same
medicine is good for fallyng out of þe mod*er* þ*a*t comeþ of
longe sitty*n*g oon a colde stoon. And make hy*m* a
fumigaciou*n* of pich*e* *and* encense j-cast on coles. And seeþ
otus o*þer* barlich*e* in a bagge, oþ*er* in many bagg*es*, *and* lei
he*m* al warme in þe man*er* of a plastr*e* boþe on þe schaar
and by-neþe vnd*er* hys ers. And þ*a*t is good boþe in
tenasmon *and* for he*m* þ*a*t ha*n* wormes. And ne ȝif hym no
st*ri*ctorie medicines tyl þe gutte be wel j-clensid of sory
hum*ur*os þ*a*t bien in hym. And aft*er* þe clensynge wiþ
clist*er*ies, orden hym þe for-seid bagg*es* in man*er*e of
plasteris. | Oþ*er*while, boþe thys sicnesse *and* tenasmon f. 130v
comyn of corupt wynd þ*a*t is in þe gutt*es*, *and* sekyn issu
and may haue no*n*, *and* þ*a*t is j-hoolden be medicines þ*a*t
co*n*sume*n* *and* wastyn sich*e* wyndes. Oþ*er*-while, it comeþ
of þe g*r*euau*n*ce of þe emoraudes *and* þa*n* it is j-heelid as þe
emeraudes bien. A special medicine *and* oyneme*n*t for þis
sicnesse is: Ȝif þe pacient bie a ma*n*, tak goot*es* talwe, *and* ȝif
he be a woma*n*, tac buck*es* talwe, *and* melt it. *And* cast þ*er*-
i*n*ne þe poudre of litarge, of ceruse, of amyde, of galles, of
balaustia, of akrene, of emathites, of bole, of sandragou*n*, of
eu*er*ich*e* of þese, j-lich*e* mych*e*. *And* wete a clowt in þis
oyneme*n*t *and* lei to his ers. *And* make hy*m* a fumigaciou*n*

1 water…garlec] *underl.* **ers…þer-inne]** *underl.* **9 boþe]** *corr. from* boþere (*er canc. twice*) **15 Oþerwhile]** *prec. by heading* Sekenesse in the ers

5 good] *in r.-h. margin:* no*ta* ben*e*

of galles, *and* psidie, *and* balaustie j-soden in reyn-wat*er*. *And* late hym sytte on an hoolid stoole þ*at* þe smoke mow smyte in-to hys ers. And afterward make hy*m* a fumigaciou*n* of colofonye *and* cow driʒt leed on cooles. But ʒif þe smoke mow nat smyte vp in-to hys ers, late wipe wel þ*at* place w*it**h* a schete. And siþe heue vp his hepis *and* sp*ri*ng vp-on þe gutte þe poudre of colofonye *and* of cow driʒt, *and* þe powdre of reed stoones þ*at* ben j-fou*n*den be-sides þe see *and* be-sides þe ryu*er*ys, *and* þe poudre of mu*m*mye, *and* of psidie, *and* of balaustie. *And* siþe pit it in-to þe gutte *and* lei w*it**h*oute*n* wermot, oþ*er* balaustia, *and* oþ*er* hoote herb*e*. And ʒif | f. 131r þe poudre wull*e* nat cleue to þe gutte, melt pich*e* *and* a-noi*n*te þe gutte þ*er*wiþ. *And* siþe sp*ri*ng on þi poudre *and* pit i*n* þe gutte. *And* late hym vse soupyng met*es* *and* laxatif met*es*, þ*at* he haue no nede to a-forcen hym to schite. And late hy*m* vsen to sitten in wat*er* þ*at* balaustie, *and* psidie, *and* sumac, *and* sich*e* oþ*er* bien j-soden i*n*ne. And late hys ers ʒoke wel þ*er*-i*n*ne *and* co*n*tinue his medicin*es* tyl he be hool.

Jn a mannes lyuere þ*er* bie*n* iij sicnesses: Oon is distemperi*n*g of þe lyuere in heete oþ*er* in coold, jn moistenesse oþ*er* in drienesse; an-oþ*er* is stoppy*n*g of þe lyuere; an þe thridde is a postym of þe lyuere. Distemperi*n*ge of þe lyuere þ*at* comeþ of hete haþ þese tokenes: bre*n*ny*n*g *and* p*ri*ckyng vnd*er* þe riʒt side, drinesse of þe tu*n*ge *and* of þe roof of þe mouþ, co*n*tinuel þirst, þe vrine is of an heiʒ colo*ur*, þe face is citryn *and* oþ*er*whiles grene. Coold þi*n*ges conforteþ hy*m* *and* hoote þi*n*ges noiʒen he*m*. He is ofte costif *and* wha*n* he schiteþ it is but litel. He wlateþ his mete, *and* slepeþ but litil. And wha*n* he slepeþ, he

4 colofonye] *corr. from* colofony*n*e **12 þe**[1]] *prec. by heading* Sekenes in the lyver*e* **19 Jn**] *2-line space left for initial*

holdeþ his mouþ hopy*n*. And o*þer*while his visage *and* his eiȝen bien infecte w*ith* a ȝelwe coloure. *And* þa*n* þei haue a gret itchy*n*ge ou*er* alle þe body *and* a scabbe. And ȝif þis diste*mp*eri*n*g be of su*m* corupt humo*ur*, þei felyn heuynesse vnd*er* þe riȝt side. And ȝif it be of colre, þe vrine is of a ful hiȝe colo*ur* w*ith* myche spume. *And* he felith*e* a smert p*ri*cchi*ng* | ache in þe leuere. *And* all*e* þe body is discolourid, f. 131v
and a-boute þe veynes þ*er* is myche reednesse *and* heete, more þa*n* in o*þer* places of þe body. And ȝif it be of blood, þe veynes be to-swolle ouere all*e* þe bodi. *And* o*þer* toknes ben a-sene þ*at* were j-teeld in þe ache of þe heed. And of sich*e* an hoote diste[m]p*er*ing*e* of þe lyuere comeþ a dropesi. And ȝif þe diste*mp*eri*n*g*e* be of coold, he feeliþ coold vnd*er* hys riȝt side, *and* his face is febelich*e* j-colourde. And ȝif þ*at* coold come of a corupt humo*ur*, he feleþ heuynesse in his lyuere, *and* na*m*ly aft*er* mete; and is face swelleþ su*m*what; *and* his vrine is discolourd; *and* he defieþ febly his mete; *and* alle his body wexiþ heuy, *and* na*m*ly aft*er* mete. His wutes bien a-stoined, *and* his heed is heuy of a gret corupt smoke þ*at* smyteþ vp in-to his heed. Hys mouþ is vnsau*er*ey *and* he is sluggy, but his sleep is trauelouse. *And* ofte-siþes þei han ryngyng in here eeren *and* scotomy, and þei ben disposid to a coold dropesi but ȝif þei be þe ra*þer* j-holpe. Tokenes of drienesse ben heuynesse in þe lyuere; þe colo*ur* of his face is j-chaungyd *and* apeired; þe lippes *and* þe tu*n*ge waxen driȝe; *and* þe cra*m*pe gooþ a-boute þe lyu*er*e; the tu*n*ge is driȝe; his vrine is thi*n*ne; his driȝt is of litel q*ua*ntite *and* drie; *and* his

4 **corupt**] *follow. by* be of su*m* corupt 7 **ache**] *prec. by heading* Sekenesse **þe leuere**] *corr. from* þeleuere 9 **more þan**] *corr. from* moreþa*n* 15 **he feleþ**] *corr. from* hefeleþ 20 **he is**] *corr. from* heis 27 **his**[1]] *follow. by canc. twice* j

body is leene. Tokenes of moistnesse ben swellinge of þe f. 132r visage; litel þirst; þe vrine is whiȝt | *and* clere, *and* oþ*er*whiles riȝt þicke, oþ*er*while menliche þicke; *and* his skyn is neische *and* his driȝt also. And ȝif þis distemp*erin*g be of flewme, þu maist j-knowe be tokenes of coold *and* of moistnesse. And ȝif it be of male*n*colie, þ*o*u maist j-know be token*es* of coold *and* of drynesse. Naþeles of male*n*colie þ*er* bie*n* special tokenes: Þe vrine is whiȝt *and* þi*n*ne, *and* he feleþ heuynesse *and* ache vnd*er* þe riȝt side, *and* grettest aft*er* mete, *and* na*m*ly wha*n* he haþ j-eten male*n*colies met*es*. *And* he feleþ gnawyng*e* *and* hurlyng a-bowtyn his leu*er*, *and* al his body is discolourd *and* heuy. And oþ*er* token*es* þ*er* ben also þ*a*t were j-teld in þe ache of þe heed. Diste[m]p*erin*g of þe lyuere þ*a*t comeþ of heete is j-heelid be medicines þ*a*t ben coold. And ȝif he haue plente of hum*ur*os þ*a*t ben enchesou*n* of þis diste[m]p*er*ing*e*, let p*ur*gen hym of þilke hum*ur*os. And furst defiȝe þe matere wiþ þe sirip of violet. *And* late hy*m* vse þeses electuaries, oþ*er*whiles oon, oþ*er*whiles anoþ*er*: diacitoniton, to restore his moistenesse þ*a*t is wasted awey w*it*h hete, diaprunys, sugre violet, t*ri*asendri, diarodon abbat*es*, rosata nouella. And ȝif his vrine wexeþ þicke *and* more þa*n* it was, ȝif hi*m* su*m* cologoge. But in þe distemp*er*ing of þe liuere þorouȝ hete, ne ȝyue hym no medicine þ*a*t scamone is i*n*ne, þei þe lyuere be stopped. But f. 132v ȝif þe sicnesse be | of oold, þu mytest ȝeue hy*m* þ[e] electuarie of þe iuys of rooses, oþ*er* oximel, oþ*er* t*ri*fera sarasenica w*it*h scamone. A special sirip*e* for hem: Tak þe root*es* of coold duretik erbis *and* þe erb*e* also, *and* coold

2 whiȝt] *interl.* h   **and**[1]] *prec. by heading* in the lyver*e*   **17 violet**] *corr. from* iviolet (i *exp.*)   **25 of**] *prec. by heading* Sekenesse   **28 and þe**] *corr. from* andþe duretik seed*es*, as of melou*n*, of cicru, of cucumer, of gourd*es*, of purselane, of letuse, of violet, of rooses, of wat*er*-lilees. *And* seeþe he*m* *and* siþe cast sugre to þe wat*er*, *and* make up þi syrip*e*. And cast þ*er*-to þe poudre of spodie, of mirabol*e* cit*ri*, *and* of reub*er*be. *And* eu*er*y morwetyde, ȝif hym þ*er*of, *and* on eui*n*tide also. And late hy*m* takyn it w*ith* þe iuys of ciceres, oþ*er* w*ith* goot*es* whey, oþ*er* wiþ wat*er* þ*at* duretik herb*e* ben sode*n* i*n*ne, oþ*er* w*ith* wat*er* þ*at* schauy*n*g of yuory is j-soden i*n*ne, *and* liuerwort, *and* hertistu*n*ge. And wha*n* þ*at* wat*er* is j-soden, cast þ*er*-to a litel vinegre þ*at* is j-maad of whiȝt wyn. Duretyk herbis ben þilke þ*at* ha*n* kynde to opene porys in a ma*n*n*es* body þ*at* be*n* j-stoppyd. And su*m*me ben hoote duretyk herb*e*, as fenel, *and* p*er*sely, radich, march, *and* þe rotis of þese ben more duretik þa*n* þe herbe. Coold duretyk ben hert*es*horn, *and* maydenher, *and* ci[c]ori, *and* ceterak. Hoote seedis þ*at* ben duretyk ben fenel seed, *and* p*er*sili seed, *and* þe seed of march, *and* of louage, *and* of anyse, *and* of ameos, *and* of anet. A-noi*n*te hy*m* w*ith*-oute*n* w*ith* popiliou*n*, *and* oile of rooses *and* of violet j-medlid to-gidere. *And* cast a litel vi*n*egre þ*er*-too oþ*er* þe gle[ire] of eyren. And | f. 133r make hym a plastre of rooses, of wat*er*-lilies, oþ*er* of þe poudre of iij sau*n*dris, *and* barly mele, *and* a litil spodie j-medlid w*ith* þe iuys of solatre, *and* a litel vi*n*egre j-warmyd *and* oile of rooses. Oþ*er* make hy*m* a plastre of spodie *and* of rooses j-medlid w*ith* þe iuys of

9 yuory] *corr. from* y*n*uory*n* **15 maydenher**] *corr. from* maydenhern (last n *canc. twice*) **16 cicori**] *corr. from* citori **21 And**] *catchword* (*in bottom margin*): make hym **make**] *prec. by heading* of the lyver*e* **25 þe**] *interl.*

12 kynde] *in l.-h. margin:* no*ta*

endyue, of morele, *and* of scariole. Anoþ*er* plastre: Take of whiȝt sau*n*dres *and* of reed rooses, *ounce semis*; of gu*m* arab*e*, of dragg*e*, of purselane seed, of spodie, *dragme* ij. Sta*m*pe he*m* w*ith* wat*er* of rooses *and* weet a clooþ þ*er*-i*n*ne, *and* ofte-siþes lei to þe liuere. And ȝif hi*m* a morwetid þe iuys of scariole, of endyue, of purslane, *and* of planteyn wiþ þe forseid sirip. Oþ*er*e medicines also þ*a*t ben good for vnkynde het*es and* feueris, be*n* good for þis sicnesse. And ȝif he be costif, make hym a clist*er*ie of bren, *and* of hockes, *and* of ly*n*seed j-soden i*n* wat*er*. Oþ*er* make hy*m* a suppositorie of scamone *and* of sugre. And diete hy*m* as me*n* þ*a*t ha*n* þe feueris. And ȝif þei ha*n* no feuerys, diete hy*m* w*ith* chekenys, *and* partriches, *and* sich*e* oþ*er* thing*es*, and ȝif hym wyn medlid w*ith* wat*er*. But þis xal nat be don but ȝif þe diste*m*pery*n*g bee oold, oþ*er* ellis þat þe heete bie nat full*e* greet. But ȝif þis distemp*er*i*n*g bie of coold, bewar of alle man*er* met*es* þ*a*t bien euel to defien, *and* fram greet met*es*, *and* fra*m* viscouse met*es*, *and* fram wyndy met*es*, *and* roostid met*es*. *And* diete hym as it was j-seed in cooldnesse of þe stomac. And ȝif he bie a riche ma*n*, late hym vse þese electuaries a-morwetide fastinge: dianthos, diaciminu*m*, f. 133v diacalamentu*m*, | þe hoote diacitonicon. And ȝif he bie a simpil ma*n*, ȝif hym diat*ri*onpip*er*ion *and* mel rooset. Also, ȝif he be a rich*e* ma*n*, ȝif hy*m* diamargaritou*n*, diacameron, diarodon of galien*es* maky*n*g oþ*er* of julians makyng. And ȝif he haue plente of flewme, lete hy*m* vsen oximel duretik. And ȝif hese sicnesse be of malencolie, ȝif hy*m* oximel sq*ui*llitik. And wha*n* þe mat*er*e is defiȝed, p*ur*ge hy*m* w*ith* a flewmagoge oþ*er* w*ith* a malogoge. And aft*er*ward make hy*m*

22 þe] *prec. by heading* Sekenesse **24 man**] *follow. by canc. twice* s a stufe of soþ*er*newode, *and* wermot, *and* mugwort, *and* m*er*che, *and* origane, *and* calamynte, *and* sauge, *and* mynte, *and* rwe, *and* horhoune, *and* lorere leues, *and* fenel. Tac of eu*er*ich*e* of þese j-lich*e* mych*e* *and* seeþ he*m* in liȝe. And late hym baþe hy*m* wel þ*er*-i*n*ne. And lat þ*at* place þ*at* is be-fore þe liu*er*e ȝoke wel in þe wat*er*. And take an handful or two of þe herb*e* *and* lei hem on þe liu*er*e in þe man*er*e of a plastre. Aft*er*ward a-noi*n*te hym w*it**h* hoote oynement*es* *and* w*it**h* hoote oiles. And in þis man*er*e þ*o*u schalt worche in simple diste*m*peri*n*g of þe lyu*er*e, þ*er*e-as þ*er* is no*n* corupt humo*ur* enchesou*n* of þ*at* diste*m*p*er*i*n*g, saue þ*at* þ*o*u xalt ȝif hy*m* no p*ur*gaciou*n*. But þu xalt vse þe same electuaries, *and* stufes, *and* plastres, in dieti*n*g, *and* oiles, *and* oynement*es*. Oþ*er* make a plastre of þe seed of fenel, of p*er*sili, march, of dauk, of carawei, j-poudrid *and* j-temprid w*it**h* þe iuys | of f. 134r mynte, of wermot, *and* of mugwort. Oþ*er* make a plastre of ysope j-soden. *And* make hy*m* a siripe of carses *and* of calamynte. Aloes j-wasschi*n* is ful p*ro*fitabil also. And eu*er*iche morwetide late hy*m* vse to drynke oximel w*it**h* wat*er* þ*at* duretik herb*e* *and* seed*es* ben j-soden i*n*ne, oþ*er* w*it**h* pyment þ*at* is j-maad w*it**h* duretik seed*es* *and* oþ*er* good spices, as gynger*e*, clowes, *and* canel.

Pyme*n*t is þus j-maad: Tak viij p*ar*ties of wyn *and* þe ix of hony þ*at* is wel despumed, *and* medle he*m* to-gidere, *and* siþe medle þ*er*-wiþ þese spic*es* j-poudrid: galingale, ging*er*, clowes, canel. *And* medle he*m* wel wiþ a sklise. *And* siþe let it renne þorow a bagge *and* kepe it. And ȝif þis diste*m*p*er*i*n*g

12 same] *corr. from* same (sa *canc.*; sa *interl.*) **15 of**[2]] *prec. by heading* of the lyver*e* **19 morwetide**] *interl.* r

22 and] *in r.-h. margin:* no*ta* **23 parties**] *in r.-h. margin:* pyment

bie of moistenesse oþ*er* of drinesse, it is nat comynly w*ith*-oute*n* distemp*er*i*n*g of heete oþ*er* of coold. *And* þ*er*-fore þ*a*t may be holpen be þ*a*t þat is j-seid be-fore, boþe here *and* in þe chapitre of horsnesse, of þe cowʒ, *and* of streitnesse of þe breest.

Dianthos is a medicine þ*a*t is good for t[i]sik, *and* for þe cardiacle, *and* for þe greuau*n*ce of þe liuere, *and* for alle man*er*e febilnesse of þe body, *and* na*m*lich*e* for febilnesse þ*a*t comeþ of long sicnesse. And it is þ*us* j-maad: Tac þe flowres of anthos, ij *pound*, *and* of þe braunches, ij *pound*; of whiʒt sau*n*dres *and* reed, *ounce* j; clowes, spik, gali*n*gale, *ounce* s*emis*; of cardamom*e*, canel, ʒedoware, *and* of note-muge, *dragme* iiij; of long pep*er*, of ging*er*, maces, lignu*m* aloes, *dragme* iij; of licoriys, *pound* s*emis*; *and* of his iuys, *dragme* f. 134v j; of sugre, | *ounce* s*emis*; of rooses, *ounce* iij; hony, q*ua*si s*emis*.

An-oþ*er* dianthos þ*a*t is moore vsed *and* is good fo[r] alle man*er* febelnesse of a mannys body: Tac of clowes, galingale, gyng*er*, spik, *and* of notemuge, *dragme* iiij; of þe floures of rooses-marine, *ounce* vj; of honi, *quantum* s*ufficit*. *And* late hy*m* eten here-of *dragme* iij at ones.

Yera-pigra of galiens makyng is good for greuaunce of þe lyu*er*e, *and* of þe heed, of eiʒen, of eeren, *and* purge*n* þe stomac. *And* ʒif þe splene be j-hardedit, it wole make hym neisch*e*. *And* it is good for þe reynes *and* for þe bladdere, *and* for þe mod*er*. *And* it is þ*us* j-maad: Tac of spik, of canel, saffren, sq*ui*nant*e*, asa*rum*, xilocassia, xilobalsamu*m*, violet, wermot, epithyme, agarik, rooses, gourde, wilde gourde, *and*

6 tisik] *corr. from* tosik **12 cardamome**] *corr. from* cardamom*eum* (u*m* *canc. twice and exp.*) **15 ounce**[1]] *prec. by heading* Sekenesse of the lyver*e*; *follow. by canc. twice and expuct.* iij of mastik, *dragme* ij; of aloes, tac þe wheiȝte of alle þe oþ*er* spices. *And* let hy*m* vsen here-of *dragme* iij. And ȝif þu wolt, ȝyue it hy*m* w*it*h pillules. Ȝyue it w*it*h sufficient diagredie.

Yerapigra of co*n*stantines makyng*e* is good to make þe siȝt clere, *and* to rekeuere þe siȝt, *and* to hoolden it. And it is good for þe stomac, *and* for þe lyuere, *and* for þe splene, *and* for he*m* þ*a*t han dissent*er*ie. *And* it purgeþ þe hum*ur*os and it is þus j-maad: Tac of mirabolan*e*, of kebuli indj, cit*ri*, of violet, of wermot, *dragme* iiij; of beller*e* emblici, cassia fistula, [e]pithime, sene, agarik, cuscute, sq*ui*nant*e*, reubarb*e*, *dragme* ij; xilocassie, spik, *and* anyse, *and* mastik, *and* xiloaloes, salge*m*me, nytre, *dragme* j; of hony, *quantum* s*ufficit*. Þis yerapigra is bet*er* for þe heed þa*n* þe toþ*er*, but þe toþ*er* is bet*er* for þe | p*ar*ties þ*a*t bien be-neþe þe mydriyf. f. 135r

Stoppyng*e* of þe lyuere is stoppy*n*g of oon of þe poor*es* of þe lyuere. There ben iiij poores of þe lyu*er*e þ*a*t mou*n* ben stoppeid. Oon is toward þe reynes þ*a*t comeþ fra*m* þe gutt*es*. An-oþ*er* is in þe ou*er* part of þe lyuere in þe gibbe. An-oþ*er* is toward þe galle. And þe iiij is in þe weie toward þe splene. And þis stoppyng comeþ of gret plente of blood, oþ*er* for þicnesse of blood, oþ*er* viscouse of þe blood. And þis comeþ oþ*er* of bloode, oþ*er* of colre, oþ*er* of flewme, oþ*er* of malencolie. Wha*n* þ*a*t weie is j-stoppid þ*a*t gooþ to þe veynes of þe guttes, þa*n* þi[lc]kene moistnesse þ*a*t þe veynes of þe guttes ȝouken ne mai nat come to þe lyuere, where-fore þ*a*t þat passeþ fra*m* þe*m* is myche *and* neische as it is in lient*er*ie. *And* gret greuaunce þei han in þe riȝt side byneþe-forþ. And þ*a*t is a comyn token of alle man*er*e stoppyng of þe lyu*er*e.

10 epithime] *corr. from* opithime **14 parties**] *prec. by heading* Stoppy*n*g of the lyver*e* **15 Stoppynge**] *2-line space left for initial* **19 is**[2]] *follow. by canc.* toward **24 þilckene**] *corr. from* þiclkene

Þe vrine is litil an of a febil colo*ur*, *and* þei slepi*n* litil. And þ*er*fore þe gutt*es* defien febilich*e*. And þe felyn gnawi*ng* *and* heuinesse be-twyn þe stomac *and* þe lyu*ere*, *and* þei be*n* þirstfull*e*.

Of þe stoppy*ng* of þe pore in þe gibbe, þese bien þe token*es*: Þe vrine is sotel *and* wateri, *and* þei felen heuynesse *and* greuau*n*ce from þe riȝt side, euene to þe ribbes *and* to rugge. And wha*n* þei goon to p*ri*uye, þei ben deliu*er*ed of litel mat*ere*. And þe ache þ*at* þei ha*n* is more scharp*e* þa*n* þe
f. 135v p*ri*ckyng*e* of nedles for streiȝt passyng of þe vrine þorow | þe smale veynes, *and* na*m*ly ȝif þe eten inflatif met*es*, as beenes, oþ*er* peeses, oþ*er* lentes, oþ*er* sich*e* bred, oþ*er* þerf, *and* sich*e* þi*n*ges.

Of stoppi*ng* of þe pore þ*at* gooþ to þe galle, þese ben þe tokenes: Colre is wyth*e*-holden i*n* þe lyu*ere*, wherefore þe vrine is of an hey colo*ur* w*ith* mych*e* spume, *and* vnd*er* þe su*n*ne is a ȝelwe colo*ur* oþ*er* a grene, for þe galle þ*at* is w*ith*-holden in þe lyu*ere*. And þei feelen p*ri*ckynges as of netles oþ*er* of nedlen vnd*er* þe riȝt side. And here face *and* here eiȝen ben j-colourid as of men þ*at* han þe ȝelwe euel of reed colre. And þei felyn ychi*ng* in here body, *and* be*n* thirstful, *and* slepen liȝttyl, *and* [han] a febel appetit. And oþ*er*while, þorow casti*ng*, þei ben deliu*er*id of colrik hum*ur*os, *and* here mowþ is bitt*er*. *And* þis is oon kynd of þe ȝelwe euel. Of stoppyng of þ*at* pore þ*at* gooþ to þe splene, þese ben þe tokenis: Þe vrine is of a swart colo*ur*, *and* oþ*er*while þicke. And þei felen miche heuynesse vnd*er* here riȝt side. And here face is of þe colo*ur* of leed or of a swart ȝelwe colo*ur*,

2 **felyn**] *follow. by canc.* gwa 10 **þe**[2]] *prec. by heading* Stoppy*ng* 15 **wythe-holden**] *corr. from* wyth*e*-holdeni (i *canc. twice*) 17 **for**] *corr. from* ffor

and al here body is ful heuy. And þei han dredful swenn*es* *and* a gret scabbe as þei it were þe mortmale. *And* here driȝt is blac. *And* þei han thenasmou*n* of heuynesse of malencolie þ*at* is in þe gutt*es*. And þis is also oon of þe spic*es* of þe ȝelwe euele. And ȝif þe lyu*er*e be distemp*er*id w*ith* eny of þe iiij hum*ur*os oþ*er* ȝif eny of þe iiij hum*ur*os be enchesou*n* of þis | stoppyng, þ*ou* maist j-knowi*n* it be þ*at* þat was j-seid in f. 136r þe laste chapitre.

For-to hele a ma*n* of þis sicnesse, me*n* must vse siche medicines þ*at* ha*n* kynde to oppyn þe pores þ*at* ben j-stoppid, and oþ*er* medicin*es* þ*at* han kynde to voide þe mat*er* a-wey þ*at* stoppeþ þe pores. And for as mych*e* as þe lyu*er*e is a nobil me*m*bir*e* *and* a worþi, it be-houeþ þ*at* his medicines ben confortabil as wel oppeny*n*g *and* p*ur*gyng. And su*m* medicines þ*er* bien þ*at* co*n*forte*n* þe lyu*er*e. Ȝif he be diste*m*p*er*id w*ith* heete, *and* openeþ þe poris þ*at* ben stoppid, *and* voidiþ a-wei þe mat*er* þ*at* stoppeþ he*m*; as rooses, *and* spodie, *and* sau*n*[d]ris, þese co*n*forteþ. An endyue, *and* scariole, *and* hertistu*n*ge, *and* maydenshere, þese co*n*forten, *and* openen, *and* p*ur*gen. Oþ*er* medicines þ*er* bien þ*at* co*n*forten, *and* openen, *and* p*ur*gen, ȝif þe diste*m*p*er*ing *and* þe stoppi*n*g bie of coold hum*ur*os, as piluole, *and* letuse, *and* coost, *and* genciane, *and* spik, *and* asa*rum*, *and* cuscute, *and* march, *and* epithime, *and* yue, boþe þilke þ*at* growen on trees *and* þilke þ*at* growen on walles. But ȝif a ma*n* wole hele oon me*m*bre of his sicnesse, he moost lo-ke wheþ*er* eny

6 of þis] *follow. by* of þis **7 stoppyng**] *prec. by heading* of the lyver **9 For-to**] *corr. from* ffor-to **12 as myche**] *corr. from* asmych*e* **18 An**] *follow. by canc.* endin **24 yue**] *corr. from* y*n*ue me*m*bre þ*a*t is nei3 be diste*m*p*er*id also. And þ*er*aft*er* þei moste worche; for 3if þe lyuere be diste*m*p*er*id oþ*er* j-stoppid, þe stomac oþ*er* þe splene mai be diste*m*p*er*id þe same tyme also. And þ*o*u xalt þa*n* 3ife þi medicines for þe lyuere to worche w*it*h-i*n*ne-forþ, *and* for þe splene w*it*h-outen-forþ. And 3if þe stomac be diste*m*p*er*id, orden þe medicines for þe stomac w*it*h-in-forþe, and for þe lyuer*e* f. 136v w*it*h-oute-forþe. And þis | schal be vnd*er*stonde 3if þe distemp*er*ing of sich*e* two me*m*bris discorden, as 3if þe oon bie of heete, þe toþ*er* of coolde.

A good rewle is a gret help*e* for þis sicnesse, and þis rewle stondeþ in many thi*n*ges: Oon is þ*a*t he baþe hi*m* nat aft*er* mete, ne walke he nat aft*er* mete myche, ne dryncke naþ*er* til þe mete þ*a*t he haþ j-ete be defied. And ne vse he nat swete mete ne swete dryncke. And vse he þe medicines þ*a*t bien j-telde in þe last chapitre, 3if þe stoppi*n*g be w*it*h diste*m*p*er*i*n*g of heete oþ*er* of coold. But specially vse he þ*a*t sirip 3if his distemp*er*i*n*g bie of heete, for þ*a*t openeþ þe stoppi*n*g. And it is p*ro*fitabil for he*m* boþe in medicines *and* in met*es* to vse p*er*silie, *and* fenel, *and* satureie, *and* sauge, and gourdis, *and* melou*n*, and þe iuys of ciceres, *and* gootes whei be hi*m*-self, oþ*er* w*it*h þe iuys of cuscute, or of scariole, oþ*er* of cicori, or of þe lasse centorie. And ofte-siþes, late hy*m* bleden at a veyne þ*a*t is j-clepid basilica for þe furst man*er* stoppi*n*g, and of þe hert veyne for þe secu*n*de, and of

2 for] *corr. from* ffor **5 with-outen-forþ**] *corr. from* w*it*h-i*n*ne (i*n*ne *exp. and* outen *interl.*) **8 schal**] *prec. by heading* Sekenesse **23 cicori**] *corr. from* scicori (c *interl.*)

1 also] *in r.-h. margin:* no*ta* **12 he**] *in l.-h. margin:* no*ta* **19 And**] *in l.-h. margin:* no*ta*

þe vey*n*ne of þe splene for þe þirde *and* for þe fourþe. But ȝif þe stoppi*n*g comeþ of coold, do as it was j-teld in þe laste chapitre. And diete hy*m* w*ith* suttyl þi*n*ges, as w*ith* carses, *and* skyrewhittes, *and* þe leues of seneuei, *and* netles, w*ith* þe brau*n*ches of radech, *and* of þe rot*es* of ellerne, *and* sich*e* oþ*er* þinges. And ȝif hym kene electuaries, as diacalamentu*m*, *and* dyatrionpip*er*ion, | *and* sich*e* oþ*er* þ*a*t bien hoote *and* f. 137r kene. And oones or ij in þe woke, ȝyf hym foure chasteyns or v j-roosted. *And* late hym ete hoot breed þe morwetyde. And but ȝif þ*o*u haue hoote bred, ȝif hym tosted bred j-weet in wyn. And þ*a*t xal kepen hym wel fram corupciou*n* of þe eyre. And also maydenhere is ful profitabil for sicnesse of þe lyu*er*e.

Aposteme of þe lyuere comeþ oþ*er*while of colre, oþ*er*while of flewme, *and* oþ*er*while of male*n*colie. Ȝif it comeþ of blood, þe ache *and* þe greuau*n*ce is vnd*er* þe riȝth*e* side. *And* he haþ comely a feu*er*e, *and* hys mouþ is swete, *and* þe white of hese eiȝen is reed, hys veynys ben fulle, *and* hys vrine is reed. Ȝif it is of colre, þ*er* is brenny*n*g *and* a scharp*e* kene ache vnd*er* þe rith side. *And* his mouþ is drei *and* bitt*er*, *and* he is þirstfull*e*. Ȝif it is of flewme, þ*er* is ache *and* greuau*n*ce vnd*er* þe riȝth*e* side w*ith* a man*er* softnesse. *And* þe face *and* all*e* þe body is of feble colo*ur*. *And* oþ*er*while, he haþ an heuy feu*er*e. And in eu*er*y posteme of þe lyu*er*e, þe vrine is troble. Ȝif it be of male*n*col*e*, þ*er* is

1 **þirde and**] *corr. from* þirde*and* 5 **ellerne**] *interl.* last l 7 **dyatrionpiperion**] *f. 137r* | trionpip*er*ion **and**[2]] *prec. by heading* of the lyvere 14 **Aposteme**] *2-line space left for initial* 15 **flewme**] *corr. from* fflewme 21 **flewme**] *corr. from* fflewme

11 **hym**] *in r.-h. margin:* no*ta*

heuynesse *and* hardnesse vnd*er* þe riȝth side, *and* drynesse w*ith*-oute*n*-forþ, *and* hese visage is of þe colo*ur* of þe erþe, *and* al þe body draweþ to þ*at* colo*ur* also. *And* oþ*er*-while þei f. 137v haue an esy fyu*ere*, *and* oþ*er*while | noon. And oþ*er*while þe posteme is in þe gibbe of þe lyu*ere*, *and* oþ*er*while in þe holwenesse þ*er*-of. Ȝif it be in þe gibbe, he feleþ hys greuau*n*ce neiȝ þe ruggebon, *and* þ*er* is swellyng a-seene. *And* he haþ greuaunce to drawe breeþ, *and* he haþ oþ*er*whil*e* a cowȝe. And vnneþe he may felen þe [t]ouchyng*e* of a ma*nnes* hand for greuance. But ȝif it be in þe holwenesse of þe lyu*ere*, he feleþ heuynesse *and* ache in þe depnesse of þe lyu*ere* *and* dou*n* to þe nauele; and he haþ gret wyl to cast, *and* oþ*er*while casteþ, *and* ȝixeþ, *and* bolkeþ. And ȝif a ma*n* pyȝt hys hand þ*er*-to, þe ach*e* waxeþ more. Ȝif þis posteme come of hoote hum*ur*os, late hy*m* blood at þe veyne of þe arme þ*at* serueþ for þe lyu*ere* *and* in þe ryȝth*e* arme. And in þe be-gynnyng of þe postym, þ*ou* xalt vse coold rep*er*cussyues to smyten a-ȝen þe mat*er* of þe posty*m*, as make a plastre of þe i*n*nere pili*n*ge of he*m*pe *and* of þe iuys of solatre, *and* ley þ*at* plastre warm on þe lyu*ere*. *And* chau*n*ge it iij or iiij siþes a dai. And a-noi*n*te þ*at* place w*ith* oile of rooses oþ*er* of violet. And late hym vse wiþ-in-for-þe f. 138r coold herb*e* in medicines, as endyue, purselane, *and* | sych*e* oþ*er*. Jn wexyng of þe posteme, vse dissolityu*es*, as barlich*e* meele j-soden w*ith* þe iuys of wermot, þ*er*-of make a plastre *and* ley þ*er*-on. But wha*n* þe posteme is ful j-waxe *and* þe mat*er* t*ur*neþ to q*uit*ure, þa*n* þe ache is moost greuouse. Þa*n* þ*ou* xalt w*ith* maturatyu*es* worche to make þe posteme ripe. Seeþe þa*n* wheete mele w*ith* oile of violet oþ*er* w*ith* freisch*e*

4 noon] *prec. by heading* Aposteem **5 þe**[1]] *interl.* **9 touchynge**] *corr. from* couchynge **23 syche**] *prec. by heading* of the lyver*e*

bot*er*e, *and* make þ*er*-of a plastre, oþ*er* of whete mele, *and* lynseed, *and* femygrek j-soden in liȝe þ*a*t ne is nat ful strong*e*. Oþ*er* in sich*e* liȝe, seeþ barly mele *and* make a plastre þ*er*of *and* w*it**h*-i*n*ne-forþe vse duretikes. Oþ*er* make a plastre of þe iuys of solatre, *and* of saundres, *and* a litel vi*n*egre, *and* of þe iuys of wermot. And wha*n* þe posteme is to-broke, þe q*ui*ture wole passe forþ wiþ hys vrine oþ*er* w*it**h* his digestiou*n*. And þa*n* mu*n*dificatifs ben good to clense þe lyuere of þ*a*t corupciou*n*, as diaprunes, sugre of violet, trifera saracenica, reubarb*e*, mylk of þe iiij coold seedys. Oþ*er* make a sirip of spikenard, *and* of hertystou*n*ge, *and* of endyue, *and* of þe iiij coold seed*es*, *and* of sugre. Oþ*er* seþe þe poudre of þe iiij coold sed*es* in wat*er* *and* clense it. *And* cast sugre þ*er*-to and siþe cast þ*er*-to þe seed of arage, letuse, p*er*sili, fenel, spikenard. *And* make | þ*er*-of a sirip. Oþ*er* ellys poudre þese f. 138v
sedys *and* do hem to þe toþ*er*. *And* make þ*er*of an electuarie *and* let hym vsen it erly *and* at mydday *and* at eue*n*. But yif þe posteme be of coold hum*urus*, lat hy*m* blood as j-said raþ*er* *and* late hym vse plastres rep*er*cussiuys as j-seid raþ*er*. But naþeles, it is bet*er* to ȝeue hym hoote duretiks boþe in sirips *and* in electuaries, as fenel seed, p*er*sely seed, march*e*, dauk. And wythouteforþe, ley plastres of dissolutyfs þ*a*t mou*n* open þe por*es* *and* t*ur*ne þe mater*e* in-to smokes *and* fumes, as of ysope, origane, centorie, rewe, celedoyn*e*, *and* sich*e* oþ*er*e. And make hym sich*e* plastres þ*a*t were j-teeld in þe posteme of þe stomac. Jn þe wexynge of þe posteme, vse plastres þ*a*t bien dissolutyues, as a plastre of wolle vnwaische j-soden in þe iuys of wermot. And wha*n* þe posteme is ful j-wexe þ*a*t þe mat*er*e draweþ to q*ui*ture, vse plastres mat*ur*atifs,

15 **þer-of**] *prec. by heading* Aposteem **Oþer ellys**] *corr. from* Oþ*er*ellys **21 fenel**] *corr. from* ffenel

as of whete meele, *and* of oile of violet, *and* hony j-medlid to-gidere. Oþ*er* make a plastre of snayles j-soden w*ith* hony, f. 139r *and* whete meele, *and* lynseed; oþ*er* | of þe rootys of affodille, *and* reysens, *and* dri3e figes j-soden in wyn, *and* li3e, *and* oile; oþ*er* of sourdowe j-soden in oile; oþ*er* of rwe j-soden w*ith* wyn *and* oile. And a-noi*n*te hym w*ith* dewte *and* popiliou*n* j-medlid to-gidere. And wha*n*ne þe poste*m* is j-broky*n*, 3yue hy*m* dianisu*m*, diasp*er*mat[ic]ou*n*, *and* diacalamentu*m*, *and* þe for-seid serip of wermot, *and* of spikenard, *and* of sich*e* oþ*er*. And 3if hy*m* myrabolan*e*, for þei ben good for boþe enchesons. *And* make hym a clist*ere* mollificatif *and* anoþ*er* mu*n*dificatif. And 3if þe mat*ere* be j-p*ur*geid be þe vrine, 3if hym wat*er* to drynke þ*at* duretik seed*es* ben j-soden i*n*ne. And 3if he be p*ur*geid þorow þe wombe, help hy*m* w*ith* þe decocciou*n* of tyme, epithyme, pollipodie, agarik, *and* sene. And vnd*er*stond in þe begynny*n*g of þese postem*us*, þe wo*m*b[e] is nei3sch*e* as þei he haad þe flux, for þe lyu*er* is vn-myty to drawe to hym moistnesse fro þe veynes of þe guttes. But in þe ende of þe posteme, a ma*n* wexiþ costif, for þa*n* þe lyu*ere* draweþ to hy*m* my3ttily moystnesse fra*m* þilke veynes. And vnd*er*stond þ*at* i*n* all*e* sicnesse of þe leu*ere*, þu xalt medle þi*n*ges þ*at* f. 139v *con*forteþ þe lyu*ere* w*ith* oþ*er* þi*n*g*us* þ*at* ben medicin*us*. |

Jn a mannes splene þ*er* bien diu*er*se sicnesse, as stoppi*n*ge, *and* swelly*n*g, hardnesch*e*, *and* neischip*e*, *and* posteme, *and* wyndnesse. And oþ*er*while he is replete of

3 **of**[1]] *prec. by heading* of the lyver*e* **4** **figes**] *corr. from* ffiges **15 hym**] *interl.* **17 wombe**] *corr. from* wo*m*bo **18 for**] *corr. from* ffor **24 Jn**] *2-line space left for initial; prec. by heading* Sekenesse

26 of] *in l.-h. margin:* replecion

hum*ur*os more þa*n* he xuld be. And he may be replete *and* full*e* of iij hum*ur*os, p*ri*ncipali of malencolie. He is ordeyned to resceyue male*n*colie þ*a*t comeþ fra*m* þe lyu*er*e, ry3t as þe bladdere vnd*er*fongeþ þe vrine; *and* þe bladdere þ*a*t cleueþ to þe lyuere vnd*er*fongeþ colre *and* galle þ*a*t comeþ fra*m* þe lyuere; and þe splene may be ful also of fleume *and* of colre. 3if it be ful of malencolie, þese bie*n* þe tokenes: Þe vrine is whi3th*e*, þi*n*ne, *and* clere, oþ*er* ell*e* swart 3elwe, oþ*er* blak, of malencolie þ*a*t is j-medlid þ*er*-wiþ þe which*e* also makeþ þe vrine þicke. *And* he feeliþ ache *and* swellyng vnd*er* þe lyft syde, *and* mech*e* hardnesse þ*er*-as þe splene liþ. And all*e* hese body is heuy *and* discolo*ur*d, *and* lene *and* feble. *And* he bolkeþ sowre, *and* hese spiti*ng* is soure *and* kene. And his face is a derk whi3t oþ*er* pale. And þe whi3t of hese ei3en ben swart 3elwe *and* þei ben t*ur*ned fra*m* þere kyndly colo*ur*. And þei fele*n* mych*e* heuynesse aft*er* | mete *and* defien febely f. 140r
here mete.

Of repleciou*n* of flewme þe tokens bien whi3t vrine *and* þicke, oþ*er* þi*n*ne, but nat clere; ache *and* hardnesse vnd*er* þe lift syde, but nat so gret as of male*n*colie. Hese bolkyng is w*it*h-oute sau*er* *and* hese spittynge also. And þe pawmes of hese hoondes ben hoote *and* þe sooles of hys feete also. And he haþ feble digestiou*n*, *and* þ*a*t þat passeþ fra*m* hym is whi3t *and* rennyng*e*, ful of spume, oþ*er* þicke w*it*h muscilages. And þe body is discolo*ur*d *and* a pale colo*ur* *and* a feble. And he wol be soon wery in goyng*e* *and* is slow in goynge, *and* more aft*er* mete þa*n* be-fore.

Of repleciou*n* of colre tokens bien: Þe vrine is of an hei3 colo*ur* *and* þi*n*ne; *and* swelli*ng*, *and* heuynesse, *and* hardnesse

14 **face is]** *corr. from* faceis **of]** *interl. and follow. by exp.* o
16 mete] *prec. by heading* of the splene

þ*er* a-boute as þe splene liyþ, wiþ heete þ*a*t is j-felid in þe depnesse of þe splene. And hese mouþ is driȝe *and* bitter*e*, *and* he is þristfull*e*. *And* he haþ gret will*e* to cast. And hese face *and* alle hese bodi is of a cit*ri*ne colo*ur*. *And* hese driȝt is citryne *and* renny*n*g, *and* oþ*er*while it is þicke. *And* hese body is lene *and* feble. *And* þis is ful hard to bien j-heelid. Neischip*e* of þe splene comeþ of flewme þ*a*t renneþ in-to hys f. 140v | pores *and* makeþ hym neisch*e*. And þe tokene here-of is þ*a*t wha*n* men touche þe place w*i*t*h* a ma*n*n*es* hand, he xal fele it alle neisch*e* vnd*er* þe fyngerys, as þei þe splene were j-t*ur*ned in-to hum*ur*os þ*a*t bien fletynge *and* neisch*e*. And þei felen also ache vnd*er* þe lyft side. And oþ*er* toknes it haþ also of þe replecioun of þe splene þ*a*t comeþ of fleume. Hardnesse of þe splene comeþ of malencolie þ*a*t is dried *and* j-harded in þe splene. And tokne þ*er*of is heuynesse in þ*a*t place þ*a*t þe splene liyþ. And þe vrine is discolo*ur*d *and* þi*n*ne, *and* oþ*er*whiles blac *and* þicke of malencolie þ*a*t is j-medlid þ*er*-wiþ. And þ*a*t makeþ a ma*n* defien euel his mete. And oþ*er*whiles fallen in-to a flux, *and* oþ*er*whiles costif. Also þis hardnesse of þe splene comeþ of viscouse flewme þ*a*t is in þe splene. And whan þe watt*ri*nesse þ*er*-of passeþ a-wey, þe re*m*nannt a-bideþ stille *and* makeþ þe splene hard. And þis hardnesse haþ þe same token*es* þ*a*t þe oþ*er* hardnesse haþ þ*a*t comeþ of malencol*e*. And hardnesse of þe splene comeþ also of colre, wha*n* þe sotile moistnesse wanysch*e* a-wei thorouȝ

4 citrine] *follow. by canc. and exp.* clo*ur* **6 ful hard**] *corr. from* fulhard **8 pores**] *prec. by heading* Aposteeme **9 place with**] *corr. from* placew*i*t*h* **13 fleume**] *corr. from* ffleume **15 is**] *follow. by canc.* hardnesse **16 liyþ**] *corr. from* liyþ*n*

7 þe] *in r.-h. margin:* neisnes **13 of**[2]] *in l.-h. margin:* hardnes hete, *and* þe gretnesse a-bideþ stille *and* wexeþ | hard. And þe f. 141r tokenes þ*er*-of bien p*ri*ckyng *and* brenny*n*ge vnd*er* þe liȝft side, *and* continuel þirst *and* bitt*er*nesse of þe mouþ, *and* cit*ri*ne colo*ur* of þe face, and þe vrine is an hiȝe colo*ur* *and* þi*n*ne. *And* he haþ a flux, *and* all*e* hese body is ȝelwe.

Stoppynge of þe splene comeþ oþ*er*-while of coold hum*ur*os, as of fleume *and* of male*n*col*e*, oþ*er*while of colre. Oþ*er*while þe stoppi*n*g is toward þe stomac, *and* þa*n* a ma*n* leueþ his appetit to mete. Oþ*er*while it is j-stoppid toward þe lyu*er*e, *and* þa*n* malencolie is w*ith*-hoolden in þe lyu*er*e *and* is j-sent forþ ou*er* al þe body. Oþ*er*while it passeþ fro þe wey þat vrine gooþ *and* makeþ þe vrine thicke. Oþ*er*while it bideþ in þilke wei, so streiȝt þ*a*t þe vrine mai nat passen þ*a*t wei but it be clensid *and* j-maad as clere *and* as þi*n*ne as eny wat*er*. Oþ*er*while þe splene is j-stoppid toward þe guttes. *And* þa*n*ne þe guttes ben j-febelid þ*a*t þei may nat wel w*ith*holden þ*a*t is w*ith*-i*n*ne hem, and so a ma*n* falleþ in-to a flux. Oþ*er*whiles þe splene is al round *and* oþ*er*while euene long*e*. Oþ*er*whiles þe splene is thicke on þe ton syde *and* þi*n*ne in þe othere side, oþ*er*while a-boue, oþ*er*while be-neþen. Oþ*er*while he is j-stoppid ou*er* eu*er*y side, oþ*er*while in su*m* side. Oþ*er*while it is j-stoppid of colre þ*a*t p*er*seþ i*n*-to þe por*es*. | f. 141v

1 **wexeþ**] *catchword* (*in bottom margin*): hard **hard**] *prec. by heading* Of the spleene 7 **fleume**] *corr. from* ffleume 13 **þilke wei**] *corr. from* þilkewei 16 **nat wel**] *corr. from* natwel 17 **a man**] *corr. from* ama*n*

6 **oþer-while**] *in r.-h. margin:* Stopping

Swellyng*e* of þe splene comeþ of hum*ur*os þ*a*t fillen þe splene *and* þ*a*t may be knowen be þat þ*a*t was j-seid in replecioun of þe splene.

Wyndynesse of þe splene comeþ of gret hum*ur*os þ*a*t ben j-genderyd of a febele hete. *And* þilke hum*ur*os letten þe wynde þ*a*t is in þe splene of hese issue. Oþ*er* it comeþ of hum*ur*os þ*a*t þorow violence dryueþ wynd in-to þe splene. *And* þ*a*t wynd makeþ þe splene gret *and* myche. And þe token here-of is of wellynge a-boute of þ*a*t wynde *and* horsynge fra*m* place to place. *And* now it comeþ, *and* now it gooþ.

Aposteme of þe splene comeþ oþ*er*while of hoote hum*ur*os *and* oþ*er*while of colde. *And* þis haþ þe same token*es* þ*a*t replecioun haþ. And also, ȝif it be of coold hum*ur*os, þei felen coold *and* ache vnd*er* þe liȝft side. Ȝif it be of heete, þei felen brenny*n*g *and* p*ri*ckyng*e* in þe liȝft side. *And* þei han a co*n*tinuel feuere.

For neischepe of þe splene ȝit it be of coold hum*ur*os, ȝif hy*m* oximel to defie þe hum*ur*os. Aft*er*ward ȝif hy*m* jerapigre g[alieni] to p*ur*gen þe hum*ur*os oþ*er* sych*e* an-oþ*er* medicine. Aft*ur* iij dai make hym a stufe of hoote herb*e*, as of origane, calamynte, horehoune, tyme, roose-marine, *and* sich*e* oþ*er*e. And þe next dai aft*er*, late hym blood vnd*er* þe ancle in þe hyndere side of þe liȝft foote. And siþe make
f. 142r hoote plastres þ*a*t ben durynge *and* | consumyng*e* þe

1 **Swellynge**] *prec. by heading* Sekenesse 2 **and**] *in l.-h. margin* 13 **of**] *follow. by canc.* hoot (ot *also exp.*) 18 **For**] *corr. from* ffor 25 **consumynge**] *prec. by heading* of the splene

1 **Swellynge**] *in l.-h. margin:* Swelling 10 **it**[1]] *in l.-h. margin:* Aposteme 17 **han**] *in l.-h. margin:* neisnes

hum*ur*os, *and* lei to þe splene, as of rwe, *and* of celydone, netles, *and* of comyn j-soden, *and* of sych*e* oþ*er*e. And late a-noi*n*te hym be-fore þe splene w*it*h warm hony, *and* sp*ri*nge þere-on þe poudre of seneuei, *and* of carse seed, *and* of comyn, *and* of sich*e* oþ*er*e.

Hardnesse of þe splene *and* stoppynge of þe splene a-corden myche in medicines, saaf þ*a*t medicines þ*a*t ben oppeny*n*g a-corden to þe stoppy*n*g of þe splene, and p*ur*gaciou*n*s *and* medicines þ*a*t ben mollitif a-corden to þe hardnesse of þe splene to make þe matere neisch*e*. And siþe þu xalt vse medicines þ*a*t bien dissolutif to dissolue þe mat*er*e *and* to drawen it a-wey þ*a*t was enchesou*n* of þe hardnesse. And vnd*er*stond þ*a*t hardnesse of þe splene is oncurabil, oþ*er* ful hard to bien j-cured, wheþ*er* it be of hete oþ*er* of coold, *and* a man haue j-had it a ȝere. Naþeles, su*m* men seyn þ*a*t it wole raþ*er* ben j-heelid aft*er* x ȝere þan aft*er* þe furst ȝere. Also wha*n* þe matere is meuy*n*g, *and* seen, *and* nat j-hyd, it is bet*er*e to bien j-heelid þa*n* ȝif it were j-hyd. Also ȝif me*n* touche þe place þ*a*t is be-fore þe splene, ȝif it be so hard þ*a*t it syncke nat vnd*er* þe fynger*es* it is incurabil. And þu xal gyf hym no laxatif medicine þorouȝ hys mouþ, ne duretik medicine, ne no me-dicine þ*a*t is ful dissolutif, neiþere w*it*h-i*n*ne, ne w*it*h-oute | tyl þu haue ȝif hym f. 142v
mollificatifs to make þe splene neisch; for ellys þe matere þ*a*t

4 þere-on] *follow. by canc. twice* hym (þere *interl.*) **14 ful hard**] *corr. from* fulhard **20 fyngeres**] *corr. from* ffynger*es* **23 tyl**] *prec. by heading* Sekenesse **24 make þe**] *corr. from* makeþe

1 of[1]] *in r.-h. margin:* no*ta* **6 Hardnesse**] *in r.-h. margin:* hardnes **20 incurabil**] *in r.-h. margin:* no*ta*

is sotel wolde vanysche a-wei *and* þe waxen hardere þa*n* he was. Ne þu xalt nat late hym blood tyl matere bie j-maad neisch*e* be mollificatifs *and* þ*a*t he bie p*ur*ged, last þe splene wexe hardere þa*n* he was. And vnd*er*stond þ*a*t þe splene is p*ur*ged þorow þe wombe, as þe lyuere is p*ur*ged þorow þe bladdere w*ith* þe vrine. And ȝif his hardnesse come of hoote hum*ur*os, ȝif hym oximel to defie þe hum*ur*os *and* on morwetyde *and* euen *and* be-fore mete. A-noi*n*te þe splene w*ith* bot*er*e *and* oile of violet oþ*er* w*ith* deute *and* froot it softly. And late hym stere wel hys lift arm as ryngyng a belle or blowyng bellies. And late hym vsen sich*e* traueile fra*m* þe tyme þ*a*t it draweþ til it be liȝt dai. *And* late hym vse to walke in hilly places morwetides tyl he swete. And ȝif hym oximel w*ith* wat*er* to drynke þ*a*t þe floures of borage *and* of violet bien j-soden i*n*ne. But late hy*m* vse before diadragant *and* dyapenydion for hys breest. And wha*n* þe splene wexeþ neisch*e*, p*ur*ge hy*m* wiþ þe electuarie of þe iuys of rooses, oþ*er* w*ith* t*ri*fera sarasenica, oþ*er* w*ith* reubarb*e*.

Electuarie of þe iuys of rooses is þus j-maad: Tak of
f. 143r sugre, j *pound and* iiij *ounce*; | *and* of þe iuys of rooses, as mych*e*; of euerich*e* of iij kyndes of saundres, *dragme* vj; of spodie, *dragme* iij; of diagredie, *ounce* j *and* iiij *dragme*; of camphore, *dragme* j. Make a sirip of þe sugre *and* of þe iuys. *And* herewiþ tempre þe poudre of þese oþ*er* þinges. And þe iij dai make hy*m* a baþ of þe leues of a vyne, *and* of

1 **þe waxen**] *corr. from* þewaxen **he was**] *corr. from* hewas 5 **þe**[1]] *interl.* 10 **as**] *follow. by canc. twice* ryn 14 **floures**] *corr. from* ffloures 15 **diadragant**] *corr. from* diadragaunt (u *exp.*) 20 **and**[2]] *prec. by heading* of the spleene

10 **And**] *in l.-h. margin:* no*ta*

turmentille, *and* of lyuerwort, hockes, violet, fenel, wermot, *and* of saleyn leu*es* in a gret q*ua*ntite. And siþe late hym reste. *And* þe next dai aft*er*, late hym blood on þe left arme in þe salutelle of þe liȝft hond, oþ*er* at þe veyne vnd*er* þe liȝft eere, *and* at þe veyne also þ*at* is vnd*er* þe ancle of þe left foot. And eu*er*ych*e* woke ȝif hym a calagoge. *And* late hy*m* drynke warm wyn þ*at* steel oþ*er* goold is j-quenchid i*n*ne, for coold þi*n*ges neyȝen þe splene. Oþ*er* make a sirip of smythys wat*er* *and* late hym drynke þ*er*of ofte-siþes w*it*h warm wat*er*. And ȝif hym of þ*at* wat*er* þ*at* iiij coold seed*es* ben j-soden i*n*ne, *and* lyuerewort, *and* maidenhere w*it*h hem. And ȝif hym diaceraseos *and* sugre of violet j-medlid to-gidere eu*er*ych*e* morwetide.

Dietynge of hem xal bien of temp*er*at met*es* *and* drynkes. *And* be þei ware of grete met*es* *and* of malencol*e* met*es*. And be-fore mete, þei xal traueil a litel, and aft*ur* mete reste hem. And late hem vse in here potage planteyn, *and* hockes, cicory, growndeswili, *and* morel, *and* mercurie, oþ*er*e j-soden be hym-self oþ*er* w*it*h fleisch*e*. And ȝif hy*m* medicin*es* | also þ*at* bien good for þe ȝelwe euel *and* for stoppyng*e* of þe lyuere þ*at* comeþ of heete. Oile þ*at* is j-maad of þe levis of myrte is good for hem. And so is a plastre j-maad of femygrek *and* hock*es*. *And* þe roote of holyhocke and þe leues *and* þe stalkes of capperys j-ete in electuaries is profitabil for þis greuau*n*n*c*e wha*n* it comeþ of heete. f. 143v

1 fenel] *corr. from* ffenel **5 foot**] *corr. from* ffoot **8 for**] *corr. from* ffor **20 also**] *prec. by heading* Sekenesse **23 femygrek**] *corr. from* ffemygrek

6 hym²] *in r.-h. margin:* no*ta* **18 and¹**] *in r.-h. margin:* no*ta* **25 of**] *in l.-h. margin:* no*ta* bene

Diacaparis is good for eu*ery* greua*n*ce of þe splene *and* of þe lyuere, boþe newe *and* oold. And ȝif þe splene is j-hardid, it makeþ hym neisch*e* a-ȝen. And ȝif it is j-dru*n*ke w*ith* wyn, it sleeþ wormes þ*a*t be*n* in a ma*n*nes wombe. And ȝif it is j-medlid w*ith* vinegre *and* j-caast in-to a ma*n*nes eere, it sleeþ þe worm*es* þ*a*t bien þ*er*-i*n*ne. And ȝif it is j-medlid w*ith* wyn *and* j-hoolden in a ma*n*n*es* mouþ, it dooþ a-wei ach*e* of þe teeþ. And ȝif it is j-meedlid w*ith* wat*er* þ*a*t rewe is j-soden i*n*ne *and* j-dru*n*ken, it makeþ a woma*n* þ*a*t is j-stopped to haue here p*ur*gaciou*n*. *And* it is þus j-maad: Take of capparis, iiij *dragme*; of sq*ui*lle, asa*rum*, centorie, piretre, pep*er*, tyme, merch, sene, gith, agrymonie, *and* of radich, *ounce* j; of hony, *quantum* s*ufficit*. Ȝyue hym þ*a*t han þe greuaunce of þe splene iiij daies here-of, but ȝif þis g*re*uaunce *and* hardnesse comeþ of coold. Oþ*er*whiles it comeþ wha*n* þe leuere is distemp*er*ed w*ith* heete and þa*n*ne it behoueþ to don redileche boþe in dieti*n*ge *and* in electuaries,
f. 144r for þe lyue[r]e wold haue coold thynges *and* þe splene | hoote. And temp*er*at medicines wole hele eu*er*e eyþere. *And* þ*er*fore oon medicine wole nat serue for þem boþe. But me*n* most vsen medicines for þe lyuere w*ith*-i*n*ne-forþ in electuaries *and* in siripis. And for þe splene, þu xal vse medicines w*ith*-outen-forþ, as plastres [and] oynement*es*. And ȝif þe lyu*er*e bie distemp*er*id w*ith* hete for þe same tyme, lei coold plastres to þe lyuere *and* hoote plastres to þe

5 j-medlid with] *corr. from* medlidw*ith* **15 greuaunce**] *follow. by canc. twice* iiij **16 þe**] *follow. by canc.* hee **18 for**] *corr. from* ffor **lyuere**] *corr. from* lyuene **19 hoote**] *prec. by heading* of the splene

18 for] *in l.-h. margin:* no*ta* p*er* gre*v*ys

splene. And a-noi*n*te þe lyuere coold oynementis *and* oiles, *and* þe splene w*ith* hoote. And furst bie a-boute to make þe splene neisch*e* w*ith* deute *and* bot*er*e, oþ*er* oile of aisches *and* briches j-medlid to-gidere, oþ*er* lynsed j-sta*m*pid *and* j-soden in botere, *and* þ*er*-of make a plastre. Oþ*er* make an oyneme*n*t of hock*es*, *and* of holyhocke, beetes, lilie rotis, *and* of oyneou*n*s j-leid in wyn *and* in oile a-iiij daies or a–v, *and* siþe j-soþin til þe wyn be co*n*sumed. And defie þe matere w*ith* oximel sq*ui*llitik oþ*er* oximel of radich. But be-fore, late hym vse diacene, oþ*er* diacaparis, oþ*er* dia-sp*er*mat[ic]on, *and* su*m* oþ*er* electuaries w*ith* oon of hem, as diarodon oþ*er* triasendri. And siþe p*ur*ge hy*m* w*ith* diacene, oþ*er* ierapigra g[alieni], oþ*er* w*ith* þe v kyndes of mirabol*e*, oþ*er* w*ith* þis special medicine: Seeþ herb*e* þ*at* bien duretik, *and* in þe same wat*er*, seeþ tyme, *and* epithime, sene, cuscute, *and* þe rynde of tamarynd*e*, *and* of aisch, *and* capparis. *And* siþe clense þ*at* wat*er* *and* cast þ*er*-i*n*ne þe poudre of mirabol*e* indj, *ounce* ij; *and* of lapis laȝuli *and* armoniac*e*, *dragme* ij. But waisch wel þe stoones bi-fore, *and* late hym drynke of þis wat*er*. And aft*er* þ*at* | he haþ vsed þis iij daies, make hym a stufe of f. 144v
hoote h*er*bis *and* duretik. And þe nexte daie aft*er*, late hym blood at þe salua[t]elle of þe leeft honde oþ*er* vnd*er* þe leeft eere. And ones a weke, ȝyf hym a clistere to p*ur*ge flewme oþ*er*e malencolie. And make plastres þ*at* bien mollitifs to make þe splene neisch*e*, as of ammoniac, myrte, *and* deute, *and* a litel vinegre j-medlid to-gidere *and* j-leid vp-on a clooþ vp-on þe splene. Oþ*er* tak drye gotus dryȝt *and* lei it al a-daiȝe in vi*n*egre. *And* siþe stampe þ*er*w*ith* ammoniac *and* þe

1 lyuere] *follow. by canc.* l **8 þe wyn**] *corr. from* þewyn **11 oon of**] *interl.* **20 he**] *prec. by heading* Sekenesse **22 saluatelle**] *corr. from* saluacelle

leeuys of whiȝt horehowne *and* mak þ*er*-of a plastre. Or make a plastre of squille j-soden *and* of a*m*moniac, oþ*er* of rwe, *and* march*e*, *and* vyne, axes, *and* wyn, *and* vinegre j-stamped to-gidere. Make a plastre *and* lei þ*er*-to. Oþ*er* make a plastre of a*m*moniac *and* of salt *and* armoniac. *And* þis is good for swelli*n*g of þe splene. And tempre þe wyn þ*at* þei drynke w*ith* wat*er* þ*at* þe roote of fenel is j-soden i*n*ne, *and* of march, *and* of p*er*sili, *and* lyu*er*wort, *and* hert*es*-tounge, *and* maidenhere, *and* filipe*n*dula, *and* ceterak, *and* pollitricu*m*, *and* adyanthos. And ȝif it be abhomynabil to drynke, do sugre þ*er*-to *and* make þ*er*-of a sirip*e*. Also late hym vse wat*er* þ*at* capparys, filip[e]ndula, *and* pentafilon ben j-soden i*n*ne. Also a plastre j-maad of turmentyne, *and* a litel oile, *and* barly mele j-medlid to-gidere on an esy feire doiþ a-wei þe hardnesse of þe splene. An-oþ*er* good plastre: Take hoote duretik seedis, *and* comyn, *and* oxes driȝt, *and* þe poudre of milie, *and* þe iuys of walwort. *And* make þ*er*-of a
f. 145r plastre. Also make hym a baaþ of hoot herbis *and* of duretik | j-soden in wat*er*. *And* wha*n* he comeþ out of þe baaþ, anoi*n*te þe place be-fore þe splene wiþ a weþeres galle, *and* lei þ*er*e a-boue wolle þ*at* was j-schore on-wasche *and* haþ ben j-dried i*n*ne þe su*n*ne. Aft*er*ward tak hony as it comeþ out of þe hony combe *and* as mych*e* of salt, as mych*e* as of hem boþe. *And* medle þese to-gidere. *And* late hym vsen of þis confecciou*n* ix daies in wexi*n*ge of þe mone þe morwetid whil he is fasti*n*g. An late hym faste til it be vndern *and* make oon of þe forseid plastres euerich*e* dai. Oþ*er* late hym drynke

3 **vyne**] *follow. by canc. twice* as **7** **fenel**] *corr. from* ffenel **9** **filipendula**] *corr. from* ffilipe*n*dula **12** **filipendula**] *corr. from* ffilipondula **19** **j-soden**] *prec. by heading* of the spleene **27** **þe forseid**] *corr. from* þeforseid

camedreos *and* camapitheos *and* make of hym a plastre also, *and* vse hem in electuar*e* also. Oile of ellerne doiþ a-wei þe hardnesse of þe splene *and* so dooþ a*m*moniac also. An oyneme*n*t to do a-wei þe hardnesse of þe splene: Tak of lynseed *and* of femigrek, *ounce* j; of þe seed of hock*es*, of wermot, *and* of cotou*n*, *ounce* s*emis*; *and* tak resynes, *and* þe roote of holy-hocke, *and* wrappe hem in herdys j-wet. *And* roost hem in hoote axen. *And* siþe stampe al þis wel to-gidere *and* do it in vi*n*egre a-dai *and* a-nyȝt, so þ*at* vn-eþes it bie wrien wiþ vi*n*egre. Amorwe do it al to-gidere, iij *pound* of oile, *and* whiȝt wyn, *and* of vinegre. But late þe to part*es* ben of oile, *and* þe iij wyn, *and* þe iiij of vi*n*egre. And cast þ*er*-to *ounce* of clene barly flo*ur* *and* seþ al þis to-gidere tyl þe wyn *and* þe wi*n*egre be consumed. *And* þa*n* wryng*e* it wel thorow a clooþ *and* cast þ*er*to wax *and* freisch*e* boter*e*, of eu*er* eiþere, *ounce* ij; of oile of violet, *ounce* s*emis*. *And* melt hem to-gidere. And kepe it for it is good for hardnesse of þe splene. And ȝif þu wolt make it good for hardnesse of þe splene þ*at* comeþ of coold, put þ*er*-to þe root*es* of sq*ui*lle, *and* of bryonye, *and* | of wilde gourdis, *and* put hem in f. 145v
vinegre w*ith* lynseed. Oþ*er* lei hem ij daies, *and* siþe boile hem w*ith* þe oþ*er*e, and at þe last do þ*er*-to *ounce* j of oile of lorere. *And* þ*er*wiþ a-noi*n*te hym eu*er*y dai be-fore þe splene. But aft*er* þ*at* þe splene is j-maad neisch*e*, it be-houeþ to haue medicines to dryen vp þe hum*ur*os of þe splene. But þu xal nat eu*er*more vse þilke medicines, but mollificatifs oþ*er*while,

5 **femigrek**] *corr. from* ffemigrek 17 **kepe it**] *corr. from* kepeit
20 **bryonye**] *corr. from* bry*n*onye **of**[2]] *prec. by heading* Sekenesse

6 **and**[2]] *in r.-h. margin:* an oynt | ment

for ellis þe splene wold be-come as hard or hardere þa*n* he was before. And for-to dryen þe splene þis is a good oinene*n*t: Tac a*m*moniac *and* melt it w*it*h vi*n*egre. *And* medle þ*er*wiþ oile of lorere, *and* wex, *and* poudre of aloes, *and* encense. *And* seeþ hem to-gidere ou*er* þe feire *and* a-noi*n*te þe splene. And aft*er*ward resolue a*m*moniac in vi*n*egre *and* medle þ*er*wiþ þe poudre of mirre, aloes, *and* cockle. *And* make þ*er*-of a plastre on a clooþ *and* lei it to his splene; þis plastre is good. Oþ*er* seeþ a*m*moniac in wyn w*it*h nytre *and* w*it*h got*es* dri3t, *and* make þ*er*-of a plastre. And make a sirip of caparis, *and* of tamarysk, *and* of filipe*n*dula, *and* of sene, *and* epithime, *and* camedreos, *and* camapitheos, *and* sticados. Seeþ al þese in þe iuys of borage *and* do þ*er*to sugre. *And* make þ*er*-of a sirip.

A posteme of þe splene is j-helid as a posteme of þe lyuere, but þe medicines must be strengere þa*n* þilke þ*at* bien j-don to þe lyu*er*e.

Wyndnesse of þe splene is j-heeled be plast*r*es, *and* oynement*es*, *and* oiles, *and* electuaries, *and* sirepis, *and* wasschi*n*ges þ*at* be*n* hoote *and* extenuatif, þ*at* is to seie, þ*at* f. 146r han | kynde to make þilke boistres wyndes more sotil þa*n* þei were. And late hym vse also medicines þ*at* bien duretik. But þu xalt vnd*er*stond þ*at* wyndnesse of þe splene comeþ oþ*er*while of wyndy met*es*, *and* þa*n* wha*n* a ma*n* etiþ siche

8 **cockle**] *interl.* last c 11 **filipendula**] *corr. from* ffilipe*n*dula
21 **kynde**] *prec. by heading* of splene **sotil þan**] *corr. from* sotilþa*n*
23 **xalt vnderstond**] *corr. from* xaltvnd*er*stond 24 **wyndy metes**] *corr. from* wyndymet*es*

1 **hardere**] *in l.-h. margin:* nota (*written with pencil*) 14 **sugre**] *in l.-h. margin:* aposto*m* (*written with pencil*) 17 **lyuere**] *in l.-h. margin:* wyndnes

met*es*, his splene is j-greuid. *And* wha*n* he leueþ siche met*es*, hese greuau*n*ce passeþ a-wei. But wha*n* þe wyndnesse comeþ of þe splene self, þa*n* a ma*n* feleþ hym-self wheþ*er* he ete sich*e* met*es* oþ*er* dooþ nat. Alle oþ*er* greuaunces of þe splene mou*n* be j-helid be þ*at* þat is j-seid here-before.

Diacene is good for all*e* sicnessis of þe heed þ*at* comeþ of malencolie. *And* it xal be take þe morwetyde fastynge in wyn. And it is good for hem þ*at* han a feble brayn, *and* for he*m* þ*at* ben for-ȝeteful, *and* for alle greuau*n*ce of þe splene þ*at* comeþ of male*n*colie, *and* a special medicine to p*ur*ge þe blood of male*n*colie. And þe best sirip þ*at* is for wodnesse þ*at* comeþ of malencolie is j-maad of þe iuys of borage, *and* sene, *and* sugre. And diasene is þ*us* j-maad: Tak of sene *ounce* iiij; of canel, of clowes, of cardamom*e*, of gali*n*gale, of maces, of lignu*m* aloes, of long pep*er*, of gyng*er*, of ȝeduar*e*, of spik, of notemuge, of ich*e* of þese, *dragme* iij. *And* su*m*me pitten þ*er*-to borage, *and* calamynte, *and* oþ*er* þi*n*ges þ*at* p*ur*gen male*n*col*e*, *and* fifti notes; *and* of brent silk, *dragme* ij; *and* of lapis laȝuli, *dragme* iij; *and* of lapis armenic*us*, *dragme* ij; *and* of sugre, *dragme* vj. Su*m*me doon as myche sene to þis confecciou*n* as of alle þe oþ*er*e þi*n*ges. Ȝyf þis to þe | pacient w*it*h wat*er* þ*at* sene haþ j-leyn i*n*ne al nyȝt. f. 146v

Diaceraseos is good for greuua*n*ce of þe stomac, *and* of þe lyuere, *and* of þe splene. *And* is þ*us* j-maad: Tak of þe juys of chiries, iiij *pound*; of dispumed hony, iij *pound*. *And* seeþ he*m* to-gidere ou*er* an esy feiȝere til it be þicke. *And*

12 borage] *corr. from* boragage **20 dragme**[2]] *follow. by canc. twice* vij **21 yf**] *follow. by canc.* hy*m* **22 pacient**] *prec. by heading* Sekenesse **j-leyn**] *corr. from* j-soden (soden *exp.*); leyn *interl.*

8 han] *in r.-h. margin:* no*ta* b*e*n*e*

þa*n* cast þ*er*-to *ounce* iij *and dragme* iiij of diagredie j-poudred; of canel j-poudred, *ounce* j; of mastik, as mych*e* as of þe poudre of þe coold seedis, *dragme* iij. Of þis ȝif a ma*n* *dragme* iij at morwe. *And* late hy*m* faste aft*er*ward til it be at myddai.

Agrippa is a good oyneme*n*t for swelli*n*g of þe splene, *and* for alle oþ*er* swelli*ng*e*s*, *and* for greuaunce of þe senewis. *And* it is þ*us* j-maad: Tak ij *pound* of þe rotis of brionie *and* of þe rote of s[icc]ide, j *pound*; *and* of sq*ui*lle, *pound* s*emis*; *and* of yrees, *ounce* iij; *and* of þe roote of filix, *ounce* ij. Waische wel al þese root*es and* stampe he*m* in iiij *pound* of oile of birch. *And* let it lie so ij daies to-gidere. Þe iij dai set it ou*er* þe feire *and* seeþ it wel til þe rot*es* wexu*n* harde. Aft*er*ward clense it *and* cast þ*er*-to xx *ounce* of wex. *And* melt he*m* to-gidere *and* kepe it.

Jn a mannes reynes oþ*er* in his kidneiren ben iij greuaunces: ache, posteme, *and* stoones. Ache comeþ oþ*er*while of coold, oþ*er*while of heete: Of heete, as of blood oþ*er* of colre; of coolde, as of flewme oþ*er* of malencolie. Þe reynes ben filled p*ri*ncipali w*it*h oon of þese hum*ur*os: w*it*h blood, colre, oþ*er* flewme; w*it*h malencolie but seldene.

Tokenes of blood ben heete in þe depnesse of þe reynes, *and* heuynesse, *and* greua*u*nce, and þe veyne þ*at* is in þe
f. 147r i*n*nere side of þe | leg vnd*er* þe ancle is ful of blood *and* þe vrine is fat *and* wel j-colo*ur*d.

Tokenes of colre ben brenny*n*g *and* p*ri*ckynge i*n* þe depnesse of þe reynes, *and* a kene ache a-boute þe reynes,

9 siccide] *corr. from* sutide **10 filix**] *corr. from* ffilix **16 Jn**] *2-line space left for initial* **19 flewme**] *corr. from* fflewme **21 flewme**] *corr. from* fflewme **24 leg**] *prec. by heading* in the Reynys **blood and**] *corr. from* blood*and* **27 kene ache**] *corr. from* keneache

and heuynesse also, *and* drynesse of þe skyn w*ith*-oute-forþ. And þe vrine is of an hiȝe colo*ur and* þi*n*ne, *and* oþ*er*whiles þicke, of colre þ*at* is j-medlid þ*er*wiþ. *And* many smale þredis ben in þe vrine, oþ*er*whiles be-neþe, oþ*er*while a-boue.

Of flewme, tokens ben coold *and* heuynesse a-boute þe reynes, *and* þe vrine is whiȝt *and* fat, *and* ȝif þe rewme is j-gloderid to-gidere a-boute þe reynes, þ*er* ben muscilages in þe vrine *and* smale white þredis.

Tokens of malencolie bie*n* þi*n*ne vrine *and* ȝelwe, oþ*er* swart ȝelwe, *and* ful of bolles. *And* oþ*er*whiles þe vrine is þicke, of malencol*e* þ*at* is j-medlid þ*er*wiþ. And þei felen mych*e* heuynesse a-boute þe reynes. *And* hem semeþ þ*at* þe place a-boute þe reynes slepeþ. And þese hum*ur*os þ*at* greuen þ*us* þe reynes oþ*er*whiles flowen fra*m* all*e* þe bodi to þe reyn*es*. *And* þe tokene here-of is al þe bodi is greued as wel as þe reynes. *And* þa*n*ne þe begynny*n*g of þe cure xal be to p*ur*ge al þe bodi of þ*at* humo*ur* þ*at* greueþ þe reyn*es*. Oþ*er*while, þe humo*ur* þ*at* floweþ to þe reyn*es* floweþ fra*m* þe heed, oþ*er*whiles fra*m* þe lyuere, oþ*er*while fra*m* þe splene. And þa*n* al þe cure xal be doon to þat membre w*ith* confortatifs *and* st*ri*ctories þ*at* may staunche þilke flowyng*e*. And ȝif þe g*re*uaunces of þe reynes bie of blood, ȝif þe ma*n* haue mych*e* blood, lat hy*m* blood in þe ryȝt arm at þe veine þ*at* s*er*ueþ to þe lyu*er*e. And siþe heele hy*m* w*ith* þe same medicin*es* | þ*at* s*er*ue*n* for colre. Furst ȝif hym diaprunis to f. 147v
defie þe mat*er*e, oþ*er*e make hym wort*es* of hock*es and* of oþ*er*e coold herbys. *And* anoi*n*te þe reynes w*ith* oile of violet *and* w*ith* fresch*e* boot*er*e. And seeþ ooten *and* solatre in wat*er*, *and* wrynge owt þ*at* wat*er*, *and* wet a clooþ þ*er*i*n*ne,

5 **flewme**] *corr. from* fflewme **25** **þat**] *prec. by heading* Sekenesse **Furst**] *corr. from* ffurst

and lei vp-on hys reynes. But ȝif þilke hum*ur*os flow nat to þe reynes fra*m* noon oþ*er* place, ȝif hym oximel to defye þilke hum*ur*os. *And* siþe ȝif hym þe electuarie of þe sirip of rooses to p*ur*gen hym of þe hum*ur*os. And ȝif he haue no gret plente of blood, p*ur*ge hy*m* w*ith* a clist*eri*e cologoge. *And* siþe make hy*m* a stufe oþ*er* a baaþ of coold herb*e*. *And* ȝyf hy*m* a drawt of wyn j-medlid w*ith* wat*er* þ*at* encense haþ j-soden i*n*ne. *And* on morwe, lat hym blede at þe veyne þ*at* is vnd*er* þe ancle in þe vttere side of þe legge. And eu*er*iche morwe oonys, late hym bloode at þe veyne in oon of þe too legg*es*, oones in þe oon leg *and* eft-sones in [þe] oþ*er*e leg, for þ*at* veyne vnd*er* þe ancle on þe i*n*nere side of þe leg serueþ for þe lyu*er*e *and* þe splene, *and* to þe modyr, *and* to þe bladdere, *and* to þe gutt*es*. But on þe vtt*er*side of þe leg he serueþ to þe reynes, *and* to þe joynt þ*at* þe legges ben teid to þe bodi, *and* for þe joynt*es* of þe chyne. And oþ*er*e medicines þ*at* were jteld for diste*m*peri*n*g of þe lyu*er*e þ*at* comeþ of heete ben good here. And ȝif þe reynes ben distemp*er*ed onlich*e* w*ith* hete *and* han naþ*er* to mych*e* blood ne colre, þei schul be j-hoolid be coold electuaries *and*
f. 148r siripis, *and* oynement*es* | *and* plasteres, w*ith*-outen p*ur*gaciou*n*s, as distemp*eri*n*g* of þe lyue*re* is. But ȝif þis greuaunce be of coold, a-noi*n*te hese reynes w*ith* deute. And ȝif þese hum*ur*os flowen fra*m* oþ*er* places þedre, make hym wortis of beet*es* *and* of carses j-soden in double wat*er*. And ȝif þe hum*ur*os ne flow nat to þe reynes fram noon oþ*er*e place, ȝyue hy*m* oximel, *and* siþe p*ur*ge hym aft*er*ward, and make hym a stufe of origane, *and* calamynte, *and* sich*e* oþ*er* hoote herbis. And wha*n* he comeþ out, lat hym drynke wyn

12 for] *corr. from* ffor **14 vtterside**] *interl. and follow. by* vitt*er*side **21 and**[2]] *prec. by heading* in the reynes

þ*a*t encense haþ ben j-soden i*n*ne, ȝif þe hum*ur*os flowen þed*re*. Ellys ȝif hym wyn þ*a*t fenel rot*es* ben soden i*n*ne. And þe nexte dai aft*er*, late hym blede vnd*er* þe ancle in þe outere side of þe leg*e*. And lat hym be cuppid *and* j-garsid on þe reynes. And aft*er*ward, a-noi*n*te hym w*ith* hony þ*a*t is dispumed *and* hoot. *And* strawe þ*er*-on þe poudre of fenel, *and* of p*er*sili, march, dauk, carawei, gyng*er*, spikenard, encense, mastik, *and* of wermot. And siþe teese cotu*n* as smalle as þu may *and* strawe it a-boue þe poudre. *And* let it ligge þ*er* tyl it falle a-wei. Also late hym etyn foxys fleisch*e* *and* a-noynte hym w*ith* his grece. *And* þ*a*t xal don hym mych*e* good. And do to hym oþ*er* medicines also þ*a*t weren j-teeld in þe distemp*er*i*n*g of þe lyu*er*e. And for as mych*e* as medicines mote passe many weis or þei comyn*n* in-to þe reynes, it be-houeþ þe*m* to haue su*m* þi*n*ge to bri*n*ge he*m* to þe reynes þ*a*t wul nat be consumed ne wastid a-wei a-noon, as opiu*m*. But vnd*er*stande riȝt as opiu*m* quencheþ a mann*es* kyndly heete, riȝt so myrre *and* baume teendiþ a ma*n*n*es* ky*n*dly heete, as oyle tendiþ *and* noryschit fer*e*. *And* þ*er*fore medle he*m* to-gidere. | f. 148v

Aposteme of þe reynes: Oþ*er*while he is in oon of hem, oþ*er*while boþe þei han postem*us*. And how-eu*er* he come, oþ*er* he is of blood, oþ*er* of colre, oþ*er* of flewme, oþ*er* of malencol*e*. Ȝif he is of blood, he feleþ hete, atche, *and*

6 fenel] *corr. from* ffenel **20 to-gidere**] *interl.* gidere] *paragraph marks are in red in folios 148v and 149r; headings are underl. in red and some initial letters are decorated in the same colour* **21 Aposteme**] *prec. by heading* Aposteem of the reynys (*underl. in red*); *2-line initial a in red; red decoration in letter p* **23 flewme**] *corr. from* fflewme

16 be] *in r.-h. margin:* no*ta* b*e*n*e*

heuynesse in þe depnesse of hese reynes, *and* hese hed akeþ, *and* he haþ wyl to caste. And hys vrine is j-lettid of hys course and oþ*er*while it is reed, oþ*er*while blodi, oþ*er*whiles it is lich*e* þe drastos of quiture of þe posteme þ*at* is j-medlid þ*er*wiþ. And he haþ ache in his chynne, and þe veyne is to-swolle þ*at* is vnd*er* þe ancle. Of colre ben þe same tokenys of greuau*n*ces, but þei ben more viole*n*t þa*n* of blood. And he feleþ brennyng *and* p*ri*tchynge in þe depnesse of þe reynes and [in] þe place a-ȝenst þe reynes. Ȝif it is of flewme, þ*er* is ache w*it*h coold, *and* w*it*h heuynesse, *and* oþ*er* toknes of flewme. Of malencol*e*, þe tokenys ben ache w*it*h gret heuynesse, *and* coold, *and* drynesse. And þ*er* is a gret difference be-twyx þis *and* colica passio, for in colica passio, þe ach*e* is vnstabil, *and* aft*er* þ*a*t a man haþ gon to p*ri*uey, hese ach*e* is a-batid *and* comynly he is costif. But þis ache is stabil *and* dureþ stille tyl þe posteme be ripe *and* broke. And ȝif þe posteme be of hoote hum*ur*os, duretik medicines sufficen to helyn hym. But medle hoote duretik w*it*h coold, þ*at* þe coold haue þe maistrei. And ȝif it be a coold posteme, late hoote duretik haue þe maystrei, boþe in siripes, *and* in electuaries, *and* i*n* plastreis. And þat þ*a*t was j-seid in þe posteme of þe lyu*er*e is good here. A good plastre to make þe poste*m* of þe reynes rype: Take hockys *and* hoolihockys, and

5 And] *red decoration in letter a* **6 Of**] *red decoration in letter o* **7 he feleþ**] *corr. from* hefeleþ **9 and**] *red decoration in letter a* **flewme**] *corr. from* fflewme **11 flewme**] *corr. from* fflewme **13 colica passio**[1]] *corr. from* colicapassio **for**] *corr. from* ffor **colica passio**[2]] *corr. from* colicapassio **15 But**] *red decoration in letter b* **ache is**[2]] *corr. from* acheis **16 þe**] *follow. by canc.* ache **22 A**] *red decoration in letter a* **23 Take**] *red decoration in letter t* **and**[2]] *catchword* (*in bottom margin*): beet*es and* violet

| betis, *and* violet, *and* seeþ hem in wat*er*. *And* siþe grynde f. 149r
hem w*ith* goose grese, hennys g*r*ece, *and* schepis talwe. Wha*n* þe posteme is of coold, a-noi*n*te þe reynes w*ith* deute *and* make a plastre of fenel seed, *and* comyn, *and* syler*e* mou*n*tayne, *and* of datis, *and* of driȝe figes j-stamped togidere w*ith* þe iuys of march *and* a litel oile, oþ*er* þe mary of a calf, oþ*er* bot*er*e, oþ*er* goce grece. And wha*n* þe poste*m* is to-broke þ*at* þu myȝt see þe quiture come out of his vrine, ȝif hym þe balles þ*at* soudenwou*n*des þ*at* ben w*ith*-i*n*neforþ þ*at* xul be toold in þe pyssyng*e* of blood. Ȝif hy*m* þilke balles w*ith* got*us* mylke oþ*er* asse mylke, and make hy*m* a plastre of barlich*e* *and* of sope. And late hym sitten in wat*er* þ*at* barly *and* hock*es* ben j-soden i*n*ne. And ȝif þe q*ui*tere be ful þicke, ȝif hym þe iuys of solatre, wermote, *and* march*e* wel j-soden *and* clensed. And aft*er*ward, ȝif hym asse mylk, for þ*at* clanseþ weel. And aft*er*ward, ȝif hym cow mylk, for þ*at* is good wheþ*er* þe wou*n*de bie w*ith*-oute or w*ith*-i*n*ne. And riȝt as þis posteme is j-heelid, so is þe posteme of þe bladdere j-heelid. And þe same toknes þ*at* þe posteme haþ a-boute þe rugge, þe same haþ þe posteme of þe bladdere a-boute þe schar*e*.

Stoones ben j-genderid in a ma*n*n*es* reynes *and* also in a mannys bladdere. And iij enchesou*n*s þ*er* bie*n* of genderi*n*ge of sich*e* stoon*es*. Oon is a viscouse mat*er*e of whom þe stoones bien j-gendered. Þe secu*n*de encheson is heete þ*at* wasteþ a-wei þe wat*r*inesse of þ*at* viscouse mat*er*e *and* turneþ þe re*m*nan*n*t in-to stoones. Þe iij enchesou*n* is þe streitnesse

1 **betis**] *prec. by heading* The stoon (*underl. in red*) **grynde hem**] *corr. from* gryndehem 2 **grece and**] *corr. from* grece*and* 7 **þe postem**] *corr. from* þeposte*m* 19 **a-boute þe**] *corr. from* a-bouteþe
22 Stoones] *2-line initial s in red; red decoration in letter t*

of þe pores *and* of þe weie þ*er* sich*e* viscouse mat*er*e xuld passe forþ-by. And oþ*er*while stoones bien j-genderid of hoote viscouse hum*ur*os, *and* oþ*er*whiles of coold. *And* f. 149v oþ*er*while þe | stoon is newe, *and* oþ*er*while oold. Of heete, toknes bie a kene p*ri*ckyng ache, *and* greua*n*nce in pissi*n*ge, *and* þe vrine is of an hiȝe colo*ur*, *and* oþ*er*whiles haþ dropes of blood oþ*er*whiles grauel, *and* þ*a*t is reed, oþ*er* grene, oþ*er* blak. Ȝif þe stoon come of coold viscouse hum*ur*os, þ*er* is gret coold a-boute þ*a*t place þ*a*t þe stoon liþ i*n*ne, *and* heuynesse, *and* greuau*n*ce. Þe vrine also is whiȝt oþ*er* swart ȝelwe, *and* þe gravel is whiȝt oþ*er* swart ȝelwe, oþ*er* of þe colo*ur* of axen. Oþ*er*while grauel is in me*nnes* wat*er* þ*a*t haue nat þe ston, as in sich*e* menn*es* wateris þ*a*t han an hoot brenny*n*g feuere oþ*er* þ*a*t han þe goutes. But þ*a*t grauel wul falle to smalle poudre ȝif it be rubbid be-twix a ma*nnes* fi*n*geris, but grauel of men þ*a*t han þe stoon is nat soo. Stoones also ben j-genderid in oþ*er* place as wel as in þe reynes or in þe bladdere, for men han stoon*es* in here stomac *and* þei ben delyuerid of hem þorow casti*n*g. Su*m* men han stoones in here gutt*es*, *and* þei be delyuerid of þem be schiti*n*g. Su*m* me*n* han stoones in oþ*er* places, as þilke þ*a*t han gout*es* a-boute here ioynt*es*, wheþ*er* it be in rugge, in legge, or in armes. Tokenes of þe stoon: Þe foot on þilke side þ*a*t þe stoon is, is a-stoneid, *and* þe rugge-boon on þ*a*t side is j-greuid. *And* þei ha*n* g*r*euau*n*ce in pissi*n*ge, *and* g*r*auel in þe vrine. And yif þe stoon bie wexi*n*g, þe vrine wex fra*m* dai to

4 stoon] *prec. by heading* Stoon **5 in**] *follow. by exp.* p*ri*ck **18 for**] *corr. from* ffor **21 Sum men**] *corr. from* Su*m*me*n*

12 Oþerwhile] *in l.-h. margin:* no*ta*

dai ful of grauel. And wha*n* þe stoon is fulwex, oþ*er* wexiþ lasse, þa*n* þe grauel wexeþ lasse in þe vrine. *And* þa*n* þe vrine wexiþ whiȝt as mylk. And þei ben j-greuid as often as þei pessyn. And þe same toknes ben of þe stoon*es* in þe reynis *and* in þe bladdare, saue þ*a*t in þe reynes, þe greuau*n*ce is behynde in þe rugge; *and* in þe bladdare it is before, in þe schare, *and* toward a mann*es* ers. A stoon þ*a*t haþ | be long f. 150r
in a ma*n* wul nat be wel j-heelid but ȝif he be kyt a-wei. A new stoon mai be helid w*i*t*h* medicines. And ȝif it be of heete, ȝif hym diaprunes þe morwetid. *And* þe euy*n*tide, ȝif hym gyngere w*i*t*h* oximel. *And* lat hy*m* take it w*i*t*h* wat*er* þ*a*t hertis-tou*n*ge, *and* mayde*n*here, *and* p*er*sile seed, *and* þe iiij coold seed*es* ben j-soden i*n*ne. Aft*er*ward, ȝif hym þe electuarie of þe iuys of rooses. And þe iij dai aft*er*, make hy*m* a baþ of m*er*curie, wermot, salwene leeues, *and* vyne leues, *and* turmentille, *and* q*ui*nquerne, sourdock*es*, burnet. And wha*n*ne he comeþ out of þe baaþ, ȝif hym þe wat*er* þ*a*t souredock, hertistu*n*ge, endyue han be soden i*n*ne. And þe next dai aft*er*, late hym blood at þe veyne vndere þe ancle in þe vttere side ȝif þe stoon bie in þe reynes, and in þe i*n*nere side ȝif he be in þe bladdere. And a-noi*n*te þe place w*i*t*h* popilion *and* vi*n*egre and lei þis plastere on: Tak sourdocke, *and* purselane, *and* þe iiij coold sedis, *and* arage, *and* sau*n*dris, *and* fenel seed, *and* p*er*sili seed. Poudre hem *and* tempere hem w*i*t*h* vi*n*eg*re* *and* w*i*t*h* wyn, oþ*er* w*i*t*h* vi*n*egre *and* þe iuys of m*er*curie. And bren hym w*i*t*h* an hoot yren in þe

1 **oþer wexiþ**] *corr. from* oþ*er*wexiþ 7 **be**] *prec. by heading* Stoon **be long**] *corr. from* belong 17 **þe water**] *corr. from* þewat*er* **þat**] *interl. and follow. by exp.* of

20 þe[1]] *in r.-h. margin:* no*ta*

ha*m*me ȝif þe stoon is in þe reynes, oþ*er* in þe i*n*nere side of þe þeiȝ ȝif he is in þe bladdere. And medle diaprunes w*ith* þe electuarie of þe iuys of rooses. And let hy*m* jche weke ete þ*er*eof þe q*ua*ntite of a chasteyn oones a woke wha*n* he gooþ to bedde. *And* þa*n* he xal nat drede how he diete hym-self. And ȝif hym a sirip of hertystu*n*ge, endyue, maydenhere, ceterac, pollitricu*m*, adianthos, *and* of þe roote of fenel, *and* of saxifrage. Seþe all*e* þese in wat*er*, *and* siþe cla*n*se þ*a*t wat*er*, *and* cast þ*er*-to sugr*e*. *And* let hy*m* take þ*er*of þe f. 150v q*ua*ntite of an he*n*neschelful w*ith* þre so | myche of warm wat*er*. And lete hym vse this fra*m* iij daies to iij daies. Also tak þe iiij coolde seedis, *and* þe seede of p*ur*selane, letuse, *and* of p*er*seli, *and* of sorel, spikenard, gali*n*gale, þe seed of saxifrage, *and* þe poudre of an hare skyn *and* his blood, *and* goot*es* mylk. Tak of all*e* þese j-lich*e* myche *and* bren hem to poudre. *And* late make rou*n*de balles of þ*a*t poudre w*ith* wat*er* of rooses of þe wheiȝte of *dragme* j. And let hym ete on of hem at a tyme *and* vsen hem fra*m* iij daies to iij daies. But ȝif it comeþ of coold, lat hym vsen oximel duretik oþ*er* oximel sq*ui*lletik. And aft*er*ward, make a baaþ of þe rot*es* of fenel, of p*er*seli, of march, of carawei, dauk, saxifrage, *and* miliu*m* solis i-soden in wat*er*. *And* lat hy*m* sitte*n* in þ*a*t baaþ vp to þe nauele. And siþe ȝif hy*m* wyn w*ith* t*ri*acle in which*e* wyn saxifrage *and* miliu*m* solis ben j-soden i*n*ne. And a-morwe, opene þe veyne þ*a*t is vnd*er* þe ancle. And ȝif þe stoon bie in his reynys, lat hy*m* vse*n* þis baaþ ofte-siþes in þe thred oþ*er* iiij age of þe moneþe. And lat hy*m* vsen þis

10 myche] *prec. by heading* Stoon **12 purselane**] *corr. from* p*ur*selbane (b *interl.*) *and follow. by interl.* a **14 an hare**] *corr. from* anhare **16 make**] *follow. by exp.* balles **20 of þe**] *corr. from* ofþe

sirip: Tac of þe juys of radich *and* of saxifrage j-liche mych*e*, *and* seeþ it ou*er* an esy fere. *And* clense it *and* put þ*er*-to sugre. Oþ*er* tac þe rot*es* of p*er*seli, march*e*, dauk, kareawei, radich, pentafilo*n*, *and* of saxifrage, *and* of breris þ*at* growen in þe feelde, burnet, *and* lange-de-beef. *And* seeþ he*m* in wat*er*, *and* pit þ*er*-to sugre, *and* make a sirip. An oyneme*n*t for þis stoon: Tac þe iuys of vitucelle, *and* of saxifrage, radich*e*, burnet, wat*er*-lilies, langdebeef, *and* medle þis iuys wiþ oile of lorere oþ*er* of su*m* hoote oile. *And* seeþ he*m* so longe tyl þe iuys be co*n*sumed a-wei. And siþe medle swynn*es* grece þ*er*wiþ *and* make þ*er*-of an oyneme*n*t. And make | a plastre of ysop*e* *and* of saxifrage jsoden to-gidere f. 151r
and leid þ*er*-on. Oþ*er* stamp þe seed of fenel, *and* of p*er*seli, march, dauk, saxifrage, careawei, radich, *and* þe gu*m*me of an yuy tree, *and* medle hem w*ith* here owne iuys. *And* make þ*er*of a plastre *and* lei vp-on þe reynys ȝif þe ston be in þe bleddere. Also bren a qwik hare *and* gras-hopperis, *and* þ*er*wiþ medle þe poudre of canel. *And* lat hy*m* vse þ*at* poudre to hys mete. Oþ*er* do a-wei þe heed *and* þe leggis of grashopp*er*is oþ*er* of cryket*es*, *and* powne he*m* in granu*m*solis *and* saxifrage to poudre. *And* lat hy*m* drynk þ*er*-of w*ith* wat*er* þ*at* pentafilon is j-soden i*n*ne *and* wyn j-medlid to-gidere. Also a fox j-ete is profitabil for þe stoon *and* his grece is good to a-noi*n*te wiþ his reynis. But medle it w*ith* þe gu*m*me of an yuy tree *and* make þ*er*of an oynement.

1 þe juys] *corr. from* þejuys **12 a**] *prec. by heading* Stoon **saxifrage jsoden**] *corr. from* saxifragejsoden **13 fenel**] *corr. from* ffenel **15 yuy**] *corr. from* y*n*uy*n* **22 inne and**] *corr. from* i*n*ne*and* **25 yuy**] *corr. from* y*n*uy*n*

23 profitabil] *in r.-h. margin:* no*ta*

And poudre of got*es* blood is good also, but feede þe goot furst fourti daies w*ith* yuy leuys *and* ȝif hy*m* whiȝt wyn to drynk. And siþe tak hese blood *and* drie it. *And* medle baume þ*er*-wiþ, oþ*er ounce* s*emis* of aloes *and* of mirr*e*, *and ounce* s*emis* of salt. *And* þis poudre wul breke þe stoon. Also take þ*at* bien in a cockys mawe j-podred *and* j-ete wol breke þe stoon *and* so wole þe sourdocke. And ȝif þe stoon be fallen down in-to þe bladdere, *and* siþe j-falle down in-to þe ȝerde *and* letteþ a ma*n* to pisse, make a baaþ of hockys *and* of bet*es and* late hym sitte þ*er*-i*n*ne vp to þe nauele. And wha*n* he comeþ oute þ*er*of, anoi*n*te þe schare be-fore þe bladdere w*ith* botere. And let piten in an enargale þorouȝ his ȝerde *and* pitte þe ston dou*n* in-to þe bladdere. *And* þere he may ligge xl ȝere w*ith*-outen pereil, but late hym vsen his
f. 151v baþi*n*ge fyue daies ar þa*n*ne þou do so. And ȝif he | mowe suffre wel, whil he setteþ in þe baþ, let hy*m* frote from his ers to his ȝerde. *And* so he may w*ith* ofte frotyng*es* make þe stoon come oute at his ȝerde. Anoþ*er*e profitabil baþi*n*g is to sitten in salt-wat*er* vp to þe brest in þe whiche salt-wat*er* saxifrage is j-soden i*n*ne, boþe þe leeu*es and* þe seed, *and* caul worten þ*at* han nat bie remeuyd siþ þei weren j-sowen. But lat þ*at* wat*er* seeþe so longe til þe half be soden a-wei *and* frote as j-saied raþ*er*. And siþe lat a-noynte hy*m* w*ith* hoote oyneme*n*t*es* oþ*er*e oiles. For-to breke þe stoon, many oþ*er* þi*n*ges ben goode, as þe ston þ*at* is in þe spou*n*ge of þe see, *and* in þe toon of an oold cok, *and* in þe bladdere of a swyn, and þe stoon þ*at* a ma*n* pisseþ j-poudred *and* j-dru*n*ke w*ith* wyn, also þe kernelus of cherystones *and* of

2 **yuy**] *corr. from* y*n*uy*n* **15** **ar þanne**] *corr. from* arþa*n*ne **mowe**] *prec. by heading* Stoon **17** **may with**] *corr. from* mayw*ith* **24** **For-to**] *corr. from* ffor-to **27** **and þe**] *corr. from* andþe plu*m*beston*es*, *and* þe seid of aisches *and* of gromyl, *and* of cicori, *and* yuy, *and* hertistu*n*ge, *and* maydenhere, *and* þe seed of gret þistelis (*and* na*m*liche of þilke þ*a*t han brede leuis *and* mycele *and* white, *and* þe seed is blak). Eu*er*iche of þese haþ vertu to breke stoones, and ȝif þei ben medlid togidere, þe v*er*tu is þe more in þe medicine. For childerne þ*a*t may nat pissen, wasche here wo*m*bis *and* frete he*m* wel w*it*h wat*er* þ*a*t march, *and* p*er*sili, *and* hockes ben soden i*n*ne. And lat hym drynk þe poudre of an hare j-brent *and* of grashopp*er*es oþ*er* of criketis j-brent. And make a plastre of saxifrage *and* of þe iuys of march *and* of swete meele, *and* lei it fra*m* his ers to his ȝerde. Þe blood of a fox j-dru*n*ken w*it*h whiȝt wyn whil þe blood is new brekeþ a stoon. And so dooþ þe iuys of lymones, for ȝif a stoon ligge in hy*m*, he wole breke þorow v*er*tu of medicine.| f. 152r

Jn a mannes bladdere *and* longi*n*ge to a mannes bladdere, þ*er* bien diu*er*se greuau*n*ces. On is clepid stranguria þ*a*t is wha*n* a ma*n* haþ gret wille to pisse, *and* pisseþ but a litel, *and* þ*a*t is dropmeele, as an euese dropeþ on an hows. An-oþ*er*e g*r*euau*n*ce þ*er* is þ*a*t is vnmensurabil passi*n*ge of vrine fra*m* a ma*n*. And þ*a*t may come*n* of greuau*n*ce of þe reyn*es*, *and* þa*n* it is j-cleped diabetes. Oþ*er*while, it comeþ of febylnesse of þe bladdere, *and* þa*n* it is j-clepid diampnes.

2 yuy] *corr. from* y*n*uy*n* **maydenhere and]** *corr. from* maydenhere*and* **6 þe medicine]** *corr. from* þemedicine **For]** *corr. from* ffor **15 vertu…medicine]** *interl. and underl.* **16 Jn]** *2-line space left for initial; prec. by heading* Stranguria **Jn…mannes[1]]** *corr. from* Jnamannes

7 and] *in l.-h. margin:* washe ther | wommbe **12 with]** *in l.-h. margin:* no*ta* be*n*e

Stranguria is oþ*er*while a sicnesse be hym-self. And he mai come of too inchesons. Oon is kene colre *and* hoot þ*at* is in þe bladdere, *and* makeþ þ*at* þe vrine droppeþ out of þe bladdere in-to þe ȝerde, riȝt as comeþ droppi*ng* in-to þe bladdere fra*m* þe reynes. And þe tokenys here-of: brenny*ng* *and* p*ri*cchi*ng*, *and* swelli*ng*e in þe ȝerde, *and* heiȝ colo*ur* of þe vrine. Oþ*er*while, it comeþ of a cold flegmatik humo*ur* þ*at* makeþ þe sicnesses laxe þ*at* ben a-boute þe necke of þe bladdere. *And* þa*n* þe vrine is descolo*ur*d *and* þicke, *and* litel in q*ua*ntite. And þe wei of þe vrine in-to þe bladdere is i-stopped, oþ*er*whiles w*ith* a stoon, oþ*er*while w*ith* a posteme, *and* oþ*er*whiles w*ith* blood þ*at* is j-gloderid to-gidere. And þa*n* it is j-helid be þe same medicines as þe stoon is *and* a posteme of þe reynes. Oþ*er*while þ*at* wei is al-to-gidere j-stopped and oþ*er*while but su*m*dele. Wha*n* þis sicnesse comeþ of a posteme, it is j-knowe be þe tokenes of þe posteme of þe reynes, saue þ*at* þis greuau*n*ce is a-boute þe schar, as þe oþ*er*e of þe reynes is be-hynde-foorþ. And þe same medicines þ*at* heelen þe toon posteme, heelneþ þe toþ*er*e. Ȝif it comeþ of þe ston oþ*er* of grauel, þu maist j-knowe it be þe token*es* þ*at* ben j-toold here-be-fore. *And* þ*at* is j-hoolpe*n* be þe same medicines þ*at* þe stoon is. And ȝif it
f. 152v comeþ of hum*ur*os þ*at* stoppen | þe wei of þe vrine, it is j-knowe be þilke gobet*es* þ*at* is a-mo*n*g þe vrine. And it is j-helid in þe same wise þ*at* þe stoon is. Ȝif strau*n*gurie come of hete, late hym blede vnd*er* þe ancle. *And* ȝif hym þe electuarie of þe iuys of rooses. And siþe baþe hym in a baþ of coold herbis. And ȝif hym eu*er*i day þe morwetid *and* at

10 þe vrine] *corr. from* þevrine **23 þe**[1]] *prec. by heading* Stranguria **24 gobetes**] *corr. from* kgobet*es* (g *interl.*) **28 eueri day**] *corr. from* eu*er*iday euene sugre violet, oþ*er* diapenidion, oþ*er* diagragantu*m* þ*a*t is coold. And let hym drynk wat*er* þ*a*t hert*es*tu*n*ge oþ*er* endyue is j-soden i*n*ne. And lat hym vsen þe sirip þ*a*t was j-teld in þe hete of þe lyuere. And anoynte hy*m* w*ith* oile of rooses oþ*er* of violet j-medlid w*ith* vinegre. And make hym a coold plastre as it haþ be teld in þe heete of þe lyu*er*e *and* of þe reynes. And þorowȝ an enargale late hy*m* vnd*er*fo*n*g woma*n*nys mylk *and* oile of violet j-medlid to-gidere. And þis is good for hoote vrine þ*a*t greueþ þe ȝerde. But ȝif þis g*r*euau*n*ce come of coold, ȝif hym oximel duretik. *And* siþe make a stufe of hoote herbis. And wha*n* he comeþ out of þ*a*t baþ, ȝif hy*m* t*r*iacle w*ith* þe iuys of my*n*te, oþ*er* wyn þ*a*t castorie is j-soden i*n*ne. And þe next dai aft*er*, late hym blood vnd*er* þe ancle and distemp*er*e t*r*iacle þorouȝ þe iuys of mynte. *And* let hy*m* resceyuen it þorouȝ an enargale. An oyneme*n*t for þis sicnesse: Tak encense, mastik, euforbe, *and* þe rote of berdane. *And* stamp*e* hem w*ith* þe grece of a cat oþ*er* of a gandere *and* rooste hym. *And* kepe þe fatnesse þ*a*t droppeþ fra*m* hym *and* medle it w*ith* reed wex. *And* þ*er*w*ith* a-noynte þe schare. Þe fleisch of a fox j-ete *and* þe grece j-vsed in þe forme of an oyneme*n*t is good for þis sicnesse *and* for coold goutes. A good sirip for þis greuau*n*ce: Tak þe roote of berdane, | mynte, *and* pyony. *And* stamp hem a litel *and* f. 153r seeþ hem in wat*er*. *And* þ*er*-to cast clene puryd hony *and* let hem vsen þis sirip. And þe same medicines ben good for þe palesei of þe bladdere *and* for þe*m* þ*a*t be-pissen þere bed. And vnd*er*stond þ*a*t þu xal nat do in here medicynes naþ*er*

12 wyn] *corr. from* w*ith*yn (*ith canc. twice*) **21 of an**] *follow. by* of an **23 mynte**] *prec. by heading* Stranguria **26 palesei**] *interl.* a

21 for] *in l.-h. margin:* no*ta*

euforbe ne scamone, but ȝif þu be a-bowte to make hym pisse. And ȝif here greua*un*ce come of febilnesse, *and* þei ben on-myty to pisse, make he*m* a baþ *and* ȝeue he*m* t*ri*acle. And anoynte þe necke of þe bladdere w*ith* hote oyneme*nt*es *and* oiles. But ȝif þere be coolde viscouse hum*ur*os in þe bladdere, ȝif hym þe medicines þ*at* were j-teld for þe stoon. For soukyng childeren þ*at* han þis sicnesse, make he*m* a baaþ ofte-siþes in wat*er* þ*at* hock*es*, *and* grou*n*d-swily, *and* yuy, *and* sich*e* oþ*er* ben j-soden i*n*ne. And late his norische ete betys, *and* arage, *and* comyn in potage tyl þe childe may pissen. But wha*n* þe child is to ȝere oold oþ*er* more, late hym drynke þe poudre of an haare j-brent *and* of grashopp*er*es oþ*er* of criket*es* also w*ith* wyn. But cast a-wei þe legg*es and* þe hedde of þe grashopp*er*es *and* of þe criket*es* also. Oþ*er*whiles, þ*er* falleþ in-to þe bladdere gret plente of vrine þ*at* streineþ þe bladdere *and* strangleþ here þ*at* þ*er* may non vrine passen out of þe bladdere. *And* þis is a ful g*re*t pena*un*ce *and* it falleþ oþ*er*-while in men þ*at* semen al hoole, oþ*er*while in men þ*at* han þe feueris. Ȝif it falle in a feuere, late baþen hym vp to nauel in wat*er* þ*at* p*er*itorie is soden i*n*ne, *and* he xal pissen a-swiþe; oþ*er* in wat*er* þ*at* wermot is j-soden i*n*ne, *and* plastre þe herbe on his schare. And þe same vertu haþ louage: He pisseþ a-noon. Oþ*er* make a f. 153v plast*re* | of fenel seed, of p*er*seli, *and* of merch j-soden in wat*er and* lei to his schare; oþere seþe march *and* bren to-gidere *and* make þ*er*of a plastere. And þis is good for he*m*

1 make hym] *corr. from* makehym **2 febilnesse**] *corr. from* ffebilnesse **7 For**] *corr. from* ffor **11 þe child**] *corr. from* þechild **19 feueris**] *corr. from* ffeueris **feuere**] *corr. from* ffeuere **24 of**[1]] *prec. by heading* Pyssyng **fenel**] *corr. from* ffenel **merch**] *corr. from* maerch (a *exp.*; e *interl.*)

þ*at* han þis greuau*n*ce *and* semen hool. *And* whiles þei baþe*n* hem, ȝif hem chiristonis kerneles j-stamped w*ith* wat*er*. Also for he*m* þ*at* han þis g*r*euau*n*ce *and* semen hool, make a plastre of louage *and* p*er*it*er*ie j-soden in wat*er* *and* lei to his schare. Oþ*er* seeþ march *and* louage in wat*er* *and* w*ith* þ*at* wat*er* medle whete bren. *And* make þ*er*of a plast*r*e *and* lei to þe schare. *And* þ*at* is good for þe stoon also.

Pyssyng of blood comeþ fra*m* w*ith*-oute-forþ, as of lepy*n*g, of fallyng, of strokys, of traueile, oþ*er* of coold eire. Oþ*er*while, it comeþ fro w*ith*-i*n*ne-forþ, as of þe lyuere, of þe splene, of þe reynes, of þe leendys, oþ*er* of þe bladdere. Oþ*er*while, it comeþ of gret ple*n*te of blood, *and* þ*at* is j-knowe be þe fulnesse of a ma*nn*es veynes. Oþ*er*while, it comeþ of keneschep*e* of þe blood *and* þe tokyn þ*er*-of is p*r*ickyng *and* heete in þe ȝeerde *and* a-boute þe ȝerd wha*n* a ma*n* pisseþ. Oþ*er*while, it is fo[r] thynschep*e* of þe blood þ*at* makeþ it to swete owt of þe veynes. *And* þa*n* þe blood is ful thy*n*ne þ*at* is j-medlid w*ith* þe vrine. And þe helpi*n*g of þese iij maneris is be medicines, as han be teeld in nose-bledyng, *and* in spitti*n*ge of blood, *and* in þe blodi flux. Wha*n* it comeþ fra*m* þe lyuere, it comeþ in gret q*ua*ntite, *and* is clene blood. *And* þei han g*r*euau*n*ce vnd*er* þe riȝt side. *And* furst þe vrine comeþ owt *and* siþe þe blood. Wha*n* it comeþ fra*m* þe splene, þei felen heuynesse *and* greuau*n*ce vnd*er* þe liȝfit side. *And* þe blood is litel in q*ua*ntite, *and* troublid, *and*

4 **louage**] *corr. from* laouage (first a *oblit.*; o *interl.*) **8 Pyssyng**] *2-line space left for initial* **9 fallyng**] *corr. from* ffallyng **strokys**] *interl.* r **19 nose-bledyng**] *corr. from* nose-bledynge (bledynge: last e *canc.*)

2 water] *in l.-h. margin:* no*ta*

male*n*coliose. Fra*m* þe reynes comeþ blood w*ith*-outen g*re*t g*re*uau*n*ce *and* it [is] litel in q*ua*ntite, but it is clere *and* j-medlid w*ith* | f. 154r þe vrine. *And* þei felen p*ri*ckyng a-boute þere reynes. Wha*n* it comeþ out of þe bladdere, þei ha*n* g*re*uau*n*ce in þe schare *and* be-neþe. *And* þe blood comeþ furst out *and* siþe þe vrine, *and* þe blood is blac. And ȝif þei pissen blood *and* q*ui*ture to-gidere, it is a token þ*at* þe bladdere is scabbid *and* haþ pymples in here, *and* namely ȝif it sti*n*ckeþ. But ȝif þe blood come fra*m* eny oþ*er* veynes, it is j-gloterid to-gidere a-loong of þe schap of a wat*er*-leche, *and* so it comeþ out w*ith* þe vrine. And oþ*er*while, it is so gret þ*at* it stoppeþ þe weie of þe vrine, *and* makeþ a ma*n* to haue þe st*ra*ngurie, *and* brengeþ a ma*n* to þe deeþ. Oþ*er*whiles, þ*er* ben wou*n*des a-boute þe reynes. *And* þa*n* a man feleþ ache þ*er*e wha*n* a ma*n* pisseþ. *And* þe vrine is oþ*er*while blodi, oþ*er*whiles j-medlid w*ith* q*ui*ture. Oþ*er*while, þ*er* ben smale bodys in þe vrine j-lyke þredis. *And* oþ*er*while þei ha*n* ichi*n*ge a-boute here ers. Ȝif it comeþ of gret plente of blood, let hym abstene hy*m* fra*m* met*es* þ*at* genderyn mych*e* blood, *and* vse met*es* þ*at* maken litel blood, as frutys and herb*e*. And ȝif þe blood comeþ fra*m* þe lyu*er*e, let hym blood in þe riȝt arme, and fro þe splene in þe lift arme, *and* fra*m* þe reyn*es* vnd*er* þe ancle in þe vttere side; and ȝif it comeþ of þe bladdere, in þe i*n*nere side of þe ancle. Ȝif it comeþ of keneschepe of þe blood, p*ur*ge hy*m* of colre w*ith* þe electuarie of þe iuys of rooses. And siþe ȝif hym coold electuaries *and* siripis, as it haþ be

1 Fram] *corr. from* ffra*m* **3 þe**] *prec. by heading* of blood **6 þe blood**] *corr. from* þeblood **9 þe blood**] *corr. from* þeblood **10 a**] *interl.* **13 þe deeþ**] *corr. from* þedeeþ

21 let] *in r.-h. margin:* no*ta* ben*e*

told in spitti*n*g of blood *and* in dissent*er*ie. But in p*ur*gaciou*n*s, ȝif hy*m* naþ*er* aloes, ne scamone, ne euforbe. Aft*er* | his p*ur*gaciou*n*, ȝif hym siche thyng*es* þ*a*t wole f. 154v stau*n*che þe bledi*n*ge, as diacodion *and* sugre of rooses, as myche as a chasteyn at oon tyme. *And* siþe ȝif hym þis sirip: Tak rooses, bole, *and* louage seed, encense, mastik, planteyn, mynte. *And* seeþ hem in reyn-wat*er* *and* cast sug*re* þ*er*-to. And þ*er*-as he feleþ ache, a-noi*n*t it w*ith* oile of rooses *and* w*ith* þe whiȝt of eyren. And lei a plastre þ*er*-on of encense, mastik, mu*m*my, sau*n*dragou*n*, *and* bole, *and* of plau*n*teyn. Sta*m*pe he*m* to-gidere *and* te*m*pere it w*ith* þe gleire of eyren. And ȝif þu see þ*a*t it is nede, make hy*m* a stufe of pentafilon, plau*n*teyn, *and* of sich*e* oþ*er* herbis. *And* lat hym sit þ*er*-i*n*ne vp to þe nauele. And late hym frote wel from þe nauele to his ȝerd. *And* let hym vsen þ*a*t ofte-siþes. And make hy*m* þis oyneme*n*t: Tak galles, *and* psidie, bole, sau*n*dragou*n*, *and* spodie, *and* sich*e* oþ*ere* st*ri*ctories *and* poudre he*m*. *And* frie he*m* w*ith* beris grece oþ*er* w*ith* su*m* oþ*ere* grece *and* clense it. And þ*er*w*ith* a-noi*n*t hy*m* þ*er*-as his moost greuau*n*ce is. And diete hy*m* *and* ȝif hy*m* oþ*er* medicin*es* ȝif it nedeþ, as it was seid in dissent*er*ie. And w*ith* þis medicines medle cicorie, oþ*er* spiknard, oþ*er* hertistu*n*ge, or maydenhere, oþ*er* þe iiij coolde sedis, oþ*er* dragagau*n*t, ȝif þe ma*n* be of flegmatik co*m*plexiou*n*. And ȝif þu suppose þ*a*t is splene be diste*m*perid w*ith* heete, put a-mo*n*g his oþ*ere* medicin*es* lyuerwort, *and* rooses, violet, *and* plu*m*bes, *and* sau*n*drys, boþe whiȝt *and* reede. *And* seeþ he*m* in tisane *and* put þ*er*-to

2 ne[2]] *follow. by* ne **3 his**] *prec. by heading* Pyssyng of blood **5 oon**] *follow. by canc.* day **7 seeþ hem**] *corr. from* seeþhem **12 make hym**] *corr. from* makehy*m* **23 flegmatik**] *corr. from* fflegmatik

ounce j of lycorys. And ȝif þu drediste of drynesse of þe breest oþ*er* of a feuer*e* etik, put to þi medicin*es* gu*m*me arabik *and* dragg*e*. And wha*n* þ*o*u seist þ*a*t þe vrine wexeþ clene, put to þi medicines co*n*firie *and* daies-eiȝe, *and* oþ*er*e f. 155r co*n*solidatifs to soude þe veyn*es* | þ*a*t ben to-broke.

A good medicine for pissyng of blood oþ*er* of quitere: Tak of þe seed of gordis, purselane, spodie, *and* of þe iuys of lycoris, *ounce* vj; of letuse seed, gu*m* arabik, hockis, rooses, anyse, dragag*e*, *and* popi seed, *dragme* iij; of þe seed of cotou*n* *and* of coynes, *dragme* ij; *and* of bole, acacie, *dragme* ij *and* s*emis*; *and* of saffren, *dragme* ij. Poudre all*e* þese *and* te*m*pre he*m* w*ith* iuys of plau*n*teyn. *And* make round balles þ*er*of *and* ȝif hym to drynke. A baaþ for þe same: Tak louage leeuys, *and* bodegar, ribwort, co*n*firie, daisie, *and* planteyn boþe þe more *and* þe lasse, *and* jp*er*i[c]on, *and* auance, *and* þe braunches of fenel, p*er*sili, v*er*uene, colu*m*byne, *and* of camomylle. Tak of eu*er*iche of þese j-liche miche, *and* seeþ he*m* in wat*er*.

A good plastre to legge on a ma*n*n*es* reyn*es* *and* on his schare in þis sicnesse: Tak of rooses, *ounce* j; of mastik, *dragme* iij; of bole, of whiȝt saundres, *dragme* s*emis*; þe ȝelkys of fyue eiren; of oyle of rooses, ij *dragme*. Medle al þese w*ith* þe iuys of þese erbis: of plau*n*teyn, co*n*firie, daisie, fenel, p*er*sili, colu*m*byne, v*er*ueyne, ribwort, ca*m*momille, *and* of aue*n*ce, of eu*er*ych*e* of þese, tak j-lich*e* mych*e* iuys; *and* of barlich*e* mele, *pound* s*emis*, *and* medle al þis to-gidere.

1 **drynesse**] *follow. by* of drynesse 5 **þat**] *prec. by heading* Diabites 11 **of**] *follow. by canc.* safre 12 **iuys**] *corr. from* yiuys (first y *canc. and exp.*) **And make**] *corr. from Andmake* 13 **A baaþ**] *corr. from* Abaaþ 15 **jpericon**] *corr. from* jp*er*iton 16 **fenel**] *corr. from* ffenel

A sirip for þis sicnesse: Tak of þe roote of fenel, p*er*sili, *and* pigle, *and* betoyne, colu*m*byne, yp*er*icon, *and* þe leeuys of plau*n*teyne *and* þe seed, *and* co*n*firie, *and* daisie, hertistu*n*ge, cicori, scariole, of eu*er*iche of þese, *ounce* j; of rooses, of licorys, of louage seed, of whiȝt saundres *and* of þe reed, *ounce* s*emis*; of dragag*e*, of gu*m*me arabik, *dragme* ij; of reysines, *ounce* s*emis*. Seeþ all*e* þese in wat*er and* cast þ*er*-to ij *pound* of sugr*e*. And eu*er*mor*e* w*ith* þe medicin*es*, loke þu medle medici*n*s þ*a*t ben mu*n*dificatif to make þe bladdere clene for drede of mor*e* perele.

Djabites is an vnmesurabil passi*n*g of vrine þ*a*t comeþ of gret drynesse of þe reynes, for wha*n* þe reynes ben ful driȝe, þei soukyn miche moistnesse of þe [v]eynys þ*a*t comeþ fra*m* þe lyuere, and þe lyuere myche of þe gutt*es*, and þe gutt*es* myche | of þe stomac *and* of þat þ*a*t is in hym-self. And þ*a*t f. 155v
moistnesse wha*n* it comeþ to þe reynes *and* fyndeþ þe wei large, passeþ swiftli to þe bladdere, *and* so passeþ forþ as it comeþ. Enchesou*n*s of þis sicnesse ben gret trauaile, to mych*e* medlyng*e* w*ith* wome*n*, cat[c]hi*n*g of a greet heete in a ma*n*n*es* bodi, oþ*er* a-noi*n*ty*n*ge a-boute þe reynes w*ith* to hoote oynement*es*, oþ*er* of a loong feuere it mai come. And oþ*er*whiles þis is a symple distemp*er*i*n*g, oþ*er*whiles it is a distemp*er*i*n*g of su*m* humo*ur* þ*a*t greueþ þe reynys. *And* ȝif it is so, þ*er* is ache, *and* heuynesse, *and* p*r*ickyng, *and* gnawyng

1 **fenel**] *corr. from* ffenel 4 **cicori**] *corr. from* cicorie (e *canc. twice*) 5 **and of**] *corr. from* andof 10 **perele**] *interl.* 11 **Djabites**] *2-line space left for initial* 12 **of þe**] *corr. from* ofþe **for**] *corr. from* ffor 13 **veynys**] *corr. from* reynys 15 **of**[1]] *prec. by heading* Diabites 18 **gret trauaile**] *corr. from* grettrauaile **to myche**] *corr. from* tomych*e* 21 **feuere**] *corr. from* ffeuere 24 **so**] *follow. by canc. twice* þat

22 **oþerwhiles**[2]] *in l.-h. margin:* þat comeþ

a-boute þe reyne. And he haþ a co*n*tinuel þurst *and* a gret appetit to pisse aft*er* þ*a*t he haþ j-dru*n*ken. But sich*e* appetit comeþ oþ*er*whiles of mych*e* drynkyng*e* of sotil wyn þ*a*t p*er*seþ þorow þe veynes *and* comeþ sone in-to þe bladdere. Oþ*er*while it comeþ of drynkyng*e* of g*r*et wyn þ*a*t þe lyu*ere* may nat wel defie for febilnesse. Oþ*er*while mych*e* pissyng comeþ of cooldnesse of þe lyu*ere* þ*a*t may nat defie þe moystnesse þ*a*t is in hym, *and* so it falleþ dou*n* to þe bladdere. But þese man*er*es of vnmesurabil pissi*n*ge ben nat diabites ne dia*m*pnes, for þei ben neiþere of þe febelnesse of þe reynes ne of þe bladdere; for wha*n* þei ben distemp*er*ed, a ma*n* xal pisse oftesiþes *and* litil at oo[n] tyme. For-te holp a ma*n* of þis g*r*euau*n*ce, men xal be a-boute to helpe þe reynes *and* to a-bate here gret heete. And yif þe diste*m*p*er*inge be of heete of su*m* humo*ur*, ȝif hy*m* oximel to defie þe humo*ur*. *And* siþe ȝif hy*m* þe electuarie of þe iuys of rooses to p*ur*gen hym of þ*a*t humo*ur*, oþ*er* w*it*h su*m* oþ*er*e cologoge. P*ur*ge hy*m* *and* þe iij dai aft*er*, make hy*m* a baþ vp to þe nauele of wat*er* þ*a*t roseen be*n* j-soden i*n*ne, *and* planteyn, letuse, f. 156r p*ur*selane, syneg*r*ene, pi*m*pinele, | violet, ribwort, *and* oþ*er* coold herb*e*. *And* seeþ w*it*h he*m* þe leeues of coyne trees, *and* of openhers trees, *and* of blak plu*m* trees, *and* of sich*e* oþ*er*e. *And* late þe pacient frote wel þ*a*t place þ*a*t greueþ hym, þ*a*t þe v*er*tu of þe herb*e* may þe raþ*er* p*er*se þorou þe porys of þe skyn. Þe next dai aft*er*, late hy*m* blood vnd*er* þe ancle w*it*h-outeforþ. Aft*er*ward ȝif hym medicines as it were but a si*m*ple distemp*eri*nge. Ȝif hy*m* diaprunis *and* sugre rooset j-

10 for] *corr. from* ffor **11 for**] *corr. from* ffor **12 oon tyme**] *corr. from* ootyme **For-te**] *corr. from* ffor-te **20 purselane**] *follow. by canc. twice* senygrene **violet**] *prec. by heading* Diabites **21 þe leeues**] *corr. from* þeleeues medlid to-gidere of þe q*ua*ntite of a chasteyn, oþ*er* dyacesarros, oþ*er* sugr*e* violet, oþ*er* t*ri*asendri, oþ*er* t*ri*arodon abbat*es*. *And* ȝif þu wolt, medle he*m* to-gidere.

Diaprunis is þus j-maad: Tak of hermodactil*e*, of manna, of violet, *dragme* x; of diagridie, of cassie, *dragme* v; of myrabol*e* cit*ri*, of kebuli indj, of be[llere] emblici, of canel, of clowes, of spik, *ounce* vj; of hony despumed, *quantum* s*ufficit*; oþ*er* of þe sirip of rooses oþ*er* of violet, þ*at* is bet*er*e. But for-to kepe þe medicine betere *and* þe lengere, make it w*it*h hony. But furst pure þ*at* hony w*it*h watere þ*at* plu*m*bes *and* violet han j-soden i*n*ne. Aft*er* þese electuaries, lat hym vse þese sirip*e*: Tak rooses, *and* leeuys of louage, *and* of an open-ers tree, *and* of a coyn tree, *and* of a mylberie tree, *and* of sich*e* oþ*er*e þ*at* were teeld in dissent*er*ie. *And* seeþ hem in wat*er* *and* make þ*er*of a sirip*e*. And þe same herb*e* j-soden *and* siþen j-stamped mak an hoot plastre. *And* lei to þe reynes. And a-no*n*cte þe reynes w*it*h coolde oiles, *and* of rosen, *and* of violet, oþ*er* of wat*er*-lilies, oþ*er*e of ma*n*drake. And lei þese plastre to þe reynes. Tak all*e* þe kynd*es* of sau*n*dris *and* spodie *and* poudre hem. *And* tak as mych*e* of barly mele *and* medle all*e* þilke w*it*h þe iuys of solatre or syng*r*ene *and* of p*ur*selane. *And* lei þe plast*r*e þ*er*-of vp-on þe reynes. But þu xalt vnd*er*stonde þ*at* þ*o*u xal nat legge eu*er*more moist medicines to þe reyn*es*, for þei wolde make þe reyn*es* ful neisch*e* *and* ful feble, | ne þ*o*u xal nat alwei vse f. 156v
driȝe medicines, but oþ*er*whiles oon *and* oþ*er*while oþ*er*e. And late hy*m* vse þis poudre in her*e* met*es*: Tak þe seed of hockys, of letuse, of purselane, *and* of plau*n*teyne, of eu*er*ich*e*, j-liche myche. *And* poudre he*m* *and* medle þ*er*w*it*h

6 bellere] *corr. from* bebli*n* **10 þat**[1]] *follow. by canc. and exp.* wat*er*
25 ne] *prec. by heading* Diampnes

as mych*e* of gu*m* arabik *and* of dragag*e* as of alle þe oþ*er*. *And* cast þ*er*-to sugre, *quantum* s*ufficit*. Lat hym vsen at oon tyme of þis poudre as myche as he may take w*ith* his twey fyngeris *and* hys thu*m*be at oon*es*. Also bore a plate of leed ful of smale hooles *and* hete it. *And* que*n*che it in vi*n*egre *and* lei it al warm to þe reines. But ley a thy*n*ne flake of cotu*n* bitwene it *and* þe skyn, *and* twies or iij renewe it a-dai. *And* be þei ware of all*e* kene met*es* þ*at* wole make he*m* þirstful. And here dieti*n*ge xal bie of coold sotele met*es*. *And* late he*m* drynke whiȝt wyn j-medlid w*ith* wat*er*, *and* be þei ware of mych*e* drynkyng. And eu*ery* monþe lat hy*m* be p*ur*ged as j-seid bi-fore. And be þei ware of pollipodie, for þ*at* oppeneþ þe veynes *and* makeþ þe blood brekyn out. *And* na*m*ly in sich*e* men þ*at* han bie liep*er*es, *and* wrastelers, *and* doeris of sich*e* oþ*er*e maistreis. For ȝif so is þe blood wol stoppe þe wei of þe vrine *and* make hy*m* to haue a st*ra*ngurie, þa*n*ne make hym a plastre of rwe [and] comy*n*n j-soden in wyn *and* oile *and* lei oon þe schare. But yif þe sicnesse comeþ of a coold a-boute þe reynes, as su*m* men seyn, ȝif hy*m* pociou*n*s of hoote medicines þ*at* ben co*n*fortatif *and* st*ri*ctorie, as is mynte *and* oþ*er*e þ*at* were j-teld in dissent*er*ie. And make a plastre of þe same *and* lei vp-on his reynes. But furste p*ur*ge hym of þe humo*ur* þ*at* is cause of þe sicnesse, and diete hym w*ith* temp*er*at hoote met*es*.

Djampnes is an vnskille-ful passinge of vrine þ*at* comeþ of defaute of þe bladdere. And þ*at* may be in too manerys:
f. 157r Oþ*er* of colre þ*at* is in þe bladdere, | *and* p*ri*ckeþ þe bladdere,

1 as myche] *corr. from* asmych*e* 15 For] *corr. from* ffor
25 Djampnes] *2-line space left for initial* 27 bladdere[1]] *catchword* (*in bottom margin*): *and* p*ri*ckeþ and] *prec. by heading* Diampnes

and makeþ þe vryne droppen out ryȝt as it comeþ to þe bladdere. And þis colre is j-medlyd w*ith* þe vryne *and* makeþ þe vryne kene *and* bytynge. Oþ*er*while, þis sicnesse comeþ of coold þ*at* febeleþ þe senewys of þe bladdere *and* makeþ þe bladdere fallen in-to a palesei. And þis falleþ come*n*ly to hem þ*at* goon barfoote *and* acoold on here body in coold wed*er*. Ȝit whan þei pissen, þei p*er*seyuen it, *and* han greuau*n*ce in þ*er* pissyng*e*. Oþ*er*whiles, þe senewys *and* þe lacertys ben so laxe þ*at* ben in þe necke of þe bladdere, þ*at* þei may not w*ith*-holden þe vrine in þe bladdere. And þa*n* passeþ þe vrine a-wei fra*m* hem þ*at* þei felen it nat, as it happeneþ in chylderen *and* in dru*n*ke men þ*at* be-pessen here bedde. And þis comeþ oþ*er*while of humo*ur*s þ*at* ben in þe senewis of þe necke of þe bladdere, for iij hum*ur*os þ*er* ben wou*n*t to be in þe bladdere þ*at* greueþ here: flewme, male*n*col*e*, *and* colre.

Tokenes of flewme ben: Þe vrine is of a feble colour*e* *and* ful of muscilages *and* of smale thy*n*ne scales, and þei han greuaunce in pyssyng*e*, *and* pisseþ droppemeele. And þ*at* is ȝif þe flewme be viscouse *and* þicke. But ȝif it be thynne, þe senewis drynken it vp, *and* þ*at* makeþ hym laxe *and* slideri. *And* þa*n* þe vrine passeþ out w*ith*-oute greuau*n*ce.

Tokenes of malencolie ben: Þe vrine is swart ȝelwe *and* ful of thynne scales. *And* þei han gret greuaunce wha*n* þei pissen *and* a-bowten here ers-hoole þei han non felynge.

Tokenes of colre ben: Þe vryne is of an heiȝ colo*ur* *and* þi*n*ne, oþ*er* þicke of colre þ*at* is j-medlid þ*er*-wiþ. *And* þei han p*ri*ckyng*e* *and* a kene ache in here bladdere, *and*

1 vryne droppen] *corr. from* vrynedroppen **10 vrine**[1]] *follow. by exp. of* **in**] *interl.* **15 flewme**] *corr. from* fflewme **19 þe flewme**] *corr. from* þeflewme

p*ri*cky*n*g in þe ȝerde wha*n* þei pissen. *And* þei han gret heete a-boute here ers-hoole.

f. 157v Diampnes þ*at* comeþ of hoot | colrik pisse is heelid as diabetes þ*at* comeþ of heete. And make hym þis confeccion þ*at* is good for hem þ*at* pissen hoot kene pisse: Tac of dragag*e*, of gu*m*me arabik, of p*ur*selane seed, of gourdys, of letuse, *dragme* iiij. Make poudere þ*er*-of *and* late hym drynken it w*ith* þe sirip*e* of rooses. But yif þis sicnesse comeþ of coold *and* of mooistnesse, ȝif hym medicines þ*at* were j-teld in dissent*er*ie, boþe in siripis, *and* in electuaries, plasteris, *and* oynement*es*, *and* baþes, for þe same medicines þa*n* stau*n*che þe flux of þe wombe, stau*n*cheþ also þe fluxes of þe bladdere, *and* of þe modere, *and* of þe emoroides. But ȝif þis comeþ of hum*ur*os þ*at* ben in þe bladdere, ȝif þe hum*ur*os ben hoote, ȝif hym oximel to defiȝe þe hum*ur*os. *And* siþe p*ur*ge hy*m* w*ith* a cologoge, oþ*er* w*ith* þe electuaries of þe iuys of rooses. But ȝif þe hum*ur*os ben coold, p*ur*ge hy*m*m w*ith* a fleu*ma*goge oþ*er* a malagoge. And þe iij day aft*er*, make hym a baaþ oþ*er* a stufe of hoote herbys. And wha*n* he comeþ out þ*er*-of, ȝif hym t*ri*acle w*ith* þe iuys of mynt oþ*er* w*ith* wyn, oþ*er* rwe oþ*er* castore han j-soden i*n*ne. And late hym vsen þis xv daies. But þ*er* ȝif þou nat hem t*ri*acle ȝif þei ben ȝonge. Also seeþ akren in wat*er* *and* w*ith* þ*at* wat*er* let hym drynken þe poudere of a booles bladd*er*. Also akren j-soden *and* j-eten ben profitabil, *and* þe wat*er* j-dru*n*ke þ*er*-to. A good plaastere j-maad þ*er*-fore is j-maad of t*ri*acle, *and* of oile, [and] of piliole j-medlid to-ged*er*e. And þese medicines ben good for þe*m* þ*at* be-pessen

3 colrik] *prec. by heading* Diampnes **6 purselane seed**] *corr. from* p*ur*selaneseed **11 for**] *corr. from* ffor **18 fleumagoge**] *corr. from* ffleu*ma*goge here bedde *and* for þe palese of þe bladdere. But ȝif þis comeþ of a sympel distemperyng of þe bladd*er* | w*ith*-outen f. 158r eny oþ*er* humo*ur* thorow coold, jt is þa*n* non neede to ȝif hym a p*ur*gacion. But do schoon on hys feete *and* kepe al hys body fra*m* coold. And a-noynte þe schare *and* þe places þ*at* ben neiȝ a-boute w*ith* hoote oyneme*nt*e*s*, as marciaton, *and* arrogon, and w*ith* hoote oyles. And make a plastre of calamynte, *and* beteyn*n* j-poudred, *and* of poudre of comyn, *and* of baies of lorere, *and* of oile of lorere j-medlid togidere. *And* al warm lei þe plastere on hys schare and anoþ*er*e be-twyn his ers-hoole *and* hys ȝerde. But oolde men ben on-curabil of þis sicnesse. And in eu*er*y coold palesei of þe bladdere, make hy*m* baþen in baþes þ*at* ben ordend for men þ*at* han þe palesie. *And* ȝif hym t*r*iacle and þe poudere of a boores bleddere j-dru*n*ken w*ith* wyn þ*at* mynte and sauge ben j-soden i*n*ne, *et cetera*.

Sjphac is a skyn þ*at* is be-twen þe guttes of a ma*n* *and* his vttere skyn. And þis skyn is oþ*er*while maad slaak þoro*ur* hum*ur*os *and* mooistnesse, riȝt as leþere wul ratche þ*at* is j-wet w*ith* wat*er*. And wha*n* þe siphac is so slak þorow þristeng of þe gutt*es*, þ*er* is swellyng*e* in þe syde of þe schaare be-side þe þeiȝ, oþ*er* in su*m* oþ*er* place of þe wombe of þe schap of an ey. And þe same man*er* swellyng*e* comeþ of a wynd. But þe slaknesse is j-knowe be þe mooistnesse of all*e* þe body, *and* of neisschep*e* of þe wombe, *and* of sich*e* oþ*er*e tokens. Wyndnesse is knowen be myche hurlyng *and* noyse of wynd in þe gutt*es*. And in þe tyme þ*at* it be

2 **þe bladder**] *corr. from* þebladd*er* **with-outen**] *prec. by heading* Siphac **13 make**] *follow. by* make **17 Sjphac**] *2-line space left for initial* **25 of**[2]] *follow. by canc. and exp.* all*e* þe body

f. 158v delyuered of sych*e* wynd in þe gutt*es*, þe swellyng | is myche seene. Oþ*er*while, þ*at* skyn is to-broke, so þ*at* þe guttes fall*e* dou*n* in-to a mann*es* cood *and* makeþ hym seme broke-balloked oþ*er* bussok þ*at* is al oon. And þis breche is oþ*er*while moore, oþ*er*while lesse. And þis breche comeþ oþ*er*while of fallyng, oþ*er*while of lepynge, oþ*er* of berynge of gret burdenys, oþ*er* of gret heeft*es*, oþ*er* of gret cryi*n*ge of a ma*n*, oþ*er* of myche wepyng*e* of childern, oþ*er* of a gret a-for-syng*e* þ*at* a ma*n* a-forseþ hym to schiten. And þ*er* is a gret difference betwen thys *and* hym þ*at* is bussok, for he þ*at* is bussok haþ ach*e* *and* greua*n*nce in his code *and* in hys stoones, but þese han swellyng*e* in þe neþ*er* party of þe schare *and* greuau*n*ce also. *And* þe swellyng*e* is in þe cood *and* nat in þe stoones. Þis sicnesse is j-heelyd be puttyng i*n*ne of þe gutte þ*at* is j-fallen in-to þe code, and siþe bi soudynge of þe siphac be medicin*es* þ*at* ben consolidatyues, þ*at* is to vnd*er*stonde, ȝif þe brech*e* be newe, for þ*at* þ*at* is oold w[u]l nat be holpen w*it*h-outen kyttynge. For slacnesse of þe siphac, loke of what humo*ur* it is be tokenes þ*at* ben j-teld here-before, *and* p*ur*ge hym of þ*at* humo*ur*. And ȝif it comeþ of wyndenesse, ȝif hym sich*e* medicynes as co*n*sumen wyndes, as it was j-told in colica passio. But ȝif þe siphac is to-broke *and* þe guttes fallen dou*n*n in-to þe cood, late hym liggen vp-riȝt *and* heuen up hese hepis, *and* putten þe guttes in a-ȝen in-to hys wombe. And siþe make þis plastre *and* lei

1 **is**] *prec. by heading* Siphac **10 for**] *corr. from* ffor **14 be**] *follow. by canc. twice* jj **16 consolidatyues**] *interl.* id **17 þe breche**] *corr. from* þebrech*e* **be newe**] *corr. from* benewe **18 be holpen**] *corr. from* beholpen **For**] *corr. from* ffor **19 of²**] *interl.* **20 here-before and**] *corr. from* here-before*and* **22 colica passio**] *corr. from* colicapassio

þer-to: Tak confirie, and | saundragou*n*, *and* mu*m*mye, *and* f. 159r ypoquyscidos, *and* a harys skyn j-soden w*ith* þe heerys *and* a ma*n*nes blood. *And* medle þese togid*ere* *and* lei hem þ*er*-as þe brech*e* is. Oþ*er* make a plastre of boole, *and* saundragou*n*, *and* mu*m*mye, *and* sumac, *and* of gu*m* arabik, *and* of galles, *and* of a lytel mastik. Poudre all*e* þese *and* medle hem w*ith* þe gleire of eiren. *And* lei it on a pece of leþere *and* lei to þe sore, and þ*er*-on lei a pece of leed *and* bynd it vp. *And* late it ligge þer*e* xl daies, for be þ*at* tyme jt wole be j-souded. And be he ware of all*e* man*er* mouynge, *and* fro traueile, of fn[e]synge, *and* wraþ, *and* couȝi*n*ge, *and* of compeny w*ith* women, and enforce he hy*m* nat to schite. And wheþ*er* þe breche be vnd*er* þe nauele oþ*er* in þe side oþ*er* vnd*er* þe schar*e*, þ*er* lei þe plastere. And whan he gooþ to p*ri*uei, let hym hoolde þ*at* place faast w*ith* his hoond, laste þe gutte falle out þ*er*-at. And diete hym w*ith* sich*e* met*es* þ*at* wole make hym neysch*e* wombed. *And* ȝif hese wombe be hard, make hym a clist*ere* mollificatif. And late hym ete aft*er* mete þe seed of p*er*seli, of anyse, *and* of march to co*n*sume þe wyndes þ*at* wole lette þe soudyng*e*. And oþ*er*whiles late hy*m* vse moist medicines, but noon erbys but it be p*er*sily oþ*er* aua*n*ce oþ*er* sich*e* oþ*er*. And brenne colu*m*bine *and and* þe flowr*e* of calamynt, *and* late hym vse þis poudre þ*er*-of to his meete. Also late hym drynk scrophularie xl daies w*ith* þe for-seid medicines, *and* reuli*n*ge, *and* þ*at* wol soude þe breche. And þe same medicines ben good for slacnesse of þe siphac. But furst p*ur*ge | f. 159v hym of þilke hum*ur*os þ*at* make þe slacnesse. *And* siþe pit in þi plaasteres myrre, *and* aloes, *and*

1 saundragoun] *prec. by heading* Siphac **2 ypoquyscidos**] *corr. from* ypoquy*n*scidos **6 and**[1]] *interl.* **7 of**[2]] *follow. by canc. twice* gleire **9 for**] *corr. from* ffor **13 þe**[2]] *interl.* **27 hym**] *prec. by heading* Siphac encense, *and* centorie. Anoþ*er* man*er* curynge of þis sicnesse *and* it is also good for hem þ*at* ben bossok, lat hem ligge in reste xl daies, þ*at* þei walken nat. Oþ*er* ȝif þei must nedys walke, make he*m* a brech oþ*er* su*m* oþ*er* byndynge beneþes, þ*at* þe guttes ne falle nat out at þe breche. And eu*ery* dai a-noynte þe place w*ith* þe oynement þ*at* is þ*us* j-maad: Tak gootys talwe *and* melt it. *And* medle þ*er*-wiþ þe iuys of þese herbys: confirie, daisie, plau*n*teyn, oxie, pentafilon, ribwort, of eu*ery*ch*e* of þese, j-lich*e* mych*e* iuys, *and* vi*n*egre, *and* of reed wyn. *And* medle hem wel to-gidere. *And* siþe cast þ*er*-to þe poudre of galles, *and* of þe blostme of hock*es* *and* of ryndys, *and* of ook akren, *and* of chasteynes, *and* of bole, *and* sau*n*dragou*n*, mastyk, nytre, mu*m*mye, *and* of borac*e*, *and* of eu*er*ich*e* of þese, j-liche mich*e*. *And* caast oile of rooses þ*er*-to, *and* medle hem to-gidere. And herewiþ a-noynte þe place. But waisch*e* it furst w*ith* wat*er* þ*at* st*ri*ctorie medicines ha*n* ben j-soden i*n*ne, but late þe wat*er* be nyȝ coold. And aft*er*ward lei þis plastere þ*er*-on: Tak of ypoquyscides, acasie, mu*m*mye, boole, galles, psidie, co*n*firie, daisie, colofonye, pich, mastik, encense, cars seed, *and* of cardomomu*m*, *ounce* s*emis*. Medle hem [with] goot*us* talwe *and* vi*n*egre ou*er* þe feire. *And* do of þis plastre in a pece of leed j-maad su*m*what holwe, *and* lei to þe soore. And þe f. 160r [beste] plastre is to þis brech*e*: Tak of amonia[c], | of galbanu*m*, of turmentille, mastik, galles, litarge, gipsum, myrt, olibanu*m*, of gret wormes þ*at* bien in þe grounde þ*at* ben angel-twaches, feern, mystelto þ*at* groweþ on ookes, aloes, aristologie boþe þe longe *and* þe rounde, colofonye,

13 mummye] *corr. from* mu*m*myn*e* **17 þe water**] *corr. from* þewat*er*
20 cars seed] *corr. from* carsseed **23 sumwhat**] *follow. by exp.* howe
24 amoniac] *f. 160r* | niaa **of²**] *prec. by heading* Siphac

pich, reed wex, bole, sandragu*n*, confirie, daisie, balaustie, spodie, acacie, mu*m*mye, of þe rynde of a þorn, *and* of þe sloo tree, *ounce* iij; *and* of ma*n*nys blood j *pound*; of goot*es* talwe, as mych*e*. *And* make it in þis wise: Take a newe weþer*es* skyn, *and* schaue of þe wulle, *and* kyt þe skyn to smale peces, *and* seeþe he*m* in wat*er* tyl þei be so tendere þ*at* þ*o*u may esylech*e* put þi fyngere thorow hem. Þa*n* wryng owt clene þe wat*er* *and* þ*er*wiþ medle þi blood *and* þi talwe. *And* cast þ*er*-to a quart of vi*n*egre, *and* as mych*e* of þe iuys of plau*n*teyn, *and* j *pound* of wex. *And* medle he*m* wel to-gidere, *and* siþe poudre all*e* þi oþ*er* þi*n*ges *and* cast hem þ*er*-to, *and* medle hem wel to-gidere. Of þis do a litel in an hou*n*des eiȝe *and* it wole drawe þe led*es* so fast to-gidere þ*at* on-neþe þu xalt opene hys eiȝe. Of þis make hy*m* a plastre *and* lei to þe soore. And make hym an electuarie of hony, of sandragou*n*, mu*m*mye, acacie, co*n*firie, daisie. *And* let hym vsen þis electuarie vij wok*es*. And xl daies, lat hym liggen stille. And ȝif he wexeþ costif, ȝif hym a clistere mollificatif. Also for breche þ*at* falleþ in-to a ma*n*n*es* breste oþ*er* in his stomac, make hym cakes of barly meele *and* of ȝelk*es* of eiren. *And* make hym drynke þe poudre | of long pilocelle, f. 160v
oþ*er* of sauge j-brent, *and* mu*m*mye, confirie, canel, þe rynde of an aisch*e*, *and* þe poudre of an oxe ters j-brent *and* j-medled w*ith* hony. And wha*n* þe guttes ben wele j-clensed, ȝif hym pillules j-maad of galbanu*m*, *and* of haar*es* her*es* j-brent, *and* of long*e* pilocelle j-medled w*ith* hony. And siþe lei þis plastere on þe breche: Tak*e* colofonye, pich, galbanu*m*, a*m*moniac, aloes, mastik*e*, mu*m*mye, olibanu*m*, *and* aristologia þe rounde, plaunteyn, roosyn, *and* wex. Sta*m*pe

21 of] *prec. by heading* Siphac **22 sauge**] *corr. from* saunge **24 wele j-clensed**] *corr. from* welej-clensed

he*m* to-gidere w*ith* an hoot eyren pestel *and* lei it on þe brech*e* w*ith*-outen eny oþ*er* þi*n*g be-twyn. And þis is good for þe breche of þe siphac. And vp-on þe plastre, lei a pulwe *and* bynde it faste. *And* lat it ligge so xxx daies. *And* eu*ery* dai late hym drynke þe poudre of astrologie boþe þe longe *and* þe rounde, *and* of galles, plau*n*teyn, of eu*er*ich*e*, j-lich*e* myche. Also tak an herbe þ*at* groweþ in wodes *and* is lich a netle, *and* is þe lengþe of a cubite oþ*er* þ*er* a-boute, *and* haþ as it were ballokstoon[e]s a-boute þe roote, *and* þe stalk þ*er*of is sqware, *and* it stynkeþ. Tak þ*er*-of *and* make þe roote clene. *And* stampe it al smal *and* tempre it w*ith* wyn. *And* ʒif hym þ*er*-of to drynken *ounce* iij whiles he is fastyng*e*. *And* let hym vsen thys iij wokes to-gidere. And be ware of costyfnesse *and* of wyndy met*es*. *And* late hym plastre þis for-seid herbe xl daies on þe breche and loke he be stille on oon place as mych*e* as he mai. And eu*er*ich*e* dai renewe hys plastere for it sowdiþ wonderefullych*e* þe breche. An-oþ*er* f. 161r plastere for þis greuau*n*ce þouʒ | þe brech*e* be of xxv ʒeere *and* þe man of xl ʒeer*e* old: Tak*e* of pich*e*, of wex, colofonie, *ounce* iij; of litarge, a*m*moniac, oppoponak, galbanu*m*, sumac, mastik, bdelliu*m*, turmentyne, serapinu*m*, radich, confirie, daisie, *ounce* j; of aristologie boþe longe *and* þe rounde, of angeltwaches, *ounce* iiij; bole, mu*m*mye, *dragme* vj; of ma*n*nes blood, *pound* j. Make it as þe raþ*er* plastere was j-maad wiþ þe weþer*es* skyn j-soden. And whane þe plastere is þicke *and* blak, þa*n* it is j-nowʒ. And wha*n* þe man haþ j-p*ur*ged hy*m* *and* j-baþed hym, lei þe plastere on his soore. And eu*ery* day late hym ete eþ*er* þe for-seid electuarie

7 **an herbe**] *corr. from* anherbe 9 **ballokstoones**] *corr. from* ballokstoonos 10 **make þe**] *corr. from* makeþe 14 **wyndy metes**] *corr. from* wyndymet*es* 18 **þe**] *prec. by heading* Satiriasis

oþ*er* of þe for-seid herbys. And ȝif it is a child þ*a*t haþ þis sicnesse, make hym lytel cakes of confirie *and* ix ȝelkys of eyren. *And* let hym eten hem in þe ix laste daies of þe wany*n*g of þe mone.

Jn a mannes ȝerde þ*er* ben diu*er*se greuau*n*ces: to myche stondyng*e* þ*a*t is clepid satiriasis, *and* flowyng of a ma*nnes* seed a-ȝens hese wille, *and* pymples, *and* swellynge, *and* cancre. Satiriasis comeþ of a gret bostuse hee[t] wynd þ*a*t falleþ dou*n* to a ma*nnes* stoon*es and* in-to hys ȝerd *and* makeþ hys ȝerde to a-ryse. And þis comeþ of no desyre, ne of no lyky*n*g þ*a*t a ma*n* haþ þ*er*-to, but w*ith* ache, greuau*n*ce, *and* swellyng. And furst þ*o*u xalt gyf hym rep*er*cussyfs, boþe in oynement*es and* in plasterys, to smyten a-ȝen þ*a*t wyndy matere, boþe a-boute þe ȝerde, *and* on þe schare, *and* on þe reynes. Anoynte þe ȝerde, *and* þe stones, þe schare, *and* reynes w*ith* oile of henbane *and* oile of mandrake. And late wassche þ*a*t membre w*ith* | coold wat*er* oþ*er* neiȝ coold, þ*a*t f. 161v salien leues ben j-soden i*n*ne, and late þe ȝerde ȝoke wele þ*er*-i*n*ne. Camphore is good also to smelle, too to drynke, *and* to beere in his hond. And late hym drynke þe sirip*e* of wat*er*-lilies. And strawe hys hows w*ith* coold herb*e and* þe leeu*es* of coold trees. And late hym wake myche, *and* faste mych*e*, *and* wele a-kelen hym. And make a plastre of p*er*sile *and* of vi*n*egre. *And* lei a-boute his ȝerde *and* on hys reynes. Oþ*er* make a plastere of oþ*er* coold herb*e* oþ*er* of opiu*m and* þe muscilage of p*er*sile j-medlyd w*ith* vinegre. Oþ*er* tak rep*er*cussyues þ*a*t schul be teld in swellyng*e* of þe stoones. And ȝif hym diaprunes *and* diacalemen[tum] j-medlid to-

5 Jn] *2-line space left for initial* **8 heet**] *corr. from* heed **17 coold**[1]] *prec. by heading* Gomorra **25 herbe**] *follow. by canc. and* **oþer**[2]] *interl.*

gidere. And make hym þis sirip: Take violet *and* þe blosteme of saly, sau*n*dres, *and* wat*er*lilies, *and* þe seed of letuse, *and* of p*ur*selane, *and* of arage. Let alle þese ligge iij nyȝt*es* in vinegre *and* siþe seeþe hem in wat*er*. *And* siþe make it vp wiþ sugre *and* cast þ*er*-to a litel ca*m*phore. And coold thyng*es* ne heleþ nat. Make hym drynk wyn þ*at* rewe is j-soden i*n*ne, oþ*er* þe iuys þ*er*of, oþ*er* wyn þ*at* comyn is j-soden i*n*ne. Also late hym ete þe seed of agn*us* cast*us* *and* make a plastere of þe leeuys.

Gomorra þ*at* is flowyng of a mann*es* seed a-ȝenst hys wille, *and* þis is of plente of blood, oþ*er* of pa-lese of þe stoones, oþ*er* of gret febelnesse of a man þ*at* may nat w*ith*-holden hys seed, oþ*er* it comeþ for þe seed is thyn *and* floweþ out redely. And ȝif it comeþ of plente of blood, þe veynes ou*er*al a ma*n*n*es* body ben ful of blood *and* to-swolle. *And* þei han likynge wha*n* þe seed passeþ a-wei fram hem. Ȝif it
f. 162r comeþ | of palesie of stoones, þei feleþ nat wha*n* þ*er* seed passeþ fra*m* þem, as men þ*at* han þe palesie of þe bladdere ne fele*n* nat wha*n* þ*er* vrine passeþ fra*m* hem. Ȝif it come of febilnesse, al þe bodi is febil, *and* leene, *and* of euel colo*ur*. Ȝif it comeþ of þi*n*neschip*e* of þe seed, it wole telle hym-self, *and* þe co*m*plexion of þe man, *and* his dietinge also. Wha*n* it comeþ of blood, late hy*m* vse to be late blood ofte-siþes vnd*er* þe i*n*nere ancle, oþ*er* of þe lyu*er* veyne of þe arme. *And* a-noynte his reyn*es* w*ith* coold oynement*es*. *And* diete hym w*ith* sich*e* met*es* þ*at* ge*n*deriþ lytel blood. Wha*n*ne it comeþ of palesie of þe stoones, ȝif hy*m* medicines þ*at* were j-teld in þe palesie of þe bladdere. Wha*n* it comeþ of

10 Gomorra] *2-line space left for initial* **16 þe**] *follow. by exp.* ceede **17 of[1]**] *prec. by heading* Gomorra **23 ofte-siþes vnder**] *corr. from* ofte-siþesvnd*er*

febelnesse, take encense, mastik, *and* mynte, *and* sau*n*dres, *and* storace, in grettere q*ua*ntite þa*n* of þe oþ*er*, *and* medle hem w*ith* þe iuys of plau*n*ten *and* w*ith* vinegre. *And* make a plastre þ*er*of, *and* lei up-on hys reynes, *and* a-boute hys ȝerde, *and* hys stoones. *And* ȝif hym oþ*er* medicynes as it was j-teld in diabetes. And ȝif hym medicines þ*at* ben confortatyf *and* st*ri*ctories, as diacodion *and* sugre rooset, *and* þe sirip of rooses, for þese que*n*che myȝtly þ*at* appetit þ*at* a man haþ to lechery. And for þis sicnesse, þ*o*u xal worche w*ith* coold medicines as þ*o*u dedist in satiriasis. Wha*n* it comeþ of þi*n*schepe, ȝif hym a sirip j-maad of iuys of mynt *and* of sugre. And w*ith* þe iuys of mynte a-noynte hys ȝerde *and* hys stoon*es*. And þis same is good to make mylk þicke þ*at* is in a woma*nn**es* tet*es*. And diete hym w*ith* met*es* þ*at* wole make þe blood þicke as whiȝt breed, *and* riȝ, *and* ȝelk*es* of eiren, *and* sich*e* oþ*er* þi*n*ges. | f. 162v And be þei ware of arage *and* of blet*es* for þei make blood þi*n*ne.

Pymples *and* postemes ben also in a mann*es* ȝerde. *And* ȝif þei be nat wele j-heelid, þei t*ur*ne in-to a cancre or in-to a feestre þ*at* is holow as a whistel or a pipe. And sich*e* postem*us* ben oþ*er*while j-hyd w*ith*-i*n*ne þe ȝerde, *and* oþ*er*whiles w*ith*-oute; *and* oþ*er*whiles þei come of heete, *and* þa*n*, as þere þei ben, þ*er* is gret heete, *and* brenny*n*g, *and* p*ri*ckyng*e*, *and* ache, *and* reednesse, *and* oþ*er*while swellinge. Oþ*er*while þei come of coold, *and* þa*n* þei felen heuynesse

7 **and**[2]] *interl.* **sugre rooset**] *corr. from* sugrerooset 10 **coold**] *follow. by canc.* sicne 12 **a-noynte**] *follow. by* a-noynte 15 **þe blood**] *corr. from* þeblood 16 **And**] *prec. by heading* Pymples 18 **Pymples**] *2-line space left for initial* 20 **feestre**] *corr. from* ffeestre

8 **þese**] *in r.-h. margin:* no*ta* b*e*ne 13 **good**] *in r.-h. margin:* no*ta*

þ*er*-a-boute, *and* coolde, *and* in boþe is greua*n*nce wha*n* þei pissen. For boþe enchesons, late hem blood vnd*er* þe ancle *and* cuppe hem on þe veynes. And make a plastre of goos grece *and* of whete meele, *and* lei it al warm to þe ȝerde, *and* ofte-siþes renewe it. And in bothen enchesou*n*s, wha*n* þe postem*us* ben j-t*ur*ned to q*ui*ture, ȝif þei ben w*it*h-i*n*neforþ, ȝif hem medicines þ*a*t ben duretik to clense þe ȝerde of q*ui*ture, laste þ*er* wax a festre in þe ȝerde. *And* þorow an enargale cast goot*es* wheiȝ in-to þe ȝerde al warm, oþ*er* medlid w*it*h dispumyd hony, *and* cast þ*er*to al warm in-to his ȝerde. Oþ*er*while þe ȝerd is to-swolle, *and* þa*n* þe ȝerd xal be baþid in warm wat*er*. Oþ*er* tak þe leues of a whiȝt thorn *and* þe smale brau*n*ches. *And* seeþe hem in wyn. *And* þ*er*wiþ waisch*e* his ȝerde *and* late hym ȝoke þ*er*i*n*ne also. And so do ij or thriȝes tyl þe swalm be a-batyd. Oþ*er* seeþe hock*es* *and* p*er*it*er*ie in wyn or in wat*er*, *and* þ*er*wiþ waisch*e* hym. Oþ*er* make a plastre of lyndseed j-powned *and* j-soden in wat*er*; oþ*er* comyn *and* þe roote of holy-hocke j-soden *and* syþe j-
f. 162rbis sta*m*ped to-gedere; oþere of driȝe benys j-soden | in wyn; oþ*er* of driȝe figes, *and* reisenes, *and* cane j-soden in swete wyn; oþ*er*e p*er*iterie *and* bren. Oþ*er* stampe lynseed *and* hocke leuys to-gidere *and* seeþe hem in wat*er*. *And* siþe cast þ*er*-to oile, *and* got*es* talwe, *and* poudre of comyn, *and* a lytel poudre touȝ cley. Oþ*er* stampe orpen *and* penywort to-gidere *and* make a plastre þ*er*-of; oþ*er* of p*er*iterie j-stamped *and* j-fried be hym-self. And let hym bleden at þe veyn þ*a*t serueþ

2 For] *corr. from* ffor **9 al warm]** *corr. from* alwarm **10 al warm]** *corr. from* alwarm **15 Oþer]** *follow. by canc.* sich*e* **17 lyndseed]** *follow. by canc.* in soden **19 in]** *prec. by heading* and postemes in the ȝerde **22 hocke leuys]** *corr. from* hockeleuys **23 comyn]** *follow. by canc. twice* of ton to þe lyuere. And ȝif þe ȝerd be j-cancrid, make þis oinement: Tak *pound* j of oold swynes grece *and* medle þ*er*wiþ *ounce* s*emis* of v*er*tegrece. *And* þ*er*wiþ a-noynte his ȝerde. Oþ*er* bren salt al to poudre, *and* þ*a*t poudre is good boþe for þe cancre of þe ȝerde *and* for þe cancre of a womans p*ri*ue membre. And so be þe leeu*es* of a þefe-þorn j-fried in grece. But wasch*e* þe ȝerd furst w*it*h vrine oþ*er* w*it*h wyn, but for no-þi*n*g w*it*h wat*er*. And aft*er* þ*a*t þ*a*t it is wel j-wassched, rubbe it wel w*it*h a clooþ *and* straw þ*er*-on þe for-seid poudre of salt, ȝif men may come ny þe cancre. Also stampe been*es* *and* seeþ hem in wyn. *And* cast þ*er*-to a litel oile *and* vi*n*egre. *And* þ*a*t is good also þ*er*fore. Oþ*er* tac an oold slowȝ of an addre *and* frie it w*it*h oile; *and* lei þ*er*-to. But ȝif þe swalm swage nat w*it*h þese medicines, slite þe ȝerde w*it*h a raso*ur* *and* late it blede su*m*what. *And* siþe lei bole *and* salt þ*er*on a litel while to stau*n*che þe bloode. And ȝif þ*er* be pympels þ*a*t wul nat brekyn, lete frete hem in sope *and* hoote wat*er* to-gidere. *And* siþe lei on hem a coole leef, oþ*er* a lilie leef, oþ*er* þe ȝelke of an ey w*it*h salt. And ȝif þei wole nat to-breke, late hy*m* rubben his ȝerde on | hys þeiȝ f. 162vbis til þei tobroken. Oþ*er* ellys open hem w*it*h a nail. And wha*n* þe quiture brekeþ out, pit þ*er*-i*n*ne þe poudre of myrre, *and* of aloes, oþ*er* mastik, *and* olibanu*m*, *and* alooes, *and* mirre j-poudreid; oþ*er* þe poudre of a schoo soole j-brent, oþ*er* of pentafilon, oþ*er* of hert*es*-horn j-brent, oþ*er* þe poudre of pympenell*e*, oþ*er* þe poudre of blew clooþ j-brent, oþ*er* of þe seed or of þe flour*es* of lappaciu*m* acutu*m*. *And* medle þ*er*-wiþ þe poudre of a mannys driȝt j-brent oþ*er* þe oile of a

6 be þe] *corr. from* beþe **10 Also**] *follow. by canc.* stampe **11 stampe**] *interl.* **20 hys**] *prec. by heading* Pymplys or aposteem of þ*e* ȝerde (yarde *written above* ȝerde *with pencil*) **21 a nail**] *corr. from* anail ma*nn*es driȝt, for þ*a*t is good for cancris. And ȝif it soudeþ nat to-gidere as it schulde, medle wiþ thi poudres su*m* of a swynnes galle *and* þe ȝelwe oyneme*n*t oþ*er* þe grene þ*a*t surgiens vsen. And ȝif it heleþ nat here-wiþ, a-nointe hym w*it*h swynes galle *and* siþe sprynge þ*er*-on þe poudre of orpyme*n*t *and* of v*er*tigrece j-brent. And ȝif þ*er* be eny deed fleisch, sta*m*pe garlek *and* lei it on eu*er*y side þ*er*of, for þ*a*t freteþ a-wei þe sori fleisch*e* *and* co*n*forteþ þe goode. And wha*n* þe sori flesch*e* is froten a-wei, anoynte hy*m* w*it*h þis oynement: Seeþ beenys *and* salt to-gidere, *and* siþe cast a-wei þe hooles of benys. *And* medle hem *and* mastik, *and* olibanu*m*, *and* ceruse, *and* wat*er* of rooses to-gidere, *and* make an oyneme*n*t þ*er*of. *And* þ*er*wiþ a-noynte þe fleisch*e*, for it wole helen hym in ij daies. And ȝif þe cancre wul nat be hoolid w*it*h medycines, kyt a-wei as meche as is j-cancrid *and* bren þe re*m*nannt w*it*h an hoot yren. And ȝif þ*er* be a festre *and* an hoole oþ*er* many hooles in þe ȝerde, hele it wiþ oyneme*n*t, ruptorie *and* w*it*h oþ*er* medicines teld in þe festre.

f. 163r |

Swellyng of þe cod *and* of his stoones comeþ oþ*er*while of hum*ur*os þ*a*t fallen a-doun in-to þe cod *and* in-to þe stoones. Oþ*er*whiles it comeþ of wynd, oþ*er*whiles of a posteme, oþ*er*while of brekyng of þe i*n*nere skyn *and* of fallyng*e* down of þe guttes in-to þe cod. And ȝif it comeþ of blood, þe veynes of þe body ben ful of blood, *and* na*m*liche þilke þa*n* ben vnd*er* þe ancle. Ȝif it comeþ of colre, þe cod is

1 for[1]] *corr. from* ffor **2 medle**] *follow. by canc. twice* þ*er* **18 þe festre**] *interl.* (festre, *corr. from* ffestre) **20 Swellyng**] *2-line space left for initial; prec. by heading* Swelly*n*g of the cod

7 garlek] *in l.-h. margin:* no*ta*

swart reed *and* brenny*n*ge for heete, *and* þ*er* is gret ache *and* p*ri*ckyng w*it*h-i*n*neforþ. 3if it is of flewme, þe cod is of pale colo*ur*, *and* mych*e* to-swolle, *and* neisch*e*, *and* heuy. 3if it be of malencolie, þe cod is to-swolle *and* ful heuy. 3if it be of wynd, þe swalm is w*it*h-outen heuynesse. 3if it be a posteme, it is oon of þe hum*ur*os *and* haþ þe same toknes þ*at* þe swelli*n*g haþ, saue þe ache is mych*e* grett*ere* *and* þe tokenes mych*e* moore violent *and* greuouse. Oþ*er*while þe swellyng comeþ of fleisch*e* þ*at* groweþ in þe cod more þa*n* þ*er* schuld. Wha*n* þis swelli*n*g comeþ of hum*ur*os, of what humo*ur* þ*at* eu*er* it be, lat hy*m* bloode in þe veyne þ*at* is vnd*er* þe ancle, *and* cuppe hym a-boue þe veynes. And siþe make coolde plastres of coold herbys j-soden in vinegre, *and* leie to þe cod to smyten a-ȝen þe hum*ur*os þ*at* ben encheson of þe swalm. Oþ*er* make a plastere of barly meele *and* of þe iuys of solatre j-medlid to-gidere. Oþ*er* stampe þe h*er*be hy*m*-self *and* leie þ*er*-too. And ȝif þe mat*ere* wul nat be smetyn a-ȝe*n*, make a plastre of barly meele, | *and* henn*es* grece, *and* oile of violet f. 163v
j-soden to-gidere *and* lei þ*er*-to. Oþ*er* make a plastre of þe crop of henbane *and* swynnes grece j-stamped to-gidere. Oþ*er* tac of þe plasteres þ*at* were j-teld in þe last chapitre. *And* þe same plasteres ben good for postem*us* of þe cod *and* of þe stoone. And ȝif þ*er* be no posteme in which*e* of all*e* þese for-seid plasteres þe likeþ, put clei *and* comyn *and* lei to þe swellyng*e*. And þese medycines s*er*uen ȝif þe swalm is of hoote hum*ur*os. But ȝif it be of coold hum*ur*os, make a stufe for þe cod of hote herb*e*. And siþe a-noynte þe cod w*it*h red

2 **flewme**] *corr. from* fflewme 11 **bloode in**] *corr. from* bloodein
18 **and**[1]] *prec. by heading* Swelly*n*g of the cod

8 **Oþerwhile**] *in r.-h. margin:* no*ta*

hony despumyd. And siþe gri*n*de þe pillyng of garlek *and* seeþe it in water*e*. *And* plastre it on þe cod *and* þ*at* wul drawe out þe hum*ur*os be smoke *and* be swety*n*g. Oþ*er* make a plastere of march *and* of clei oþ*er* of louage j-soden in wyn, oþ*er* of p*er*it*er*ie, oþ*er* of netlyn j-stamped *and* j-het wele in an erþen pot wele j-stopped a-boue w*it*h-outen eny oþ*er* liquor*es*. Oþ*er* make a plastere of rooses j-drie, *and* of drie figes, *and* of millefoil, *and* of hou*n*dys driȝt j-soden in whiȝt wyn. And þis is good wheþ*er* þe swalm come of heete oþ*er* of coold. Oþ*er* tak þe dust of a smythes gry*n*dyngstoon *and* medle it w*it*h vinegre. *And* make þ*er*-of a plastre, but a-noynte þe cod be-fore ȝif þe swalm comeþ of heete. Oþ*er* seeþe fenel seed, *and* þe seed of p*er*sele, dauk, march, f. 164r caraway, comyn, | anyse in watere. And in þ*at* wat*er* weete wolle þ*at* is vn-waisch*e* *and* lei to swalm. Ȝif it comeþ of coold hum*ur*os oþ*er* of wynd also, þe slewȝ of an addre j-friȝed in oile is good for þis sicnesse. And so bien broken *and* soden in vinegre *and* in hony *and* j-plastred on þe swalm. And ȝif þis greua*n*nce be oold *and* þe ma*n* be ful of hum*ur*os, ȝif þe swalm comeþ of blood, late hym oftesiþes bleden vnd*er* þe ancle. And ȝif it come of eny oþ*er* humo*ur*, p*ur*ge hym w*it*h su*m* oþ*er* medicine þ*at* a-cordeþ þ*er*-to. And late hym ofte-siþes be j-cupped a-boue þe buttokes. And ȝif it be a posteme, lei þ*er*to þese for-seid plastres, furst rep*er*cussifs to smyten þe matere a-ȝen; and ȝif it wole nat, lei þ*er*-to dissolutyfs, and ȝif þe matere vanysch*e* nat a-wei but wexeþ rype *and* brekeþ. Ȝif þe posteme is w*it*h-outen þe

5 netlyn] *follow. by canc. and exp.* vn **j-stamped]** *interl.* j **13 fenel]** *corr. from* ffenel **14 comyn]** *catchword* (*in bottom margin*): anysy in **anyse]** *prec. by heading* Swelly*n*g of the cod **24 þese]** *corr. from* þ*er*ese (*er canc.*) **furst]** *corr. from* ffurst

cod, hele it vp as oþ*er* postem*es* ben j-heelid. But ȝif þe posteme be w*it**h*-i*n*ne þe cod, ȝif hym electuaries *and* sirepis þ*at* han ben j-teeld here-before to clense þe cod of q*ui*ture, ȝif it wole nat be clensid w*it**h*-oute. Oþ*er* ȝif þe posteme wexeþ hard w*it**h*-i*n*ne, þ*o*u miste sclytte þe cod *and* let out þe q*ui*ture. And ȝif þ*er* ben posteme oþ*er* fleisch*e* growyng*e* on eny of þe stoon*es*, schaf it a-wei w*it**h* a raso*ur*. And ȝif þe ston be hard *and* sound, late hym a-bide stille. And ȝif he roote eny-thi*n*g, kit hym of *and* siþe heele up þe wounde. But ȝif þe cod be to-swolle of bresyng*e*, make a plastre of oile, *and* t*ur*mentyne, *and* of barly meele *and* lei þ*er*-to. And ȝif þe bresyng*e* is oold, make a plastre | of beenys, *and* of f. 164v comyn, *and* of hony. Oþ*er* ȝif þe place is reed, breke beenes *and* seeþ hem in vinegre *and* lei þ*er*to. And ȝif þe place is nat reed, seeþ hem in wyn. Su*m*men slitten þe cod *and* letteþ þe humo*ur* gon out *and* siþe heliþ vp þe wounde. Also for swellyng *and* ache of þe cod: Tak pollipodie *and* grynd it w*it**h* got*us* talwe til þe herbe be riȝt smalle j-ground. *And* lei þ*er*-of a-broode on an hoot tyl-stoon. *And* lei to hys me*m*bre *and* chaunge it ofte-siþes. *And* ȝif þe swalm be harde, late þe membre ȝoke in warm salt-wat*er*.

Jn a ma*n*n*es* ers ben diu*er*se sicnesses. Oon is of þe emoroides. Oþ*er* þ*er* bien as figes, *and* buyles, *and* clystes in þe ers. Emoroides ben v veynes þ*at* come to þe ers to delyuere þe body of sori malencolies blood þ*at* wole noiȝe oþ*er* me*m*bris. And oþ*er*-while þese veynes blede to mych*e*, oþ*er*whiles þei ben to haard j-stopped, and oþ*er*whiles þei ben to-swolle. *And* þ*at* swalm oþ*er*while is w*it**h*-i*n*ne,

12 plastre] *in bottom margin:* a of[1]] *prec. by heading* Sekenesse **13** of] *interl.* **22** Jn] *2-line space left for initial* **23** figes] *corr. from* ffiges buyles] *corr. from* buy*n*les oþ*er*while is w*it*h-oute. Swellyng*e* of þese veynes comeþ oþ*er*while of drast*es* of þe blood þ*at* falleþ down to þe veynes mouþes *and* stoppeþ hem, oþ*er* of þilke blod þ*at* stoppeþ hem, oþ*er* of þicnesse of þe sky*n*, oþ*er* of brenny*n*g þ*at* men brende hem wha*n* þei flowede*n* to mych*e*. And wha*n* þe blood [n]e mai nat haue his issue as it schuld haue, it t*ur*neþ a-ȝen to þe lyuere *and* disposeþ a man to þe dropesi. Stoppyng*e* *and* w*it*hholdy*n*g of blood co*m*y of þe same enchesons. And oþ*er*while, þei ben all*e* to-stopped, and oþ*er*while su*m* ben j-stopped *and* su*m* ben vnstopped. f. 165r Mych*e* flowyng*e* of þese veynes comeþ | oþ*er*while in certen tymes, as þe flowi*n*g of blod þ*at* comeþ to women oones in a moneþ. And sich*e* flowy*n*g of þese veynes ne xal nat be j-stau*n*chid bi medicines, for þei wole hem-self cesse of bledyng. Also wha*n* it is nede, þei wole blede. But wha*n* þe bledyng*e* is to mych*e*, it is good to staunche*n* it. *And* siche fluxes comeþ of gret plent of blood, oþ*er* of keneschip*e* of þe blood, oþ*er* of thynschep*e* of þe blood, oþ*er* of febelnesse, as oþ*er* fluxes doon. And þis flowyng*e* comeþ to a ma*n* wha*n* he is xl ȝeere oold; to sich*e* men þ*at* han t*ra*uailed myche in here youthe, oþ*er* han t*ra*ualeid myche w*it*h oþ*er*e p*ar*ties of here bodi. And oþ*er*while þe blood þ*at* floweþ fra*m* hem is reed, cleere, *and* hoot in þe flowynge. And þese ben tokenes of keneschep*e* of þe blood. Oþ*er*-while it is blak *and* þicke. *And* þ*at* is token of male*n*colie þ*at* is i*n*ne þe blood. Oþ*er*while it is þi*n*ne *and* renny*n*g, *and* þ*at* is token of sotylte

6 ne] *corr. from* me **11 comeþ**] *f. 165r* | meþ **oþerwhile**] *prec. by heading* in the ers **14 for**] *corr. from* ffor **23 þe**] *follow. by canc. and exp.* fla

26 is[2]] *in l.-h. margin:* no*ta*

of blood. Oþ*er*while it is ȝelwe, *and* þ*a*t is token of flewme *and* colre j-medlid to-gid*er*e. Þese colo*ur*s of þe blood ben þ*us* j-know: Do su*m* of þe blood in a lynney clooþ *and* waisch*e* a-wei þe blood, *and* þe clooþ woil be of sych*e* a colo*ur* as þe blood is. And yif he blede mych*e* at a tyme, *and* blede ofte-siþes, *and* þe veynes of hys legg*es* *and* of his thies ben ful of blood, þa*n* þis flowyng*e* comeþ of plent[e] of blood. Ȝif it comeþ co*n*tinuel-lych*e* *and* litel, *and* febeleþ a man, *and* greueþ hym in þe flowyng*e*, þa*n* it comeþ of febelnesse. Tokenes of w*it**h*-hooldyng of blood þ*a*t xul flowen ben heuynesse a-boute þe reynes, *and* jchynge of þe buttokk*es*, *and* of þe | rugge, *and* of þe schaar, *and* þei han greuau*n*ce whan þei schiten, *and* þei han heed-ache, *and* pale colo*ur* of face. For flowi*n*g of þis blood ȝif it comeþ of gret plente of blood, let hym blede wel at þe lyuere weyn of þe arm. And ȝif it comeþ of oþ*er* hum*ur*os, ȝif hym a p*ur*gacion. But ȝif hym noon aloes ne oþ*er*e medicine þ*a*t is ful oppeny*n*ge, but su*m* oþ*er*e cologog*e* or fleu*ma*goge. Siþe make hym a baaþ as jt was j-teld in dissent*er*ie. *And* aft*er*, oppen þe veyne þ*a*t is vnd*er* þe vtt*er*e ancle. And siþe make hym suppositories *and* fumygaciou*n*s as in disse*n*terie. And late hym drynke a-morwe *and* on eue þe juys of millefoile j-medlid w*it**h* warm wyn, *and* plast*r*e þe herbe to his ers. Oþ*er* tak an herbe þ*a*t is like leek *and* haþ a whiȝt flowr *and* a sauor of garlek. Sta*m*pe it w*it**h* must oþ*er* new ale *and* lat

f. 165v

6 blede ofte-siþes] *corr. from* bledeofte-siþes **7 plente**] *corr. from* plento **8 and litel**] *corr. from and*litel **10 with-hooldyng**] *corr. from* w*it**h*hat-hooldyng (hat *exp.*) **þat**] *interl.* **12 þe**[1]] *in bottom margin:* b **rugge**] *prec. by heading* Sekenesse **14 For**] *corr. from* ffor **15 weyn**] *interl.* e **of þe**] *corr. from* ofþe **18 fleumagoge**] *corr. from* ffleu*ma*goge **21 fumygaciouns**] *corr. from* ffumygaciou*n*s

hym drynk þ*er*-of eu*er*ych*e* morwetyd. And make hym a fumigacion of kalendula *and* of leek j-soden in wyn, oþ*er* of kalendula, *and* leek, *and* planten j-soden in wat*er*e. Leek j-eten oþ*er* j-dru*n*k openeþ þe veynes; but ȝif it be plasterid w*it**h*-oute, he stoppeþ þe veyne. Also make hym a pocion of whiȝt hore-howne, *and* aua*n*ce, *and* millefoil, *and* plau*n*teyn j-sta*m*ped a litel to-gidere *and* soden in wyn. And make hym a poudre to etyn of clowes, *and* femygrek, *and* canel, *and* sych*e* oþ*er*e co*n*fortabil þi*n*ges. An oyneme*n*t for þe eme-roides: Tak þe poudre of leek seed j-brent *and* of litarge j-brent, *and* medle hem w*it**h* oile of lynseed. *And* þ*er*-wiþ a-noynte þe emeroides ȝif þe soore is w*it**h*-oute þe ers. And ȝif
f. 166r it is w*it**h*-i*n*ne, wete a weke in þe | oynement *and* pit it in-to þe soore. And so þ*o*u xal do be alle man*er* oynement*es* þ*a*t ben for þis sicnesse. Anoþ*er* oynement: Tac croppis of ellern *and* of mylberi tree *and* stampe hem as þei þ*o*u woldest make sauce of hem. *And* siþe tempere hem vp w*it**h* oile of ȝelk*es* of eyren in þe manere of an oynement. Oþ*er* tac þe poudre of acacie, *and* of brent leed, *and* of ceruse, *and* þe poudre of bole, *and* of coporose, *and* of psidie. *And* te*m*pre it w*it**h* vinegre *and* w*it**h* þe iuys of pentafilon. Oþ*er* tac þe poudre of amtymonye, of litarge, of ceruse, *and* of leed. Let hem all*e* ben j-brent *and* temp[r]e he all*e* w*it**h* oile of lynseed. *And* make an oynement. But ar þa*n* he be a-noynted w*it**h* þis oyneme*n*t oþ*er* w*it**h* eny of þe oþ*er*, make hym a fumygacion

2 fumigacion] *corr. from* ffumigacion **5 of whiȝt**] *corr. from* ofwhiȝt **8 femygrek**] *corr. from* ffemygrek **9 An oynement**] *corr. from* Anoyneme*n*t **13 oynement**] *prec. by heading* in the ers **25 fumygacion**] *corr. from* ffumygacion

3 leek] *in l.-h. margin:* no*ta*

of softe j-soden in wyn. *And* late hym sitte in þe herbe tyl þe herbe wexe coold. And siþe a-noynte þe emeroides w*ith* þe oynement. Also tak betoyne, of eg*re*moyne, of mynt, millefoile, mugwort, plau*n*tei*n*, strauberiwise, of eu*e*rich*e* of þese, m*anipulum* j; of pep*er*, *ounce* s*emis*; of wyn, *quantum* s*ufficit*. Seeþ all*e* þese in þe wyn *and* late hym drynke þe wyn ix daies fasti*n*g. Also stampe celidoine, *and* pentafilon, *and* horehowne, *and* lat hy*m* drynk hem w*ith* stale ale. And oþ*er* medicines þ*at* bien good for dissent*er*ie *and* lient*er*ie ben good for þis sicnesse. And bie þei ware of malencolies met*es*. And afor-se þei nat hem to schyte. And bie þei ware of met*es* þ*at* wole open þe endys of þe veynes, as ben kene metis, *and* comyn. And fro medicines þ*at* ben openy*n*g as aloes, *and* scamone, *and* pollipodie, *and* sich*e* oþ*er*. For whiþholdyng*e* of þis blood *and* swellyng of þe veynes, furst | f. 166v purge hym w*ith* su*m* medicine þ*at* is openy*n*g, as aloes oþ*er* scamone, oþ*er* w*ith* wat*er* þ*at* pollipodie haþ be soden i*n*ne. Siþe make hym a baaþ of yp*er*icon, *and* march, *and* p*er*it*er*ie, *and* gorst, horhowne, pollicarie, *and* sich*e* oþ*er* herb*e* j-soden in wat*er*. Oþ*er* tac hym a p*ur*gacion ȝif þu wult of tyme, *and* epithime, *and* sene, *and* myrabol*e* indj, of lapis laȝuli. Poudre all*e* þese *and* lat hym drynk þe poudre w*ith* wat*er* þ*at* borage is j-soden i*n*ne. And siþe late hym blede vnd*er* þe ancle in boþe sydes *and* on boþe legg*es*. And a-noon aft*er*, make hym a fumygacion of comyn salt, *and* nytre, *and* of salge*m*me,

1 **of**] a *blank space has been left follow. by* of 2 **þe emeroides**] *corr. from* þeemeroides 14 **For**] *corr. from* ffor 16 **purge**] *prec. by heading* Sekenesse 21 **myrabole**] *follow. by canc. twice* mde 24 **boþe**[1]] *corr. from* boþere (*er canc.*)

15 **whiþholdynge**] *in r.-h. margin:* medicyn*e* | for w*ith*hol | dy*n*g

and of piliole, *and* of euforbe, *and* of comyn, *and* of siler*e* mou*n*tayn, j-poudred *and* j-soden in wyn in a stopped vessel. And lat þe fume here-of come þorou a pipe to þe emeroides. *And* þe same dai late hym be cupped on þe reynes. And late hy*m* vsen diacalamentu*m* oþ*er* diat*ri*onpip*er*ion. And eu*er*y dai þe morwetid lat hym drynk warm wyn þ*at* pep*er* haþ be soden i*n*ne, *and* on euentide also. Oþ*er* make hym a fumigacion of moylen, *and* calamy*n*te, *and* wermot, *and* euforbe j-soden in liȝe *and* pep*er* þ*er*-wiþ. Oþ*er* vp-on an hoot querne cast wyn *and* let þe smoke þ*er*of come to his ers þorow a pipe. Oþ*er* make a plastre of figes, *and* strawe þe plastre w*ith* poudre of calamynte *and* of siler mou*n*tayne, *and* lei þ*er*-to. *And* a-boue lei a lynnen clowt j-wet in þe gleire of eiren. *And* lat it ligge þ*er*-to til it be driȝe, *and* þa*n* drawe it violently a-wei. Oþ*er* tac þe roote of a softe *and* p*ri*cke it al a-bowt w*ith* þe poynt of þi knyffe. *And* do it in wyn þe poudre of pep*er*, *and* of comyn, *and* a litel scamone. *And* al a nyȝt lei þ*at* roote in þ*at* wyn *and* siþe lei it to þe f. 167r emeroides. Oþ*er* ȝif hym smal lymaile of | yren in electuaries *and* þ*at* wole open hem. Also wha*n* þei swellen, wheþ*er* þei aken or naut aken, make a stufe of whiȝt wyn þ*at* hoot herb*e* ben j-soden i*n*ne, as wermot, *and* piliole, *and* rwe, *and* sauge, calamynte, *and* whiȝt horhowne. *And* late set þ*er* ou*er* his ers on a stool ful of hooles. Oþ*er* make hy*m* a plastre of p*er*it*er*ie j-stamped a litel *and* friȝed in his owne iuys. And w*ith* þese medicines, oþ*er* þei wull*e* driȝen vp oþ*er* þei wull*e* oppen. Oþ*er* tac þe poudre of bole, *and* of sau*n*dragou*n*, mastik, olibanu*m*, *and* medle hem w*ith* þe gleire of eiren. *And* lei it on a ly*n*nen clooþ *and* do þ*at* to þe emeroides. *And* let it

11 **figes**] *corr. from* ffiges 19 **yren**] *prec. by heading* in the ers
24 stool ful] *corr. from* stoolful

ligge þ*er* til it be dri3e *and* þa*n* pulle it sodeynly a-wei. *And* þe emeroides wole open 3if þei were late j-stopped. Oþ*er* make a plastre of whete, *and* of þe iuys of lappaciu*m* acutu*m*, oþ*er* of þe poudre of elebor*us* nig*er*, oþ*er* of spurge sed, oþ*er* of þe roote of jary j-clensed *and* j-put in a ma*n*n*es* ers makeþ þe veynes bleden. And 3if þe emeroides ben to-swolle of flewme, tac þe poudre of a blew lynnen clooþ j-brent, *and* of a got*es* hoorn j-brent, *and* psidie j-brent, *and* sp*ri*ng þe poudre on hem. But late hym furst waische*n* hem w*it*h his owne vrine. Oþ*er* bren a pyn-appel *and* sp*ri*ng þe poudre on hem. And make hym a fumigaciou*n* of calamynte, *and* origan, *and* laua*n*dere, *and* kalen-dula, *and* of salt-nitre j-soden in wat*er* *and* lat þe fume þ*er*-of come*n* in-to is ers. Oþ*er* seeþ leek *and* siþe stampe it w*it*h got*es* grece. *And* lei it on þe emoroides *and* it wole a-bate þe swalm of hem. But vnd*er*stonde wha*n* þu xal staunche þe flux of þe emeroides, þu | most leue oon or too open, oþ*er* ell*e* þe man my3te falle f. 167v
in-to a dropesie.

Figis ben whi3te bleynes *and* neisch*e* in a mann*es* ers. *And* oþ*er*while þei ben euen longe, *and* oþ*er*-while þei be round. Oþ*er*while þei ben w*it*h-i*n*ne þe ers, oþ*er*while þei be w*it*h-oute. 3if þei ben w*it*h-i*n*neforþ, tak a rauenh*us* herte *and* got*us* horn*es* *and* make poudre of hem. *And* late hy*m* vse þ*at* poudre boþe in met*es* *and* in drynkes. And make poudre of alym *and* of ook applen *and* sprynge on þe figis. Blake boiles in þe ers ben incurabil as su*m*men sen, but 3if þu wult

6 **þe emeroides**] *corr. from* þeemeroides 17 **most**] *prec. by heading* Sekenesse in the ers 19 **Figis**] *corr. from* ffigis 25 **figis**] *corr. from* ffigis

6 **to-swolle**] *in r.-h. margin:* medicyn if | þey be*n* of flew[me]

bynde hem faste w*ith* a sylken thred *and* late hem hongen tyl þei fallen a-wei. Postem*us* þ*at* bien in a mann*es* ers ben j-heelid w*ith* an oyneme*nt* j-mad of oile of rooses *and* of ceruse j-medlid to-gidere, oþ*er* of leed j-brent *and* litarge j-medlid w*ith* þe ȝelke of an ey. Brent leed is þ*us* j-maad: Melt leed in an erþen vessele *and* stere it w*ith* a grene haselen ȝerde. *And* it wole turne to blac poudre. And who þ*at* haþ sich*e* a posteme, ne inforsche he hym nat to schite. And bie he ware þ*at* he be nat costyf. *And* ȝif he be, make hys wombe neysch*e* w*ith* a mollificatif clistere. For cleuynge of þe ers þ*at* comeþ of hoote kene hum*ur*os, a-noi*n*te hym w*ith* þe oile of eyren, oþ*er* of rooses, oþ*er* w*ith* þe iuys of lilie roote, oþ*er* w*ith* freisch*e* bot*er*e, oþ*er* w*ith* lard j-medlid w*ith* bot*er*e, oþ*er* w*ith* oile of whete, oþ*er* w*ith* þe white of an ey. Laus c*r*eatoris amen.

9 he ware] *corr. from* heware **10 For**] *corr. from* ffor **14 þe white**] *prec. by* þe whiþ

5 Brent] *in l.-h. margin:* no*ta* ben*e*

Notes

39,2 humo*urs*] Mediaeval science, and especially medicine, was governed by the theory of the four humours and qualities, which had already appeared in the Hippocratic writings. The theory was finished by Aristotle, approved by Galen, and refined in mediaeval Jewish and Arab works. The four humours included *blood* (blood), *fleume* (phlegm), *colere* (yellow bile), and *malencolye* (black bile). The four qualities, *hoot* (hot), *coold* (cold), *drie* (dry), and *moyst* (wet), were applied to objects depending on either an extreme degree or on the dominance of one of them, 'when considered in relation either to the state of good proportion within the object's genus or to any other object of comparison' (Singer 1997: 266).

It was believed that the Universe was composed of the following four elements which, in turn, had different qualities (in brackets): fire (hot and dry), air (hot and wet), water (cold and wet), and earth (cold and dry). The humours were also present in the human body and, on the basis of their prevalence, a person could be *colryk* (choleric), *fleumatik* (phlegmatic), *malencolic* (melancholic), or *sanguyn* (sanguine); each type of individual had a different "complexion". A direct link was established between the Universe macrocosm and the human body microcosm. Good health was the result of reaching equilibrium amongst the four humours.

The influential *Secretum secretorum*, a mediaeval encyclopaedic treatise on a wide range of topics, ascribes the conservation of health to two main factors: 'First that a man vse convenient metes accordyng to his age, to the seson and tyme of the yere, and to the custume of his nature, that is to sey, that he vse such metes and drynkes with the which he hath be brought forth before, the which confermed his nature, þat is to say, that accordeth with his complexion. Secondly, that he be purged of all superfluous and corruptif humours.' (Manzalaoui 1977: 50).

The theory also leant on a set of analogies with the number four; they included, for instance, the ages of man: *chyldhood* (childhood), *ȝouþe* (youth), *manhood* (manhood), and *elde* (old age), or the seasons of the year: *ver* (spring), *somer* (summer), *heruest* (autumn), and *wynter* (winter).

39,3 body] The *Liber de diversis medicinis* divides the human body into three main "parties" and "membres": 'the hert, the lyu*er*, the harnes, and ilkane of thies hase his place whare he may put owt his sup*er*flueties and are called in phiseke emu*n*datoria eor*um*. The clensynge place of þe hert is vnder þe armes, the clensy*n*g place of þe lyu*er* is by-twix þe thee & þe body, and þe clensyng place of þe harnes es vnder þe ere & vndir þe throtte' (Ogden 1938: 51–52).

39,26 V*ersus*] This word introduces the Latin text. Amongst other meanings, a *verse* denotes a specific sentence or passage from a prose treatise.

41,15 Vnde] Another way of introducing the Latin passage.

43,27 wynt*er*] By synecdoche: year(s).

46,21 colo*ur*...signys] For the mediaeval physician, uroscopy was possibly the most basic of all skills. The practitioner could evaluate the state of the digestion of patients, which was the focal process to mediaeval physiology, by examining their urine. The practice of uroscopy did not involve touching the patient, and was readily shown by means of medical texts and coloured illustrations. The study of urine could also resolve dubiety about pregnancy and virginity (Getz 1990: 12).

The essential guide for analysis was the colour, texture, smell, and, occasionally, even taste of the urine. The results were then adapted to the humoural schema, and diagnosis and prognosis postulated upon variations of age, sex, and time of the patient's birth (Gottfried 1986: 177).

47,10 dietinges] The importance of diet was emphasised by Galen, who thought that if a cure could be achieved by means of dietary habits, the patient should refrain from pharmacological prescriptions. He developed the "thinning diet", an up-to-date and engaging description of a low-fat, low-calorie diet (Singer 1997: 305–324).

57,19 Jn…24 of[1]] The gynaecological material is not present in all the extant versions of the Middle English Gilbertus. In the case of *H509*, information for the treatment of sicknesses specific to women is dispersed throughout the text, although the complete treatise on diseases of women held in other manuscripts, such as *H307*, is missing.

Religion also exerted influence on obstetrics, illustrated for instance by the variety of material devices to invocate the help of safeguarding saints available. Women usually went on pilgrimages to shrines before giving birth in order to get metal badges, which then they wore. An example of this is provided by the Norfolk mystic Margery Kempe, who travelled to Cologne in 1433 to worship a piece of "owr Ladys smokke", thought to succour women in childbirth (she had had fourteen children by then). This type of objects represented powerful symbols of fertility in an age when inability to engender a healthy child brought discredit on women of all social classes (Rawcliffe 2004: 303).

57,26 bokys] Medical writings in Middle English medical prose can be categorised in a number of ways, each having its limitations. The next classification follows the one outlined by Voigts and McVaugh (1984: 19–24). Verse and prose represent the first distinction. Verse functions as a mnemonic aid, as it enables recalling the virtues of herbs, a list of bloodletting veins, or a dietary need. Works in prose are much more numerous; Robbins (1970: 395) classified them by subject matter: diagnosis, prognosis, and therapeutics. One of the problems posed by this categorisation has to do with works that may contain the three elements.

Medical texts can also be ranked on the basis of the intended audience: lay people, highly trained physicians or surgeons, and village healers. The limitation is that it is not always possible to establish for whom the book was planned.

Another possible sorting of Middle English prose medical texts is in terms of their origin: academic medicine or popular remedy-book. These would constitute the ends of a continuum, being possible for some text-types (uroscopic, for example) to take up an intermediate point. This approach may be closer than others to the mediaeval understanding of the texts. Remedy-books, which correspond to the older and broader category, mainly contain treatment for diseases or symptoms, deriving from works such as Macer's *De virtutibus herbarum* or the Salernitan *Antidotarium Nicolai*. The usual organisation is a *de capite ad pedem* structure. Several of these remedy-books have been edited by Ogden (1938), Dawson (1934), or Henslow (1972).

Academic medicine consists of English translations of learned Latin medicine whose original authors were ancient, Arabic writers, or mediaeval university masters. Amongst them are the surgeries of William of Saliceto, Roger of Salerno, Henry of Mondeville, Lanfranc, Guy de Chauliac, John Arderne, or Gilbertus Anglicus. It is within this category that *H509* could be included.

57,26 philosophie] This refers to natural philosophy, the mediaeval study of nature and the universe comprising both theoretical and experimental science.

58,16 But…20 good] Late mediaeval doctors had access to two different traditions of medical theory, training, and practice. One of them was classical (chiefly Greek) and derived from the works of Hippocrates and his school at Cos, and from Galen. Much of this Greek body of works did not reach Western Europe during the early Middle Ages, but found a flourishing way to the Islamic world, from where it re-entered the West in the twelfth century. By this time, Arabic authors had supplemented it with glosses and commentaries. Some of these authors, particularly Avicenna, Albucasis, and Rhazes, became authorities in their own right. The larger part of this Greek-based and Arabic-improved corpus was theoretical. Remedies were founded on the Greek humoural theory; changes in diet and the use of drugs were key elements for healing. These treatments were hardly effective given the imprecision of mediaeval pharmacy.

The second tradition stemmed from folk medicine, thus being more practical. It was especially strong in England and several reasons may account for this: England's remoteness, the relative non-existence of the classical tradition in mediaeval English culture, and also the recommendation of Anglo-Saxon leeches that they should deal directly with their patients. Leeches, who used drugs and performed surgery as well, developed a less complete clinical tradition that functioned as an alternative to the Greek theoretical one. However, the Greek model overpowered much of the vernacular tradition, as it was adopted by English universities. But it did linger on amongst surgeons, barbers, and village leeches. Some English monasteries, mainly those of the Benedictines, also kept to it (Gottfried 1986: 7–8).

Both traditions seem to be present in the text of *H509*: the author refers to both "bokys of philosophie", which would cover a theoretical framework, and to "þe leche", which would represent a more empirical practice of medicine.

59,3 he[2]...8 wylle] One of the recurrent hallmarks of mediaeval medicine is the strong connection to religion, which had an impact on the practice of medicine. The life of patients and outcome of operations were thought to be decided by God, and not men. Thus references to God are common in mediaeval medical texts. The following instance is taken from the *Liber de diversis medicinis* (Ogden 1938: 54): 'thurgh þe grace of God he sal be helpede of þis sekenes'. In *H509*, there are several references to God (see f. 14r, f. 57r, or f. 97r, for example). Similar invocations are also common in GUL MS Hunter 503 and GUL MS Hunter 513.

Gottfried (1986: 10) remarks the important role that ecclesiastical authorities had in the universities, where physicians were trained. They also maintained supervising functions over the corporations of other types of practitioners, especially the confraternities (socio-religious societies set up within most guilds). Furthermore, Christian tenets impinged upon the philosophy of medicine. The fact that the soul was considered more important than the body was related to what could be taught, preventing the advancement of medical specialities like anatomy and physiology in the universities.

Slack (1979: 254) notes that 'the clergy's contribution to the literature was particularly large. The study of medicine had flourished among members of religious orders in the Middle Ages, and it is not surprising to find among the most successful authors of the early sixteenth century, Thomas Moulton, a Dominican, Andrew Boorde, once a Carthusian, and Paynel, once an Austin friar'.

60,23 haþ] Reading taken from *H307*.

63,12 me*n*strua] *De secretis mulierum*, which had been falsely ascribed to Albertus Magnus, establishes the inception of menstruation at the age of thirteen; most other mediaeval writers concede that the age for this was thirteen or fourteen (Bullough and Campbell 1980: 324). In the treatise on the diseases of women held in *H307*, the age is somewhat earlier: 'þey han suche purgaciou*n*s fro þe tyme off xij wynt*er* age in to þe age of fifty wy*n*ter; neþeles su*m* wy*m*men han it leng*er*' (ff. 149v–150r).

67,5 seeþ] Hieatt (1998: 138–139) remarks that there is still a great deal to be done in the study of mediaeval culinary vocabulary. Culinary terms are employed in *H509* for the making of recipes. Hieatt provides the example of the verb *sēthen* ('to seethe'), which may not have had strictly the same meaning as *boil* in early English, as in some contexts, it seems to mean *simmer*.

70,5 browes] The word *bries* (*MED breu*) also appears in *H509*. As for *browes* (*MED brŏue*), this word has two meanings: the eyebrow and the eyelid; *bries* only refers to the eyebrow.

71,6 aloes] Trevisa (Seymour *et al.* 1975–1988: 905–907) makes a distinction between *aloes* ('a tree wiþ good smelle and bredeþ in Ynde') and *aloe* ('fruyt of a certein herbe þat hatte aloe [...]. Also of aloe is þre kynde, *citrinum*, *epaticum*, and *caballinum* [...]. And þese þre manere kyndes beþ dyvers in goodnesse, for *caballinum* is good, *epaticum* is bettre, and *citrinum* is best...'. In the text, the term employed throughout is *aloes*, although, in one instance at least, it refers to the herb: *aloes epatik*. However, other copies consulted of the Middle English Gilbertus also show *aloes*, suggesting that this was the term generally used. It is difficult to determine (when the term occurs without pre- or post-modification) if reference is made to the herb or the tree, as both of them had medicinal uses.

72,9 delices] The medicinal recipes against ailments and illnesses could be made in different ways depending on the wealth of the patient and on whether he or she could afford the ingredients (see also ff. 109r/v; f. 133r). Sometimes details of the constitution of the sick person were added to this (see f. 116v).

82,19 floures] This refers to the menstrual flow. The expression "women in their flowers" is found in the treatise *De passionibus mulierum*, attributed to Trotula, the famous midwife from Salerno. This is possibly the earliest and most well-known of the mediaeval gynaecological texts and it is customarily dated to the second half of the eleventh century (Bullough and Campbell 1980: 323). In it, the menstrual flow is believed to be responsible for regulation of the female temperament. Whereas in men the prevailing heat is kept under control by sweat, the immoderate moistness in women is purged by 'the menses that are commonly called flowers, for, just as trees do not bear fruit without flowers, likewise women without flowers are unable to fulfil their function of conception' (Jacquart and Thomasset 1988: 71). The same idea is expressed in *H307*: 'We schulen vndirstonde þat wy*m*me*n* han lesse hete in her body þan men *and* more moistnesse for defaute of hete þat schulde drye her humours and her moistnesse. But neþeles, kynde haþ ordeyned wy*m*men a purgaciou*n* at certeyn tymes of bledyng to make her bodyes cleene and hool fro siknesse' (f. 149v).

166,8 basilica] Large vein of the arm initiating from the elbow and discharging into the axillary vein. It has received this name from its presumed great importance; the right and left basilic veins were formerly thought to be in direct communication with the liver and the spleen respectively (*OED*).

185,18 feuere etik] A continuous or recurring, wasting fever (said to result from ulcers, the "stone", faulty diet, emotional disturbances, etc., but especially associated with tuberculosis) (*MED*).

190,20 fisycyens] Galen stated that 'the learned physician was the best of all possible advisors on any subject, the optimal counselor, who could dispense savoir-faire on both the health of the soul and of its companion on this earth, the body. The marks of the good advisor were his dignity, his gravity, and his independent income. In short, he was a gentleman and a philanthropist, uninterested in material gain and devoted to a life of leisure and contemplation' (Getz 1990: 14).

Physicians represented the social and, to some degree, professional elite amongst doctors, whereas surgeons carried the stigma of being craftsmen, which implied the idea that they were less proficient than physicians. Physicians were university-trained, surgeons were not. Universities emphasised the difference between the *medicus* (the artisan or craftsman) and the *magister medicinae* (the scholarly physician).

200,1 suffocacyou*n*...mode*r*] From *suffocatio* (or *prefocatio*) *matricis*, a Latin translation of an expression found in Greek and Arabic. It is explained by the Hippocratic idea of a uterine displacement, in which the womb was linked with the upper parts of the body (Jacquart and Thomasset 1988: 173–177).

203,28 a[1]...lytil[2]] This is not a mistake of duplication by the scribe of *H509* because the same expression is used in other copies (*H307*; MS Wellcome 537).

206,11 blody fluxe] Term used for stomach ailments, often applied specifically to intestinal dysentery. The following remedy is offered in a fifteenth-century English version of *Materia medica*, a collection of tracts and recipes on various subjects that was a common text for doctors: 'For the bloody flux. Take yarrow and waybread and stamp them in a mortar, and take the juice of them and fair flour of wheat and temper them together and make a cake and bake it in ashes and make the sick to eat it as hot as he may suffer it. *Probatum est.*' (Dawson 1934: 46).

218,1 calami*n*te] There are a number of possibilities concerning the meaning of this word, as supplied by the *MED*. First, it can refer to *calamīn* (an ore of zinc, cadmia, calamine; most likely, both zinc carbonate and the hydrous silicate of zinc). It can make reference to *calaminte* as well, a member of the genus *Calamintha*, chiefly the common calamint (*C. officinalis*) or the round-leaved mint (*Mentha rotundifolia*). The term *calaminte* is also used to denote a resin from the storax tree (*Styrax officinalis*), a kind of storax.

243,21 Tak…acacie] Reading taken from *H307*.

324,24 beste] Reading taken from *H307*.

Glossary

The objective of this glossary is to be a complement and aid for a better understanding of the edited text and to supply all the different spellings and forms of content words, which may be of dialectal and/or lexical interest. Therefore, it gathers all major words used in the text, namely nouns, adjectives, verbs, and adverbs. Due to the multiple spellings of a single word, the entry found in the *MED* has been adopted for the headword;[10] a number between brackets refers to the specific entry, with a different sense, collected in that dictionary. When two or more parts of speech are possible for the same headword, they have been grouped under the same heading if they have a related meaning; otherwise, they have been arranged in different entries. Headwords are printed in bold type, as well as terms or phrases within entries, in which the headword is indicated by a swung dash (~). The order of entries is alphabetical with *þ* placed after *th* and *ȝ* after *y*.[11]

Headwords not found in the *MED* are signalled with "ø", in such cases either the most frequently occurring form in the text has been

10 Sometimes the terms provided as entries in this glossary appear as sub-entries in the *MED*. Such is the case, for instance, of *oxe(s eie*, which is recorded under *oxe*. With compounds, on several occasions, the first element is a main entry in the dictionary, whereas the second is a sub-entry, such as *dīacitōnicon* (prefix *dīa* + *citōnicon*).

11 With hyphens or blank spaces between two elements of the same headword, the ordering adopted follows the convention of the *MED*, where those elements are not taken into account for alphabetical arrangement (for example, **al togeder** appears after *alteratīf* and not after *ākorn* in the glossary); the same applies to word occurrences.

selected or the reconstruction with a likely form is rendered; those marked with an asterisk ("*"), not included in the *MED* either, are taken from Getz (1991). The entry is followed by the corresponding part of speech, which is italicised. In some entries, information about the particular lexical field of the term is provided (MED., ZOOL., SURG., etc.); this normally follows the *MED*. Then the translation (modern equivalent or cognate) is offered; when the word is polysemous, the different meanings that it can have in the text are supplied.[12] The *MED* and the *OED* have been taken as the main references for this purpose. If the term exists in Present-Day English but it is an obsolete one, a synonym is provided on most occasions. In addition, when the term is not clear or has changed its meaning with regard to Present-Day English, a brief definition is supplied. For botanical terms, the equivalent is given first and then, where possible, their genus, species, and botanical family are included.[13] A question mark (?) preceding an equivalent or definition means that it is not totally clear. The last type of information furnished in the entries consists of the different spellings or forms of a lemma (word tokens), which are followed by the number of occurrences in decreasing order of frequency (and alphabetically when they have the same frequency). Emendations in word tokens are marked by square brackets, following the method used in the edited text.

12 The exception are botanical terms since most of them can make reference to the plant or tree, as well as to its flower, fruit, seed, etc. Instances of this are *cardamome*, which can denote the spice or the plant, *carewei*, a term used both for the plant and for its fruit or seed, or *ellebre*, which can be employed to mean the plant and its root.

13 The resource consulted for the purpose has been the *USDA PLANTS Database* (available at <http://plants.usda.gov/java/>, as it provides standardised and modern bibliographic information about plant names.

A

abāten *v.* to abate
a-bate (5×), *a-baten* (3×), *a-batyd* (2×), *a-batyn* (2×), *abate* (1×), *abateþ* (1×), *a-batid* (1×)
abāting *ng.* abating
a-batyng (1×)
abhomināble *adj.* abominable
abhomynabil (1×)
abhominăciŏun *n.* loathing, nausea
abhominacioun (5×), *abhominacion* (2×)
abīden *v.* to abide
a-bideþ (4×), *a-byde* (3×), *a-bide* (1×), *a-bidynge* (1×)
āble *adj.* able
able (1×)
abŏundaunce *n.* abundance
habundaunce (8×)
abŏundaunt *adj.* abundant
habundaunt (6×)
abŏute(n *adv.* about
a-bowte (8×), *a-boute* (7×), *a-bowt* (2×), *abowte* (1×), *a-bowten* (1×), *a-bowtyn* (1×)
abŏve(n *adv.* above
a-boue (20×), *a-bouen* (2×), *a-bouyn* (1×), *a-bove* (1×)
abrōd(e *adv.* *(1)* out
a-brood (4×), *a-broode* (1×)
absteinen *v.* to abstain
absteyne (7×), *abstene* (2×), *absteine* (1×), *absteyn* (1×)
abstinence *n.* abstinence
abstinence (5×)
acācia *n.* acacia: (a) genus *Mimosa*, fam. *Fabaceae*; (b) MED. gum made from the juice of green plums or sloes
acacie (12×), *acacia* (2×), *acasie* (2×), *[acacie]* (1×), *accacie* (1×)
acces(se *n.* attack, seizure of any disease
accesse (13×)
accōrd *n.* accord
a-cord (1×)
accōrden *v.* to accord
a-corden (6×), *a-cordyng* (4×), *a-cordeþ* (3×), *acorden* (1×), *a-cordyn* (1×), *a-cordynge* (1×)
āche *n.* *(1)* ache
ache (172×), *ac[h]e* (1×), *aches* (1×), *atche* (1×)
acōld *adj.* cold
acoold (1×)
acorus *n.* sweet flag (*Acorus calamus*, fam. *Acoraceae*)
accorun (1×), *acorus* (1×)
adai *adv.* by day
a-dai (3×), *a-day* (3×), *aday* (1×)
adama(u)nt *n.* diamond
audemaunt (1×)
adden *v.* to add
adde (1×)
***adiantos** *n.* adiantum, maidenhair fern (*Adiantum capillus-veneris*, fam. *Pteridaceae*)
adianthos (1×), *adyanthos* (1×)
adŏun *adv.* downwards
a-down (10×), *a-doun* (7×)
affodil *n.* ramson (*Allium ursinum*, fam. *Liliaceae*)
affodille (5×)
affōrcen *v.* to force

a-forcen (1×), *afor-se* (1×), *a-forseþ* (1×), *aforseþ* (1×), *a-forsyng* (1×)
affōrcing *ng.* effort
a-forsyng (1×), *a-for-synge* (1×)
affraien *v. (1)* to disturb
a-ferd (1×), *a-fraiȝen* (1×)
Affricān *n.* African
affr[i]cane (1×)
afōr(e *adv.* before
a-fore (2×)
afōr(e-seid *ppl.* aforesaid
adj.: *a-for-seid* (2×), *a-fore-seyd* (1×), *a-for-seyd* (1×); *adv.*: *a-for-seyd* (1×)
afōrn-seid *ppl.* aforesaid
a-forn-seid (1×)
after *adv.* after
after (13×), *aftur* (10×)
after-ward *adv.* afterwards
afterward (32×), *afturward* (13×), *after-ward* (3×), *afterwarde* (1×), *aftyr-ward* (1×)
agarik(e *n.* agaric (*Polyporus officinalis*, fam. *Polyporaceae*)
agarik (5×), *agaric* (1×), *agarice* (1×), *agar[ike]* (1×), *agaryk* (1×)
agasten *v.* (*ppl.*) **agast**, aghast
a-gast (1×)
āğe *n.* age
age (11×), *ages* (3×)
agnus castus *n.* agnus castus (*Vitex agnus-castus*, fam. *Verbenaceae*)
agnus castus (1×)
agrest *n.* uncultivated, wild plant
agresta (1×)
***agrippa** *n.* kind of ointment
agrippa (1×)
agū(e *adj.* acute (fever)
ague (1×), *agues* (1×)

air *n. (1)* air
eire (5×), *eyr* (4×), *eir* (2×), *eiȝyr* (1×), *eyre* (1×)
akēlen *v.* to cool off
a-kelen (1×), *akelyn* (1×)
āken *v.* to ache
akeþ (13×), *aken* (4×), *ake* (2×)
āking *ng.* & *ag.* aching
ng.: *akyng* (4×), *akynge* (3×), *akyngge* (2×), *a[k]inge* (1×); *ag.*: *akynge* (1×)
ākorn *n.* acorn
akren (3×), *akrene* (1×)
āle *n.* ale, beer
ale (6×)
Alexandrīn *adj.*[14] Alexandrian
alexandrinum (1×)
alfīta *n.* barley meal
alfice (1×)
al-gāte(s *adv.* always
algatis (2×), *algate* (1×), *algatys* (1×)
alīche *adv.* alike
a-leche (1×), *a-lyche* (1×)
***alipiados** *n.* [see **laurel**]
alipiades (1×)
alma(u)nde *n.* almond (*Amygdalus communis*, fam. *Rosaceae*)
alemaundes (10×), *almaund* (4×), *alemaund* (2×), *alemaundys* (2×), *alemandis* (1×), *alemaunde* (1×), *alemaundis* (1×), *alemaunt* (1×), *allemaund* (1×)
alōe(s *n.* aloe (fam. *Aloaceae*)
aloes (41×), *alloes* (1×), *alooes* (1×)
~ **ci(co)trinum**
aloes cicatryn (1×)
~ **epatīk**, opaque, liver-coloured

14 Only recorded as a noun in the *MED*.

form of Socotrine aloes
aloes epatik (1×)
al-ōnelī *adv.* solely
aloonly (1×)
alōng *adv.* along
a-long (1×), *a-loong* (1×)
alsō *adv.* also
also (246×), *al-so* (15×)
alteratīf *n.* alterative medicine (promoting alteration in quality: hot-cold, moist-dry)
alteratyfs (1×)
al togeder *adv.* completely; *phr.* all together
adv.: alto-gedere (1×); *phr.: al to-gidere* (3×), *al to-gedere* (1×)
alūm *n.* alum
alym (5×)
al-wei *adv.* always
alway (1×), *alwei* (1×)
ambrōse *n.* ambrose, wild sage, wood germander (*Teucrium scorodonia*, fam. *Lamiaceae*)
ambrose (1×)
amēnden *v.* to cure
a-mendid (1×)
ameos *n.* bishop's weed (*Ammi majus*, fam. *Apiaceae*)
ameos (15×)
amidŏun *n.* crushed hulled wheat
amyde (28×), *amide* (3×)
amōmum *n.* amomum (any of a variety of aromatic plants of the *Zingiberaceae* fam.)
amonie (4×), *a-mome* (1×), *amome* (1×), *amonye* (1×)
amorwe(n *adv.* in the morning
a-morwe (5×), *a-morewe* (1×), *amorowen* (1×), *amorwe* (1×)
ampte *n.* ZOOL. ant
empte (1×)
anacardus *n.* marking nut (*Semecarpus anacardium*, fam. *Anacardiaceae*)
anacardy (1×)
analempsie *n.* form of epilepsy
analempsie (5×), *analempcie* (1×)
anclē *n.* ankle
ancle (22×)
anēt(e *n.* dill (*Anethum graveolens*, fam. *Apiaceae*)
anet (15×), *anete* (2×)
angel-twacche *n.* ZOOL. earthworm
angel-twaches (1×), *angeltwaches* (1×)
anger *n.* anger
angur (2×), *anger* (1×)
angrī *adj.* angry
angry (2×)
angwisshe *n.* anguish
angwische (1×)
anientishen *v.* to weaken
anentesep (1×)
anight(es *adv.* by night
a-nyȝt (4×), *a-niȝth* (2×), *a-niȝt* (1×), *a-nytȝ* (1×), *a-nyȝth* (1×)
anīs *n.* anise (*Pimpinella anisum*, fam. *Apiaceae*)
anyse (37×), *anise* (4×), *anis* (1×), *anysy* (1×)
an-ōn *adv.* at once
a-noon (8×), *a-non* (1×)
answēre *n.* answer
answere (1×)
answēren *v.* to answer
answere (1×)

***ant(h)os** *n.* [see **rōs-marīn(e**]
anthos (2×), *anthes* (1×)
antimōnie *n.* MED. & ALCH. antimony
antymonye (4×), *amtymonye* (1×), *antemonye* (1×), *antimonye* (1×), *antymonie* (1×)
apeiren *v.* to make worse
apeiriþ (2×), *apeired* (1×), *a-peireþ* (1×), *a-peirid* (1×), *a-peyr* (1×), *appeirid* (1×)
apeiringe *ng.* worsening
a-peiryng (1×)
***apium ranarum** *n.* celery-leafed crowfoot (*Ranunculus sceleratus*, fam. *Ranunculaceae*)
apium ranarum (1×)
apoplexie *n.* apoplexy
apoplexie (9×), *appoplexie* (2×), *a-poplexie* (1×), *apoplexis* (1×)
apostēm(e *n.* abscess
posteme (66×), *postym* (56×), *postemus* (18×), *postemys* (8×), *aposteme* (6×), *postem* (5×), *postemes* (5×), *apostym* (4×), *apostem* (1×), *p[o]steme* (1×), *postim* (1×), *postteme* (1×), *postymus* (1×)
apostolicon *n.* antiseptic ointment
apostolicon (1×)
appel *n.* (a) apple (*Pyrus malus*, fam. *Rosaceae*); (b) ANAT. & MED. **~ of the eie**, eyeball
appel (6×), *applen* (4×), *applys* (3×)
ap(p)etīt *n.* appetite
appetit (16×), *appetyt* (4×), *appetite* (1×), *appetitys* (1×)
apprōpren *v.* to be appropriate
appropred (1×)

aquila *n.* type of chemical
aquilleie (1×)
Arabī *n.* Arabia [see also **gŏmme**]
arabye (1×)
arāğe *n.* orache (genus *Atriplex*, fam. *Chenopodiaceae*)
arage (10×)
arēchen *v.* *(2)* to retch
arecheþ (1×)
argālia *n.* urethral catheter
enargale (4×)
arīsen *v.* to arise
a-riseþ (1×), *a-ryse* (1×), *aryssen* (1×), *a-ryst* (1×)
aristologīe *n.* plant of the *Aristolochiaceae* fam.; **~ rōtŏunde, ~ (the) rŏund(e**, round-leaved birthwort (*Aristolochia rotunda*); **~ (the) lōng**, elongated
aristologia rotunda (2×), *aristologia þe rounde* (1×), *aristo[logie] long, þe round* (1×), *aristologie longe, þe rounde* (1×), *aristologie rounde* (1×), *aristologie þe longe, þe rounde* (1×), *aristol[ogie] þe rounde* (1×), *aristologie þe rounde* (1×)
arm *n.* arm
arme (16×), *arm* (4×), *armes* (3×)
armoniak *n.* ammonia
ammoniac (10×), *armoniac* (2×), *ammoniak* (1×), *amonia[c]* (1×), *armoniace* (1×), *armoniak* (1×)
arm-pit *n.* armpit
arm-pittys (1×)
aromatik *adj.* aromatic
aromatik (2×), *aroma[ti]c* (1×), *aromatyk* (1×)
āron *n.* cuckoo-pint or wake-robin

(*Arum maculatum*, fam. *Araceae*)
aaron (1×)
arraien *v.* to arrange
araie (1×)
***arrogon** *n.* kind of ointment
arrogon (2×)
ărs *n.* anus
ers (40×)
arwe *adj.*[15] threatening
arw (1×)
ashāmen *v.* to feel shame
a-schamyd (1×)
asīde *adv.* aside
a-syde (2×)
asken *v.* to ask
askeþ (1×), *axeþ* (1×)
aslant(e *adv.* at an angle
a-slont (1×)
asp(h)alt *n.* native asphalt
aspalte (1×)
asse *n.* ZOOL. ass
asse (8×)
assh(e *n. (1)* European ash (*Fraxinus excelsior*, fam. *Oleaceae*)
aische (2×), *aischen* (2×), *aisches* (2×), *aisch* (1×), *ase* (1×)
asshe *n. (2)* ashes
axen (7×), *askys* (3×), *askes* (2×), *axes* (2×), *askyn* (1×), *axene* (1×), *haschen* (1×)
as(s)wāğen *v.* to alleviate
a-swage (2×), *a-swagen* (1×), *a-swageþ* (1×), *a-swagyn* (1×)
astŏned *adj.* stunned
a-stoined (1×), *a-stoneid* (1×), *stoneied* (1×)

15 Only recorded as a noun in the *MED*.

astŏnen *v.* to stun
a-stoneyen (1×)
astrologīe *n.* [see **aristologīe**]
astrologie þe longe, þe rounde (1×), *þe longe astrologe* (1×)
°**aswīth(e** *adv.* very much
a-swiþe (1×)
***athanasia** *n.* type of electuary
athanasia (4×), *athanasie* (1×)
athurst *adj.* thirsty
a-þurst (1×)
at ōnes *adv.* at once
at onys (3×), *at oones* (1×)
atrament *n.* (a) black pigment or ink; (b) vitriol
atrament (2×), *atrement* (1×)
atter-cop(pe *n.* ZOOL. spider
attircoppe (1×)
atwin(ne *adv.* apart
a-twynny (1×)
atwō *adv.* in two
a-two (2×)
aumbre *n.* (a) ambergris; (b) resin amber (fossil)
amber (1×), *[a]mber* (1×)
availen *v.* to avail
a-vayle (1×)
avence *n.* wood avens (*Geum urbanum*, fam. *Rosaceae*)
auence (8×), *auance* (4×), *auannce* (1×)
aventen *v.* (a) to release (winds); (b) to let blood
a-uentisid (1×)
°**Avicen** *n.* Avicenna
Auycen (1×)
awēden *v.* to become enraged
awhood (1×)

awei *adv.* away
a-wey (52×), *a-wei* (31×), *a-way* (3×), *a-wey* (2×), *awey* (2×)
awei-ward *adv.* away
a-weyward (2×)
ayēn *adv.* again
a-ȝen (9×), *a-ȝeen* (2×), *a-ȝeyn* (2×)
azarabacca(ra *n.* asarabacca, hazelwort (*Asarum Europaeum*, fam. *Aristolochiaceae*)
asarum (7×), *asari* (1×), *aȝarum* (1×)

B

bācīn *n.* basin
bacyn (4×), *basyn* (1×)
bagge *n. (1)* bag
bagge (16×), *bagges* (2×)
bagge-ful *n.* bagful
baggeful (1×)
bai(e *n.* bay (laurel) (*Laurus nobilis*, fam. *Lauraceae*)
baies (9×), *bayes* (1×) [see also **oil(e**]
bak *n.* back
bac (1×), *bakke* (1×)
bāken *v.* to bake
j-bake (1×), *j-baken* (1×)
bal *n.* (a) ball; (b) MED. pill
balles (9×), *bolles* (3×), *balle* (1×), *belles* (1×)
balaustia *n.* balausta (fruit of pomegranate)
balaustia (8×), *balaustie* (6×), *bala[u]stia* (1×), *balustia* (1×)
ballok-stōn *n.* testicle
ballokstoon[e]s (1×)
bār *adj.* bare
bare (2×)
barbŏur *n.* barber(-surgeon)
barbours (1×)
bār-fōt *adj.* barefoot
barfoote (1×)
barlī *n.* barley (genus *Hordeum*, fam. *Poaceae*)
barly (24×), *barliche* (16×), *barlyche* (10×)
basilic(a *n.* basilic vein
basilica (3×)
basilicon *n. (1)* basil (genus *Ocymum*, fam. *Lamiaceae*)
basilicon (3×)
bath *n.* bath
baaþ (27×), *baþ* (9×), *baþes* (3×), *baþe* (1×)
bāthen *v.* to bathe
baþe (8×), *baþen* (5×), *bathyn* (2×), *bathynge* (1×), *baþid* (1×), *baþin* (1×), *j-baþed* (1×)
bāthing *ng.* bath(ing)
baþinge (7×), *baþing* (1×)
baume *n.* (a) balm (*Melissa officinalis*, fam. *Lamiaceae*); (b) ointment containing balm
baume (7×), *bawme* (6×)
bēche *n.* European beech (*Fagus sylvatica*, fam. *Fagaceae*)
beche (2×), *beches* (1×)
bed *n. (1)* bed
bedde (8×), *bed* (2×), *beed* (1×)
bedegar *n.* bedeguar (gall or excrescence on a rosebush or eglantine)
bodegar (1×)

bedellium *n.* (a) tree of the genus *Commiphora*; (b) gum resin of such trees
bedellie (2×), *bdellium* (1×), *bedellium* (1×), *bodellie* (1×)
bēf *n.* beef (meat)
beef (2×)
bēing *ng.* existence
beynge (2×)
belle *n. (1)* bell
belle (1×), *bellies* (1×)
belle *n. (3)* opium poppy (*Papaver somniferum*, fam. *Papaveraceae*)
belle (1×)
ᵒ**bellerici emblici** *n.* type of myrobalan
bellere emblici (1×), *be[llere] emblici* (1×), *bellerici emblici* (1×)
bēm *n.* beam
beemes (1×)
bēn *v.* to be
is (1769×), *bien* (482×), *bie* (476×), *be* (348×), *ben* (314×), *was* (71×), *were* (41×), *js* (27×), *by* (6×), *been* (5×), *bi* (5×), *weren* (4×), *weryn* (4×), *[ben]* (3×), *[is]* (3×), *werun* (3×), *arn* (2×), *bee* (2×), *bye* (2×), *byn* (2×), *wore* (2×), *bein* (1×), *beyn* (1×), *beynge* (1×), *i[s]* (1×), *ys* (1×)
bēn(e *n. (1)* bean (*Vicia faba*, fam. *Fabaceae*)
beene (7×), *beenes* (6×), *beenen* (5×), *beenys* (4×), *benys* (3×), *been* (2×), *bene* (2×), *benen* (1×), *bienen* (1×)
berberie *n.* European barberry (*Berberis vulgaris*, fam. *Berberidaceae*)
berbere (1×)
bērd *n. (1)* beard
beerd (1×)
***berdane** *n.* great burdock (*Arctium lappa*, fam. *Asteraceae*)
berdane (2×)
bēren *v. (1)* to bear
bere (2×), *beryng* (2×), *beere* (1×), *bore* (1×), *j-bore* (1×)
bēring *ng.* bearing
berynge (1×)
ᵒ**berule** *n.* water parsnip (*Berula erecta*, fam. *Apiaceae*)
berule (1×)
best *adj. sup.* best
best (10×), *beste* (4×), *beest* (1×), *[best]* (1×)
bēst(e *n.* beast
beest (4×), *beste* (2×), *beestis* (1×), *best* (1×), *bestes* (1×)
bēte *n. (1)* red beet (*Beta vulgaris*, fam. *Chenopodiaceae*), white beet (*B. cicla*, fam. *C.*)
beetes (10×), *betes* (5×), *beetis* (3×), *betys* (2×), *b[e]etis* (1×), *betis* (1×), *bietes* (1×)
betein(e *n.* betony (*Betonica officinalis*, fam. *Lamiaceae*)
beteyne (4×), *betoyne* (3×), *beteynn* (1×)
bēting *ng. (1)* & *ag. (1)* beating
ng.: betyng (1×); *ag.: betyng* (1×)
bettre *n.*, *adj.*, & *adv.* better
n.: betere (1×); *adj.: betere* (7×), *beter* (6×), *betyr* (3×), *bettere* (1×); *adv.: betere* (3×), *beter* (1×)
bicche *n.* ZOOL. female of dog, bitch
biche (1×)
bicǒmen *v.* to become

be-come (1×), *bicomeþ* (1×)

bīden *v.* to remain
bideþ (1×)

bifallen *v.* to come about
be-falleþ (1×)

bifōre(n *adv.* before
bi-fore (18×), *be-fore* (13×), *bie-fore* (10×), *by-fore* (8×), *before* (4×), *bifore* (2×), *be-for* (1×)

bifōre(n-said *adv.* beforesaid
bi-fore-seid (1×), *byforeseyd* (1×)

biginnen *v.* to begin
be-gyn (2×), *begynne* (2×), *begynnyth* (2×), *bi-gynnyth* (2×), *be-gynne* (1×), *begynneþ* (1×), *be-gynnythe* (1×), *biegynne* (1×), *bygynne* (1×)

biginning(e *ng.* beginning
begynnyng (11×), *be-gynnyng* (3×), *bygynnyng* (2×), *be-gynning* (1×), *be-gynnynge* (1×), *bi-gynnyng* (1×), *bigynnyng* (1×), *by-gynnynge* (1×)

bihīnde-fōrth *adv.* from behind
be-hynde-foorþ (1×), *byhynde-forþe* (1×)

bihīnde(n *adv.* behind
be-hynde (4×), *by-hynde* (2×), *bi-hynde* (1×)

bihōven *v.* to behove; **(it) bihoveth**, it is necessary
be-houeþ (7×), *behoueþ* (2×), *bihoueþ* (2×), *behoued* (1×), *bie-houeþ* (1×), *byhoueþ* (1×)

bīl(e *n. (2)* (a) festering sore; (b) swelling
buyles (2×), *boiles* (1×), *buyle* (1×), *bylys* (1×)

bīnden *v.* to bind
bynd (3×), *bynde* (2×), *byndeþ* (1×), *byndyn* (1×)

binding(e *ng.* binding
byndynge (1×)

binēth(e-fōrth *adv.* lower down
by-neþeforþ (2×), *be-neþe-foorthe* (1×), *be-neþe-forþ* (1×), *byneþe-forþ* (1×), *by-neþe-forþe* (1×), *by-neþeforþe* (1×)

binēthe(n *adv.* beneath
by-neþe (7×), *byneþe* (3×), *be-neþe* (2×), *be-neþen* (2×), *by-neþen* (2×), *byneþen* (2×), *beneþes* (1×), *bie-neþe* (1×), *bineþe* (1×)

binimen *v.* to take away
be-nemeþ (2×), *by-nemeþ* (1×)

binŏmen *v.* to dull
by-[n]o[m]en (1×)

bipissen *v.* to urinate
be-pessen (2×), *be-pissen* (1×), *be-pyssed* (1×)

birch(e *n.* (a) European birch (*Betula alba*, fam. *Betulaceae*); (b) mastic tree (*Pistacia lentiscus*, fam. *Anacardiaceae*)
birch (1×), *birche* (1×), *briches* (1×)

birthen *n.* burden
burdenys (1×)

bisīnesse *n.* business
bysynesse (1×)

bis-malwe *n.* marsh mallow (*Althaea officinalis*, fam. *Malvaceae*)
bismalue (3×), *bismalues* (1×)

bīten *v. (1)* to bite
biten (2×), *bitiþ* (1×), *j-bete* (1×), *j-byte* (1×)

bitēn *v. (2)* to tug or pull at (sth.)
bieten (1×)

bī-tīme *adv.* on time
be-tyme (1×), *be-tymes* (1×), *by-tymes*

(1×)

bīting *ng.* biting; *ag.* sharp
ng.: bityng (1×); *ag.: bytynge* (3×), *bytyng* (2×), *bitinge* (1×), *bitynge* (1×), *bytinge* (1×)

bitōknen *v.* to be a symptom of sth.
be-tokeneþ (5×), *be-tokneþ* (2×), *betokneþ* (1×), *be-tokyn* (1×), *be-tokynneþ* (1×), *be-tokynth* (1×), *bie-tokeneþ* (1×), *bitoknyng* (1×)

bitter *adj.* bitter
bitter (10×), *bittere* (10×), *bytter* (7×), *bitere* (2×), *bittyr* (1×), *bitur* (1×), *byttere* (1×)

bit(t)erhēde *n.* bitterness
bytturhed (1×)

bit(t)ernesse *n.* bitterness
bitternesse (6×), *bytternesse* (1×)

bitwēne *adv.* in between
be-twyn (1×), *bi-twene* (1×), *by-twynne* (1×)

bladdre *n.* (a) bladder; (b) blister
bladdere (55×), *bleddere* (6×), *bladdare* (2×), *bladder* (2×), *bleddre* (2×), *bladdre* (1×), *bladdres* (1×), *bladdris* (1×), *bledder* (1×)

ᵒ**bladdrī** *adj.* unsubstantial
bladdry (1×)

ᵒ**bladdrish** *adj.* unsubstantial
bladdrische (2×)

blāk *adj.* black
blac (32×), *blak* (20×), *blake* (10×)

blākish *adj.* blackish
blackysche (3×)

blāknes(se *n.* blackness
blacnesse (5×), *blaknesse* (1×)

blaunchen *v.* to remove the hull (of almonds, etc.) after soaking in hot water
blaunched (1×), *blaunchid* (1×), *j-blaunched* (1×)

blaunk *adj.* white
blank (1×)

blēden *v.* to bleed
blood (31×), *blede* (24×), *bleden* (8×), *bledyn* (3×), *bloode* (2×), *bledeþ* (1×), *bledin* (1×), *bleede* (1×), *bleediþ* (1×)

blēdinge *ng.* bleeding
bledyng (9×), *bledinge* (4×), *bledynge* (3×), *bleding* (2×)

blein(e *n.* inflammatory swelling; blain
bleynes (3×), *bleynys* (2×), *bleyne* (1×), *bleynis* (1×), *bleynnys* (1×)

blēre-eied *adj.* bleary-eyed
blere-eiȝed (2×)

blēren *v.* *(1)* to have watery or rheumy eyes
blereid (2×), *blered* (1×), *blerid* (1×)

ᵒ**blēreshipe** *n.* bleariness
blereschipe (1×)

bleu *adj.* blue
blew (2×), *blw* (1×)

blite *n.* herb; garden beet
bletes (2×), *blites* (2×)

blōd *n.* *(1)* blood
blood (302×), *blod* (2×), *bloode* (2×), *bleed* (1×), *blode* (1×)

ᵒ**blōdful** *adj.* full of blood
blodful (1×)

blōdī *adj.* bloody
blodi (2×)
~ **flux**, dysentery
blodi flux (4×), *blody fluxe* (1×)

blōd-lēting(e *ng.* bloodletting

blood-letyng (2×), *blood-latyng* (1×), *blood-latynges* (1×), *blood-letinge* (1×), *blood-letynge* (1×), *blood-letyngus* (1×)

blosme *n.* blossom

blosmes (2×), *blosteme* (1×), *blostme* (1×), *blostmes* (1×)

blouen *v. (1)* to blow

blowe (1×), *bloweþ* (1×), *blowith* (1×), *blowyng* (1×)

blouing *ng. (1)* blowing

blowyng (1×)

bocche *n.* swelling

boche (4×), *bochches* (1×), *botche* (1×), *bot[c]hys* (1×)

bōdī *n.* body

body (132×), *bodi* (11×), *bodys* (4×), *bodies* (1×)

bōdīlī(ch *adj.* physical

bodyly (2×)

boillen *v.* to boil

boile (2×), *boyle* (1×)

boistres *adj.* boisterous

boistres (1×), *boistrus* (1×), *bostuse* (1×)

boistrŏusnesse *n.* boisterousness

boistirnesse (1×)

bōk *n. (1)* book

bokys (2×)

bōle *n. (1)* ZOOL. bull

boles (8×), *bole* (2×), *bolys* (2×), *booles* (2×), *boole* (1×)

bōl(e *n. (3)* red astringent earth, Armenian bole

bole (33×), *boole* (1×)

~ armoniak

bole armoniac (2×), *boole arm[oniac]* (1×)

bolken *v.* to belch; to vomit

bolkeþ (3×), *bolken* (1×), *bolkyng* (1×)

bolking *ng.* belch(ing); vomiting

bolkyng (13×), *bolkynges* (3×), *balkynges* (1×), *bolkynge* (1×), *bolkyngys* (1×)

bōn *n. (1)* bone

bonys (4×), *boon* (2×), *bon* (1×), *boones* (1×)

bonair(e *adj.* gentle

bonere (1×)

bōr *n.* ZOOL. boar

beris (1×), *boor* (1×), *boores* (1×)

borāğe *n.* borage (*Borago officinalis*, fam. *Boraginaceae*)

borage (17×)

bōras *n.* borax

borace (3×), *berace* (1×), *boras* (1×)

bōrd *n.* board

boord (2×), *bord* (1×)

botme *n.* bottom

botme (5×)

bŏuen *v. (1)* to bow

bowen (1×), *boweþ* (1×), *bowyng* (1×)

bŏugh *n.* bough

bowes (2×), *bowe* (1×), *wowes* (1×)

box *n. (2)* box

box (1×)

braien *v. (2)* to crush

j-braied (1×)

brain *n.* brain

brayn (48×)

brākinge *ng. (2)* vomiting

brakyng (3×), *brakynge* (1×)

brān *n.* bran

bren (14×), *bryn* (10×), *bran* (2×), *breen* (1×), *brem* (1×)

bras *n.* brass

bras (4×)
brāsen *adj.* made of brass
brasen (2×)
braunch *n.* branch
braunches (4×), *braunche* (1×)
brēch *n.* surgical girdle
brech (1×)
brēch(e *n.* breaking; fracture
breche (16×), *briche* (1×), *bryche* (1×)
brēd *n. (1)* bread
breed (13×), *bred* (6×), *bried* (1×)
brēden *v. (3)* to develop
j-bred (1×)
breiding(e *ag.* upbraiding
braydyng (1×)
brēken *v.* to break
breke (14×), *brekeþ* (12×), *j-broke* (5×), *brekyn* (4×), *j-brokyn* (3×), *broken* (2×), *j-broken* (2×), *br[e]ke* (1×), *brekyng* (1×), *broke* (1×)
brēkinge *ng.* breaking
brekyng (3×), *brekynge* (3×)
brennen *v.* to burn
j-brent (44×), *bren* (9×), *brent* (6×), *brenne* (4×), *brend* (2×), *brennyng* (2×), *breen* (1×), *brende* (1×), *brenneþ* (1×), *bur[n]* (1×), *j-brend* (1×)
brenninge *ng.* & *ag.* burning
ng.: brennyng (10×), *brennynge* (1×); *ag.: brennyng* (7×), *brennynge* (3×)
brēr *n.* (a) prickly plant; (b) blackberry (*Rubus fruticosus*, fam. *Rosaceae*), dewberry (*R. caesius*, fam. *R.*)
breris (1×)
brēst *n. (1)* thorax, chest
breste (41×), *breest* (28×), *brest* (23×), *breeste* (3×)
brēst-bōn *n.* breastbone
brestbon (1×)
brēth *n. (1)* breath(ing)
breeþ (13×), *breþ* (8×)
brēthen *v. (1)* to breathe
breþen (2×), *breþinge* (2×), *breþeþ* (1×), *breþin* (1×), *j-brethid* (1×)
brēthinge *ng.* breathing
breþing (9×), *breþinge* (5×), *breþynge* (1×)
brid *n.* ZOOL. bird
briddes (3×), *birdys* (1×)
brīd(e *n. (1)* young woman
breidus (1×)
brid-līm *n.* birdlime
byrdlym (2×)
bright *adj.* bright
briȝt (2×)
brightnesse *n.* brightness
briȝtnesse (1×)
brim-stōn *n.* sulphur
brymston (2×), *brenston* (1×)
brīn *n.* eyebrows; eyelids
bries (10×), *briȝes* (2×)
bringen *v.* to bring
browt (3×), *browȝt* (2×), *brynge* (2×), *bryngeþ* (2×), *brengeþ* (1×), *bringe* (1×), *brouth* (1×), *brouȝt* (1×), *bryng* (1×), *j-browt* (1×), *j-browȝt* (1×)
brīonīe *n.* common bryony (*Bryonia dioica*, fam. *Cucurbitaceae*)
brionye (2×), *brionie* (1×), *bryonye* (1×)
brīsen *v.* to bruise
bresyd (1×), *brise* (1×), *bryse* (1×), *j-brisud* (1×)
brīsinge *ng.* bruising

bresynge (2×), *brysynge* (1×)
bristel *n.* bristle, stiff hair
brustles (1×)
brōd *adj.* broad
brede (1×), *brode* (1×), *broode* (1×)
broke-balloked *adj.* having scrotal hernia
broke-balloked (1×)
broth *n.* broth
broþ (2×), *brooþ* (1×), *broþes* (1×), *broþþes* (1×)
brŏue *n.* eyebrow; eyelid
browes (2×), *browys* (1×)
brŏun *adj.* brown
brown (3×)
brŏunish *adj.* brownish
brownysche (1×)
brŏunnes *n.* brownness
brownnesse (1×)
bukke *n.* ZOOL. (a) male goat; (b) male deer
bucke (1×), *buckes* (1×)
bulten *v.* *(1)* to sift
bulte (1×), *j-bulted* (1×)
burblen *v.* to bubble
burblyng (1×)
burnēt *n.* *(2)* great burnet (*Sanguisorba officinalis*, fam. *Rosaceae*), garden burnet (*Poterium sanguisorba*, fam. R.), common pimpernel (*Anagallis arvensis*, fam. *Primulaceae*)
burnet (3×)
burnishen *v.* to burnish
burnyschyd (1×)
°**bussok** *adj.* ?suffering from hernia
bussok (3×), *bossok* (1×)
buter(e *n.* butter
botere (28×), *boter* (2×), *botyr* (2×), *bootere* (1×), *boture* (1×)
buttok *n.* buttock
buttokes (1×), *buttokkes* (1×)

C

cacchen *v.* to catch
catche (4×), *j-cauȝt* (2×), *cauȝt* (1×)
cacching *ng.* catching
cachinge (1×), *cat[c]hing* (1×), *catchinge* (1×)
cāke *n.* cake
cakes (3×)
calamīn *n.* calamine
calamina (3×), *calamyna* (3×), *calamyne* (1×)
calaminte *n.* *(1)* member of the genus *Calamintha*, fam. *Lamiaceae*: common calamint (*C. officinalis*); round-leaved mint (*Mentha rotundifolia*)
calamynte (33×), *calamynt* (4×), *calaminte* (3×)
calamus aromaticus *n.* fragrant herb
calamus aromaticus (6×), *calame aromatik* (1×), *calamy aromat[ik]* (1×)
calcāne *n.* heel bone (os calcis)
calcance (1×)
calf *n.* *(1)* ZOOL. calf
calf (2×)
callen *v.* to call
callen (1×)
***camapiteos** *n.* ground pine (*Ajuga chamaepitys*, fam. *Lamiaceae*)
camapitheos (2×)

camedris *n.* common or wall germander (*Teucrium chamaedrys*, fam. *Lamiaceae*)
camedreos (6×)
camomille *n.* camomile (*Anthemis nobilis*, fam. *Asteraceae*)
camamille (4×), *camomille* (3×), *camomylle* (2×), *cammamille* (1×), *cammomille* (1×)
candel *n.* candle
candele (1×)
cāne *n.* sugar cane (*Saccharum officinarum*, fam. *Poaceae*)
cane (1×)
cānel *n. (1)* cinnamon (*Cinnamomum zeylanicum*, fam. *Lauraceae*)
canel (50×)
canicūlēr *adj.* dog days (from late July to early September)
caniculere (2×)
canker *n. (1)* cancer; ulcer
cancre (9×), *cancris* (2×), *cankre* (2×), *canker* (1×), *kankere* (1×)
cankren *v.* to become cancerous
j-cancrid (3×)
capar *n.* European caper (*Capparis spinosa*, fam. *Capparidaceae*)
caperis (2×), *capparis* (2×), *caparis* (1×), *caperus* (1×), *capparys* (1×), *cappery*s (1×)
capitel *n.* type of strong lye
capitelle (3×)
cāpŏun *n.* ZOOL. capon
capoun (4×), *caponys* (1×)
caprifoile *n.* European honeysuckle (*Lonicera periclymenum*, fam. *Caprifoliaceae*)
caprifolie (1×)

carabe *n.* fruit of carob tree (*Ceratonia siliqua*, fam. *Fabaceae*)
carabe (3×), *cara[b]e* (1×), *carabie* (1×)
cardamome *n.* cardamom (*Elettaria cardamomum*, fam. *Zingiberaceae*)
cardamome (12×), *cardamomum* (5×), *cardomomum* (3×), *cardomome* (2×), *cardame* (1×), *cardamo[me]* (1×)
cardiācle *n.* pain about the heart
cardiacle (21×)
carewei *n.* caraway (*Carum carui*, fam. *Apiaceae*)
carawey (8×), *caraway* (5×), *carawei* (5×), *carewey* (2×), *careaway* (1×), *careawei* (1×), *careawey* (1×), *carwey* (1×), *kareawei* (1×)
***carpobalsamum** *n.* balm (*Balsamodendron opobalsamum*, fam. *Burseraceae*)
carpobalsame (1×), *carpobalȝamum* (1×), *ca[r]pobalȝamum* (1×)
cās *n.* case
caas (1×)
cassia *n.* cassia (fam. *Fabaceae*)
cassie (3×)
~ **fistūla**, pods (also pulp) of purging cassia (*Cassia fistula*, fam. *F.*)
cassia fistula (13×)
~ **lignea**, cassia bark
cassia lignea (3×)
casten *v.* to cast; to vomit
cast (139×), *caste* (36×), *casten* (9×), *j-cast* (9×), *casteþ* (6×), *castyn* (4×), *castiþ* (2×), *caast* (1×), *castist* (1×), *castyng* (1×), *j-caast* (1×)
casting *ng.* casting; vomiting

castyng (4×), *castynge* (4×), *casting* (3×), *castinge* (2×)

castōrie *n.* MED. dried perineal glands of beaver or their secretion
castore (23×), *castorie* (6×), *castory* (2×), *castori* (1×)

cat *n.* ZOOL. cat
cat (1×)

catalempsī *n.* catalepsy
catalempsie (4×), *cathalempsie* (2×), *cathalemsie* (1×), *catolempsie* (1×)

cathimia *n.* ore containing gold or silver
cathmia (2×), *cathmye* (2×)
~ **arğenti**, lead or zinc ore containing silver
cathmie argente (1×)

caudrŏun *n.* kettle, cauldron
caudroun (1×)

caul *n.*, **cōl** *n.* *(1)* cabbage, kale, mustard, or some other plant of the genus *Brassica*, fam. *Brassicaceae*
caul (3×), *coole* (2×), *cale* (2×), *cool* (2×)
wīld(e ~, wild mustard, charlock
wyld caule (1×), *wyld cool* (1×)
~ wort = caul
coole wortes (1×), *coole wurtys* (1×)

caumfre *n.* camphor (*Camphora officinarum*, fam. *Lauraceae*)
camphore (13×), *camfer* (1×), *camphere* (1×), *ca[m]phore* (1×)

cause *n.* cause
cause (8×), *causes* (4×)

causōn *n.* PATHOL. chronic fever
causon (1×)

celidoine *n.* *(1)* greater celandine (*Chelidonium majus*, fam. *Papaveraceae*)
celedoyne (3×), *celidoine* (2×), *celydonie* (2×), *cellidonie* (1×), *celydone* (1×), *celydoyne* (1×)

centorīe *n.* common centaury (*Centaurium umbellatum*, fam. *Gentianaceae*)
centorie (17×)
lēs(se ~, yellow centaury (*Chlora perfoliata*, fam. *G.*)
lasse centorie (2×), *lesse centorie* (1×)

centrum galli *n.* wild clary (*Salvia verbenaca*, fam. *Lamiaceae*)
centre galli (1×), *centrum galli* (1×)

certain *adj.* certain
certeyn (5×), *certen* (2×)

cerūse *n.* white lead
ceruse (20×)

cēsen *v.* to cease
cesseþ (6×), *cesse* (3×), *cessen* (3×), *cessyn* (2×), *ceessen* (1×), *ceessiþ* (1×), *ceesythe* (1×), *cessyng* (1×), *sesse* (1×)

ceterak *n.* fern, prob. scale fern (*Ceterach officinarum*, fam. *Polypodiaceae*)
ceterak (3×), *ceterac* (1×)

chaf *n.* straw (refuse of grain)
chaf (2×)

chanel *n.* tube
chanel (1×)

chapītre *n.* chapter
chapitre (21×), *chapetre* (2×)

chaude-pis(se *n.* urinary disease
chaudepisse (1×)

chaumbre *n.* chamber
chaumbre (1×)

chaunğen *v.* to change
chaunge (2×), *j-chaungyd* (1×)

chaunğinge *ng.* changing

chaungyng (1×), *chaungynge* (1×)
chēke *n.* jaw; cheek
chekys (10×), *cheke* (7×), *checkys* (1×), *cheken* (1×), *chekyn* (1×)
chēre *n. (1)* face
chere (2×)
cherī *n.* cherry (*Prunus cerasus*, fam. *Rosaceae*)
cheries (1×), *chiri* (1×), *chiries* (1×), *chiry* (1×), *chyry* (1×)
cherī-stōn *n.* stone of a cherry
cherystones (1×), *chiristonis* (1×)
cherlok *n.* wild mustard, charlock (*Brassica arvensis*, fam. *Brassicaceae*)
karlooc (1×)
ches-bolle *n.* poppy or its seed pod [see **popī(e**]
chise-bolles (1×)
chēse *n.* cheese
chese (2×)
chest(e *n.* chest
chest (1×)
chesteine *n.* chestnut (*Castanea sativa*, fam. *Fagaceae*)
chasteyn (5×), *chasteynes* (3×), *chasteyns* (3×), *casteyn* (1×), *chesteynes* (1×)
cheuen *v. (1)* to chew
chewe (3×), *chiewe* (3×), *chiew* (2×), *chew* (1×), *chewyn* (1×), *chiewen* (1×), *j-chewyd* (1×)
cheuinge *ng.* chewing
chewynge (1×)
chiken *n.* ZOOL. chicken
chekens (2×), *chekenys* (2×), *chike* (2×), *chekenes* (1×), *chekun* (1×), *chekyn* (1×), *chicken* (1×), *chikenes* (1×), *chyken* (1×)
chiken-mēte *n.* scarlet pimpernel (*Anagallis arvensis*, fam. *Primulaceae*)
chikemete (1×)
chīld *n.* child
child (8×), *childe* (3×), *childeren* (3×), *children* (3×), *childes* (2×), *chyldren* (2×), *childern* (1×), *childerne* (1×), *childrun* (1×), *childryn* (1×), *chylderen* (1×)
chīldhōd *n.* childhood
childhood (5×), *chyldhood* (2×)
°**chimole** *n.* astringent remedy
chimole (1×)
chin *n.* chin
chyne (5×), *chine* (1×), *chyn* (1×), *chynne* (1×)
chinke *n.* asthma or whooping cough
chynke (1×), *chynnckes* (1×)
cicer *n.* chick-pea (*Cicer arietinum*, fam. *Fabaceae*)
ciceres (4×)
cicorēa *n.* chicory (*Cichorium intybus*, fam. *Asteraceae*); heliotrope
cicori (2×), *cicorie* (2×), *ci[c]ori* (1×), *[ci]cori* (1×), *cicory* (1×)
ciperus *n.* galingale (*Cyperus longus*, *Cyperaceae*)
ciperi (1×)
cīren *v.* to impregnate with wax or sealing compound, to waterproof
cyred (1×)
cirurğīe *n.* surgery
surgery (1×)
cirurğien *n.* surgeon
surgiens (1×)
citōnie *n.* quince (*Cydonia oblonga*, fam. *Rosaceae*)

citonyes (15×), *ci[t]onyes* (3×), *cytonies* (3×), *citonye* (2×), *cy[t]onyes* (2×), *citone* (1×), *cytonie* (1×)

*citre *n.* [see **saf(f)rǒun**]
citre (11×), *cicru* (1×), *citeres* (1×), *citri* (1×)

°**citri** *adj.* type of myrobalan: green fruit of *Terminalia citrina*, fam. *Combretaceae*
citri (7×), *ci[tri]* (4×)

citrīn(e *adj.* reddish yellow
citrine (8×), *citryne* (4×), *citryn* (2×), *cytrine* (1×)

clarifīen *v.* to clarify
clarifie (2×), *clarefyen* (1×), *j-clarefied* (1×)

clauing *ng.* clawing
clawynge (1×)

clei *n.* clay
cley (3×), *clei* (2×), *clay* (1×)

clēne *adj.* & *adv.* clean
adj.: *clene* (35×), *cleene* (2×); *adv.*: *clene* (1×)

clēnen *v.* to clean
clene (2×)

clensen *v.* to cleanse
clense (48×), *j-clensyd* (10×), *clanse* (7×), *j-clensed* (6×), *j-clensid* (5×), *clensyn* (3×), *clanseþ* (2×), *clansiþ* (2×), *clenseþ* (2×), *clensid* (2×), *cle[n]se* (1×), *clensed* (1×), *clens[e]n* (1×), *clen-seþ* (1×), *clensyd* (1×), *cl[e]nsyn* (1×), *clensyng* (1×), *j-clansed* (1×), *j-clansyd* (1×)

clensing *ng.* cleansing
clensynge (4×), *clansynge* (3×), *clansyng* (2×), *clensyng* (1×)

clēpen *v.* to call
j-clepid (28×), *clepid* (11×), *j-clepyd* (7×), *clepyd* (6×), *clepe* (3×), *clepiþ* (2×), *clepen* (1×), *clepith* (1×), *clepyn* (1×), *j-cleped* (1×)

clēr *adj.* clear
clere (17×), *cleere* (5×), *cleer* (2×)

clēren *v.* to clear
cleriþ (2×), *clereþ* (1×)

clēven *v.* *(1)* to adhere
cleueþ (5×), *cleue* (3×), *cleuen* (1×), *cleuyde* (1×)

clēving(e *ng.* *(1)* & *ag.* *(1)* sticking
ng.: *cleuynge* (6×), *cleuyng* (5×); *ag.*: *cleuynge* (1×)

clīmbing *ng.* climbing
climbynge (1×)

clistēr *n.* MED. clyster
clystes (1×)

clistēri(e *n.* MED. clyster
clisterie (27×), *clisteries* (8×), *clistere* (7×), *clisteres* (2×), *clystere* (2×), *clistre* (1×), *clysterie* (1×)

clok(ke *n.* clock
clok (4×), *clook* (1×)

clōsen *v.* to close
closed (2×), *closeþ* (2×), *j-closed* (2×), *clonsynd* (1×), *closen* (1×)

clōth *n.* cloth
clooþ (43×), *clowt* (8×), *cloothe* (2×), *cloþ* (2×), *cloþis* (1×), *cloutys* (1×), *clowte* (1×), *clowth* (1×) [see also **horned clōth**]

clō(ve *n.* *(2)* clove (*Caryophyllus aromaticus*, fam. *Myrtaceae*)
clowes (32×), *clewes* (1×), *clowys* (1×)

coconode *n.* seed of spurge laurel
coconydie (1×)

cod *n.* *(1)* scrotum

cod (20×), *cood* (3×), *code* (2×)
coin *n. (2)* [see **citōnie**]
coyn (1×), *coyne* (1×), *coynes* (1×)
cok *n. (1)* ZOOL. cock
cockys (1×), *cok* (1×)
cokkel *n.* corn cockle (*Agrostemma githago*, fam. *Caryophyllaceae*); darnel (*Lolium temulentum*, fam. *Poaceae*)
cockyl (2×), *cockle* (1×), *cookyl* (1×)
cōl *n. (2)* charcoal; mineral coal
colys (4×), *coles* (3×), *colees* (1×), *cooles* (1×)
colagog *n.* & *adj.* medicine promoting the discharge of bile
n.: cologoge (7×), *calogoge* (2×), *calagoge* (1×), *[c]alogoge* (1×), *colagoge* (1×), *colo[go]ge* (1×); *adj.: cologoge* (1×)
cōld *n.* & *adj.* cold
n.: coold (131×), *cold* (3×), *coolde* (3×), *colde* (1×); *adj.: coold* (236×), *coolde* (26×), *colde* (6×), *cold* (5×), *coldere* (1×)
cōlden *v.* to grow or make cold
cooldyd (1×), *j-cooldid* (1×)
cōldnesse *n.* coldness
cooldnesse (14×), *coldnesse* (6×)
°**colera rubea** *n.* red choler
colera rubea (1×)
colerik *adj.* choleric
colric (21×), *colrik* (9×), *coleric* (2×), *colryc* (2×), *colryk* (2×), *colericus* (1×), *colerik* (1×), *colrick* (1×)
colia(u)ndre *n.* coriander (*Coriandrum sativum*, fam. *Apiaceae*)
coliaundre (2×), *coliaundyr* (1×)
cōlīs *n.* strained, clear meat broth
colyis (6×), *coliys* (1×)
*__collica passio__ *n.* illness of the colon
colica passio (8×), *collica passio* (1×)
collides *n.* form of dysentery
colides (1×)
collīrie *n.* collyrium
collirie (16×), *colliries* (13×), *colirie* (1×), *coliries* (1×), *collire* (1×), *colliry* (1×)
colofōnie *n.* colophony (resin obtained by distilling turpentine)
colofonye (8×), *colofyne* (2×), *colofonie* (1×)
cōlon *n. (2)* large intestine or colon (including the rectum)
colon (2×)
coloquint(ide *n.* colocynth (*Citrullus colocynthis*, fam. *Cucurbitaceae*)
coloquintida (1×)
cŏlŏur *n.* colour
colour (58×), *coloure* (10×), *colours* (3×), *colowr* (3×)
cŏlŏuren *v.* to colour
j-colourd (1×), *j-colourde* (1×), *j-coloured* (1×), *j-colourid* (1×), *j-colurd* (1×)
cŏlŏuring *ng.* colouring
colourynge (1×)
colre *n.* choler, bile
colre (141×), *colere* (2×)
columbīne *n.* columbine (*Aquilegia vulgaris*, fam. *Ranunculaceae*)
columbyne (3×), *columbine* (2×)
cōmb *n.* comb
combe (2×), *komb* (1×)
cŏmen *v.* to come
comeþ (546×), *come* (112×), *comen*

(15×), comyn (9×), *comyth* (2×), *comy* (1×), *comyng* (1×), *comynge* (1×), *comynn* (1×), *comyþe* (1×), *comyȝt* (1×), *kome* (1×)

cŏmfort *n.* comfort
confort (1×)

cŏmfortāble *adj.* MED. strengthening
confortabil (13×), *confortabyl* (6×)

cŏmfortatīf MED. *n.* invigorating food or medicine; *adj.* invigorating
n.: confortatyues (6×), *confortatifs* (5×), *confortatyuus* (1×), *confortatyuys* (1×); *adj.: confortatyf* (2×), *confortatif* (1×)

cŏmforten *v.* MED. to strengthen
confortep (15×), *conforte* (7×), *conforten* (5×), *confort* (3×), *confortyn* (3×), *conforted* (1×), *confortest* (1×)

cŏmīn *n.* cumin (*Cummin cyminum*, fam. *Apiaceae*)
comyn (44×), *comynn* (1×)

commūn(e *adj.* common
comyn (9×)

commūnelī *adj.*[16] common; *adv.* commonly
adj.: comynly (1×); *adv.: comynly* (7×), *comely* (6×), *comenly* (1×), *comly* (1×), *comonly* (1×), *comyly* (1×), *comynlyche* (1×)

cŏmpaignīe *n.* (a) company; (b) sexual intercourse
company (1×), *compeny* (1×), *cumpany* (1×), *cumpeny* (1×)

cŏmpaignīing *ng.* sexual intercourse
cumpenyinge (1×)

cŏmpās *n.* circle
compase (1×)

compassiŏun *n.* compassion
compassioun (1×)

°**complexif** *adj.* complex
complexif (1×)

complexiŏun *n.* constitution
complexioun (12×), *complexion* (11×), *complexiouns* (1×)

compŏuned *ppl.* PHARM. composed of ingredients having different medicinal properties
componed (9×)

conceiven *v.* to conceive
conceyuyd (2×), *conceyuyng* (2×), *conseiuyd* (1×)

condiciŏun *n.* condition
condicions (1×)

confecciŏun *n.* concoction
confeccion (2×), *confeccioun* (2×)

cŏnferīe *n.* comfrey (*Symphytum officinale*, fam. *Boraginaceae*)
confirie (17×), *confirye* (1×), *confyri* (1×)

confūsiŏun *n.* confusion
confusion (1×)

conğēlen *v.* to coagulate
congelyd (2×), *j-congeled* (1×)

conglūtinatīf *adj.* MED. having the property of closing wounds by producing a glutinous substance
conglutynatif (1×)

cŏngre *n.* ZOOL. conger, marine eel
congur (1×)

cŏnnen *v.* to know
kan (1×), *kunne* (1×)

conserven *v.* to conserve

16 Only recorded as an adverb in the *MED*.

conserue (1×)
consolidatīf MED. *n.* medicine promoting cicatrization or closing of a wound; *adj.* having such properties
n.: consolidatyues (6×), *consolidatifs* (5×), *consolidatyfs* (1×); *adj.: consolidatyues* (1×)
ºConstantīn *n.* Constantinian
constantines (1×)
constrictīf MED. *n.* medicine thickening and thus detaining the discharge of bodily fluids; *adj.* having such properties
n.: constructyues (1×); *adj.: constrictif* (1×)
consūmen *v.* to consume
consumed (5×), *consumen* (3×), *consume* (2×), *consumeþ* (1×), *consumid* (1×), *consumyd* (1×), *consumynge* (1×)
continūēl *adj.* continual
continuel (11×)
continūel(l)ī *adv.* continually
continueliche (3×), *continuel-lyche* (1×), *continuellyche* (1×), *contin[u]elyche* (1×)
continūen *v.* to continue
continue (2×)
contrārie *n.* & *adj.* contrary
n.: contrarie (1×); *adj.: contrarie* (4×), *contrary* (1×)
cǒntrē(e *n.* country
contrey (1×), *cuntrees* (1×)
cop *n.* tip (of the nose)
coppe (2×)
coperōse *n.* metallic sulphate; vitriol
coperose (4×), *coporose* (1×)
corāl *n. (1)* coral
coral (11×)
corigiōle *n.* prob. common knotgrass (*Polygonum aviculare*, fam. *Polygonaceae*)
corigiole (1×)
cōrn *n.* corn (of pepper)
corn (1×), *cornes* (1×)
cornēr *n. (1)* corner (of the eye)
cornere (1×), *corneris* (1×)
corrōsīf MED. *n.* substance which destroys organic tissue by corrosive action; *adj.* having such properties
n.: corrosyues (7×), *corosyues* (6×), *corosifs* (1×), *corrosifs* (1×), *corrosiues* (1×), *corrosyuus* (1×), *corrosyuys* (1×); *adj.: corrosyf* (3×), *corosif* (1×), *corrysifs* (1×)
corrupciǒun *n.* corruption
corupcioun (9×), *corupcion* (7×), *corupciouns* (1×)
corrupten *v.* to corrupt
corupt (1×)
ºcorupt *adj.* corrupt
corupt (92×), *corrupt* (1×), *corupte* (1×)
cost *n. (3)* costmary (*Chrysanthemum balsamita*, fam. *Asteraceae*)
coost (8×), *cost* (4×)
costīf *adj.* costive
costyf (13×), *costif* (12×), *coostif* (2×)
costīfnes(se *n.* costiveness
costifnesse (1×), *costyfnesse* (1×)
cotidiān *adj.* MED. intermittent, quotidian (fever)
cotidian (4×), *cotidianes* (1×), *cotidians* (1×), *cotidyan* (1×)

cotŏun *n.* cotton (*Gossypium*, fam. *Malvaceae*)
cotun (5×), *cotoun* (4×), *cootun* (1×), *coton* (1×)
cŏu *n.* ZOOL. cow
cow (6×), *cowe* (1×), *kow* (1×)
cough *n.* cough(ing)
couȝe (49×), *couȝ* (3×), *cowȝ* (3×), *cowȝe* (3×), *couȝes* (2×), *couȝwe* (2×), *kow* (2×), *cowys* (1×), *kouȝe* (1×)
coughing *ng.* coughing
cowȝyng (3×), *couȝinge* (1×), *couȝwinge* (1×), *couȝwynge* (1×), *couȝynge* (1×), *cowȝwinge* (1×), *cowȝwynge* (1×)
cŏurs *n.* course
cours (6×), *course* (1×)
cŏveiten *v.* to covet
coueit (1×), *coueityng* (1×), *coueyt* (1×)
cŏveitŏus *adj.* covetous
coueitouse (1×), *coueitows* (1×)
cŏvenāble *adj.* appropriate
couenable (1×), *couenabyl* (1×)
cŏveren *v.* *(1)* to cover
keuere (1×), *keuereþ* (1×), *keuerid* (1×), *keueryn* (1×)
crab(be *n.* *(1)* ZOOL. crab
crabbes (4×), *crabbe* (1×)
craft *n.* *(1)* craft
craft (3×)
crampe *n.* *(1)* violent contraction of muscles, spasm; disease with such characteristics
crampe (4×), *cramp* (1×), *cramppe* (1×)
crēmen *v.* *(2)* to foam, to froth
cremed (1×)
crēpen *v.* to creep
crepyn (1×)
crēping *ng.* & *ag.* creeping
ng.: creping (1×); *ag.: creping* (1×)
cresse *n.* plant of the *Brassicaceae* fam., esp. common watercress (*Nasturtium officinale*) and garden cress or garden peppergrass (*Lepidium sativum*)
carses (10×), *carse* (3×), *carsen* (2×), *karses* (2×), *cars* (1×), *car[s]es* (1×), *karsen* (1×)
crī(e *n.* cry
cry (1×)
crīing *ng.* crying
cryinge (3×), *cryyng* (2×), *criynge* (1×)
criket *n.* ZOOL. cricket
criketes (2×), *criketis* (1×), *cryketes* (1×)
crŏme *n.* crumb of bread
crummes (3×), *crummys* (2×)
crop *n.* any part of a medicinal herb except the root
crop (1×), *croppes* (1×), *croppis* (1×)
croue *n.* ZOOL. crow
crowe (1×), *crowes* (1×)
cruste *n.* crust of bread
crust (1×)
cūbit(e *n.* measure of length (usu., eighteen inches)
cubite (1×)
cūcŏmer *n.* cucumber (*Cucumis sativus*, fam. *Cucurbitaceae*)
cucumer (1×)
culver *n.* ZOOL. dove
culuere (3×)
cuppe *n.* MED. cupping glass
cuppe (1×)

cuppen *v.* SURG. to bleed (sth.) by means of a cupping glass
cuppid (4×), *cuppe* (3×), *cuppen* (3×), *j-cupped* (3×), *cuppyd* (2×), *cupped* (1×), *j-cuppid* (1×), *j-cuppyd* (1×)
cūre *n. (1)* cure, treatment
cure (5×), *cures* (2×)
cūren *v. (2)* to cure
j-cured (1×)
cūring *ng.* curing
curynge (1×)
cuscūte *n.* dodder (*Cuscuta epithymum*, fam. *Cuscutaceae*)
cuscute (6×)
cutten *v. (1)* to cut
kyt (9×), *j-kyt* (3×), *kit* (1×)
cuttinge *ng.* cutting
kyttynge (1×)
ºcyclamen *n.* cyclamen (fam. *Primulaceae*)
ciclamen (1×)

D

dai *n.* day
daies (56×), *day* (25×), *dai* (23×), *days* (2×), *daie* (1×), *daiȝe* (1×), *dayes* (1×)
daies-īe *n.* (a) European daisy (*Bellis perennis*, fam. *Asteraceae*); (b) comfrey (*Symphytum officinale*, fam. *Boraginaceae*)
daisie (8×), *daie-eiȝe* (1×), *daies-eiȝe* (1×), *daisye* (1×), *dayes-eiȝe* (1×)
damascēne *n.* damson (*Prunus damascena*, fam. *Rosaceae*)
damascenes (1×)
dāte *n. (1)* fruit of the palm tree, date (*Phoenix dactylifera*, fam. *Palmae*)
dates (2×), *datis* (1×), *datys* (1×)
dauk(e *n.* wild carrot (*Daucus carota*, fam. *Apiaceae*)
dauk (14×), *dawk* (1×)
declināciŏun *n.* decline
declinacion (1×)
dēcocciŏun *n.* medicinal preparation made by boiling
decoccioun (2×), *decocciouns* (1×)
dēcrēsen *v.* to decrease
decrescyng (1×)
dēd *adj.* dead
deed (4×), *dede* (1×), *deede* (1×), *deid* (1×)
dēde *n.* deed
dedisse (1×)
dēdlī *adj.* deadly
dedly (1×)
dēf *adj.* deaf
deef (1×)
dēfaut(e *n.* lack
defaute (11×), *defaut* (1×)
dēfīen *v. (2)* to digest (food, drink)
defie (12×), *defied* (9×), *defiȝe* (6×), *defien* (4×), *defieþ* (4×), *defiȝed* (4×), *defiȝen* (3×), *defye* (2×), *defeeþ* (1×), *defeid* (1×), *defieȝen* (1×), *defiȝinge* (1×), *defyed* (1×), *defyen* (1×), *defyyd* (1×)
dēfnes(se *n.* deafness
deefnesse (9×), *defnesse* (1×)
deien *v.* to dye
j-died (1×)
deintē *n.* fine food or drink
deinteys (1×), *deynteis* (1×)
dēl *n. (2)* part

del (1×)
dēlen *v.* to have sexual intercourse
dalt (1×)
delicāt *adj.* delicate
delicat (2×)
dēlīce *n.* [see **deintē**]
delices (1×)
dēliveraunce *n.* delivery
delieueraunce (2×), *delyueraunce* (2×)
dēliveren *v.* to deliver
delyuere (8×), *delyuered* (4×), *delyuerid* (4×), *deliuerid* (3×), *delyueryn* (3×), *delyueryd* (2×), *deliuered* (1×), *delyuereþ* (1×), *delyuerithe* (1×), *delyueriþ* (1×), *diliuerid* (1×)
demigraine *n.* hemicrania
demygrayn (1×), *domigrayn* (1×)
dēp *adj.* deep
depe (2×), *deep* (1×), *dee[p]* (1×)
dēparten *v.* to depart
departe (1×), *departed* (1×), *departen* (1×), *departeþ* (1×), *departyd* (1×)
dēpnes(se *n.* inner part of the body or of a bodily organ
depnesse (12×)
dēpūten *v.* to allot
depute (1×)
derk *adj.* dark
derk (8×), *derke* (2×)
derknes(se *n.* darkness
dercnesse (2×), *derknesse* (2×)
dēsiccatīve *n.* MED. medicine promoting dryness
desiccatyfs (1×)
dēsīr *n.* desire
desire (2×), *desyre* (2×)
dēsīren *v.* to desire
desyre (2×), *desire* (1×), *desireþ* (1×), *desiriþ* (1×)
dēsīringe *ng.* desiring
desyryng (1×)
dēspūmed *ppl.* of honey: clarified
dispumed (6×), *despumed* (5×), *despumyd* (2×), *dispumyd* (2×)
dēstroien *v.* to destroy
destreiȝen (3×), *destrie* (3×), *distreiȝe* (2×), *destreiȝed* (1×), *destriȝe* (1×), *destriȝen* (1×), *destruen* (1×), *destryen* (1×), *distreyed* (1×), *distreyen* (1×), *distroy* (1×), *j-distriȝed* (1×)
dēstroiinge *ng.* destroying
destreyng (1×)
dēstrucciŏun *n.* destruction
destruccion (1×)
dēterminen *v.* to determine
determynd (1×)
dēth *n.* death
deeþ (11×), *deþ* (1×)
deu *n.* dew
dew (1×)
deute *n.* kind of salve
deute (10×), *dewte* (7×)
dēvel *n.* devil
deuelus (1×)
dīabēte *n.* diabetes
diabetes (3×), *diabites* (1×), *djabites* (1×)
dīacalamentum *n.* MED. drug made of calamint
diacalamentum (8×), *diacalemen[tum]* (1×)
dīacameron *n.* MED. compound drug
diacameron (2×)
***dīacap(p)aris** *n.* MED. electuary made of capers

diacaparis (2×)

dīacastōrie *n.* MED. drug made of castoreum

dycastore (1×)

***dīaceraseos** *n.* MED. electuary made of cherries

diaceraseos (2×), *dyacesarros* (1×)

dīaciminum *n.* MED. drug made of cumin

diaciminum (2×), *dyacymynum* (2×), *diacymynum* (1×), *dyacyminum* (1×)

dīacitōnicon *n.* MED. drug made of quince

diacitoniton (2×), *diacitonyton* (2×), *dyacitonyton* (2×), *diacitonicon* (1×), *dyacitonycon* (1×)

dīacodion *n.* MED. drug made of poppies

diacodion (5×), *dia[c]odioun* (1×), *diaconidion* (1×), *dyacodion* (1×)

dīadragantum *n.* MED. drug made of gum tragacanth

diadragante (2×), *diagragantum* (2×), *diadragant* (1×), *diadragantoun* (1×), *diadragantum* (1×), *diadragaunt* (1×)

dīadrağğē *n.* MED. sweet medicinal preparation

diadrage (2×)

dīagredie *n.* MED. diagrydium (drug made of scammony and used as a laxative)

diagredie (5×), *diagridi* (1×), *diagridie* (1×)

dīalanga *n.* MED. drug used for sciatica

dialange (1×)

dīamargariton *n.* MED. drug made of pearls

diamargariton (3×), *diamargaritoun* (1×)

dīameron *n.* MED. drug made of mulberries

diameron (1×)

***diampnes** *n.* disease of the urinary bladder provoking excessive urination

diampnes (3×), *djampnes* (1×)

dīanisum *n.* MED. electuary made of aloes and tansy

dianisum (1×), *dyanysum* (1×)

dīantos *n.* MED. drug made of rosemary

dianthos (3×), *dian[t]hes* (1×), *[di]anthos* (1×)

*~ **muscate**, with musk added

dyanthos muscate (1×)

dīapapaver *n.* MED. drug made of poppies

diapapauer (3×), *diapapauere* (2×), *diapapauar* (1×)

dīapenidion *n.* MED. sweet drug used to relieve coughing

diapenidion (7×), *diapenydion* (2×), *dyapenydion* (2×), *dyapenidion* (1×), *dyapenydyon* (1×)

***dīapigamum** *n.* MED. electuary made of rue

diapigamum (2×)

***dīapiretrum** *n.* MED. electuary made of pellitory

diapiretron (1×), *diapiretrum* (1×)

***dīaprassium** *n.* MED. electuary made of horehound

diaprassion (1×), *diaprassium* (1×)

dīaprūnis *n.* MED. drug made of plums

diaprunes (4×), *diaprunis* (3×), *diaprunys* (1×)

dīarīa *n.* diarrhoea
djarria (1×)

dīarodon *n.* MED. drug made of roses
diarodon (3×), *dyarodoun* (1×)
~ **abbatis**
diarodon abbates (2×), *diaradon abbatis* (1×), *diarodon abbatis* (1×)

***dīarris** *n.* MED. electuary made of iris
diarris (2×), *diarres* (1×)

dīasenē *n.* MED. drug made of senna
diacene (5×), *diasene* (1×)

dīaspermaticon *n.* MED. drug made from seeds
diaspermat[ic]on (5×), *dia-spermat[ic]on* (1×), *diaspermat[ic]oun* (1×), *dyaspermat[ic]on* (1×)

dīatrionpiperion *n.* MED. drug made of three kinds of peppers
diatrionpiperion (4×), *dia[tri]onpiperion* (1×), *diatrion[piperion]* (1×), *diatrionpiperon* (1×), *dyatrionpiperion* (1×)

dīazinziberis *n.* MED. drug made of ginger
dyaȝinȝiber (1×)

dīen *v.* to die
deiȝe (2×), *deyinge* (1×), *diȝe* (1×)

dīēten *v.* to regulate the diet for purposes of health
diete (13×), *dieten* (4×), *dietid* (3×), *dietyd* (2×), *dietyn* (1×), *dietyng* (1×), *dyete* (1×)

dīēting *ng.* regulation of the diet for purposes of health
dietyng (17×), *dietinge* (5×), *dietinges* (2×), *dieting* (1×), *dietynge* (1×), *dietynges* (1×), *dietyngis* (1×)

difference *n.* difference
difference (4×)

dīğestīf *adj.* digestive
digestyf (1×)

dīğestiŏun *n.* digestion
digestioun (6×), *digestion* (5×)

dighten *v.* to prepare
j-diȝt (1×)

dīmidia *n.* half
dimidia (5×)

dimnes *n.* dimness (of the eyes)
dymnesse (1×)

dīnen *v.* *(2)* to dine
dyne (1×)

discolŏuren *v.* to discolour
discolourd (5×), *descolourd* (1×), *discoleryd* (1×), *discolourid* (1×)

discolŏuring *ng.* discolouring
discoloring (1×)

discōrden *v.* to differ
discorden (2×)

discreciŏun *n.* discretion
discrecyon (1×)

discrēt(e)lī *adv.* judiciously
discretely (1×), *dis[c]retely* (1×)

disēse *n.* disease
desesis (1×)

dish *n.* dish
disch (1×)

dispōsen *v.* to dispose
disposed (1×), *disposeþ* (1×), *disposid* (1×), *disposyd* (1×)

dispōsiciŏun *n.* disposition
disposicioun (2×), *disposicion* (1×)

dissenterie *n.* dysentery
dissenterie (29×)
dissolūtīf MED. *n.* medicine producing dissolution or dissipation of a morbid condition; *adj.* having such properties
n.: dissolutyues (11×), *dissolutyfs* (2×), *dis[solutyues]* (2×), *dissolityues* (1×), *dissolutiues* (1×), *dissolutiuus* (1×); *adj.: dissolutif* (2×), *dissolutyues* (2×), *dissolitif* (1×), *dissolutyfs* (1×)
dissolven *v.* to dissolve; PHYSIOL. & MED. to reduce or waste; to weaken
dissoluen (6×), *dissolued* (4×), *dissolue* (3×), *dissolueþ* (3×), *dissoluyd* (1×)
distemperaunce *n.* PHYSIOL. morbid condition due to the imbalance of humours or qualities
distemperaunce (3×)
distemperen *v.* PHYSIOL. to be upset by imbalance of humours or qualities
distemperid (10×), *distempered* (4×), *distempere* (1×), *distemperyd* (1×)
distemperinge *ng.* PHYSIOL. improper balance of humours or qualities
distempering (18×), *distemperinge* (4×), *distemperyng* (4×), *diste[m]peringe* (2×), *diste[m]pering* (1×)
distillen *v.* to distil
distille (3×), *distilled* (1×)
distǒurbaunce *n.* disturbance
disturbacion (1×)
ditain(e *n.* (a) dittany of Crete (*Origanum dictamnus*, fam. *Lamiaceae*); (b) white dittany (*Dictamnus albus*, fam. *Rutaceae*)
ditanndre (1×), *dyteyn* (1×)
dīūretik MED. *n.* medicine capable of promoting urination; *adj.* inducing or promoting urination
n.: duretik (2×), *duretikes* (1×), *duretiks* (1×); *adj.: duretik* (19×), *duretyk* (4×)
dīvers(e *adj.* diverse
diuerse (26×), *di-uerse* (2×), *diuersse* (1×)
dīversitē *n.* diversity
diuersite (34×)
doctǒur *n.* doctor of medicine
doctours (1×)
dodden *v.* to shear or shave
dodden (1×)
dōer(e *n.* one who performs an action
doeris (1×)
dogge *n.* ZOOL. dog
dogge (2×)
dōing(e *ng.* performance of an action
doyng (1×), *doynge* (1×)
dominācīǒun *n.* domination
dominacion (1×), *dominacyon* (1×)
dōn *v. (1)* to do
do (122×), *doiþ* (18×), *doon* (17×), *don* (8×), *dooþ* (8×), *j-doon* (4×), *doeþ* (2×), *doo* (2×), *j-do* (2×), *j-don* (2×), *dede* (1×), *dedist* (1×), *dide* (1×), *done* (1×), *doost* (1×), *doþ* (1×)
dǒuble *adj.* double
double (4×), *dowble* (3×)
dǒun *adv.* down
down (27×), *doun* (23×), *dounn*

(1×), *downe* (1×), *downn* (1×), *j-down* (1×)
dŏun-right *adv.* face down
doun-riȝt (1×)
dŏun-ward *adv.* downwards
downward (8×), *dounward* (2×)
dragaunce *n.* dragonwort (*Dracunculus vulgaris*, fam. *Araceae*)
dragance (1×)
dragaunt *n.* (a) gum tragacanth; (b) some kind of vitriol
dragagant (9×), *dragagante* (6×), *dragagaunt* (4×), *dragagantum* (2×), *dragagannt* (1×), *dragaga[n]te* (1×), *dragagaunte* (1×)
drağğē *n.* *(2)* sweet medicinal preparation
dragage (33×), *dragge* (15×), *drage* (1×)
dragme *n.* dram (unit of apothecary's weight of one eighth of an ounce)
dragme (308×)
drast *n.* dregs
drastes (2×), *drastys* (2×), *drastos* (1×), *drestys* (1×)
drastī *adj.* like dregs
drasty (2×)
drauen *v.* to draw
drawe (13×), *draweþ* (9×), *drawen* (6×), *drawyng* (5×), *drawyn* (4×), *draw* (2×), *j-drawe* (1×)
draught *n.* draught (of liquid)
drawt (2×)
drauing(e *ng.* drawing
drawyng (1×)
drēd(e *n.* dread
drede (6×), *dreed* (1×)
drēdeful *adj.* dreadful; afraid
dredful (4×), *dredfulle* (2×)
drēden *v.* to dread
drede (3×), *drediste* (1×), *dredyng* (1×)
drēmen *v.* *(2)* to dream
dremyng (1×)
drēming *ng.* *(2)* dream(ing)
dremyng (1×)
drīe *n.* *(1)* dryness; *adj.* *(1)* dry
n.: driȝe (1×); *adj.: driȝe* (69×), *dryȝe* (6×), *drye* (5×), *drie* (4×), *dry* (3×), *drei* (1×)
drīen *v.* *(1)* to dry
driȝe (12×), *j-dried* (5×), *drie* (4×), *drieþ* (4×), *dryen* (2×), *dryeþ* (2×), *dried* (1×), *driȝed* (1×), *driȝen* (1×), *drye* (1×), *dryyt* (1×), *j-drie* (1×)
drīenes(se *n.* dryness
drinesse (23×), *drynesse* (15×), *drienesse* (7×), *driȝenesse* (1×)
drīing *ng.* *(1)* drying
dryinge (1×)
drink(e *n.* drink
drynk (9×), *dryncky*s (7×), *drynkys* (7×), *drynke* (6×), *drynkes* (6×), *dryncke* (4×), *dryncke*s (3×), *drynck* (2×), *drync* (1×)
drinken *v.* to drink
drynke (41×), *drynk* (22×), *dryncke* (21×), *drinke* (6×), *drynken* (6×), *j-drunke* (6×), *j-drunken* (5×), *dryncky*n (4×), *drynkyn* (3×), *j-drunk* (3×), *drincke* (2×), *drync* (2×), *drynck* (2×), *drinck* (1×), *drinckyng* (1×), *drinkyn* (1×), *drunke* (1×), *drunken* (1×), *dryncky*ng (1×), *drynkeþ* (1×), *j-drunck* (1×), *j-*

drunkyn (1×)
drinkinge *ng.* drinking
drynkynge (5×), *drynckynge* (3×), *drynckyng* (1×), *drynkyng* (1×), *drynkynges* (1×)
drit *n.* excrement
driȝt (25×), *drit* (11×), *dryt* (4×), *dryȝt* (4×), *dirt* (1×), *dryȝth* (1×)
drīven *v.* to drive
dryueþ (3×), *driuen* (1×), *dryue* (1×), *dryuen* (1×)
drŏnke-leu(e *adj.* addicted to drink, habitually drunk
drunklew (1×)
drŏnken *ppl.* drunk
drunken (1×)
drōpe *n. (1)* drop
drope (7×), *dropes* (3×), *dropis* (2×)
drōpe-mēl(e *adv.* by drops
dropmeele (1×), *droppemeele* (1×)
dropesī(e *n.* dropsy
dropesi (3×), *dropesie* (1×), *dropesy* (1×), *dropisies* (1×), *dropsy* (1×)
droppen *v.* to drop
droppeþ (4×), *dreppynge* (1×), *dropeþ* (1×), *droppen* (1×), *dropping* (1×), *j-dropped* (1×)
drōs *n.* dross
drosse (1×)
dul *adj.* dull
dul (2×), *dulle* (2×)
dullen *v.* to dull
j-dulled (1×)
°**dulshipe** *n.* dullness
dulschipe (1×)
dūren *v.* to last
dureþ (5×)
dūring *adj.* lasting
duryng (1×), *durynge* (1×)
dūst *n.* dust
dust (4×)
dwellen *v.* to dwell
duellyng (1×), *dwelle* (1×)
dwellinge *ng.* dwelling
dwellynge (1×)

E

eft-sōne(s *adv.* soon after
eft-sones (2×), *eftsones* (1×), *eft-sonys* (1×)
ēgre *adj.* sour
egre (1×)
egremoine *n.* European agrimony (*Agrimonia eupatoria*, fam. *Rosaceae*)
egremoyne (7×), *agrymonie* (1×), *egremonie* (1×), *egremony* (1×), *egremonye* (1×)
ei *n. (1)* egg
eyren (31×), *ey* (27×), *eiren* (12×), *eiryn* (1×), *eiȝe* (1×), *eyn* (1×)
eie *n. (1)* eye
eiȝen (125×), *eiȝe* (78×), *eiȝyn* (2×), *eyȝen* (1×)
eie-lid *n.* eyelid
eiȝeledys (2×), *eeiȝlidis* (1×), *eiȝe-ledis* (1×)
ei-shel *n.* eggshell
ey-schelle (1×)
ēk *adv.* also
eke (1×)
elboue *n.* elbow
elbow (4×)
ēlde *n.* old age
elde (5×), *eld* (1×)

ēl(e *n. (3)* ZOOL. eel
eel (6×), *eelys* (1×), *elys* (1×)
***electarie** *n.* squirting cucumber (*Ecballium elaterium*, fam. *Cucurbitaceae*)
electarie (1×)
ēlectūārie *n.* electuary (medicine in which the ingredients are combined with honey or syrup to form a paste)
electuaries (46×), *electuarie* (29×), *alectuarie* (2×), *electuare* (2×), *electuaryes* (2×), *electuaris* (1×), *electuarys* (1×), *ellectuarie* (1×)
element *n.* element
elementes (6×), *element* (1×), *elementus* (1×)
ellebre niger *n.* black hellebore (*Helleborus niger*, fam. *Ranunculaceae*)
eleborus niger (7×)
eller(n *n.* European elder (*Sambucus nigra*, fam. *Caprifoliaceae*); dwarf elder (*S. ebulus*, fam. *C.*)
elerne (3×), *ellerne* (3×), *ellern* (1×)
elles *adv.* else
ellys (8×), *ellis* (2×)
elm(e *n.* wych elm (*Ulmus montana*, fam. *Ulmaceae*); common elm (*U. campestris*, fam. *U.*)
elm (1×)
ematīte(s *n.* (a) hematite, red iron ore; (b) bloodstone, heliotrope
emachites (6×), *emathites* (3×), *emathite* (2×)
emblici *n.* type of myrobalan [see **mirabolān**]
emblice (1×)
emoroid(es *n.* hemorrhoids
emeroides (8×), *emoroides* (4×), *emeraudes* (1×), *emeraudis* (1×), *emerawdes* (1×), *eme-roides* (1×), *emoraudes* (1×)
emplāstre *n.* plaster
emplastre (3×), *emplastres* (2×), *enplastre* (2×), *em-plaistris* (1×), *enplastris* (1×)
emptī *adj.* empty
empti (1×)
encens *n.* incense
encense (41×), *encence* (1×), *incense* (1×)
enchēsŏun *n.* cause (of disease)
enchesouns (22×), *enchesoun* (16×), *encheson* (8×), *enchesons* (5×), *enche-souns* (1×), *inchesons* (1×)
enclōsen *v.* to enclose
enclosid (2×), *enclosyd* (2×)
encrēsen *v.* to increase
encrescep (3×), *encresce* (2×), *encrescyn* (2×)
encrēsing *ng.* increase
encressyng (1×)
ēnde *n. (1)* end
ende (10×), *endys* (4×)
endīve *n.* wild lettuce (*Lactuca virosa*, fam. *Asteraceae*)
endyue (17×)
enemī *n.* enemy
enemy (1×)
enfōrcen *v.* to exert force
enforcep (2×), *enforce* (1×), *inforsche* (1×)
enfōrcing *ng.* exerting of force
enforsynge (1×)
enğendren *v.* PHYSIOL. & MED. to produce

engenderid (2×), *engendrid* (1×), *engendryn* (1×)

enointen *v.* MED. to apply a healing unguent or medicine
a-noynte (81×), *a-nointe* (29×), *anoynte* (12×), *anointe* (6×), *a-noint* (4×), *a-nointest* (3×), *a-noncte* (3×), *a-noynt* (3×), *a-noynted* (3×), *a-nointist* (2×), *a-noyntest* (2×), *anointed* (1×), *anoncte* (1×), *[a-noynte]* (1×), *an-oynte* (1×), *a-noynten* (1×), *a-noyntynge* (1×)

enointing *ng.* MED. application of a healing unguent or medicine; healing ointment or salve
a-nointynge (1×), *a-nointyngys* (1×), *a-noyntinges* (1×), *a-noyntyng* (1×), *a-noyntynges* (1×)

entraille(s *n.* viscera, entrails
entrailes (4×)

entren *v.* to enter
entre (2×)

enviŏus *adj. (1)* envious
enuyous (1×)

epilencie *n.* epilepsy
epilencie (19×)

epithīme *n.* thyme dodder (*Cuscuta epithymum*, fam. *Cuscutaceae*)
epithime (7×), *epithyme* (3×), *ephitime* (1×), *[e]pithime* (1×)

ēre *n. (1)* ear
eere (79×), *eeren* (34×), *eeres* (8×), *eeris* (8×), *eeryn* (2×), *eerys* (2×), *ieeres* (1×)

ērlī *adv.* early
erliche (1×), *erly* (1×)

ērn *n. (1)* ZOOL. eagle
heron (1×)

ērthe *n. (1)* earth
erþe (14×)

ērthen *adj.* earthen
erþen (5×), *erþenne* (1×)

ēse *n.* ease; health
eese (2×), *ese* (2×)

ēsē *adj.* convenient; gentle
esy (34×), *ese* (1×)

ēsen *v.* to ease
j-esyd (2×), *esid* (1×)

ēsīlī *adv.* easily
esily (4×), *esyly* (3×), *esile* (1×), *esiliche* (1×), *esyleche* (1×), *esyli* (1×), *esyliche* (1×)

ēst *n.* east
est (4×)

ēstward *adv.* eastwards
estward (2×)

ēst-wīnd *n.* wind blowing from the east
estwynd (1×)

esula *n.* esula (*Euphorbia uralensis*, fam. *Euphorbiaceae*)
esula (2×)

ēten *v.* to eat
ete (31×), *j-ete* (14×), *etyn* (10×), *eten* (8×), *j-etyn* (7×), *eteþ* (4×), *etiþ* (4×), *j-eten* (3×), *eete* (2×), *y-eten* (1×)

etīk *n. (2)* & *adj. (2)* MED. hectic (fever)
n.: etik (4×); *adj.: etik* (5×)

ēting(e *ng.* eating
etyng (6×), *etynge* (3×)

euforbia *n.* officinal spurge (*Euphorbia resinifera*, fam. *Euphorbiaceae*)
euforbe (21×), *euforbbe* (1×), *heuforbie*

(1×)
eufrāse *n.* euphrasy (*Euphrasia officinalis*, fam. *Scrophulariaceae*)
eufrace (12×), *eufrase* (2×), *eufras* (1×), *eufrasie* (1×)
ēve(n *n.* evening
eue (7×), *euene* (7×), *euen* (2×), *even* (1×)
ēven *adj.* even; *adv.* evenly
adj.: euene (1×); *adv.: euene* (5×), *euen* (1×)
ēvenlī *adj.* equal
euenly (1×)
ēve(n-sōng *n.* evening
euensong (1×)
ēve(n-tīde *n.* evening
euentide (2×), *euentyd* (1×), *euetid[e]* (1×), *eue-tyd* (1×), *euintide* (1×), *euyntid* (1×), *euyntide* (1×), *euyn-tyde* (1×)
ēver *adv.* ever
euer (9×), *euere* (2×), *euyr* (1×)
ever-euch-thing *n.* everything
eueriche-þing (1×)
everi-thing *n.* everything
euery-þing (1×)
ēver-mō(r *adv.* always
euermore (10×), *euer-more* (5×)
ēves *n.* eaves
euese (1×)
***exage** *n.* twelve pennyweight, six oz. Troy
exage (4×)
exaumple *n.* example
exaumpyl (1×)
excess *n.* excess
excesse (2×)
expērience *n.* experience
experience (1×)
expulsīf *n.* expulsive medicine (having power to expel or eliminate)
expulsiue (1×)
°**extenūātīf** *adj.* having power to make thin
extenuatif (1×)

F

fāce *n.* face
face (25×)
failen *v.* to fail
fayle (1×), *foileþ* (1×)
fair *adj.* fair
fair (1×), *feire* (1×), *feyer* (1×), *feyr* (1×)
falewī *adj.* reddish or brownish yellow
felawe (1×)
fallen *v.* to fall
falleþ (38×), *fallen* (24×), *falle* (23×), *fallyn* (4×), *fallyng* (4×), *j-fallen* (4×), *j-falle* (2×), *falliþ* (1×)
fallinge *ng.* & *ag.* falling
ng.: fallyng (13×), *fallynge* (2×), *falling* (1×), *fallynges* (1×); *ag.: fallyng* (1×)
fals *adj.* false
fals (1×)
falslī *adv.* falsely
falsly (1×)
fāren *v.* to travel
fareþ (1×)
fast(e *adv.* fast
fast (6×), *faste* (4×), *faast* (1×)
fasten *v.* *(1)* to fasten

fasse (1×), *j-fassyd* (1×)
fasten *v. (2)* to fast
faste (3×), *fastinge* (3×), *fastyng* (3×), *fasting* (2×), *fastynge* (2×), *fast* (1×)
fasting(e *ng. (2)* fasting
fastyng (7×), *fastinge* (1×), *fastynge* (1×)
fāt *adj.* fat
fat (8×), *fate* (1×)
fatnes(se *n.* fat
fatnesse (12×), *fat-nesse* (1×)
fattī *adj.* fatty
fatty (2×)
fēble *adj.* feeble
feble (44×), *febyl* (5×), *febil* (3×), *feblere* (3×), *febel* (1×), *febele* (1×), *fe-ble* (1×)
fēblen *v.* to enfeeble
j-feblyd (3×), *febeleþ* (2×), *febleþ* (2×), *j-feblid* (2×), *febeliþ* (1×), *febelyn* (1×), *j-febelid* (1×), *j-febelyd* (1×)
fēblenesse *n.* feebleness
feblenesse (20×), *febilnesse* (9×), *febelnesse* (6×), *febylnesse* (6×)
feblī(che *adv.* feebly
febeliche (2×), *febely* (2×), *febiliche* (1×), *febly* (1×), *feblysche* (1×)
fecche *n.* vetch (used as a measure of small quantity)
fetche (2×), *feche* (1×), *fuch* (1×), *veche* (1×)
fēden *v.* to feed
fedeþ (2×), *fede* (1×), *feede* (1×), *j-feed* (1×)
feith *n.* faith
feiþ (1×)
fēld *n.* field
feelde (1×), *feeldys* (1×), *feldis* (1×)
fēlen *v. (1)* to feel
feleþ (21×), *felen* (16×), *fele* (9×), *felyn* (7×), *feelyn* (3×), *j-fele* (3×), *feelen* (2×), *feeliþ* (2×), *feele* (1×), *felithe* (1×), *feliþ* (1×), *felt* (1×), *felun* (1×), *j-feeliþ* (1×), *j-feleþ* (1×), *j-felid* (1×), *j-felyn* (1×)
fēling(e *ng. (1)* feeling
felyng (4×), *feelinge* (1×), *felynge* (1×)
felt *n.* felt (fabric)
felt (1×), *felte* (1×)
fenel *n.* fennel (*Foeniculum vulgare*, fam. *Apiaceae*)
fenel (92×), *fenelle* (1×)
fēnigrēk *n.* fenugreek (*Trigonella foenum-graecum*, fam. *Fabaceae*)
femygrek (23×), *femigrek* (4×), *femy-grek* (1×)
fērdful *adj.* inclined to fear
ferdful (1×)
fērn *n. (1)* any member of the order *Filicales*, fern
feern (1×)
fērs *adj.* fierce, bold
fers (1×), *ferus* (1×)
ferting *ng.* farting
farting (1×)
fēsaunt *n.* ZOOL. pheasant
fesauntʒ (1×)
fēstre *n. (1)* fistula, fistulous wound
festre (5×), *feestre* (1×)
fēstringe *ng.* festering
festrynge (1×)
fether *n.* feather
feþere (2×)
fēver *n.* fever
feuere (77×), *feueres* (11×), *feuerys*

(5×), *feuer* (3×), *feueris* (3×), *fyuere* (2×)
fige *n.* (a) fig (*Ficus carica*, fam. *Moraceae*); (b) MED. **fige(s** piles or hemorrhoids
figes (16×), *figges* (7×), *figis* (2×), *fig* (1×), *fige* (1×), *figge* (1×), *fyges* (1×)
fighten *v.* to fight
fiteþ (1×), *fyte* (1×)
fighting(e *ng.* fighting
fytynges (1×)
filago *n.* prob. cudweed (*Gnaphalium uliginosum*, fam. *Asteraceae*)
filago (2×)
filipendula *n.* dropwort (*Spiraea filipendula*, fam. *Rosaceae*)
filipendula (2×), *filip[e]ndula* (1×)
fillen *v.* to fill
filleþ (4×), *fille* (2×), *fillen* (2×), *filled* (1×), *fyllyd* (1×)
filth *n.* filth
filþe (2×)
fīnden *v.* to find
fynde (2×), *fyndeþ* (1×), *j-founden* (1×), *j-foundyn* (1×)
finger *n.* finger
fynger (4×), *fingeris* (1×), *fyngere* (1×), *fyngeres* (1×), *fyngeris* (1×), *fyngerys* (1×), *fyngre* (1×), *fyngres* (1×), *fyngris* (1×), *fyngur* (1×)
fīr *n.* fire
fier (9×), *feyr* (8×), *feir* (5×), *feire* (5×), *fyer* (5×), *fere* (4×), *feer* (3×), *fiere* (3×), *fyere* (3×), *feere* (1×), *feirys* (1×), *feiȝere* (1×), *fer* (1×), *feyren* (1×)
fīrī *adj.* fiery
feire (1×)
fish *n.* ZOOL. fish
fischȝ (5×), *fische* (3×), *fysch* (3×), *fisches* (2×), *fisch* (1×), *[f]ischȝ* (1×), *fysche* (1×), *fyschȝ* (1×)
flāke *n.* *(2)* layer
flake (1×)
flank(e *n.* flank
flancke (2×), *flanke* (1×)
flēsh *n.* flesh
fleische (19×), *flesche* (9×), *fleisch* (4×), *fleischȝ* (1×), *flesch* (1×), *fleschȝ* (1×)
flēshlī(ch *adj.* fleshy
fleischly (1×)
flēting *ag.* *(1)* flowing
fletynge (1×)
fleumagog *n.* phlegmagogue (drug for purging excess phlegm)
fleumagoge (5×), *flewmagoge* (2×)
fleumatīk *n.* pathological excess of phlegm; *adj.* phlegmatic
n.: *fleumatica* (1×); *adj.*: *fleumatic* (8×), *fleumatik* (8×), *flegmatik* (2×), *fleumatyk* (2×), *fleumatike* (1×), *flewmatik* (1×)
fleum(e *n.* phlegm
flewme (111×), *fleume* (30×), *flewmes* (1×)
flex *n.* flax (*Linum usitatissimum*, fam. *Linaceae*)
filix (1×), *flax* (1×)
flīe *n.* *(1)* ZOOL. any insect that flies
flee (1×), *fliees* (1×), *flien* (1×), *flye* (1×)
flīen *v.* to fly
fleen (1×), *fleeþ* (1×)
flouen *v.* to flow
floweþ (11×), *flowen* (9×), *flow* (3×),

flowe (3×), *floweden* (1×), *flowynge* (1×), *j-flowed* (1×)

flouing *ng.* flow(ing)
flowyng (16×), *flowynge* (10×), *flowing* (2×), *flowinge* (1×)

flŏur *n. (1)* (a) flower; (b) menstrual flow
floures (13×), *flowres* (2×), *flewr* (1×), *flour* (1×), *flowr* (1×), *flowre* (1×)

flŏur *n. (2)* flour
flour (2×), *flowre* (1×)

flŏur-de-līce *n.* fleur-de-lis (genus *Iris*, fam. *Iridaceae*)
flourdeliȝ (1×)

flux *n.* flow
flux (56×), *fluxes* (7×), *fluxe* (2×) [see also **blōdī**]

fnēsen *v.* to sneeze
fnese (9×), *fn[e]se* (1×), *fneseþ* (1×), *fnesynge* (1×)

fnēsing *ng.* sneezing
fnesinge (1×), *fn[e]synge* (1×)

fōl-hardī *adj.* foolhardy, foolishly daring
ful-hardy (1×)

fōlīe *n.* folly
foly (1×)

***folii** *n.* leaves of trees of the cinnamon fam. (*Lauraceae*)
folie (2×), *folium* (2×), *folii* (1×), *folij* (1×)

folk *n.* folk
folk (14×), *folkes* (1×)

folwen *v.* to follow
folewеþ (2×), *folowеþ* (2×), *folewen* (1×), *folweþ* (1×)

fōm *n.* foam
fome (1×), *foom* (1×)

fōmen *v.* to foam at the mouth, to slaver
fomen (1×)

fōmī *adj.* foamy
fomy (2×)

forbrennen *v.* to burn up
forbrent (1×)

fordōn *v.* to destroy
for-doþ (2×)

fōr(e-said *ppl.* aforesaid
for-seid (24×), *forseid* (11×), *for-seyd* (7×), *forseyd* (6×)

fōr(e-saien *v.* to say previously
for-seid (1×)

fōrhēd *n.* forehead
forheed (6×), *foreheed* (5×), *for-heed* (5×), *fore-heed* (4×), *for-hed* (3×), *forhed* (1×)

fōrme *n.* form
forme (4×)

forsōth *adv.* indeed
for-soþe (2×)

fōrth *adv.* forth
forþ (7×)

fōrth-bī *adv.* past, alongside
forþ-by (1×)

forwelked *ppl.* withered
forwelkyd (1×)

foryētful *adj.* forgetful
for-ȝeteful (1×), *forȝetefulle* (1×), *for-ȝetful* (1×), *for-ȝytful* (1×)

foryētfulness(e *n.* forgetfulness
forȝetfulnesse (1×)

ᵒ**foryēveri** *adj.* forgiving
for-ȝeuery (1×)

fōt *n.* foot
feet (16×), *fete* (3×), *feete* (2×), *foot*

(2×), *foote* (2×)
fŏul *n.* ZOOL. fowl
foulys (1×)
fŏundement *n.* (a) bottom, base; (b) ANAT. lower extremity of rectum, anus
foundement (9×), *fundement* (5×), *fondement* (1×), *founde-ment* (1×), *fundament* (1×)
fox *n.* ZOOL. fox
fox (3×), *foxis* (1×), *foxys* (1×)
frēnd *n.* friend
frend (1×)
frēndful *adj.* friendly
frendful (1×), *frendfulle* (1×)
frenesīe *n.* frenzy
frenesie (4×), *frenesi* (3×), *frenesy* (1×), *frenesye* (1×)
frenetīk *adj.* frantic
frentik (3×), *frentic* (1×), *frentyk* (1×), *frentyke* (1×)
frēsen *v.* to freeze
for-frosen (1×)
frēsh *adj.* fresh
freische (4×), *freischȝ* (3×), *fresche* (3×), *freisch* (1×)
frēten *v. (1)* MED. to corrode, to destroy
frete (12×), *freten* (4×), *freteþ* (4×), *fretyn* (2×), *fretyt* (1×), *j-frete* (1×)
frētere *n.* corrosive substance
freteres (1×)
frēting MED. *ng. (1)* corrosion or destruction of bodily tissue; *ag.* gnawing (pain)
ng.: fretynge (1×); *ag.: fretyng* (2×), *fretynge* (1×)
frīen *v. (3)* to fry
frie (3×), *fried* (2×), *j-fried* (2×), *j-friȝed* (2×), *j-fryid* (2×), *friȝed* (1×), *fryed* (1×)
frōten *v.* to rub
frote (7×), *froten* (3×), *froot* (1×), *frotyn* (1×), *j-froted* (1×), *y-froted* (1×)
frōtinge *ng.* rubbing
frotynges (1×)
fruit *n.* fruit
fruyt (3×), *frutys* (2×), *fruytis* (2×), *fruȝt* (2×), *frutes* (1×), *fruytes* (1×), *fruȝth* (1×), *frytis* (1×)
frumentē *n.* frumenty (potage made of boiled hulled grain mixed with milk)
fur-mente (1×), *furmente* (1×)
ful *adj.* & *adv.* full
adj.: ful (38×), *fulle* (8×), *full* (1×), *fullere* (1×); *adv.: ful* (119×), *fulle* (4×)
ful-fillen *v.* to fill
fulfilyeþ (1×)
fullī *adv.* fully
fullyche (1×)
fulnes(se *n.* (a) fullness; (b) MED. repletion of humours, plethora
fulnesse (6×)
ful-waxen *ppl.* full-grown
fulwex (1×)
fūme *n.* (odorous) smoke, vapour
fume (10×), *fumes* (4×)
fūmetēre *n.* fumitory (*Fumaria officinalis*, fam. *Fumariaceae*)
fumytre (2×)
fūmigāciŏun *n.* MED. suffumigation
fumigacioun (15×), *fumigacion* (3×),

fumigaciouns (3×), *fumygacion* (3×), *fumygacioun* (2×), *fumigacyouns* (1×), *fumygaciouns* (1×)
further *adj.* & *adv.* further
adj.: forþere (1×), *furþere* (1×); *adv.: for-þer* (1×)

G

Gābrīel *n.* Archangel Gabriel
Gabriel (1×)
gaderen *v.* to gather
j-gaderid (3×), *gadere* (2×), *gaderid* (1×), *gaderyth* (1×), *j-gaderyd* (1×)
gaderinge *ng.* MED. & SURG. gathering of corrupt humours
gaderyng (2×)
galanga *n.* [see **galingāle**]
galange (1×)
galban(e *n.* galbanum (gum resin obtained from certain plants of the genus *Ferula*, fam. *Apiaceae*)
galbanum (14×)
Galien *n.* Galen
g[alieni] (2×), *galienes* (1×), *galieni* (1×), *galiens* (1×)
galingāle *n.* galingale (*Alpinia galanga* or *officinarum*, fam. *Zingiberaceae*)
galingale (12×), *galyngale* (3×), *galynggale* (2×), *galinge* (1×)
galle *n. (1)* gall
galle (37×), *galles* (7×)
galle *n. (3)* oak gall (excrescence on an oak leaf)
galles (16×), *gallos* (1×)
***gallia muscata** *n.* medicine containing musk
gallia muscata (1×), *gallie muscate* (1×)
gallitricum *n.* [see **centrum galli**]
gallitricum (1×)
gandre *n.* ZOOL. gander
gandre (3×), *gandderis* (1×), *gandris* (1×)
gardin *n.* garden
gardyns (1×)
gargarisme *n.* MED. gargle
gargarisme (17×), *gargarismes* (1×), *gargarismis* (1×), *gargarismus* (1×), *gargarysme* (1×), *gargorisme* (1×)
gār-lēk *n.* garlic (*Allium sativum*, fam. *Liliaceae*)
garlek (8×), *garlec* (3×)
garsen *v.* SURG. to make cuts or incisions in order to let blood; to scarify
garsyd (2×), *garsen* (1×), *garsyn* (1×), *j-garsid* (1×)
garsinge *ng.* SURG. scarification
gar-synge (1×), *garsynge* (1×)
ğelē *n.* jelly
gelee (1×)
ğenciān(e *n.* yellow gentian (*Gentiana lutea*, fam. *Gentianaceae*)
genciane (5×), *gencian* (1×)
ğendren *v.* to produce
j-genderid (8×), *genderiþ* (2×), *genderid* (1×), *genderyn* (1×), *genderythe* (1×), *gendreþ* (1×), *gendriþ* (1×), *gendryd* (1×), *j-gendered* (1×), *j-genderyd* (1×), *j-gendrid* (1×), *j-gendryd* (1×)
ğendringe *ng.* production
genderinge (1×)

ğenerāllī *adv.* generally
generaly (1×)
ğenerātīf *adj.* productive
generatyf (1×)
gēten *v. (1)* to get
get (1×)
gīle *n. (3)* treachery
gyle (1×)
ğinğivere *n.* ginger (*Zingiber officinale*, fam. *Zingiberaceae*)
gynger (38×), *gyngere* (5×), *ginger* (4×), *ȝinȝibere* (1×)
ğipsum *n.* gypsum
gipsum (1×)
girdel *n.* belt
gerdyl (1×)
gith *n.* black seed (*Nigella sativa*, fam. *Ranunculaceae*)
gith (3×)
glād *adj.* glad
glad (3×), *glaad* (1×)
glādlī *adv.* gladly
gladly (1×)
gladnes(se *n.* gladness
gladnesse (2×)
glaire *n.* white of an egg, albumen
gleire (12×), *gleyre* (3×), *gleir* (1×), *gle[ire]* (1×), *gleyr* (1×)
glas *n.* glass
glas (4×), *glos* (2×)
glāsen *adj.* made of glass
glassen (1×)
glāsī *adj.* of phlegm: thick, viscid, and glass-coloured
glasi (5×)
glet *n.* mucus
glat (6×), *glet* (1×)
gleu *n.* glue
glew (1×)
glouinge *ag.* glowing
glowyng (3×), *glowynge* (1×), *glowȝyng* (1×)
gnauen *v.* (a) to gnaw; (b) ANAT. & MED. to corrode (organic tissue)
gnawe (2×), *gnawyn* (1×)
gnauing(e *ng.* (a) gnawing; (b) MED. corrosion (of organic tissue)
gnawyng (5×), *gnawing* (1×), *gnawinges* (1×), *gnawynge* (1×)
gobet *n.* lump; medicinal pellet
gobetes (3×), *gobet* (1×), *gobetis* (1×), *gobettes* (1×)
gobetmēle *adv.* bit by bit
gobet-mele (1×), *gobetmele* (1×)
God *n. (1)* God
god (3×), *goddes* (1×), *goddus* (1×), *goddys* (1×)
gōd *n. (2)*, *adj.*, & *adv.* good
n.: good (2×); *adj.: good* (292×), *goode* (12×), *gode* (2×); *adv.: good* (1×)
gōdnes(se *n. (2)* goodness
godenesse (1×)
gōld *n.* gold
goold (12×), *gold* (1×), *goolde* (1×)
gōme *n. (3)* flesh surrounding the teeth, gums
gomes (7×), *gomys* (4×)
gŏmme *n.* gum
gumme (12×)
~ **Arabī**, ~ **Arabīk**, gum from certain species of acacia [see **acācia**]
gum arabik (14×), *gumme arabik* (14×), *gum arabe* (6×), *gumi arabe* (4×), *gumme arabe* (4×), *gumi arabik* (1×), *gumy arabik* (1×)

*__gomorra__ *n.* uncontrolled flow of sperm
gomorra (1×)

gōn *v.* to go
gooþ (16×), *go* (9×), *goon* (7×), *goiþ* (4×), *gon* (3×), *goo* (3×), *goynge* (3×), *goþ* (2×), *goyng* (2×), *gooithe* (1×)

gorst *n.* gorse (*Ulex europaeus*, fam. *Fabaceae*)
gorst (2×)

gōs *n.* ZOOL. goose
goce (1×), *goos* (1×), *goose* (1×)

gōstlī *adj.* spiritual
gostly (1×)

gōt *n.* ZOOL. goat
gootes (12×), *gotes* (9×), *gotus* (7×), *goot* (5×), *gotys* (4×), *gootys* (3×), *gootis* (2×), *gootus* (2×), *gotis* (2×)

gŏurd(e *n.* *Cucurbitaceae* fam.: (a) cucumber (*Cucumis sativus*); (b) colocynth (*Citrullus colocynthis*); (c) gourd (*Lagenaria vulgaris* or *siceraria*); (d) water-melon (*Citrullus vulgaris*)
gourdys (16×), *gourde* (9×), *gourdes* (9×), *gourdis* (8×), *goorde* (2×), *gordis* (1×), *gou[r]de* (1×)

gŏute *n.* *(1)* gout
goutes (5×), *goute* (2×)

grāce *n.* God's grace
grace (2×)

grain *n.* (a) grain; (b) spice, esp. seed of *Amomum meleguetta*, fam. *Zingiberaceae*
greyns (7×), *greins* (6×), *greynes* (3×), *greynys* (2×), *greyn* (1×), *greynnis* (1×)

ºgranumsolis *n.* [see **grŏmil**]
granumsolis (1×)

grāpe *n.* *(1)* grape (*Vitis vinifera*, fam. *Vitaceae*)
grapys (2×), *grapes* (1×)

gras *n.* red clover (*Trifolium pratense*, fam. *Fabaceae*)
iij-leuyd gras (1×)

gras-hoppere *n.* ZOOL. grasshopper
grashopperes (4×), *grashopperis* (2×), *gras-hopperes* (1×), *gras-hopperis* (1×)

gravel *n.* gravel
grauel (9×), *gravel* (1×)

grēne *adj.* green
grene (20×)

grēnish *adj.* greenish
grenysche (1×)

grennen *v.* to grin
grenyng (1×)

grēs(e *n.* grease
grece (32×), *greces* (1×), *grese* (1×)

grēt *n.*, *adj.*, & *adv.* great
n.: grete (1×); *adj.: gret* (151×), *greet* (17×), *grete* (12×), *grettere* (6×), *gretter* (3×), *grettest* (2×), *gretere* (1×), *grette* (1×), *grett[e]re* (1×), *grettyr* (1×); *adv.: gret* (2×)

grēt-hēded *adj.* having a large head; ?stubborn
gret-hedid (1×)

grētnes(se *n.* quantity
gretnesse (2×)

grēvaunce *n.* sickness; injury
greuaunce (150×), *greuaunces* (33×), *greuance* (17×), *greuannce* (9×), *greuances* (4×), *greuannces* (3×), *greuauncee* (1×), *greuauncis* (1×), *greuauncys* (1×), *greuaunnce* (1×),

greuuance (1×), *greuuances* (1×), *greuuaunces* (1×), *grewance* (1×)

grēven *v.* to injure; to afflict
greueþ (13×), *j-greuyd* (7×), *j-greued* (3×), *j-greuid* (3×), *greuyd* (2×), *greue* (1×), *greued* (1×), *greuen* (1×), *greuueþ* (1×), *greuyn* (1×), *greuyth* (1×)

grēvǒus *adj.* serious, severe
greuouse (12×), *greuous* (6×), *greuouce* (1×), *greuows* (1×)

grēvǒustē *n.* heaviness
greuoste (1×), *greuouste* (1×)

grīnden *v. (1)* to grind
j-ground (3×), *grinde* (1×), *grinden* (1×), *grynd* (1×), *grynde* (1×), *gryndeþ* (1×), *j-grond* (1×)

grīnd-stōn *n.* millstone
gryndyngstoon (1×)

grinten *v.* to grind (one's teeth)
grynteþ (1×)

grǒmil *n.* common gromwell (*Lithospermum officinale*, fam. *Boraginaceae*)
gromyl (1×)

grouen *v.* to grow
groweþ (7×), *growen* (3×), *grow* (2×), *growe* (1×), *growyng* (1×), *growynge* (1×), *growyth* (1×)

grǒund *n.* ground
ground (7×), *grounde* (3×), *grownd* (1×)

grǒunde-swilie *n.* European groundsel (*Senecio vulgaris*, fam. *Asteraceae*)
groundeswily (1×), *ground-swily* (1×), *groundyswily* (1×), *growndeswili* (1×)

grūel *n.* gruel
grwel (2×), *grewel* (1×)

gut *n.* gut
guttes (101×), *gutte* (19×), *guttys* (6×), *gut* (4×)

gutta rosacea *n.* pustules on the face or body
gutta rosacea (1×), *gvtta rosacea* (1×)

H

hakken *v.* to hack, to chop into small pieces
j-hacked (1×)

half *n.* & *adv.* half
n.: half (11×); *adv.: half* (1×)

halm *n.* straw
halm (1×)

halven-dēl(e *n.* half portion of anything
halfendel (1×)

hamme *n. (1)* part of the human leg which is behind the knee
hamme (1×)

happenen *v.* to happen
hapneþ (3×), *happeneþ* (2×)

hard *adj.* hard; firm
hard (33×), *harde* (5×), *hardere* (3×), *haard* (1×)

harde *adv.* tightly
harde (2×)

harden *v.* to harden
j-hardid (2×), *hardid* (1×), *hardyd* (1×), *j-harded* (1×), *j-hardedit* (1×), *j-hardyd* (1×)

hard-hōlden *v.* to hold hard
hardholdynge (1×)

hardī *adj.* bold

hardy (2×)
hardīnes(se *n.* bravery
hardinesse (1×)
hardnes(se *n.* (a) hardness; (b) MED. morbid hardening or hardness of a bodily substance, tissue, or structure
hardnesse (31×), *hardnesche* (1×)
hāre *n.* ZOOL. hare
hare (11×), *haare* (2×), *haares* (1×), *harys* (1×)
harm *n.* harm
harm (4×), *harme* (1×)
harming(e *ng.* harm
harmyng (1×)
harsk *adj.* harsh
harsche (1×)
hāselin *n.* made of hazel
aselyn (1×), *haselen* (1×)
hāstī(e *adj.* hasty
hasty (2×)
hāstīlī(e *adv.* hastily
hastiliche (1×)
hāven *v.* to have
haþ (191×), *han* (161×), *haue* (129×), *haaþ* (16×), *hadden* (6×), *j-haad* (5×), *hast* (4×), *haast* (2×), *[haþ]* (2×), *j-had* (2×), *j-haþ* (2×), *haad* (1×), *haan* (1×), *hadde* (1×), *haiþ* (1×), *[han]* (1×), *hanne* (1×), *haste* (1×), *hath* (1×), *hathe* (1×), *haþe* (1×), *hauynge* (1×)
hēd *n. (1)* head
heed (186×), *hed* (7×), *hedde* (1×), *heede* (1×), *heedes* (1×)
hēd-āche *n.* headache
heed-ache (4×), *heedache* (3×), *hed-ache* (2×), *hedache* (2×)
heft *n.* weight
heeftes (1×)
heigh *adj.* high
heiȝ (6×), *hiȝe* (6×), *hey* (2×), *heiȝere* (1×)
height(e *n.* height
heyȝte (1×)
hei-hōve *n.* ground ivy (*Nepeta hederacea*, fam. *Lamiaceae*)
heihoue (4×), *heyhoue* (2×)
hēle *n. (1)* health
heele (1×)
hēlen *v. (1)* to heal
hele (20×), *j-heelid* (14×), *j-helyd* (14×), *j-heelyd* (12×), *heele* (7×), *j-helid* (7×), *heelid* (6×), *heelyd* (6×), *heleþ* (4×), *helyd* (4×), *heelen* (3×), *helen* (3×), *helid* (3×), *helyn* (3×), *heeliþ* (2×), *heeled* (1×), *heelneþ* (1×), *hel[e]d* (1×), *heleeþ* (1×), *heliþ* (1×), *helyng* (1×), *holeþ* (1×), *hoolid* (1×), *hoolyd* (1×), *j-heleed* (1×), *j-holyd* (1×), *jhoolid* (1×)
hēlen *v. (2)* to cover
heled (1×)
hēling(e *ng. (1)* healing
helyng (3×), *heelyng* (1×), *helynge* (1×)
help *n.* help
helþ (3×), *helþe* (1×)
helpen *v.* to help
helþeþ (8×), *helþe* (7×), *holþen* (5×), *j-holþen* (5×), *holþyn* (4×), *j-holþe* (4×), *helþ* (2×), *j-holþyn* (2×), *helþyn* (1×), *holþ* (1×), *hoolþyn* (1×), *j-hoolþen* (1×)
helpinge *ng.* improvement
helþing (1×)

hemlok(e *n.* hemlock (*Conium maculatum*, fam. *Apiaceae*)
hemlok (1×)
hemp *n.* hemp (*Cannabis sativa*, fam. *Cannabaceae*)
hemp (1×), *hempe* (1×)
hemp-sēd *n.* hempseed
hempseed (1×)
hen *n. (1)* ZOOL. hen
hen (8×), *henne* (7×), *heen* (3×), *hennes* (3×), *hennys* (3×), *hennus* (1×)
***henbane** *n.* henbane (*Hyoscyamus niger*, fam. *Solanaceae*)
hennebane (9×), *henbane* (7×)
°**henshelleful** *n.* measure of volume
henneschelful (1×), *henschel-ful* (1×)
hēr *n.* hair
heeris (7×), *heer* (3×), *heere* (3×), *herys* (3×), *heerys* (2×), *here* (2×), *heeres* (1×), *heres* (1×), *heris* (1×), *hers* (1×)
hēr *adv.* here
here (19×)
hēr-after *adv.* hereafter
here-after (1×)
hēr-after-wārd *adv.* hereafter
here-aftur-ward (1×)
hērbe *n.* herb
herbe (55×), *herbys* (28×), *herbis* (27×), *erbis* (2×), *erbys* (2×), *erbe* (1×)
hēr-bifōre(n *adv.* previously
here-be-fore (5×), *here-before* (4×), *here-bi-fore* (1×)
hērd(e *n. (3)* coarse part of flax
herdys (1×)
hēred *ppl.* haired
j-heeryd (2×)
hēren *v.* to hear
here (1×)
hēr-for *adv.* for this reason
here-fore (2×)
hērī *adj.* hairy
heery (2×)
hērīnesse *n.* hairiness
herynesse (1×)
hēring(e *ng.* hearing
heryng (2×), *heringe* (1×), *herynge* (1×)
hēr-in(ne *adv.* herein
here-inne (1×)
hermodactiles *n.* dried root, prob. that of an Asiatic plant (*Colchicum luteum*, fam. *Colchicaceae*)
hermedactile (1×), *hermodactile* (1×), *hermodactiles* (1×)
hēr-of *adv.* hereof
here-of (28×)
hert *n.* ZOOL. male red deer, hart
hertes (5×), *hert* (1×), *hertys* (1×)
herte *n.* heart
herte (33×), *hert* (20×), *hertes* (1×), *hertys* (1×)
hertes-horn *n.* (a) horn or antler of a hart; medicinal substance derived from burning the horn; (b) some kind of plant
hertes-horn (5×), *herteshorn* (1×), *hertyshorn* (1×)
hert(es-tŏnge *n.* hart's-tongue fern (*Phyllitis scolopendrium*, fam. *Aspleniaceae*)
hertistunge (6×), *hertes-tounge* (1×), *hertestunge* (1×), *hertistonge* (1×), *hertis-tounge* (1×), *hertystounge* (1×),

hertystunge (1×)
hēr-tō *adv.* hereto
here-to (1×)
hervest *n.* autumn
heruest (8×)
hēr-with *adv.* in addition to this
herewiþ (4×), *here-with* (2×)
hēte *n. (1)* heat
heete (131×), *hete* (62×), *heet* (1×), *heetes* (1×), *heetus* (1×), *hetes* (1×)
hēten *v.* to heat
heete (4×), *hete* (3×), *heetyn* (2×), *hetyn* (2×), *j-hat* (2×), *heet* (1×), *heeteþ* (1×), *j-het* (1×), *yhat* (1×)
hētenes *n.* hotness
hetnesse (1×)
hētinge *ng.* heating
heetyng (1×)
hēven *n.* heaven
heuyn (1×)
hēven *v.* to lift up
heuyn (2×), *heue* (1×), *heuen* (1×), *heueþ* (1×)
hēvī *adj.* heavy
heuy (25×), *[h]euy* (1×)
hēvīen *v.* MED. to afflict with disease
heuyeþ (1×), *j-heuyed* (1×)
hēvīnes(se *n.* heaviness; disease
heuynesse (56×), *heuinesse* (1×), *heuynesche* (1×), *heyuynesse* (1×)
hīden *v.* to hide
j-hyd (3×), *hideþ* (2×), *hiden* (1×), *hyd* (1×), *y-hid* (1×)
hider-wārd *adv.* in this direction
hidurward (1×)
hīen *v.* to act quickly
hie (1×)
hil(le *n.* hill
hillys (1×)
hillī *adj.* hilly
hilly (1×)
hīnder *adj. (1)* back
hyndrere (6×), *hendrere* (2×), *hindre* (1×), *hyndere* (1×)
hipe *n.* hip
hepis (2×)
hok(ke *n. (1)* any of several plants of the related genera *Malva* and *Althaea*, fam. *Malvaceae*; esp. common mallow (*Malva sylvestris*) and marsh mallow (*Althaea officinalis*)
hockes (34×), *hockys* (16×), *hocke* (6×), *hockis* (1×)
hōlden *v. (1)* to hold
hoolde (5×), *holden* (3×), *holdyn* (3×), *hoolden* (3×), *holdeþ* (2×), *j-holdyn* (2×), *j-hoolden* (2×), *helde* (1×), *helden* (1×), *heldist* (1×), *hold* (1×), *holde* (1×), *holdiþ* (1×), *hoold* (1×), *hooldyn* (1×), *j-holde* (1×), *j-holden* (1×), *j-hoold* (1×)
hol(e *n. (1)* husk
hooles (2×)
hōl(e *n. (2)* hole
hoole (7×), *hooles* (4×), *hole* (2×), *holys* (2×)
hōl(e *adj. (2)* healed, healthy
hool (11×), *hole* (1×), *hoole* (1×)
hōl(e *adv.* wholly
hool (3×)
holen *v. (1)* to peel
j-hool (1×)
hōlen *v. (2)* to make a hole
hooled (1×), *hoolid* (1×)
hōlī *adj. (2)* holy

hooly (2×)

hōlī-hok(ke *n.* marsh mallow (*Althaea officinalis*, fam. *Malvaceae*)

holy-hocke (7×), *holyhocke* (4×), *holy-hockes* (1×), *hoolihocke* (1×), *hoolihockyn* (1×), *hoolihockys* (1×), *hooly-hocke* (1×), *hoolyhockys* (1×)

hōlsǒm *adj.* wholesome

holmsome (1×), *holsomere* (1×)

holwe *adj.* hollow

holow (2×), *holwe* (2×), *holewe* (1×)

holwenes(se *n.* hollowness

holownesse (4×), *holwenesse* (2×), *hollownesse* (1×), *holwnesse* (1×)

hōnd(e *n.* hand

hondys (7×), *hond* (5×), *hand* (4×), *hondes* (2×), *hoond* (2×), *honde* (1×), *hondis* (1×), *hoondes* (1×), *hoondis* (1×), *hoondys* (1×)

hōndful *n.* handful (as a measure)

handful (1×), *hanful* (1×)

hōndling(e *ng.* handling

handlynge (1×)

hōngen *v.* to hang

hangen (3×), *hange* (1×), *hangeþ* (1×), *hongen* (1×)

hǒnī *n.* honey

hony (128×), *honi* (1×)

~ **rōsēt**, MED. mixture of hony and roses

hony roset (3×)

hōpeful *adj.* hopeful

hapfulle (1×)

hōr *adj.* gray (esp. of hair or beard)

hoor (1×)

hōr(e-hǒune *n.* horehound (*Marrubium vulgare*, fam. *Lamiaceae*); **whīt ~**

horehowne (10×), *horehoune* (4×), *horhowne* (4×), *horhoune* (2×), *hore-howne* (1×)

horn *n.* (a) horn; (b) SURG. vessel used in phlebotomy

hornes (4×), *horn* (3×), *hoorn* (1×)

***horned clōth** *n.* ANAT. cornea

horned clooþ (1×)

ºhornen *v.* SURG. to bleed (sth.) by means of a horn

j-horned (1×)

hors *n.* ZOOL. horse

horsys (1×)

hors-elne *n.* horseheal, elecampane (*Inula helenium*, fam. *Asteraceae*)

horsel (4×), *horshel* (2×), *horsheel* (1×)

horsinge *ng.* rushing about noisily [cf. *MED*]

horsynge (1×)

hōsnes(se *n.* hoarseness

horsnesse (11×), *hoorsnesse* (3×), *hoosnesse* (3×)

hōt *adj.* hot

hoot (133×), *hoote* (106×), *hote* (15×), *hattere* (1×), *hee[t]* (1×), *hoo[t]* (1×), *hootte* (1×), *hot* (1×), *j-hoot* (1×)

hōten *v. (1)* to name

hatte (4×), *hite* (1×), *hiȝt* (1×)

hōtnes(se *n.* PHYS. & MED. dominant hot quality

hootnesse (2×), *hotnesse* (1×)

hǒund *n.* ZOOL. hound

houndys (5×), *hound* (2×), *houndes* (2×)

hǒundes-tǒnge *n.* hound's-tongue (*Cynoglossum officinale*, fam.

Boraginaceae)
houndestonge (7×)
hŏure *n.* hour
houres (9×), *houre* (2×), *howres* (1×)
hŏus *n.* house
hows (6×)
hōven *v. (1)* to hover
houeþ (2×), *houe* (1×)
hōven *v. (2)* to need, to be necessary
houeþ (1×)
hūğelī *adv.* hugely
hugely (1×)
hūmŏur *n.* ANAT. one of four fluids (blood, phlegm, choler, melancholy) which form and nourish the body
humours (155×), *humour* (99×), *humuros* (86×), *humures* (16×), *humoures* (4×), *humurus* (3×), *humurs* (2×), *humorys* (1×), *humoure* (1×), *humoureres* (1×), *humur* (1×)
hurling(e *ng.* rumbling of the stomach or the bowels
hurlyng (4×), *hurlinges* (1×), *[h]urlyng* (1×), *hurlynge* (1×)
hurten *v.* to hurt
hirteþ (1×)
hurting(e *ng.* (a) hurting; (b) wound; disease
hurtyng (2×), *hertynge* (1×), *hirtynge* (1×), *hyrtyng* (1×)

I

īdelnes(se *n.* idleness
ydelnesse (1×)
***iera** *n.* purging electuary
iera (1×)
~ **fortissima**, purging electuary
iora fortissima (1×)
īles-pīl *n.* ZOOL. hedgehog
ylspil (1×)
ilīche *adv.* alike
j-liche (28×), *j-lyche* (22×), *i-liche* (1×), *iliche* (1×), *j-lyke* (1×), *ylyche* (1×)
īlik passio *n.* intestinal disorder due to obstruction in the ileum, colic
jlica passio (1×)
iliŏun *n.* ileum (portion of the small intestine which opens into the caecum)
jlion (1×)
incommoditē *n.* sickness
incomodites (1×)
incūrāble *adj.* incurable
incurable (8×), *incurabil* (2×), *incurabile* (1×), *in-curable* (1×), *on-curabil* (1×), *oncurabil* (1×)
Inde *adj. (1)* type of myrobalan: ripe fruit of *Terminalia citrina*, fam. *Combretaceae* [cf. *MED*]
indj (7×), *inde* (1×), *indi* (1×), *ind[i]* (1×), *ynde* (1×)
indīğestiŏun *n.* indigestion
indigestion (1×)
indignāciŏun *n.* irritation of the stomach
indignacion (1×)
indispōsed *ppl.* diseased
indisposed (1×)
°**indorum** *adj.* of India
indorum (1×)
infecciŏun *n.* infection
infeccioun (4×), *infeccion* (1×),

infeccions (1×), *jnfeccion* (1×)
infecten *v.* to infect
infect (2×), *infecte* (1×)
inflātīve *adj.* of food: causing swelling, producing wind
inflatif (1×)
infūse *adj.* infused
infuse (3×)
inmōst *adj.* innermost
inmast (1×)
inne *adv.* in
inne (32×), *in* (1×)
inner(e *adj.* inner
innere (8×), *inn[e]re* (1×)
*__innibes__ *n.* common jujube (*Zizyphus jujuba*, fam. *Rhamnaceae*)
innibes (7×), *inimbes* (5×)
inough *adv.* enough
j-now (7×), *j-nowȝ* (1×)
inscīsīf *adj.* MED. & SURG. having the property of dissolving viscous, thick, or heavy humours
inscisif (1×)
instrūment *n.* instrument
instrumentes (2×)
in-wārd *adv.* inwards
in-ward (1×), *inward* (1×), *inwarde* (1×)
iperīcon *n.* St.-John's-wort (*Hypericum perforatum*, fam. *Clusiaceae*)
ypericon (2×), *jperi[c]on* (1×), *ypericoun* (1×)
ipoquistidos *n.* hypocistis (pharmaceutical preparation made from the thickened juice of the parasitic plant *Cytinus hypocistis*, fam. *Cytinaceae*)
ypoquyscidos (2×), *ipoqwyssides* (1×), *jpoquisides* (1×), *ypoquyscides* (1×), *ypo-quyscidos* (1×)
īren *n.* iron
yren (4×), *eyren* (3×)
īreos *n.* Florentine iris (*Iris florentina*, fam. *Iridaceae*)
yreos (6×), *yrees* (2×), *yren* (1×)
īsōpe *n.* *(1)* hyssop (*Hyssopus officinalis*, fam. *Lamiaceae*)
ysope (32×), *jsope* (2×), *isope* (1×)
issūe *n.* (a) defecation; (b) discharge
issu (3×), *issue* (2×)
ivel *n.* disease; *adj.* evil
n.: *euel* (5×), *euele* (3×), *e[uel]* (1×), *euelys* (1×); *adj.*: *euel* (18×), *euyl* (3×), *euele* (2×)
īvī *n.* European ivy (*Hedera helix*, fam. *Araliaceae*)
yuy (7×), *iuen* (1×), *yue* (1×)
īvorī(e *n.* & *adj.* ivory
n.: *yuer* (1×), *yuory* (1×); *adj.*: *yuory* (2×)

J

jacinct(e *n.* jacinth (precious stone)
jacinctus (1×)
jarus *n.* [see **āron**]
jary (1×)
jaunīs *n.* jaundice
jaundes (1×)
jera-logodiōn *n.* purgative medicine
yeralogodion (1×)
jera-pigra *n.* hiera picra, a purgative containing aloes
yerapigra (3×), *ierapigra* (2×),

jerapigra (1×), *jerapigre* (1×), *yera-pigra* (1×)
jera-ruffini *n.* purgative medicine
ierarufa (1×)
joi(e *n.* joy
ioy (1×), *ioye* (1×)
joinen *v. (1)* to join
ioynen (1×)
joint *n. (1)* joint between bones
ioyntes (2×), *ioint* (1×), *joynt* (1×), *joyntes* (1×)
jubbe *n.* upper convex surface of the liver
gibbe (4×)
ᴓ**Jūlian** *n.* Julian
julians (1×), *julij* (1×)
jūniper *n.* juniper (*Juniperus communis*, fam. *Cupressaceae*)
iuniperi (1×)
jūs *n.* juice
iuys (301×), *juys* (4×), *juse* (1×)

K

ᴓ**kalendula** *n.* pot marigold (*Calendula officinalis*, fam. *Asteraceae*)
kalendula (2×), *kalen-dula* (1×)
kebulus *n.* type of myrobalan: fruit of *Terminalia chebula*, black myrobalan
kebe (2×), *kebule* (2×), *kebuli* (2×), *ke[be]* (1×), *[k]ebule* (1×), *kebulle* (1×)
kēlen *v.* to quench (thirst); to cool
j-kelyd (2×), *kele* (1×), *keleþ* (1×)
kēmben *v.* to comb
kemben (1×), *kembeþ* (1×), *kymbe* (1×)
kēne *adj.* sharp
kene (36×)
kēnshipe *n.* fierceness
keneschipe (6×), *keneschepe* (3×), *keneschip* (3×), *keneschype* (1×)
kēp *n.* attention, heed
kepe (2×)
kēpen *v.* to keep
kepe (12×), *kep* (2×), *keep* (1×), *kepen* (1×), *kepeþ* (1×), *kept* (1×), *kepyn* (1×)
kide *n.* ZOOL. kid, young of a goat
kydes (1×), *kydis* (1×)
kide-nēre *n.* kidney
kydeneyren (2×), *kidneiren* (1×)
kīnde *n.* kind
kynde (24×), *kyndes* (12×), *kynd* (6×), *kende* (1×), *k[i]ndys* (1×)
kīnd(e *adj.* kind
kynde (1×)
kīndelī *adj.* natural, necessary to life; *adv.* naturally
adj.: kyndly (10×), *kyndlyche* (6×), *kyndeliche* (1×), *kyndely* (1×), *kyndelyche* (1×); *adv.: kyndly* (5×)
kirnel *n.* kernel; seed
kerneles (3×), *kernelus* (1×), *kyrnelys* (1×)
kissen *v.* to kiss
kyssid (1×)
knāve *n. (1)* boy
knaue (2×)
knē *n.* knee
knees (1×)
knēden *v.* to knead
j-knede (1×)
knīf *n.* knife

knyf (1×), *knyffe* (1×)
knokken *v.* to pound
knocke (1×)
knotte *n.* knot, knob
knot (1×), *knotte* (1×)
knouen *v.* to know
know (34×), *j-knowe* (17×), *j-know* (10×), *knowe* (6×), *knowen* (4×), *knoweþ* (2×), *j-knowin* (1×), *knowyn* (1×)
knouing(e *ng.* knowing
knowyng (1×)

L

lacerte *n.* muscle
lacertys (2×), *lacertes* (1×)
lādanum *n.* resin obtained from a plant of the genus *Cistus*, fam. *Cistaceae*
lapdanum (3×)
ladder(e *n.* ladder
laddres (1×)
lakken *v.* to lack
lac (1×), *lacken* (1×), *lackeþ* (1×)
lakking(e *ng.* lack
lackynge (1×)
lange-de-bēf *n.* bugloss (*Anchusa officinalis*, fam. *Boraginaceae*)
langdebeef (1×), *lange-de-beef* (1×), *langedebeef* (1×),
lapacia acutum *n.* any of certain docks or dock-like plants
lappacium acutum (2×)
***lapis armenicus** *n.* copper sulfate
lapis armenicus (2×), *lapis armonicus* (2×)
lapis lazuli *n.* lapis lazuli (semi-precious stone)
lapis lazuli (4×)
lap-wink(e *n.* ZOOL. (a) hoopoe; (b) lapwing
lapwyng (1×), *lapwynke* (1×)
lārd *n.* lard
lard (3×)
lārğe *adj.* large
large (2×)
last(e *adj.* & *adv.* last
adj.: last (6×), *laste* (4×); *adv.: last* (2×), *laste* (1×)
lasten *v.* *(1)* to last
lasteþ (2×), *lastiþ* (1×)
lāt(e *adj.* & *adv.* late
adj.: late (4×); *adv.: late* (1×)
lāter(e *adv.* later
lattere (2×)
Lātīn *n.* Latin
latyn (2×)
latŏun *n.* copper alloy, latten
latun (1×)
laughen *v.* to laugh
lauȝeþ (1×), *lawyng* (1×), *lawȝeþ* (1×)
laughing(e *ng.* laughing
lawyng (1×)
laump(e *n.* lamp
lampes (1×)
launcel(e *n.* ribwort plantain (*Plantago lanceolata*, fam. *Plantaginaceae*)
launceolum (1×)
laurel *n.* spurge laurel (*Daphne laureola*, fam. *Thymelaeaceae*)
laureole (1×), *lorel* (1×)
laurer *n.* laurel tree, bay tree (*Laurus*

nobilis, fam. *Lauraceae*)
lorere (29×), *lorer* (2×), *lore[re]* (1×), *lorerer* (1×)

lavender(e *n. (2)* lavender (*Lavandula officinalis*, fam. *Lamiaceae*)
lauendre (3×), *lauandere* (1×)

laxātīf *n.* & *adj.* laxative
n.: laxatif (2×); *adj.: laxatif* (12×)

lax(e *adj.* lax
laxe (7×)

lēche *n. (3)* physician, surgeon
leche (5×), *lechys* (1×)

lēche-craft *n.* art or science of medicine/surgery
lechecraft (1×)

lecherī(e *n.* sexual intercourse
lecherie (1×), *lechery* (1×), *letchery* (1×)

lecherŏus *adj.* lascivious
lechours (1×), *letchours* (1×)

lēd *n.* lead
leed (16×)

lēf *n. (1)* leaf
leues (19×), *leeues* (16×), *leeuys* (11×), *leef* (6×), *leuys* (6×), *leuis* (1×), *levis* (1×)

leg *n.* leg
legges (6×), *leg* (5×), *leggis* (3×), *legge* (2×), *lege* (1×), *leggus* (1×)

lei(e *n. (1)* (a) lye; (b) MED. & SURG. solution used for cleansing wounds, removing dead tissue, etc.
liȝe (11×), *lyȝe* (1×)

leien *v. (1)* to apply
lei (111×), *ley* (51×), *leie* (21×), *leggen* (11×), *j-leid* (10×), *legge* (7×), *j-leyn* (5×), *leid* (5×), *j-leyd* (2×), *liggen* (2×), *leist* (1×), *leiþ* (1×), *leiȝe* (1×), *lej* (1×), *l[e]y* (1×), *liþ* (1×), *lyggen* (1×), *y-leid* (1×)

lēk *n.* leek (*Allium porrum*, fam. *Liliaceae*)
leek (17×), *leekes* (1×)

ᵒ**lencro-peper** *n.* type of pepper [see **peper**]
lencropiper (1×)

lēnd(e *n.* loins
leendys (2×), *leendis* (1×), *lendes* (1×), *lendus* (1×), *leyndys* (1×)

lēne *adj. (1)* lean
leene (8×), *lene* (7×)

lēnenes(se *n.* leanness
lennesse (1×)

ᵒ**lēneshipe** *n.* leanness
leneschipe (4×), *leeneschipe* (1×)

length(e *n.* length
lengþe (1×)

lēnītīf *n.* & *adj.* MED. laxative
n.: lenetif (1×), *lenytyues* (1×); *adj.: lenytif* (1×)

lent *n.* lentil (*Ervum lens*, fam. *Fabaceae*)
lentes (4×)

lēpen *v.* to leap
leepiþ (1×)

lēpere *n.* one who jumps
lieperes (1×)

lēping(e *ng.* leaping
lepyng (3×), *lepynge* (2×), *leeping* (1×), *lepingus* (1×)

lēsen *v. (4)* to lose
lese (4×), *lesyn* (3×), *liese* (2×), *leesen* (1×), *leesyn* (1×), *liesen* (1×), *lieseþ* (1×), *liesyn* (1×)

lēsing(e *ng. (3)* losing
lesyng (3×), *leesyng* (2×), *liesyng* (2×),

lessyng (1×)

lēs(se *n. (2)* sth. that is smaller in size; *adj.* & *adv.* less

n.: lasse (3×); *adj.: lasse* (9×), *lesse* (2×); *adv.: lasse* (5×)

lēten *v.* to let

let (206×), *late* (199×), *lat* (156×), *lete* (19×), *lettep* (7×), *letten* (6×), *lette* (3×), *j-let* (1×), *j-lete* (1×), *j-lettid* (1×), *j-lettyd* (1×), *la[t]* (1×), *le[t]* (1×), *letyng* (1×)

lether *n.* leather

lepere (3×), *leipere* (1×), *leper* (1×)

lēting(e *ng.* letting

lettyng (1×), *letyng* (1×)

letuse *n. (1)* lettuce (*Lactuca sativa*, fam. *Asteraceae*)

letuse (26×)

lēven *v. (1)* to leave

leue (9×), *leuep* (4×), *leeue* (2×), *leef* (1×), *leuyn* (1×), *leuyng* (1×)

lēven *v. (2)* to have leaves [see **gras**]

lēving(e *ng. (1)* leaving

leuyng (1×)

licium *n.* MED. & SURG. medicinal powder made from dried juice of certain plants

licium (8×)

licorīs *n.* liquorice (dried root of *Glycyrrhiza glabra*, fam. *Fabaceae*)

lycorys (12×), *licoryis* (7×), *liquorys* (7×), *licorys* (6×), *lycoryis* (3×), *liquoryis* (2×), *lycoris* (2×), *licoriys* (1×), *liquorik* (1×), *liquoris* (1×), *liquoriys* (1×), *lyquorys* (1×)

licŏur *n.* liquor

licour (4×), *lycour* (3×), *liquore* (1×), *liquores* (1×)

lid *n.* eyelid

ledes (1×), *ledys* (1×)

līen *v. (1)* to lie

ligge (14×), *liggen* (12×), *lip* (9×), *lize* (2×), *j-loyn* (1×), *legge* (1×), *leggen* (1×), *leggyn* (1×), *ley* (1×), *lie* (1×), *liep* (1×), *liggep* (1×), *lithe* (1×), *liye* (1×), *liyp* (1×), *liypn* (1×), *lizen* (1×), *lyep* (1×), *lygge* (1×), *lyggyn* (1×), *lyip* (1×)

līenterīa *n.* lientery (a form of diarrhoea)

lienterie (5×), *lienteries* (1×), *ljentirie* (1×)

līf *n.* life

liyf (1×), *lyuys* (1×)

lift *adj.* left

lyft (11×), *lizft* (10×), *lift* (8×), *left* (3×), *leeft* (2×), *lifte* (1×), *lizfit* (1×)

light *n.* light; *adj. (1)* bright

n.: lizt (3×); *adj.: lizt* (2×)

light *adj. (2)* light (in weight, etc.)

lizt (3×), *lyzt* (3×)

lighten *v. (1)* to light

j-liztid (1×), *lizt* (1×)

lighten *v. (2)* to relieve

j-liztid (1×), *j-lizttyd* (1×), *liztep* (1×), *lizttep* (1×)

lightlī *adv.* lightly

liztly (6×), *liztlyche* (3×), *lizttyl* (1×)

lightnes(se *n. (1)* light

lithnesse (1×)

lignum alōes *n.* lign-aloes (*Aquilaria agallocha*, fam. *Thymelaeaceae*)

lignum aloes (11×), *ligni aloes* (1×)

līk *adj.* alike

lick (1×), *lik* (1×), *liyk* (1×), *lyik*

(1×), *lyk* (1×), *lyke* (1×)
līken *v. (1)* to like
likeþ (3×)
līken *v. (2)* to be comparable (to sth.)
j-lickynd (1×), *lickened* (1×)
līking(e *ng. (1)* liking
likynge (2×), *lykyng* (2×), *lykynge* (1×)
līknen *v. (2)* (*ppl.*) **likned**, similar
lycnyd (1×)
līknes(se *n.* likeness
licnesse (1×), *lycnesse* (1×)
lilīe *n.* Madonna lily (*Lilium candidum*, fam. *Liliaceae*)
lilie (6×), *lilye* (2×), *lilies* (1×), *lily* (1×)
līm *n. (2)* lime
lym (3×), *lyme* (2×)
līmaille *n.* metal filings
lymaile (6×), *lymail* (1×)
limon *n. (1)* lemon (*Citrus limon*, fam. *Rutaceae*)
lymones (1×)
līnen *adj.* linen
lynnen (9×), *lynen* (4×), *lynenne* (1×)
linet *n.* lint made from linen, used for dressing wounds
lynet (4×)
līnī *adj.* made from flax
lynney (1×)
līn-sēd *n.* seed of flax, linseed
lynseed (25×), *lynsed* (5×), *lyndseed* (1×), *lyn-seed* (1×)
lip(pe *n. (1)* lip
lippes (11×), *lyppes* (1×), *lyppis* (1×)
liquid(e *adj.* liquid
liquide (1×)
lisping(e *ag.* lisping
lypschyng (1×)
litarğe *n.* lead monoxide, litharge
litarge (9×)
litarğī(e *n.* lethargy
litargie (5×), *litarge* (4×), *ljtargie* (1×)
lītel *n.*, *adj.*, & *adv.* little
n.: lytil (8×), *litel* (6×), *lytyl* (3×), *lityl* (2×); *adj.: lytil* (32×), *litel* (21×), *lytyl* (15×), *litil* (9×), *lityl* (8×), *lytel* (8×), *lytul* (3×), *lytille* (1×); *adv.: lytil* (10×), *litil* (6×), *lityl* (4×), *litel* (3×), *lytyl* (3×), *lytel* (2×), *litul* (1×)
lītellīe *adv.* gradually
lytly (2×)
lith *n. (1)* (a) joint of the body; (b) limb
lizte (41×), *lizt* (12×), *lyte* (1×)
liven *v. (1)* to live
leueþ (1×), *leuyng* (1×), *lyueþ* (1×)
liver(e *n. (1)* liver
lyuere (103×), *liuere* (6×), *leuere* (5×), *lyuer* (2×), *leuer* (1×), *lyue[r]e* (1×)
~ **vein(e**, basilic vein
lyuere weyn (1×)
liver-wort *n.* liverwort (*Marchantia polymorpha*, fam. *Marchantiaceae*)
lyuerwort (3×), *liuerwort* (1×), *lyuerewort* (1×)
living(e *ag.* living, alive
leuyng (1×)
lōf *n. (2)* loaf
loof (3×)
lōken *v. (2)* to look
loke (16×), *lokyng* (4×), *lo-ke* (1×), *lokyd* (1×)

lōmb *n.* ZOOL. lamb
lambren (2×), *lambes* (1×)
lōn(e *adj.* alone
alone (1×)
lōng *adj. (1)* long
long (28×), *longe* (5×), *lengere* (1×), *longa* (1×), *longae* (1×), *longao* (1×), *loong* (1×)
lǒnge *n.* lung
lunges (10×), *lungys* (6×), *lunge* (2×)
lōnge *adv.* long
longe (20×), *long* (2×), *lenger* (1×)
longen *v. (3)* to belong
longen (1×), *longinge* (1×)
lōrdship(e *n.* MED. predominance of a bodily humour or quality
lordschipe (1×)
lōsen *v. (2)* to lose
j-lost (2×), *loost* (1×), *lost* (1×)
lōth *adj.* loath
looþ (1×), *loþ* (1×)
loue *adj.* low
lowere (1×)
lǒus(e *n.* ZOOL. louse
luys (1×), *lyis* (1×)
lǒv-āche *n.* lovage (*Levisticum officinale*, fam. *Apiaceae*)
louage (16×), *loueache* (3×), *louache* (2×), *loueage* (2×)
lǒven *v. (1)* to love
louen (2×), *loueþ* (1×), *louyd* (1×), *louyn* (1×), *louyng* (1×)
lupīne *n.* white lupine (*Lupinus albus*, fam. *Fabaceae*)
lupines (3×), *lupynes* (2×)
lust *n.* lust
lust (1×)

M

***macedo** *n.* alexanders (*Smyrnium olusatrum*, fam. *Apiaceae*)
macedo (1×)
***macematicon** *n.* cabbage juice [see **caul**]
macematicon (1×)
ºMacer *n.* Macer
macer (3×)
mācis *n.* (a) aril or outer covering of the nutmeg used as a spice; (b) gum mastic
maces (11×), *mace* (1×), *masys* (1×)
º**macro-peper** *n.* plant of the fam. *Piperaceae*
macropiper (2×)
mader(e *n.* madder (*Rubia tinctorum*, fam. *Rubiaceae*)
madur (2×), *mader* (1×)
magnēs *n.* variety of magnetite; loadstone
magnes (1×)
maide-chīld *n.* girl child
maide-child (1×), *mayd-chyld* (1×)
maiden *n.* young woman
maydenesse (1×), *maydyn* (1×)
maiden-hēr *n.* maidenhair fern (either *Adiantum capillus-veneris*, fam. *Pteridaceae* or *Asplenium trichomanes*, fam. *Aspleniaceae*)
maidenhere (5×), *maydenhere* (5×), *maydenhern* (1×), *maydenshere* (1×), *maydynhere* (1×)
maistrī(e *n.* mastery
maistre (1×), *maistrei* (1×), *maistreis* (1×), *maystrei* (1×)

maithe *n.* stinking camomile (*Anthemis cotula*, fam. *Asteraceae*)
maiþen (1×), *mayþen* (1×)

majorane *n.* marjoram, sweet marjoram (*Origanum majorana*, fam. *Lamiaceae*)
maiorane (7×)

māken *v.* *(1)* to make
make (425×), *j-maad* (112×), *makeþ* (94×), *mak* (41×), *maad* (33×), *maken* (30×), *mad* (3×), *j-mad* (2×), *makest* (2×), *makyng* (2×), *jmaad* (1×), *[maad]* (1×), *ma-ken* (1×), *makeþ* (1×), *makun* (1×), *makyst* (1×)

māking(e *ng.* making
makyng (3×), *makynge* (2×)

maladī(e *n.* disease
maledies (1×)

***malagoge** *n.* medicine used to purge melancholy
malagoge (3×), *malogoge* (1×)

malard(e *n.* ZOOL. (wild) duck, drake
malard (1×)

malencolī(e *n.* melancholy, black bile; *adj.* melancholic, dominated by black bile
n.: malencolie (108×), *malencole* (10×), *malencolye* (3×), *malencoly* (1×); *adj.: malencolie* (4×), *malencolies* (2×), *malencole* (1×), *malencolys* (1×)

malencolik *adj.* [see **malencolī(e** *adj.*]
malencolicus (1×), *malencolik* (1×)

malencoliŏus *adj.* [see **malencolī(e** *adj.*]
malencolies (4×), *malencoliose* (1×), *malencoliouse* (1×)

malīce *n.* malice
malice (2×), *malicie* (1×)

malwe *n.* common mallow (*Malva sylvestris*, fam. *Malvaceae*); marsh mallow (*Althaea officinalis*, fam. *Malvaceae*)
malues (2×), *malue* (1×)

man *n.* man
man (271×), *men* (130×), *mannes* (109×), *mannus* (46×), *mannys* (21×), *manes* (2×), *manus* (2×), *mennes* (2×), *manna* (1×), *manys* (1×)

mandrag(e *n.* either of two Old World mandrakes (*Mandragora vernalis* or *officinarum*, fam. *Solanaceae*)
mandrake (3×), *mandrage* (1×)

manēr(e *n.* manner
maner (69×), *manere* (64×), *maneres* (35×), *manerys* (6×), *maneris* (5×), *maners* (1×)

manhēd(e *n.* manhood
manhood (5×)

mānia *n.* mania
manya (1×)

manipulum *n.* handful
manipulum (9×)

manna *n.* natural exudates from trees and shrubs
manna (3×)

marble-stōn *n.* marble
marbelstoon (1×)

marciatŏun *n.* kind of ointment for bones, joints, etc.
marciaton (6×)

margarīt(e *n.* pearl
margarites (2×)

margĕrī(e *n.* pearl
margeri (2×)
marwe *n. (1)* marrow
mary (3×), *mari* (1×)
mastik *n.* mastic (*Pistacia lentiscus*, fam. *Anacardiaceae*)
mastik (74×), *mastic* (4×), *mastyk* (3×), *mastike* (1×)
mātēr(e *n.* matter
matere (48×), *mater* (32×), *materie* (1×)
mātrīs *n.* uterus, womb
matrice (3×)
mātūrātīf MED. *n.* maturative remedy (promoting suppuration); *adj.* maturative
n.: maturatyues (2×), *maturatif* (1×), *maturatyfs* (1×); *adj.: maturatif* (1×), *maturatifs* (1×)
maue *n.* stomach
maw (4×), *mawe* (3×), *mawhe* (1×)
maunğer *n.* manger, feeding trough for animals
mangeer (1×)
mēd(e *n. (1)* mead
meeþ (7×)
medicīnāble *adj.* medicinal
medicinable (2×), *medicinabyl* (1×)
medicīn(e *n.* medicine
medicines (133×), *medicine* (47×), *medicynes* (33×), *medicyne* (8×), *medycines* (7×), *medicinys* (4×), *medycynes* (3×), *medicyns* (2×), *medycine* (2×), *me-dicine* (1×), *medicinis* (1×), *medicins* (1×), *medicinus* (1×), *medicyines* (1×), *medycyne* (1×)
medlen *v.* to blend, to mix
medle (144×), *j-medlid* (74×), *j-medlyd* (37×), *j-medled* (6×), *medlid* (6×), *medlyd* (4×), *j-medelyd* (3×), *medele* (3×), *medelyd* (2×), *y-medlid* (2×), *y-medlyd* (2×), *j-medeled* (1×), *j-medelid* (1×), *j-meedlid* (1×), *j-meedlyd* (1×), *medl[e]* (1×), *medled* (1×), *medlee* (1×), *y-medled* (1×)
medling(e *ng.* mixture; mixing
medelyng (5×), *medlyng* (3×), *medlynge* (1×)
mēk *adj.* docile, meek
meke (2×)
mēl *n. (2)* meal
meel (1×), *mele* (1×)
°**melano-peper** *n.* black pepper
melanopiper (2×)
mēle *n. (1)* meal made by grinding grain; flour
mele (34×), *meele* (14×)
mēle *n. (3)* apple
meele (1×)
melilōte *n.* common melilot (*Melilotus officinalis*, fam. *Fabaceae*)
mellilot (6×), *mellilet* (2×)
melissa *n.* balm (*Melissa officinalis*, fam. *Lamiaceae*)
mellise (1×)
mellicrāte *n.* hydromel (mixture of honey and water)
mellicrate (4×)
mēlŏun *n.* musk melon (*Cucumis melo*, fam. *Cucurbitaceae*)
meloun (17×), *melone* (1×)
mel rōsēt *n. (1)* + *adj.* MED. mixture of honey and roses
mel rooset (1×), *mel roset* (1×)
melten *v.* to melt

melt (9×), *melte* (1×), *molten* (1×)

membre *n.* limb
membre (19×), *membris* (9×), *membres* (2×), *membrys* (2×), *membir* (1×), *membire* (1×)

memithe *n.* yellow horned poppy (*Glaucium flavum*, fam. *Papaveraceae*)
memythe (2×), *memyth* (1×), *m[e]myth* (1×), *me-mythe* (1×), *me-my[t]he* (1×)

mēne *n. (3)* mean, sth. between two extremes; *adj. (2)* in a middle state between two extremes
n.: mene (2×), *meene* (1×); *adj.: mene* (1×)

mēne *adj. (1)* inferior
meene (1×), *mene* (1×)

mēnēlī *adv. (1)* slightly
menliche (1×)

mēnğen *v.* to mix, to mingle
j-meynd (3×), *menge* (1×), *mengyd* (1×)

menstrūe *n.* MED. & SURG. menstruation
menstrua (1×)

mentastrum *n.* horsemint (*Mentha sylvestris*, fam. *Lamiaceae*)
men[t]astre (1×)

merch(e *n.* celery (*Apium graveolens*, fam. *Apiaceae*)
march (41×), *marche* (12×), *merch* (4×), *mark* (1×), *merche* (1×)

Mercurī(e *n.* all-good (*Chenopodium bonus-henricus*, fam. *Chenopodiaceae*)
mercurie (8×)

mēre *n. (1)* ZOOL. mare
mare (1×)

mēsel *adj.* afflicted with leprosy
mesel (1×), *meseles* (1×)

mēte *n. (1)* food
mete (97×), *metes* (94×), *metys* (21×), *metis* (20×), *meete* (2×)

mēten *v. (2)* to feed
mete (1×)

mēting(e *ng. (4)* meeting
metinge (1×)

mēvāble *adj.* movable
meuabyl (1×)

mēven *v.* to move
meue (1×), *meueþ* (1×), *meuyd* (1×), *meuyn* (1×), *meuyng* (1×), *mevith* (1×), *moueþ* (1×)

mēving(e *ng.* moving
meuyng (4×), *meuynge* (2×), *meuy[n]ge* (1×), *mevynge* (1×), *mouyng* (1×), *mouynge* (1×)

***miclete** *n.* type of electuary
myclete (5×), *miclete* (1×)

mid-dai *n.* midday
mydday (5×), *myddai* (1×)

middel *n.* & *adj.* middle
n.: medle (1×), *medyl* (1×), *myddel* (1×), *myddele* (1×), *mydel* (1×), *mydil* (1×), *mydle* (1×), *mydlyn* (1×), *mydyl* (1×); *adj.: mydle* (2×), *medil* (1×), *mydil* (1×), *mydyl* (1×)

mid-night *n.* midnight
mydnyth (3×), *mydnyȝt* (3×), *mydniȝt* (1×), *mydnyt* (1×), *mydnyȝth* (1×)

mid-rif *n.* ANAT. diaphragm
mydrif (8×), *mydryf* (4×), *mydriyf* (1×)

mid-sŏmer *n.* midsummer
mydsomer (1×), *mydsomere* (1×)

mid-ward *n. (1)* middle
mydward (1×), *mydwardys* (1×)

Mīghel *n.* Michael, the Archangel
mihel (1×)
might *n.* might
myȝth (1×)
mightī *adj.* mighty
myty (1×)
mightlī *adv.* mightily
myȝtly (1×), *myȝttily* (1×)
mīlde *adj.* mild
myld (1×), *mylde* (1×)
mīle *n. (2)* millet
milie (1×)
mil-foil(e *n.* milfoil, yarrow (*Achillea millefolium*, fam. *Asteraceae*)
millefoile (3×), *mille-foil* (2×), *millefoil* (1×)
***mil(i)um solis** *n.* [see **grŏmil**]
milium solis (2×)
milk *n.* milk
mylk (69×), *mylke* (7×), *milk* (6×), *meylk* (1×), *milke* (1×), *mykil* (1×)
milking(e *ng.* milking
mylkynge (1×)
milne-stōn *n.* millstone
myll[n]e-stoon (1×)
milt(e *n.* spleen
mylt (2×), *mylte* (1×)
mīnd(e *n. (1)* mind
mynde (4×), *mende* (1×)
ministrāciŏun *n.* agency, mediation
mynistracion (1×)
minte *n. (1)* plant of the genus *Mentha*; esp. common spearmint (*Mentha viridis*, fam. *Lamiaceae*)
mynte (46×), *mynten* (11×), *mynt* (6×), *myntes* (5×), *myntene* (3×), *mynnten* (1×), *myntis* (1×), *myntyn* (1×)
mirabolān *n.* fruit of several species of *Terminalia* [see also **citri** & **indi**]
mirabole (7×), *mirabe* (6×), *myrabole* (5×), *myrabolane* (4×), *mirabolane* (3×), *myrabe* (1×)
mīrī *adj.* swampy
myry (1×)
mirī(e *adj.* merry
mery (1×)
mirre *n.* MED. myrrh (gum resin from the tree *Commiphora abyssinica* and related species)
mirre (30×), *myrre* (11×)
mirt(e *n.* (a) myrtle (*Myrtus communis*, fam. *Myrtaceae*); (b) MED. concoction containing its berries
myrte (5×), *myrtes* (5×), *myrt* (1×), *myrtys* (1×)
mirth(e *n.* joy
myrthe (2×), *murþe* (1×)
mirtille *n.* MED. preparation from the berries or leaves of the European myrtle [see **mirt(e**]
myrtelles (2×), *myr[t]elle* (1×), *myrtille* (1×), *myrtilles* (1×), *myr[t]illes* (1×)
misseien *v.* to insult
misseieþ (1×)
mistel-tō *n.* mistletoe (*Viscum album*, fam. *Viscaceae*)
mystelto (1×)
mistērī(e *n. (1)* mystery
mysterys (1×)
misturning *ng.* distortion
mysturnyng (1×)
mītigāciŏun *n.* mitigation
mytigacioun (1×)
mītigātīf MED. & SURG. *n.* soothing preparation, palliative; *adj.* soothing,

lenitive
n.: mytigatifs (5×), *mitigatyues* (3×), *mytigatyues* (3×), *mitigatifs* (1×), *myt[i]gatifs* (1×); *adj.: mytigatif* (2×), *mitigatif* (1×), *mitigatyues* (1×), *mytigatifs* (1×)

mōder *n.* ANAT. & MED. uterus, womb
moder (14×), *modere* (1×), *moderis* (1×), *modyr* (1×)

moile *n.* pudding
moylen (1×)

moist(e *adj.* moist
moist (48×), *moyst* (8×), *moiste* (3×), *moost* (1×)

moistenes(se *n.* moistness
moistnesse (27×), *moystnesse* (4×), *moistenesse* (3×), *mooistnesse* (3×), *moostnesse* (1×)

moistūr(e *n.* moisture
moisture (2×), *moysture* (1×)

mōld(e *n. (2)* top or crown of the head
molde (1×)

mollificātīf MED. *n.* softening medicine, ointment; *adj.* softening
n.: mollificatifs (4×), *mollificatif* (1×), *mollyficatifs* (1×); *adj.: mollificatif* (4×), *mollificatyf* (1×)

mollitīf *n.* & *adj.* [see **mollificātīf**]
n.: mollityues (2×), *mollytiuus* (2×), *molitifs* (1×), *mollityf* (1×), *mollytifs* (1×); *adj.: mollitif* (2×), *mollitifs* (1×), *mollytif* (1×)

mōn(e *n. (1)* moon
mone (4×)

mōng(e *n.* mixture of legumes/grains
monge (1×)

mŏnk *n.* monk
monkes (1×)

mōnth *n.* month
monþe (3×), *monþes* (3×), *moneþ* (2×), *moneþe* (1×)

mōr(e *n. (1)* root
mores (2×)

mōr(e *n. (3)* sth. that is larger in size; *adj.* & *adv.* more
n.: more (4×); *adj.: more* (18×), *moore* (1×); *adv.: more* (69×), *moore* (4×), *mo* (1×), *moo* (1×)

morel *n. (1)* black solanum, belladonna (*Solanum nigrum*, fam. *Solanaceae*)
morel (2×), *morele* (1×)

mor-mal(e *n.* dry-scabbed ulcer
mortmale (1×)

morphēa *n.* skin disease characterised by leprous or scurfy eruptions, morphea
morfeu (1×)
rēd ~, morphea originating from choler or blood and characterised by reddish scurf
reed morphees (1×)

mōrtēr *n. (1)* mortar
mortere (5×), *morter* (2×)

mortreues *n.* COOK. dish of thick consistency made with pounded and boiled chicken
mortrewys (1×)

mōrwe *n.* morning
morwe (9×), *morow* (2×), *morowe* (1×)

mōrwe-tīde *n.* dawn
morwetyd (7×), *morwetid* (5×),

morwetyde (5×), *morwetide* (3×), *morewetyd* (1×), *moreȝtyde* (1×), *morwetied* (1×), *morwetides* (1×), *morwetydes* (1×)

mōst *adv.* most
moost (16×)

mōt *n. (1)* speck, particle
motus (1×)

mōten *v. (2)* must
most (18×), *moost* (13×), *moste* (8×), *must* (7×), *mote* (5×), *moten* (5×), *mot* (3×), *muste* (3×), *maist* (1×), *moist* (1×), *moot* (1×), *moyst* (1×), *[m]ust* (1×), *mytest* (1×)

mouen *v. (3)* may
may (104×), *mai* (21×), *mow* (18×), *maist* (17×), *mown* (14×), *moun* (13×), *myȝtest* (12×), *myȝt* (9×), *mowe* (8×), *mowen* (7×), *mytest* (5×), *miȝtest* (3×), *miȝt* (2×), *myȝte* (2×), *miste* (1×), *mitest* (1×), *mowun* (1×), *mytist* (1×), *myȝtist* (1×)

mŏulen *v.* to grow mouldy
j-mouled (1×)

mŏuntain(e *n.* mountain
mountayn (3×), *mountayne* (3×), *montane* (1×), *montayne* (1×), *mounteyn* (1×)

mŏus *n.* ZOOL. mouse
mouse (1×)

mŏuth *n.* mouth
mouþ (104×), *mowþ* (8×), *mouþe* (4×), *mowth* (4×), *mouþes* (1×), *mowþe* (1×)

much(e *adv.* much
myche (156×), *meche* (5×), *miche* (4×), *mechil* (1×), *mechyl* (1×)

mug-wēd *n.* mugwort (*Artemisia vulgaris*, fam. *Asteraceae*)
mugweed (1×)

mug-wort *n.* [see **mug-wēd**]
mugwort (4×)

mul-berī(e *n.* mulberry tree (genus *Morus*, fam. *Moraceae*)
mylberie (2×), *mylberi* (1×)

multitūde *n.* multitude
multitude (1×)

mummie *n.* substance taken from embalmed corpses
mummye (14×), *mummy* (1×)

mundificātīf MED. & SURG. *n.* cleansing substance; *adj.* cleansing
n.: *mundificatifs* (6×), *mundificatyues* (3×), *mundificatyf* (1×), *mundificatyfs* (1×); *adj.*: *mundificatif* (6×)

muscadel(le *n.* sweet wine made from muscat grapes
muscate (1×)

mūscilāğe *n.* (a) thick, gelatinous substance obtained from the seeds or roots of certain plants; (b) ANAT. viscous body fluid
mussilage (9×), *muscilage* (7×), *muscilages* (4×)

musk *n.* musk
musk (6×)

must *n.* juice of grapes, must
must (1×)

mustard *n.* black mustard (*Brassica nigra*, fam. *Brassicaceae*); white mustard (*B. alba*, fam. *B.*)
mustard (1×)

N

nāddre *n.* ZOOL. adder
addre (4×)
nail *n.* nail
nayl (2×), *nail* (1×), *nailes* (1×), *nayles* (1×), *naylys* (1×)
nāme *n.* name
name (2×)
nām(e)lī *adv.* namely
namly (30×), *namlyche* (6×), *namely* (4×), *namliche* (3×), *nameliche* (1×), *namelyche* (1×), *namlye* (1×)
nāmen *v.* to name
namyd (1×)
narw(e *adj.* narrow
narwe (2×)
°**narweshipe** *n.* narrowness
narweschipe (1×)
nātūrāl *adj.* natural
naturel (7×)
nātūrāllī *adv.* naturally
naturellyche (1×)
nātūr(e *n.* nature
nature (6×)
nausea *n.* nausea
nausea (1×)
nāvel(e *n.* navel
nauele (17×), *nauel* (1×), *naule* (1×)
nēd(e *n. (1)* need
nede (1×), *neede* (1×)
nēd(e)ful *adj.* needful
needful (2×), *nedeful* (1×), *nedful* (1×)
nēd(e)lī *adv. (2)* necessarily
nedlyche (1×)
nēden *v. (2)* to need
nedeþ (12×), *nede* (2×), *neede* (1×), *nyeden* (1×)
nēdes *adv.* necessarily
nedys (2×)
nēdle *n.* needle
nedles (2×), *nedele* (1×), *nedlen* (1×)
neigh *adv.* near
neiȝ (5×), *neyȝ* (1×), *nyȝ* (1×)
neighen *v. (1)* to harm
neyȝen (3×), *neyeþ* (1×)
°**neishipe** *n.* softness of texture
neischipe (2×), *neischepe* (1×), *neisschepe* (1×)
nekke *n.* neck
necke (18×), *neck* (2×), *nek* (1×)
~ **pit**, depression over the jugular notch at the base of the neck
necke-pyt (3×), *necke-piȝt* (1×), *neck-piȝt* (1×)
nēp *n. (2)* turnip (*Brassica rapa*, fam. *Brassicaceae*)
neep (1×)
nept(e *n.* catnip, catmint (*Nepeta cataria*, fam. *Lamiaceae*)
nepte (1×)
nēr *adv. (2)* near
nere (1×)
nēr-the-lēs *adv.* nevertheless
narþelees (3×), *narþeles* (2×), *nerþeles* (1×)
nēshe *adj.* soft in texture
neische (30×), *nesche* (3×), *neysche* (2×), *neesche* (1×), *neisch* (1×), *neiȝsche* (1×)
nēshenes(se *n.* softness in texture
neischenesse (1×)
nēstril *n.* nostril
nestrilles (3×), *nostrelle* (1×)

ne-the-lēs *adv.* nevertheless
naþeles (12×)
nether(e *adj.* lower
neþer (8×), *neþere* (2×), *neþerer* (1×)
nethermōst *adj.* lowest
neþermost (1×)
netle *n.* nettle (plant of the genus *Urtica*, fam. *Urticaceae*)
netlen (6×), *netle* (4×), *netles* (4×), *netlene* (1×), *netlyn* (1×)
rēd ~, red dead-nettle (*Lamium purpureum*, fam. *Lamiaceae*)
reed netlen (2×), *reed netlees* (1×), *reed netles* (1×)
neue *n.* & *adj.* new
n.: newe (1×); *adj.: newe* (12×), *new* (4×), *nwe* (1×)
neulī *adv.* newly
newly (1×)
nēver *adv.* never
neuer (4×), *neuere* (2×)
nēver-mōr(e *adv.* never again
neuer-more (1×)
next(e *adj.* & *adv.* next
adj.: next (8×), *nexte* (3×); *adv.: next* (1×)
niğella *n.* (a) fennel-flower (*Nigella sativa*, fam. *Ranunculaceae*); (b) one of two plants: corn cockle (*Agrostemma githago*, fam. *Caryophyllaceae*) or darnel (*Lolium temulentum*, fam. *Poaceae*)
nygille (2×), *nigelle* (1×), *nygelle* (1×)
night *n.* night
nyȝt (11×), *nyȝth* (4×), *niȝth* (2×), *niȝtes* (1×), *niȝtis* (1×), *nytes* (1×), *nyȝte* (1×), *nyȝtes* (1×)
nightin-gāle *n.* ZOOL. nightingale
nyȝtyngale (1×)
nītre *n.* native sodium carbonate, natron
nytre (11×), *nitre* (4×)
nōble *adj.* noble
nobil (2×)
noien *v.* to harm
noiȝeþ (2×), *noiȝe* (1×), *noiȝen* (1×), *noyȝe* (1×)
noiful *adj.* harmful
neyful (2×), *noyful* (1×)
noise *n.* noise
noyse (7×), *noise* (2×)
nol *n.* back of the head; nape
nolle (3×)
nōlī mē tangere *n.* skin disease of the face
noli me tangere (2×)
nō-mōre *adv.* no more
na-more (1×)
nōn *n.* noon
noon (11×)
norīce *n.* wet nurse
norische (1×)
norishen *v.* to nourish
j-norisched (1×), *j-noryschid* (1×), *noriscep* (1×), *norische* (1×), *norischeþ* (1×), *norisschyd* (1×), *norysche* (1×), *noryschet* (1×), *noryschit* (1×), *noryschynge* (1×)
norishing(e *ng.* nourishing
norsching (1×)
north *n.* north
north (3×), *northe* (2×)
northen *adj.* northern
northen (1×)
northen-wīnd *n.* wind blowing from the north
norþenewynd (1×)

north-ward *adv.* northwards
northward (1×)
nōse *n. (1)* nose
nose (39×), *noose* (7×)
nōse-thirl *n.* nostril
nosethrilles (2×), *nose-þirles* (2×), *nose-þrille* (2×), *nose-thrilles* (1×), *nose-þrilles* (1×)
nostrille *n.* nostril
nostrilles (5×), *nostrille* (1×), *nostrylle* (1×)
not *adv.* not
nat (258×), *not* (25×), *naut* (2×), *nawt* (2×), *naȝthe* (1×), *nowt* (1×)
nŏte *n. (1)* nut
notes (6×), *note* (5×), *noote* (2×), *nootes* (1×), *notys* (1×)
nōte-mug(e *n.* nutmeg (*Myristica fragrans*, fam. *Myristicaceae*)
notemuge (11×), *note-muge* (2×), *notemuges* (2×)
nŏu *adv.* now
now (12×), *j-now* (2×)

O

obtalmīa *n.* ophthalmia
obtalmie (5×), *obtalmye* (3×)
occupāciŏun *n.* occupation
ocupacion (1×), *ocupaciowns* (1×)
ōcimum *n.* basil (*Ocimum basilicum*, fam. *Lamiaceae*)
oȝimi (1×), *oȝimum* (1×), *oȝymi* (1×)
oculus christī *n.* wild clary (*Salvia horminoides*, fam. *Lamiaceae*) or wild sage (*S. verbenaca*, fam. *L.*)
oculus xristi (2×)

of *adv.* off
of (8×)
oft(e *adv.* often
ofte (15×), *oft* (1×)
often *adv.* often
often (1×)
often-sīthes *adv.* often
often-siþes (2×), *oftyn-siþes* (2×), *often-syþes* (1×), *oftyn-seþes* (1×)
often-tīme *adv.* often
oftyn-tyme (1×)
often-tīmes *adv.* often
often-tymes (1×)
ofte-sīthe *adv.* often
ofte-siþe (1×)
ofte-sīthes *adv.* often
ofte-siþes (29×), *oftesiþes* (3×), *ofte-syþes* (3×), *oftesyþes* (1×)
ofte-tīme *adv.* often
ofte-tyme (3×)
ofte-tīmes *adv.* often
ofte-tymes (2×)
oil(e *n.* oil
oile (184×), *oyle* (17×), *oiles* (13×), *ooile* (3×), *oyles* (2×), *ooile* (1×), *oyl* (1×)
~ **de bai(e**, bay oil
de bay (2×)
~ **de olive**, olive oil
de olyue (3×), *de oliue* (2×)
oinement *n.* ointment
oynement (45×), *oynementes* (25×), *oynementis* (3×), *anoynement* (2×), *oynnement* (2×), *a-noyntement* (1×), *oinement* (1×), *oinenent* (1×), *onymentes* (1×)
oinyon *n.* (a) common onion (*Allium cepa*, fam. *Liliaceae*); (b) sea

onion or squill (*Urginea maritima*, fam. *L.*)
oynouns (5×), *onyouns* (3×), *onyoun* (2×), *onyons* (1×), *oynen* (1×), *oyneouns* (1×), *oyneuns* (1×), *oynnouns* (1×), *oynonun* (1×), *oynoun* (1×)

ōk(e *n.* (a) British oak (*Quercus robur*, fam. *Fagaceae*); (b) evergreen or holm oak (*Q. ilex*, fam. *F.*)
ook (7×), *ookes* (2×), *ookys* (2×), *okes* (1×)

ōld(e *adj.* old
oold (26×), *old* (8×), *oolde* (4×), *eld* (2×), *olde* (2×), *eeld* (1×), *elde* (1×), *hold* (1×), *hoold* (1×)

olibane *n.* aromatic gum resin; frankincense
olibanum (22×), *olybanum* (1×)

olive *n.* [see **oil(e**]

omfacinum *n.* sap or oil of unripe grapes or olives
onyfacie (1×)

on *adv. (1)* on
on (1×)

ōnes *adv.* once
oones (9×), *ones* (8×), *onus* (1×), *oonys* (1×)

ōnlī *adv.* only
only (2×), *oonly* (2×)

ōpen *adj.* open
open (5×), *opene* (3×), *hopyn* (1×)

ōpen-ars *n.* fruit of the medlar tree (*Mespilus germanica*, fam. *Rosaceae*)
openers (2×), *open-ers* (1×), *openhers* (1×)

ōpenen *v.* to open
open (5×), *opene* (4×), *oppyn* (4×), *openeþ* (3×), *oppeneþ* (3×), *openen* (2×), *oppen* (2×), *opened* (1×)

ōpening(e *ag.* opening
openyng (2×), *oppenyng* (2×), *oppenynge* (1×)

ōpenlī *adv.* openly
openly (1×)

opium *n.* analgesic and soporific medicine derived from juice from the seed-pod and leaves of the opium poppy (*Papaver somniferum*, fam. *Papaveraceae*)
opium (28×)

opobalsamum *n.* sap of the balm of Gilead (*Commiphora meccanensis*, fam. *Burseraceae*)
opobalȝamum (1×)

opopanak *n.* medicinal gum derived from the juice of *Opopanax chironium*, fam. *Apiaceae*
oppoponak (2×), *opoponac* (1×), *oppopanac* (1×)

ordeinen *v.* to prepare
orden (2×), *ordeyne* (2×), *ordeine* (1×), *ordend* (1×), *ordeyned* (1×), *ordyyne* (1×)

ordūr(e *n.* excrement
ordure (6×)

orīgane *n.* wild marjoram (*Origanum vulgare*, fam. *Lamiaceae*)
origane (22×), *origan* (7×)

orīganum *n.* [see **orīgane**]
origanum (1×)

°**oriyn** *n.* rust; stone in the bladder
oriyn (1×)

orobus *n. (1)* bitter vetch (*Vicia orobus*, fam. *Fabaceae*)
orobus (2×), *orobȝ* (1×)

orpiment *n.* arsenic trisulphide, orpiment
orpement (8×), *orpiment* (1×), *orpyment* (1×)
orpin *n.* orpine (*Sedum telephium*, fam. *Crassulaceae*)
orpyn (2×), *orpen* (1×)
os sepie *n.* *(2)* calcareous internal shell of cuttlefish
os sepie (3×)
ōte *n.* oat (*Avena sativa*, fam. *Poaceae*)
ooten (3×), *oote* (1×), *otus* (1×)
ōther-whīle *adv.* sometimes
oþerwhile (204×), *oþer-while* (15×), *oþerwile* (3×), *eiþer-whyle* (1×), *oþerwhilee* (1×), *oþer-whyle* (1×), *oþerwhyle* (1×), *oþerwyle* (1×)
ōther-whīles *adv.* sometimes
oþerwhiles (97×), *oþer-whiles* (7×), *oþerwiles* (3×)
ōther-wīse *adv.* otherwise
oþerwyse (1×)
ouen *adj.* own
owne (6×)
ŏunce *n.* ounce
ounce (165×), *oʒ* (1×)
ŏut(e *adv.* out
owt (45×), *out* (43×), *oute* (5×), *owte* (5×), *outere* (1×), *vt* (1×)
ŏutmōst *adj. sup.* outermost
vtmast (1×)
ŏutputtinge *ag.* **the ~ vertū**, the expulsive capability of the body
owt-pyttynge (1×)
ŏutre *adj.* outer
vttere (7×)
ŏutwārd(e *adv.* outwards
owtward (3×), *outeward* (1×), *outward* (1×)
ōven *n.* oven
ouene (3×), *ouen* (1×)
ōver *adj.* upper
ouer (11×), *ouere* (5×), *ouerere* (1×)
ōver-al *adv.* overall
oueral (4×), *ouerall*e (2×), *ouer-alle* (1×)
overcŏmen *v.* to overcome
ouer-come (3×), *ouercome* (3×)
ōvermōst *adj. sup.* uppermost
ouermoost (1×)
overmuche *adv.* excessively
ouer-myche (1×)
overplentēvŏus[17] *adj.* superabundant
ouerplentiuus (2×), *ouerpletiuus* (1×)
ōvet *n.* fruit
ofete (2×)
oxe *n.* ZOOL. ox
oxe (3×), *oxes* (1×)
oxe(s eie *n.* marguerite (*Chrysanthemum leucanthemum*, fam. *Asteraceae*)
oxie (1×)
***oxifistula** *n.* tamarind's bark [see **tamarinde**]
oxifistula (2×)
oximel *n.* oxymel (medicinal preparation of vinegar and honey, often with other herbal ingredients); **~ compŏuned**, oxymel composed of several ingredients besides vinegar and honey; **~ dīūretik**, oxymel that induces urination;

17 The form recorded in the *MED* is **plentēvŏus**.

simple ~, oxymel made of proper proportions of vinegar and honey; **~ squillītik**, oxymel containing squill
oximel (55×), *oxymel* (1×)

P

pācient(e *n.* patient
pacient (13×), *pacyent* (1×)
paire *n. (1)* pair
peyre (1×)
pāl(e *adj.* pale
pale (24×)
pālenes(se *n.* paleness
palenesse (1×)
palesī(e *n.* palsy
palesie (17×), *palesei* (3×), *palasie* (2×), *pa-lese* (1×), *palese* (1×), *palesye* (1×)
palat(e *n.* uvula
palet (1×)
pālish *adj.* pale
palysche (1×)
panne *n. (1)* pan, cauldron
panne (1×)
pappe *n.* breast
pappe (1×), *pappes* (1×)
paralisī(e *n.* paralysis
paralisis (1×)
parchemīn *n.* parchment
parchemyn (1×)
pāreles *n.* parings (of fruit)
pareles (1×)
part *n.* part
part (19×), *partes* (5×), *parte* (3×)
parten *v.* to divide
parte (4×)
pārtī(e *n.* part
party (23×), *parties* (9×), *partys* (2×), *parteys* (1×), *parti* (1×), *partie* (1×), *partis* (1×), *partye* (1×)
partrich(e *n.* ZOOL. partridge
partriches (5×), *partriche* (2×)
passen *v.* to pass
passeþ (29×), *passe* (8×), *passen* (5×), *passyng* (3×), *passyd* (2×), *passyn* (2×), *j-passed* (1×), *j-passid* (1×), *passed* (1×), *passiþ* (1×)
passe-nēpe *n.* parsnip (*Pastinaca sativa*, fam. *Apiaceae*)
pasnep (1×)
passing(e *ng.* passing
passinge (2×), *passyng* (2×), *passing* (1×)
pasternāk *n.* [see **passe-nēpe**]
pastinake (1×)
paum(e *n.* palm (of the hand)
pawmes (2×), *paume* (1×), *pawme* (1×)
pēce *n.* piece
pece (7×), *peces* (1×), *piece* (1×)
pein(e *n.* pain
peyn (1×)
peltre *n.* (a) common pellitory (*Parietaria officinalis*, fam. *Urticaceae*); (b) **~ of spain**, pellitory of Spain (*Anacyclus pyrethrum*, fam. *Asteraceae*)
peletre (5×)
penaunce *n.* penance
penaunce (1×)
pēnide *n.* barley sugar
penydes (15×), *penides* (2×)
penī wort *n.* pennywort (*Cotyledon umbilicus*, fam. *Crassulaceae*)

peny-wort (1×), *penywort* (1×)
penta-filon *n.* European cinquefoil (*Potentilla reptans*, fam. *Rosaceae*)
pentafilon (11×)
peper *n.* pepper (*Piper nigrum*, fam. *Piperaceae*)
peper (53×)
perceiven *v.* to perceive
perseyue (1×), *perseyuen* (1×)
pērcen *v.* to pierce
persep (2×), *ipersed* (1×), *j-perceed* (1×), *perse* (1×), *perseep* (1×), *persip* (1×), *perssep* (1×), *persyng* (1×)
perche *n. (1)* ZOOL. perch (freshwater fish)
perche (1×)
pēre *n. (1)* pear (*Pyrus communis*, fam. *Rosaceae*)
perees (1×), *peres* (1×), *perys* (1×)
perīl *n.* peril
perile (2×), *pereel* (1×), *pereil* (1×), *perel* (1×), *perele* (1×)
perilŏus *adj.* perilous, dangerous
perilouse (10×)
peripleumonīe *n.* MED. inflammation of the lungs
peripleumonie (4×), *peripleumonye* (2×), *peripleumonys* (1×), *peripleumuonie* (1×)
peritōrī(e *n.* pellitory of the wall (*Parietaria officinalis*, fam. *Urticaceae*)
periterie (12×), *peritorie* (6×)
pērl(e *n. (2)* pearl
perles (2×), *periles* (1×)
perselī *n.* common or garden parsley (*Petroselinum crispum*, fam. *Apiaceae*)
persili (14×), *persilie* (14×), *persile* (8×), *persily* (7×), *perseli* (6×), *persillie* (6×), *persely* (3×), *persilye* (3×), *perseile* (1×), *persele* (1×)
persicārīe *n.* one of the species of *Polygonum*, fam. *Polygonaceae*; esp. peachwort (*P. persicaria*) or water-pepper (*P. hydropiper*)
persicarie (2×)
pēse *n.* pea (*Pisum sativum*, fam. *Fabaceae*)
peesen (1×), *peeses* (1×), *pese* (1×), *pesen* (1×), *peses* (1×), *pesun* (1×)
pestel *n.* pestle (instrument used to grind materials in a mortar)
pestel (2×), *pestele* (1×)
pestilence *n.* pestilence
pestilence (1×)
petrōlēum *n.* petroleum
petroile (1×), *petroley* (1×)
***peusadanum** *n.* hog's fennel (*Peucedanum officinale*, fam. *Apiaceae*)
peusadan[um] (1×)
philosophīe *n.* natural science
philosophie (1×)
phisicien *n.* physician
fisycyens (1×)
pich(e *n. (1)* wood tar
piche (5×), *pich* (3×)
pī(e *n. (2)* pie
pye (1×)
***pigami** *n.* rue seed [see **rūe**]
pigamy (1×), *pygamy* (1×)
pigge *n.* ZOOL. pig
piȝe (3×), *pigges* (1×)
pigle *n.* European stitchwort or great starwort (*Stellaria holostea*, fam. *Caryophyllaceae*)
pigle (1×)

pīk(e *n. (2)* ZOOL. pike fish
pyke (1×)
pilen *v. (1)* to peel
pile (1×)
pīling(e *ng.* rind, peeling
pilinge (1×), *pillyng* (1×)
pilocelle *n.* mouse-ear hawkweed (*Hieracium pilosella*, fam. *Asteraceae*)
pilocelle (2×)
pilule *n.* pill, pellet
pillules (29×), *pilulees* (4×), *piliulees* (2×), *pilules* (1×), *puleles* (1×), *pullulees* (1×), *pullules* (1×), *pululees* (1×), *pylulees* (1×)
pīment *n.* sweetened, spiced wine
pyment (2×)
pimpernel(e *n.* one of several plants, esp. great and salad burnets (*Sanguisorba officinalis* and *Poterium sanguisorba*, fam. *Rosaceae*), burnet saxifrage (*Pimpinella saxifraga*, fam. *Apiaceae*), and pimpernel (*Anagallis arvensis*, fam. *Primulaceae*)
pimpinele (1×), *pympenelle* (1×), *pymperenelle* (1×)
pimple *n.* swelling
pymples (8×), *pemples* (1×), *pimples* (1×), *pympels* (1×), *pympil* (1×)
pīn-appel *n.* pine cone; ~ **kirnel**, pine nut
pyn-appel (5×)
pīn(e *n. (2)* pine nut
pynes (5×), *pynees* (1×)
pionē *n.* plant of the genus *Paeonia*, esp. male or entireleaved peony (*P. mascula*, fam. *Paeoniaceae*) and common peony (*P. officinalis*, fam. *P.*)
pionie (2×), *pyony* (2×), *pyonye* (2×), *pionye* (1×), *pyonie* (1×)
pīpe *n. (1)* pipe, tube
pipe (5×), *pypes* (1×)
piretrum *n.* pellitory (of Spain) (*Anacyclus pyrethrum*, fam. *Asteraceae*); pellitory of the wall (*Parietaria officinalis*, fam. *Urticaceae*)
piretre (25×), *peretre* (1×), *pyretre* (1×)
pis(se *n.* urine
pisse (7×)
pissen *v.* to urinate
pissen (9×), *pisse* (6×), *pissep* (6×), *pessyn* (1×), *pissed* (1×), *pyssynge* (1×)
pissing(e *ng.* urination
pissinge (3×), *pissyng* (2×), *pyssyng* (2×), *pissynge* (1×), *pyssynge* (1×)
plāce *n.* place
place (53×), *places* (23×), *placys* (1×)
plantein(e *n.* plant of the plantain fam. (*Plantaginaceae*): ~ **the mōre**, great plantain (*Plantago major*); ~ **the lēsse**, ribwort plantain (*P. lanceolata*)
plaunteyn (42×), *plaunteyne* (16×), *planteyn* (9×), *plaunten* (4×), *plauntein* (2×), *plantein* (1×), *planten* (1×), *planteyne* (1×)
plāstre *n.* MED. plaster
plastre (156×), *plastres* (26×), *plastere* (18×), *plaistere* (4×), *plasteres* (4×), *plasteris* (3×), *plaastere* (1×), *plaasteres* (1×), *plaastre* (1×), *plaistre* (1×), *plasterys* (1×), *plastreis* (1×), *plastr[e]s* (1×)
plāstren *v.* MED. to cover with a plaster

plastre (12×), *j-plastred* (9×), *j-plaistred* (1×), *plasterid* (1×), *plastrid* (1×)

plāt(e *n.* plate
plate (1×)

pleinen *v.* to complain
pleynen (1×)

plentē *n.* plenty; *adj.* plentiful
n.: plente (36×), *plent* (1×), *plent[e]* (1×); *adj.: plente* (1×)

plentēful *adj.* plentiful
plentiful (1×)

plentēvŏus *adj.* plentiful
plentiuus (5×), *ple[n]tiuus* (2×), *plenteuous* (1×), *plenteuouse* (1×), *plentiuosse* (1×), *plentiuouse* (1×), *plentuouse* (1×)

plēsen *v.* to please
j-plesyd (2×)

pleuresī *n.* pleurisy
pleuresie (12×), *pleuresy* (1×), *pleuresye* (1×), *pluresie* (1×)

plŏume *n.* plum (*Prunus domestica*, fam. *Rosaceae*)
plumbes (7×), *plummes* (4×), *plombes* (1×), *plum* (1×), *plumbe* (1×), *plumbys* (1×)

plum *n.* lead (metal)
plum (1×)

***pocio muscata** *n.* electuary containing musk
pocio muscata (1×)

pōciŏun *n.* potion
pocion (1×), *pocioun* (1×), *pociouns* (1×)

podagre *n.* MED. gout in the foot, podagra
podagre (1×)

pointe *n. (1)* point
poynt (3×)

poisonen *v.* to poison
j-poysend (1×)

policārī(e *n.* fleabane (*Pulicaria dysenterica*, fam. *Asteraceae*)
pollicarie (1×)

polipodī(e *n.* polypody (*Polypodium vulgare*, fam. *Polypodiaceae*)
pollipodie (6×), *polipodie* (4×), *polie* (1×)

ø**pollitricum** *n.* haircap-moss (*Polytrichum commune*, fam. *Polytrichaceae*)
pollitricum (2×)

pōme *n.* fruit of any kind
pomyis (1×)
~ **citrīn(e**, citron (*Citrus medica*, fam. *Rutaceae*)
pome citrine (1×)

pōme-garnet(e *n.* pomegranate (*Punica granatum*, fam. *Punicaceae*)
pome-garnade (1×), *pomegarnade* (1×), *pome-garnadis* (1×), *pomegarnat* (1×), *pomgarnad* (1×), *pomme-garnade* (1×)

popī(e *n. (1)* opium poppy (*Papaver somniferum*, fam. *Papaveraceae*) or any of the varieties of this plant; **blāk ~**, variety of opium poppy with black seeds; **rēd ~**, red poppy; **whīt ~**, variety of opium poppy with white flowers
popi (7×), *popy* (7×), *popie* (1×), *popye* (1×)

pōpiliŏun *n.* ointment based on poplar leaves or buds
popilion (8×), *popilioun* (2×)

porciŏun *n.* portion
porcion (2×), *porcioun* (2×)
pōre *n. (1)* pore
pores (12×), *porys* (8×), *pore* (3×), *poores* (2×), *poris* (2×), *poures* (2×)
pork(e *n.* pork
pork (2×)
portulāke *n.* purslane (*Portulaca oleracea*, fam. *Portulacaceae*)
portulake (15×)
pōse *n.* catarrh
pose (17×)
potāğe *n.* potage, thick soup
potage (4×)
pot(e *n. (1)* pot, vessel
pot (3×), *poot* (1×), *pottys* (1×)
pŏudre *n. (1)* powder
poudre (155×), *poudere* (9×), *powdre* (9×), *poudres* (5×), *pouder* (2×), *pouderes* (1×), *pouderis* (1×), *poudrys* (1×), *powdres* (1×)
pŏudren *v.* to powder
poudre (27×), *j-poudred* (12×), *j-poudrid* (6×), *j-poudryd* (2×), *j-podred* (1×), *j-pouderid* (1×), *j-poudreid* (1×), *j-powdred* (1×), *poudere* (1×), *poudred* (1×), *y-poudered* (1×)
pŏuēr(e *n.* power
powere (1×)
pŏund(e *n. (1)* pound
pound (81×), *pownd* (4×), *pounde* (2×), *powund* (2×)
pŏunen *v.* to pulverize
powne (8×), *j-powned* (4×), *pownne* (2×), *powned* (1×)
pŏus(e *n.* pulse
pouse (15×)
preciŏus(e *adj.* precious
preciouse (1×)
preien *v. (1)* to pray
preie (1×), *prey* (1×)
preiēr(e *n. (2)* prayer
preieres (1×)
priken *v.* to prick
prickeþ (3×), *pricke* (1×)
priking(e *ng.* & *ag.* pricking
ng.: *prickyng* (14×), *prickynge* (9×), *pricching* (2×), *prechyng* (1×), *pricchyng* (1×), *pric[k]inge* (1×), *prickynges* (1×), *pritchynge* (1×); *ag.*: *prickyng* (1×), *prickynge* (1×)
principāl *adj.* principal
principal (6×)
principālli(e *adv.* principally
principaly (4×), *principali* (2×), *princypaly* (1×)
privē *n.* privacy; *adj. (1)* private
n.: *priuei* (2×), *pryuei* (2×), *preuye* (1×), *priuey* (1×), *priuye* (1×); *adj.*: *priue* (2×), *preuy* (1×)
privētē *n.* privacy
priuyte (1×)
prōfitāble *adj.* profitable
profitabil (30×), *profitable* (26×), *profitabyl* (14×), *profitabile* (2×), *profytabil* (2×), *profitabel* (1×), *profytable* (1×), *profytabyl* (1×)
prōfit(e *n. (1)* profit
profite (1×), *profiȝt* (1×)
prōfiten *v.* to profit
profiteþ (2×)
prōpre *adj.* proper
propre (1×)
prōpretē *n.* property
propirtees (2×), *propirteys* (2×), *propirtes* (1×)

prŏud *adj.* proud
proud (2×), *prowd* (1×)
psidie *n.* rind, bark, blossoms of pomegranate (tree) (*Punica granatum*, fam. *Punicaceae*)
psidie (11×)
psīlōtre *n.* depilatory ointment
psilotrum (1×)
pūliol *n.* pennyroyal (*Mentha pulegium*, fam. *Lamiaceae*)
piliole (18×), *puliole* (2×), *piluole* (1×), *pilyole* (1×)
pullen *v.* to pull
pullen (5×), *pulle* (4×)
pulville *n.* surgical pad or dressing
pulwe (1×)
purcelan(e *n.* [see **portulāke**]
purselane (24×), *purslane* (2×), *porcelane* (1×), *pursylane* (1×)
pūren *v.* to purify
puryd (3×), *pure* (1×), *purid* (1×)
purgāciŏun *n.* MED. purgation
purgacioun (27×), *purgaciouns* (13×), *purgacion* (12×), *purgacions* (1×), *purga-cioun* (1×), *purgacyouns* (1×)
purğen *v.* *(1)* MED. to purge
purge (44×), *purgen* (37×), *purgeþ* (14×), *j-purged* (5×), *purged* (5×), *purgyn* (4×), *j-purgeid* (3×), *j-purgyd* (2×), *purgeid* (2×), *j-purgid* (1×), *pu[r]geþ* (1×)
purğing(e *ag.* MED. purging
purgyng (1×)
putten *v.* to put
pit (23×), *put* (20×), *pyt* (12×), *j-pit* (5×), *pitte* (2×), *piȝt* (2×), *j-piȝt* (1×), *j-put* (1×), *piten* (1×), *pitten* (1×), *pitteþ* (1×), *putten* (1×), *puttyng* (1×), *pyȝt* (1×)

Q

°**quādruplen** *v.* to quadruple
quadrapliеþ (1×)
quail(e *n.* ZOOL. quail (migratory bird)
quaile (1×), *quayle* (1×)
quāken *v.* to quake
quakeþ (4×), *quake* (1×)
quāking(e *ng.* quaking
qwakyng (1×)
quantitē *n.* quantity
quantite (46×)
***quantum sufficit** *adv.* as much as necessary
quantum sufficit (37×)
quartain(e *adj.* quartan (fever)
quarteyn (2×), *quarteins* (1×)
quart(e *n.* quart
quart (1×), *quar[t]* (1×)
quartēr(e *n.* quarter
quarter (1×)
°**quasi** *adv.* almost
quasi (1×)
quēd(e *n.* *(1)* evil, wickedness
qweed (1×)
quenchen *v.* to quench
quenche (7×), *j-quenchid* (4×), *j-qwenchid* (2×), *quenched* (2×), *quencheþ* (2×), *j-quenchyd* (1×), *quenchid* (1×), *quenchyn* (1×)
quērn(e *n.* *(2)* quern, mill
querne (2×)
quibibe *n.* Java peppercorn, cubeb (*Piper cubeba*, fam. *Piperaceae*)

quibibes (4×), *quybibes* (3×), *quybib[e]s* (1×)
quīk *adj.* quick
quyk (2×), *quwyk* (1×), *qwik* (1×), *qwyck* (1×)
quinquinervīe *n.* ribwort plantain (*Plantago lanceolata*, fam. *Plantaginaceae*)
quinquerne (1×)
quitter(e *n.* pus
quiture (30×), *quitere* (3×), *quytere* (1×)
quitteren *v.* to form pus, to suppurate
quitereþ (1×)
quittering *ng.* suppuration
quituring (1×), *quituryng* (1×)

R

radich(e *n.* radish (*Raphanus sativus*, fam. *Brassicaceae*)
radich (23×), *radiche* (11×), *radech* (1×), *radik* (1×), *radych* (1×), *radyche* (1×)
rai(e *n.* *(2)* thread; streak; *adj.* striped
n.: ray (1×); *adj.: ray* (1×)
raisīn *n.* raisin
reysyns (4×), *reisenes* (3×), *reisynes* (1×), *reysens* (1×), *reysines* (1×), *reysynes* (1×)
ram *n.* ZOOL. ram, male sheep
ram (1×)
rāpe *n.* *(3)* turnip (*Brassica rapa*, fam. *Brassicaceae*) or rape (*B. napus*, fam. *B.*)
rapes (1×)
°**Raphael** *n.* Raphael
Raphael (1×)
raskinge *ng.* spitting, hawking
raskyng (1×)
rāsŏur(e *n.* razor
rasour (2×)
rāther(e *adv.* rather
raþer (14×), *raþere* (10×)
rau(e *adj.* raw
rawe (4×), *raw* (3×)
rāven *n.* ZOOL. raven
rauenhus (1×)
ravīning *adj.* ravening
rauenyng (1×)
rēal *adj.* *(1)* royal
ryal (1×)
receit(e *n.* reception
receit (1×), *r[e]ceit* (1×)
receiven *v.* to receive
receyuen (4×), *resceyue* (3×), *receyve* (1×), *receyued* (1×), *receyuyn* (1×), *resceyuen* (1×), *resceyueþ* (1×), *resceyuid* (1×), *reseiueþ* (1×), *reseyue* (1×), *reseyuen* (1×), *reseyuyth* (1×)
rēchen *v.* *(1)* to stretch
ratche (1×)
rēching(e *ng.* *(2)* belching; retching
rechyng (1×), *rechynge* (1×)
recoveren *v.* *(2)* to recover
rekeuere (1×)
rēd *adj.* red
reed (87×), *reede* (8×), *red* (1×), *ryede* (1×)
rēden *v.* *(1)* to read
rad (1×)
rēdīlī *adv.* *(2)* readily
redely (1×), *redileche* (1×)

rēdish(e *adj.* reddish
reedysche (1×)
rēdnes(se *n.* redness
reednesse (15×), *rednesse* (5×), *redynesse* (1×)
reğendren *v.* to cause to grow again
regendrieþ (1×)
regnen *v.* to reign, to rule
regnþ (6×), *regne* (3×), *regnen* (3×), *regneþ* (2×), *regnyng* (2×), *regniþ* (1×), *reugne* (1×)
regning(e *ng.* predominance
regnyng (1×)
rein *n. (1)* rain
reyn (3×), *reynys* (1×)
~ **wāter**, rainwater
reyn-water (15×), *reynwater* (2×)
reine *n. (2)* (a) kidney; (b) loins, flanks
reynes (77×), *reynys* (8×), *reynis* (2×), *reines* (1×), *reyne* (1×), *reyns* (1×)
relenten *v.* to dissolve
j-relentid (1×)
relēven *v.* to relieve
releue (1×)
remedī(e *n.* remedy
remedi (1×), *remedie* (1×)
remenaunt *n.* remnant
remnannt (3×), *remnawnt* (2×), *remnaunt* (1×)
remēven *v.* to remove
remeuyd (1×), *re[m]ewid* (1×)
reneuen *v. (1)* to renew
renewe (6×), *renew* (3×)
rennen *v. (1)* to run
renne (3×), *renneþ* (2×), *j-runne* (1×), *ren* (1×), *rennen* (1×)
renning(e *ng. (1)* producing of a bodily discharge; discharge; *ag. (1)* running
ng.: rennyng (2×); *ag.: rennyng* (3×), *rennynge* (1×)
repenten *v.* to repent
repenteþ (1×), *repentyng* (1×)
repercussīf MED. *n.* medicine that disperses pathological concentrarions of humours; *adj.* having such power, thus reducing swelling or inflammation
n.: repercussyues (14×), *repercussiues* (2×), *repercussiuus* (1×), *repercussiuys* (1×), *repercussyfs* (1×); *adj.: repercussif* (3×), *repercussifs* (1×), *repercussiues* (1×), *repercussyues* (1×)
replēciŏun *n.* MED. & PHYSIOL. condition of being full of blood, humours, or fluids; pathological overabundance of humours
replecion (6×), *replecioun* (6×)
replēte *adj.* MED. & PHYSIOL. full (of blood, humours, etc.)
repleet (11×), *replet* (8×), *replete* (2×)
repressen *v.* to repress
repressid (1×)
rēsīn(e *n.* resin
resynes (5×)
resolven *v.* to dissolve
resolue (6×), *resolued* (4×), *resoluyd* (4×), *resoluen* (1×), *resolvyng* (1×)
rēsŏun *n. (2)* reason
reson (2×), *resoun* (1×)
rēst(e *n. (1)* rest
reste (4×), *reeste* (2×), *rest* (2×)
reste-boef *n.* restharrow (*Ononis repens*, fam. *Fabaceae*)
restaboues (1×), *restabouis* (1×)

rēsten *v. (1)* to rest
reste (2×), *rest* (1×), *restyn* (1×)
restōren *v.* to restore
restoreþ (2×), *restore* (1×), *restorithe* (1×), *restoryn* (1×)
restreinen *v.* to restrain
restreyne (1×)
retentīf *n.* capacity to retain nourishment
rotentif (1×)
retenūe *n.* retention[18]
retenues (1×)
reuain *n.* second growth of grass or hay in a season
raueyne (1×)
reule *n.* MED. & SURG. instruction for cure
rewle (2×)
reulen *v.* MED. & SURG. to cure
rewle (1×), *rewlid* (1×)
reuling(e *ng.* MED. medical regimen
reulinge (1×)
reume *n.* MED. (a) watery fluid or humour conceived as draining from the higher parts of the body, and capable of causing diseases; secretion, flux; (b) catarrh
rewme (21×)
reupontic *n.* prob. root of a kind of rhubarb (*Rheum rhaponticum*, fam. *Polygonaceae*)
reuponte (1×)
ribaudī(e *n.* lechery
rybawdys (1×)
rib(be *n. (1)* rib
rybbys (2×), *ribbes* (1×), *ribbys* (1×)

18 Different meaning in the *MED*.

rib(be *n. (2)* ribwort (*Plantago lanceolata*, fam. *Plantaginaceae*)
reube (2×)
rib(bewŏrt *n.* [see **rib(be** *n. (2)*]
ribwort (4×)
rīche *adj.* rich
riche (4×)
rīe *n.* rye (*Secale cereale*, fam. *Poaceae*)
riȝe (1×), *rye* (1×)
riğğe *n.* back
rugge (8×), *rugh* (1×), *rygge* (1×)
riğğe-bōn *n.* (a) spine; (b) vertebra
riggeboon (1×), *ruggebon* (1×), *rugge-boon* (1×)
right *adj.* right
riȝt (26×), *riȝth* (2×), *riȝthe* (2×), *rith* (1×), *ryȝt* (1×), *ryȝthe* (1×)
right(e *adv.* very
riȝt (41×), *riȝth* (4×), *ryt* (4×), *ryȝt* (4×), *rythe* (1×)
rīnd(e *n. (1)* rind
rynde (15×), *rynd* (4×), *ryndes* (2×), *ryndys* (2×)
ring *n.* ring
ryng (7×)
ringen *v. (2)* to ring (a bell)
ryngyng (1×)
ringing(e *ng.* sensation of ringing in the ear
ryngyng (3×), *ryngynge* (3×), *rynginge* (2×)
rīpe *n. (1)* reaping; *adj.* ripe
n.: ripe (1×); *adj.: ripe* (11×), *rype* (4×)
rīpen *v. (1)* to ripen
ripen (1×)
rīs *n. (2)* rice (*Oryza sativa*, fam. *Poaceae*)

riys (2×), *rizs* (2×), *riz* (1×)
rīsen *v.* to rise
ryse (3×), *riseþ* (2×), *rysyn* (1×), *rysynge* (1×)
rīsing(e *ng.* & *ag.* rising
ng.: risyngus (1×); *ag.: rysyng* (1×)
rivelen *v.* to become wrinkled
ryuelyd (1×)
rivēr(e *n.* river
ryueres (2×), *ryuere* (1×), *ryuerys* (1×)
rōche *n. (3)* ZOOL. European roach (freshwater fish)
roche (1×)
rŏdī *adj.* reddish
rody (1×), *ruddy* (1×)
rōf *n.* roof
roof (3×)
rolle *n.* roll
rolles (1×)
rolling(e *ng.* rolling
roulyng (1×)
°**rōpi** *adj.* ropy, viscous
ropi (1×)
***roris ciriacy** *n.* oak flowers [see **ōk(e**]
roris ciriacy (1×)
***rosata nouella** *n.* electuary made from roses
rosata nouella (2×), *rosa[t]a nouella* (1×)
rōse *n. (1)* rose (genus *Rosa*, fam. *Rosaceae*)
rooses (77×), *roses* (67×), *rosees* (40×), *rose* (3×), *roose* (2×), *roseen* (1×), *rosen* (1×), *rosyn* (1×), *rosys* (1×)
rōsēt *adj.* made of a distillation of red or white roses, coloured and flavoured with roses [see **hŏnī**, **mel rōsēt**, & **sugre**]
rōsī *adj.* rosy
rosey (1×)
rōsīn(e *n.* rosin (distillate of turpentine)
roosyn (1×)
rōs-marīn(e *n.* rosemary (*Rosmarinus officinalis*, fam. *Lamiaceae*)
roose-marine (1×), *rooses-marine* (1×), *rosemarine* (1×)
rōsten *v.* to roast
j-rosted (7×), *j-rostyd* (4×), *rooste* (3×), *rostyd* (3×), *roost* (2×), *roostid* (2×), *roste* (2×), *rostid* (2×), *j-roosted* (1×), *j-roostid* (1×), *j-rostid* (1×), *rost* (1×), *rosteed* (1×)
rōt *n.* rot
roote (1×)
rōte *n. (4)* root
roote (29×), *rote* (18×), *rotes* (10×), *rootes* (9×), *rotis* (4×), *rootis* (3×), *rootys* (3×), *rotys* (1×)
rōten *v. (1)* to rot
roted (4×), *roote* (3×), *rotyng* (2×), *j-roted* (1×), *j-rotyd* (1×), *rootid* (1×), *rote* (1×), *roten* (1×), *roteþ* (1×), *rotyd* (1×)
rōtennes(e *n.* (tooth) decay
rotenesse (1×), *rotennesse* (1×)
rough(e *adj.* rough
rowz (1×)
roughnes(se *n.* hoarseness
rowznesse (3×), *rownesse* (1×)
rŏund(e *adj.* round
round (7×), *rounde* (4×)
rūbarbe *n.* rhubarb (*Rheum officinale* or *palmatum*, fam. *Polygonaceae*)

reubarbe (9×), *reubarb* (1×), *reuberbe* (1×), *rubarbe* (1×)

rubben *v.* to rub
rubbe (4×), *rubben* (2×), *rubbid* (1×)

rūe *n.* common rue (*Ruta graveolens*, fam. *Rutaceae*)
rwe (27×), *rewe* (22×), *rew* (6×)

ruptōrī(e *n.* MED. & SURG. caustic or escharotic medicine
ruptorie (1×)

S

sādlī *adv.* fully
sadly (1×)

saf(f)rŏun *n.* saffron crocus (*Crocus sativus*, fam. *Iridaceae*)
saffren (7×), *safrun* (5×), *safroun* (3×), *saffrun* (1×), *safren* (1×)

sāl armoniak *n.* ammonium chloride, sal ammoniac
sal armoniac (5×)

sāl-ğemme *n.* rock salt
salgemme (6×), *sal-gemme* (3×), *salt-gemme* (1×)

sāl-nītre *n.* naturally occurring salt, prob. sodium carbonate
sal-nitre (1×), *salnitre* (1×), *salt-nitre* (1×)

salou(e *n.* willow (genus *Salix*, fam. *Salicaceae*)
salie (1×), *saly* (1×)

salouen *adj.* of the willow tree
saleyn (2×), *saleyne* (1×), *salien* (1×), *salwene* (1×), *salyen* (1×)

°**salouish** *adj.* sallowish
salewysch (1×)

salt *n. (1)* salt; *adj.* salty
n.: salt (33×), *saalt* (1×); *adj.: salt* (28×), *salte* (1×)
~ **armoniak**, ammonium chloride, sal ammoniac
salt armoniac (2×)
~ **fleum(e**, phlegm mixed with choler, salt phlegm
salt flewme (11×), *salt fleume* (2×)

salten *v.* to salt
salt (2×), *j-salted* (1×)

saltish *adj.* salty
saltysche (1×)

saltnes(se *n.* saltiness
saltnesse (1×)

salt-wāter *n.* (a) sea water; (b) salted water
salt-water (9×)

salvatel *n.* ANAT. vein between the ring finger and little finger of the right hand
salua[t]elle (1×), *salutelle* (1×)

sām(e *adj.* same
same (69×)

sāmŏun *n.* ZOOL. salmon
samonus (1×)

samsūchon *n.* elder (*Sambucus nigra*, fam. *Caprifoliaceae*)
sansuke (5×), *samsuke* (2×)

sandal(e *n.* sandalwood (species *Santalum*, fam. *Santalaceae*)
sendel (1×)

sāndī(e *adj.* sandy
sondy (1×)

san-dragŏun *n.* red juice or resin of the dragon tree (*Dracaena draco*, fam. *Agavaceae*)
sandragoun (15×), *saundragoun* (9×),

sandragun (3×), *saundragun* (3×), *sancdragoun* (2×), *samdragoun* (1×), *sanedragun* (1×), *sangedragoun* (1×)
sanguinārī(e *n.* shepherd's purse (*Capsella bursa-pastoris*, fam. *Brassicaceae*)
sanguinarie (5×)
sanguin(e *adj.* sanguine
sanguyn (6×), *sanguin* (3×)
sanguinitē *n.* consanguinity
sanguinite (1×)
sanicle *n.* sanicle (*Sanicula europaea*, fam. *Apiaceae*)
sanicle (1×)
sape *n. (1)* new wine boiled to a syrup
sape (5×)
sāp(e *n. (2)* sap of a tree
sap (2×)
sarcocol(le *n.* Persian gum
sarcocolle (11×)
satiriasis *n.* satyriasis
satiriasis (3×)
satureie *n.* savory (*Satureja hortensis*, fam. *Lamiaceae*)
satureie (2×), *saturie* (1×)
sauce *n.* sauce
sause (2×), *sauce* (1×), *sauces* (1×)
sauflī *adv.* safely
sauely (1×)
sauğe *n.* sage (*Salvia officinalis*, fam. *Lamiaceae*)
sauge (24×)
saun-de-ver(e *n.* saline scum cast up over glass after vitrification, sandiver
sandeuer (1×)
saundre *n.* [see **sandal(e**]
saundres (16×), *saundris* (8×), *saundrys* (8×), *saundrees* (1×), *saun[d]ris* (1×)
sāven *v.* to protect
sauep (2×), *j-sauyd* (1×), *sauyn* (1×)
sāve-nāp(e *n.* towel
sauenap (1×)
sāverei(e *n.* plant of the genus *Satureja*, fam. *Lamiaceae*
sauerey (3×), *saueray* (1×), *sauereie* (1×)
savīn(e *n.* savine (*Juniperus sabina*, fam. *Cupressaceae*)
sauyne (4×)
sāvŏur *n.* savour
sauer (1×), *sauor* (1×), *sauour* (1×)
sāvŏuren *v.* to savour
j-sauered (1×), *j-saueryd* (1×), *sauerid* (1×)
sāvŏurī(e *adj.* savoury
sauery (1×)
saxifrağe *n.* saxifrage, any plant of the genus *Saxifraga*, fam. *Saxifragaceae*
saxifrage (12×)
scab(be *n.* scab
scabbe (3×), *scabbys* (3×)
scabben *v.* to scratch
scabbid (1×)
scābiŏus(e *n.* any of the plants of the genus *Scabiosa*, fam. *Dipsacaceae*
scabiose (1×), *scabyouse* (1×)
scalden *v.* to scald, to burn
scaldyng (1×)
scalding(e *ag.* scalding
scaldyng (1×)
scāle *n. (1)* (a) hull of grain; (b) flake

scales (5×), *scalees* (1×)
scālen *v. (1)* (*ppl.*) **scaled**, having scales, scaly
scalyd (2×), *scaled* (1×)
scamōnī(e *n.* scammony (*Convolvulus scammonia*, fam. *Convolvulaceae*)
scamone (19×), *scamonye* (1×)
scāpen *v. (1)* to escape
scapen (1×)
scariol(e *n.* any of several plants associated with lettuce, esp. prickly lettuce (*Lactuca scariola*, fam. *Asteraceae*) or corn sowthistle (*Sonchus arvenis*, fam. *A.*)
scariole (12×)
scārsnes(se *n.* insufficiency
scarsnesse (1×)
sclīce *n.* MED. spatula
sklice (2×), *sklise* (1×)
scŏme *n.* scum
scome (1×)
scorpiŏun *n.* ZOOL. scorpion
scorpion (1×)
scotōmīe *n.* dizziness and dimness of sight
scotomye (2×), *scotomie* (1×), *scotomy* (1×)
scŏuren *v. (2)* to scour
scoryd (1×)
scrōphulārīe *n.* plant or herb of the genus *Scrophularia*, fam. *Scrophulariaceae*
scrophularie (1×)
scul(le *n.* skull
skulle (1×)
scurf *n.* scaly disease of the skin
scorff (1×)
sē *n. (1)* sea
see (11×)
sebesten *n.* Assyrian plum (*Cordia myxa*, fam. *Boraginaceae*)
sebestem (1×)
sēd *n.* seed
seed (153×), *seedes* (8×), *seedis* (8×), *sedis* (4×), *sedys* (3×), *sede* (2×), *sedes* (2×), *seid* (2×), *sed* (1×), *seede* (1×), *seedys* (1×)
sēgğe *n. (2)* privy, latrine; **gōn to ~**, to void the bowels or bladder
sege (3×), *seege* (1×)
seien *v. (1)* to say
seie (11×), *j-seid* (11×), *seid* (10×), *sey* (7×), *say* (5×), *seyn* (5×), *seyd* (3×), *j-seed* (2×), *seist* (2×), *j-seyd* (1×), *j-seyn* (1×), *said* (1×), *saied* (1×), *seiþ* (1×), *seyde* (1×), *seyden* (1×), *seye* (1×)
seint(e *n.* saint
seint (3×)
sēlde *adj.* infrequent; *adv.* seldom
adj.: selde (1×); *adv.: seld* (1×)
sēlden(e *adv.* seldom
selden (2×), *seldene* (1×), *seldom* (1×), *syldan* (1×)
sēlden(e-whanne *adv.* rarely
selde[n]e-whanne (1×)
sēmelī *adj.* seeming
semelyche (1×), *semlyche* (1×)
sēmen *v. (2)* to seem
semeþ (10×), *semen* (4×), *seme* (3×), *semyn* (2×)
°**semis** *n.* half
semis (84×)
sēn *v. (1)* to see
seen (6×), *seeþ* (5×), *see* (4×), *a-seene*

(2×), *a-sene* (2×), *sen* (2×), *j-seeþ* (1×), *j-seie* (1×), *j-sie* (1×), *j-sien* (1×), *se* (1×), *seen* (1×), *seene* (1×), *seest* (1×), *seyn* (1×), *sie* (1×), *sye* (1×)

senden *v. (2)* to send
j-sent (2×), *sent* (2×)

senē *n. (1)* powdered leaves or pods of senna (genus *Cassia*, fam. *Fabaceae*)
sene (21×)

sen(e)vei *n.* plant of the genus *Brassica*, fam. *Brassicaceae*, prob. black mustard (*B. nigra*) or white mustard (*B. alba*)
seneuey (13×), *seneuei* (3×)

serāpīnum *n.* sagapenum (medicinal gum prob. derived from the plant *Ferula persica*, fam. *Apiaceae*)
serapinum (2×), *serap[inum]* (1×), *serepinum* (1×)

serpentārī(e *n.* prob. dragonwort (*Dracunculus vulgaris*, fam. *Araceae*)
serpentarie (1×)

serven *v. (1)* to serve
serueþ (5×), *seruen* (4×), *serue* (1×), *seruyn* (1×)

servīs(e *n.* service
seruices (1×)

sestern(e *n.* cistern
sisterne (1×)

setewāl(e *n.* long zedoary (*Curcuma zedoaria*, fam. *Zingiberaceae*)
ȝedwarie (2×), *ȝedeware* (1×), *ȝedoare* (1×), *ȝedoware* (1×), *ȝeduare* (1×), *ȝedware* (1×), *ȝoduale* (1×)

sēthen *v. (1)* to boil, to seethe
j-soden (198×), *seeþ* (93×), *seþe* (26×), *seeþe* (17×), *soden* (16×), *j-sode* (6×), *seþ* (6×), *j-sodyn* (4×), *seþen* (3×), *jsoden* (2×), *sodyn* (2×), *y-soden* (2×), *i-soden* (1×), *j-seden* (1×), *j-seeþ* (1×), *j-sooden* (1×), *j-soþin* (1×), *seþeþ* (1×), *siþe* (1×), *ysode* (1×)

sēthing(e *ag.* boiling
seþing (1×)

setten *v.* to sit
set (12×), *setten* (1×), *setteþ* (1×), *settyn* (1×)

seurlī *adv.* surely
surely (1×)

shāmeful(le *adj.* ashamed
schamfulle (1×)

shāp(e *n.* shape
schap (3×), *schaap* (2×)

shāpen *v.* to shape
j-schapen (1×)

shār(e *n. (2)* pubic region, groin
schare (19×), *schaar* (5×), *schaare* (1×), *schar* (1×)

sharp *adj.* sharp; ~ **fēver**, high fever
scharp (19×), *scharpe* (5×)

sharpen *v.* to sharpen
scharpeþ (1×)

sharpnes(se *n.* sharpness
scharpnesse (7×)

shāven *v.* to shave
schaue (4×), *j-schaud* (1×), *schaaf* (1×), *schaf* (1×)

shāving(e *ng.* scraping; ~ **of guttes**, intestinal tissue discharged with the stool
schauynge (5×), *schauyng* (3×)

shel(le *n.* shell

schelle (2×), *schelles* (2×)
shēp *n.* ZOOL. sheep
schepis (9×), *scheep* (1×), *scheepis* (1×), *schepe* (1×), *schepys* (1×), *scheyp* (1×)
shēphērdes-purs *n.* [see **sanguinārī(e**]
scheperdis-purs (1×), *scheperdis-purse* (1×), *scheperdus-purs* (1×), *scheperdys-purs* (1×)
shēphērdes-yērd *n.* teasel (*Dipsacus pilosus* or *sylvestris*, fam. *Dipsacaceae*)
scheperdes-ȝerde (2×), *scheperdys-ȝardese* (1×), *scheppardes-ȝerde* (1×)
shēre *n. (1)* pair of scissors or shears
scherys (1×)
shēren *v.* to shear
j-schore (5×), *j-schoore* (1×), *j-[shoren]* (1×), *schore* (1×)
shēte *n. (2)* sheet
schete (2×)
sheuen *v. (1)* to show
schewe (1×), *schewyd* (1×), *schewyn* (1×)
shīning(e *ng.* & *ag.* shining
ng.: schinnyng (1×); *ag.: schynnyng* (1×), *schynyng* (1×), *schynynge* (1×)
shīr(e *adv.* brightly
schyre (1×)
shīten *v.* to defecate
schite (8×), *schiteþ* (3×), *schiten* (2×), *schiȝt* (2×), *schyte* (2×), *schiting* (1×)
shō *n.* shoe
scho (1×), *schoo* (1×), *schoon* (1×)
short *adj.* short
schort (5×)
shortlī *adv.* shortly
schortly (1×)
shrinken *v.* to shrink
schrynckeþ (1×), *schrynkeþ* (1×)
shulder *n.* shoulder
schulder (1×), *schulderyn* (1×), *schuldres* (1×), *schuldris* (1×), *schuldrys* (1×)
shulder-blād(e *n.* shoulder blade
schulder-blad (1×), *schuldre-blades* (1×), *schuldyrbladys* (1×), *xulder-blad* (1×)
shulen *v. (1)* shall
xal (161×), *xalt* (49×), *xul* (46×), *xuld* (32×), *schal* (7×), *xullen* (7×), *xulde* (5×), *schuld* (4×), *schulde* (4×), *schullen* (4×), *scholde* (3×), *schul* (3×), *schulle* (2×), *xulden* (2×), *xuldyn* (2×), *xullyn* (2×), *schalt* (1×), *scholdest* (1×), *schullin* (1×), *schullyn* (1×), *xa[l]* (1×), *xulle* (1×)
sīcamŏur(e *n.* sycamore (*Ficus sycomorus*, fam. *Moraceae*)
sicamour (1×), *sichomour* (1×)
siccidis *n.* ?wild cucumber (*Echinocystis lobata*, fam. *Cucurbitaceae*)
s[icc]ide (1×)
sīde *n.* side
syde (47×), *side* (39×), *sydes* (6×), *sydys* (5×), *sydis* (3×), *sidis* (1×)
sight(e *n.* sight
siȝt (13×), *siȝte* (2×), *syth* (1×)
°**signa febris** *n.* type of fever
signa febris (1×)
sīgne *n.* sign
signes (37×), *signys* (7×), *signe* (6×), *signis* (1×), *signus* (1×), *syngnes* (1×)
significāciŏun *n.* symbol, sign
significaciouns (1×)

sīk *n.* & *adj.* sick
n.: seke (1×), *sike* (1×), *syk* (1×); *adj.: siyk* (8×), *syk* (5×), *syik* (2×), *seik* (1×), *seke* (1×), *sekerest* (1×), *seyk* (1×), *sik* (1×), *sike* (1×), *syyk* (1×)

sīken *v. (1)* to be ill
sekyn (1×)

sīking(e *ng.* laboured or difficult breathing
sikynge (1×)

sīk-man *n.* patient
sicman (2×), *sike-man* (1×), *sik-man* (1×), *syke-man* (1×)

sīknes(se *n.* sickness
sicnesse (222×), *sicnesses* (24×), *siknesse* (4×), *sicnessys* (3×), *sicnessis* (2×), *syknesse* (2×), *sekenesse* (1×), *siccnesse* (1×), *sicnese* (1×), *siknesses* (1×)

sīlence *n.* silence
silence (1×)

*****siler(is)** *n.* sesely (genus *Seseli*, fam. *Apiaceae*)
silere (4×), *sylere* (2×), *sileos* (1×), *siler* (1×), *sileris* (1×), *silery* (1×), *silore* (1×), *syleos* (1×)

silk(e *n.* silk
silk (3×)

silken *adj.* silken
sylken (1×)

silver *n.* silver
syluere (1×)

simphite *n.* [see **cǒnferīe**]
symphite (2×), *simphite* (1×)

simple *adj.* simple
symple (9×), *simple* (3×), *sympel* (3×), *sympil* (2×), *simpel* (1×), *simpil* (1×), *sympille* (1×)

sincopis *n.* PATHOL. syncope
syncopis (3×), *sincopis* (2×)

sineu *n.* sinew
senewys (6×), *senewis* (4×), *senewes* (1×)

singen *v.* to sing
syngeþ (2×), *syngyng* (1×)

singing(e *ng.* singing
synggyng (1×)

singrēne *n.* houseleek (*Sempervivum tectorum*, fam. *Crassulaceae*)
syngrene (16×), *singrene* (2×), *synegrene* (2×), *synngrene* (1×)

sinken *v.* to sink
syncke (1×), *synckeþ* (1×), *synke* (1×)

sinne *n.* sin
synne (1×)

sinoch *n.* unintermittent fever
sinochus (1×)

siphac *n.* peritoneum
siphac (6×), *sjphac* (1×)

sirup *n.* MED. syrup
sirip (89×), *siripis* (10×), *siripe* (9×), *sirrip* (6×), *siripes* (3×), *sirepis* (2×), *sirypis* (2×), *serip* (1×), *sirips* (1×), *siripys* (1×), *sirripis* (1×), *sirryp* (1×), *siryp* (1×), *surripis* (1×), *syrip* (1×), *syripe* (1×)

*****sisymbre** *n.* hedge mustard (*Sisymbrium officinale*, fam. *Brassicaceae*)
sisymbre (1×)

sīth *n.* time
siþes (6×), *siþis* (1×), *syþes* (1×)

sitten *v.* to sit
sitten (6×), *sitte* (5×), *sittyn* (3×),

[sete] (1×), *sit* (1×), *sittyng* (1×), *sytte* (1×)

sitthe *adv.* afterwards
siþe (172×), *siþþe* (55×), *siþ* (5×), *syþe* (3×), *syþþe* (2×)

sitthen *adv.* afterwards
siþen (1×), *syþþen* (1×)

skil *n.* skill
skyl (1×)

skim *n.* impure foam that rises to the surface as a result of boiling
skym (1×)

skimming *ng.* [see **skim**]
skymmyng (1×)

skin *n. (1)* skin
skyn (27×), *skynnes* (9×), *skynes* (1×)

skīrwhīt(e *n.* (a) parsnip or water-parsnip (*Pastinaca sativa*, fam. *Apiaceae*); (b) white pepper (*Eruca s.*, fam. *Brassicaceae*)
skyrewhittes (1×)

slak *adj.* slack
slaak (1×), *slak* (1×)

slaknesse *n.* slackening
slacnesse (3×), *slaknesse* (1×)

slēn *v.* MED. & SURG. to destroy; to kill
sleeþ (9×), *slee* (6×), *j-slawe* (3×), *sleen* (2×), *j-slaw* (1×), *sleinge* (1×), *sleþ* (1×)

slēp *n.* sleep
sleep (22×), *sleepe* (1×), *slep* (1×), *slepe* (1×)

slēpen *v.* to sleep
slepe (7×), *slepeþ* (3×), *slepyn* (2×), *sleped* (1×), *slepen* (1×), *slepin* (1×), *slepte* (1×)

slēpful *adj.* sleepy; lethargic
sleepfulle (1×), *slepful* (1×)

slēpī *adj.* sleepy
slepy (1×)

slēping(e *ag.* sleeping
slepyng (2×)

sleuthe *n.* sloth
slouþe (3×), *sleuþe* (2×), *slowþe* (1×)

sliderī *adj.* slippery
slideri (2×), *slyderere* (1×)

slitten *v.* (a) to split; (b) to make an incision
sclytte (1×), *slite* (1×), *slitten* (1×), *sliȝt* (1×), *slyt* (1×)

slō *n.* sloe (*Prunus spinosa*, fam. *Rosaceae*)
sloon (2×), *sloo* (1×)

slŏmbering(e *ng.* sleep
slombringe (1×)

slou *adj.* slow
slow (8×), *slowe* (1×)

slough *n. (2)* scale of an adder
slewȝ (1×), *slowȝ* (1×)

sloulī *adv.* slowly
slowly (1×)

slounes(se *n.* slowness
slownesse (1×)

sluggī *adj.* sluggish
sluggy (1×)

smāl *adj.* small
smale (29×), *smal* (23×), *smalle* (4×)

smālnes(se *n.* thinness, smallness
smalnesse (1×)

°**smālshipe** *n.* thinness, smallness
smalschipe (1×)

smel *n.* smell
smel (1×)

smellen *v.* to smell

smelle (7×), *smellyn* (3×), *smellen* (1×), *smelleþ* (1×), *smellyng* (1×)
smelling(e *ng.* & *ag.* smelling
ng.: smellyng (2×), *smellynges* (2×); *ag.: smellyng* (8×), *smellynge* (4×), *smelling* (1×)
smert *adj.* painful, sore
smart (1×), *smert* (1×), *smerte* (1×)
smerten *v.* to suffer pain
smerte (3×), *smertyn* (1×)
smerting(e *ng.* & *ag.* aching; itching
ng.: smertyng (4×), *smertynge* (2×), *smartyng* (1×); *ag.: smertyng* (1×)
smīlen *v.* to smile
smylyng (1×)
smīten *v.* to strike
smyte (6×), *smyten* (4×), *smyteþ* (2×), *smytyn* (2×), *smetyn* (1×)
smith *n.* blacksmith
smythes (1×), *smythys* (1×), *smyþes* (1×), *smyþis* (1×)
smīting(e *ng.* striking
smytynge (4×), *smytyng* (3×), *smytinge* (1×)
smōke *n.* smoke
smoke (37×), *smokes* (4×), *smokys* (1×)
smōkī *adj.* smoky
smoky (1×)
smōth(e *adj.* smooth
smoþe (1×)
smōthenes(se *n.* smoothness
smoþenesse (1×)
snail *n.* zool. snail
snail (3×), *snayles* (3×)
snou *n.* snow
snow (1×)
sō *adv.* so
so (126×), *soo* (6×)
sodein *adj.* sudden
sodeyn (3×), *soden* (2×)
sodeinlī *adv.* suddenly
sodenly (4×), *sodenlyche* (1×), *sodeynly* (1×)
soft(e *n.* mullein (*Verbascum thapsus*, fam. *Scrophulariaceae*; *Asarum europaeum*, fam. *Aristolochiaceae*)
softe (2×)
soft(e *adj.* soft
soft (3×), *sooft* (2×), *softe* (1×)
softlī *adv.* softly
softly (5×)
softnes(se *n.* softness
softnesse (3×), *sooftnesse* (1×)
sōken *v.* to soak
ȝoke (5×), *ȝokyn* (2×), *j-soke* (1×), *sokyn* (1×), *sowkyn* (1×), *ȝouken* (1×)
solatrum *n.* any of several herbs of the genus *Solanum* (fam. *Solanaceae*), esp. black solanum, belladonna
solatre (19×)
sōle *n.* (a) sole (of foot, shoe); (b) ZOOL. sole fish
sooles (3×), *sole* (1×), *soles* (1×), *solus* (1×), *solys* (1×), *soole* (1×)
sŏm-dēl *adv.* partly
sumdel (3×), *sumdele* (1×), *sumdelle* (1×)
sŏmer *n. (1)* summer
somer (11×)
sŏmer-tīme *n.* summertime
somer-tyme (1×)
sŏm-tīme *adv.* sometimes
sumtyme (13×)
sŏm-what *adv.* somewhat

sumwhat (17×), *sumqwhat* (1×), *sumwat* (1×), *sumwhaȝt* (1×)

sōne *adv.* soon
sone (20×), *soone* (2×), *so[n]e* (1×), *soon* (1×)

sŏnne *n.* sun
sunne (29×)

sōpe *n. (2)* soap
sope (6×), *sopees* (1×), *sopys* (1×)

sopēr(e *n. (1)* supper, meal
sopere (1×), *soperes* (1×), *soperis* (1×)

sōr(e *n. (1)* pain, sore; *adj. (2)* aching
n.: soore (11×), *sore* (5×), *soor* (2×); *adj.: sore* (2×)

sōre *adv.* bitterly
sore (3×)

sorel *n.* sour dock, sorrel (*Rumex acetosa*, fam. *Polygonaceae*) or wood sorrel (*Oxalis acetosella*, fam. *Oxalidaceae*)
sorel (2×)

sōrī *adj.* (a) causing pain; (b) poor in quality
sori (3×), *sory* (3×)

sorwe *n.* sorrow
sorow (12×), *sorwe* (5×), *sorowe* (1×)

sotil *adj.* (a) sharp; (b) light
sotyl (10×), *sotel* (3×), *sotil* (3×), *suttyl* (2×), *sotele* (1×), *sotile* (1×)

sotilnes(se *n.* thinness (of blood)
sotylnesse (1×)

sotiltē *n.* thinness (of blood)
sotylte (4×)

souden *v. (1)* to heal by promoting cicatrization or knitting
soude (3×), *souden* (3×), *soudeþ* (2×), *j-souded* (1×), *soud[i]þ* (1×), *sowde* (1×), *sowden* (1×), *sowdiþ* (1×)

souding(e *ng.* healing or knitting of a wound or fracture
soudynge (2×)

sŏue *n. (2)* ZOOL. sow, female swine
sowes (1×)

souen *v. (1)* to sow
j-sowen (1×)

sŏuken *v.* to suck
souken (2×), *soukyn* (1×)

sŏuking(e *ag.* sucking
soukyng (2×), *sokynge* (1×), *sowkyng* (1×)

soul(e *n.* soul
soule (1×), *sowle* (1×)

sŏund(e *adj.* healthy; strong
sound (2×)

sŏuping(e *ag. (1)* liquid, soft
soupyng (2×)

sŏur *adj.* sour
soure (18×), *sowre* (11×), *sowr* (10×), *sour* (2×)

sŏur-dokke *n.* sorrel (*Rumex acetosa*, fam. *Polygonaceae*)
sourdocke (2×), *sourdockes* (1×), *soure-dock* (1×)

sŏur-dough *n.* leaven
sourdouȝ (1×), *sourdowe* (1×)

sŏurnes(se *n.* sourness
sournesse (1×)

sŏuth *n. (2)* south
sowth (2×), *south* (1×), *souþ* (1×)

sŏuthern(e-wōde *n.* southernwood (*Artemisia abrotanum*, fam. *Asteraceae*)
sopernewode (2×), *soupernewode* (2×), *sotherne-woode* (1×), *souperwode* (1×)

sŏuthward *adv.* southwards
sowthward (1×)

sŏuth-wīnd *n.* wind blowing from

the south
souþwynd (1×)
soverain *adj.* sovereign
souereyn (2×), *soueren* (1×)
Spain(e *n.* Spain
spayne (3×)
sparplen *v.* to sprinkle
j-sparlied (1×), *j-sparplid* (1×)
spēch(e *n.* speech
speche (3×)
speciāl(e *adj.* special
special (17×), *speciale* (1×), *specialle* (1×)
speciāllī *adv.* specially
specially (1×), *specialy* (1×)
spēken *v.* to speak
speke (6×), *spekyn* (4×), *spoke* (2×), *spoken* (2×), *spokyn* (2×), *j-spoke* (1×), *j-spoken* (1×), *speken* (1×), *spekynge* (1×)
spēking(e *ng.* speaking
spekyng (1×)
spek(ke *n.* speck
speckys (1×)
spēten *v.* to spit
spete (6×), *spetyn* (4×), *spitte* (2×), *speet* (1×), *speteþ* (1×), *spit* (1×), *spottyn* (1×), *spyttyt* (1×)
spēting(e *ng.* spitting; spittle
spetyng (27×), *spetynge* (5×), *spetinge* (2×), *speting* (1×)
speuen *v.* to vomit
spewe (1×)
speuing(e *ng.* vomit(ing)
spewynge (2×), *spuynge* (1×), *spwyng* (1×)
***spica celtica** *n.* spike celtica (*Valeriana celtica*, fam. *Valerianaceae*)
spica celtica (1×)
°**spicassie** *n.* type of plant
spiccassie (1×)
spīce *n. (1)* spice
spices (10×), *spicis* (1×), *spises* (1×)
spīcerī(e *n.* spice
spicerie (1×), *spiceries* (1×), *sp[i]cery* (1×)
spīk(e *n. (2)* valerianaceous plant, prob. *Valeriana officinalis*, fam. *Valerianaceae*
spik (30×)
spīkenard *n.* spikenard (*Nardostachys jatamansi*, fam. *Valerianaceae*) [also **spīk(e** *n. (2)*]
spikenard (5×), *spicnard* (2×), *spiknard* (1×), *spyknard* (1×)
spinache *n.* spinach (*Spinacia oleracea*, fam. *Chenopodiaceae*)
spinage (1×)
spirit *n.* spirit
spiritys (4×), *spirites* (2×), *spiritis* (2×), *spiritus* (1×), *spirytis* (1×), *spirytys* (1×), *spritys* (1×)
spiritūāl *adj.* **~ membres**, respiratory organs, esp. the lungs
spiritual (4×)
spitten *v. (1)* to spit
spittyn (1×)
spitting(e *ng.* spitting; spittle
spittyng (8×), *spyttyng* (4×), *spittynge* (2×), *spyttynge* (2×), *spiting* (1×), *spitting* (1×), *spittinge* (1×), *spytyng* (1×)
splēn(e *n.* spleen
splene (110×), *spleen* (1×)
spōdium *n.* powder derived from ashes of ivory or other substances

spodie (29×), *spodye* (1×)
spōn *n.* spoon
spon (1×)
spōn-ful *n.* spoonful
sponefulle (6×), *sponeful* (2×)
sponğe *n.* sponge
spounge (2×), *sponge* (1×)
spot *n. (1)* spot
spottes (1×)
spōtel *n.* saliva, slaver
spotyl (8×), *spotel* (2×), *spotil* (2×)
sprenten *v.* to leap
j-spreynt (3×), *j-sprent* (2×), *j-spreynd* (1×)
springen *v.* to sprinkle
spring (9×), *springe* (3×), *sprynge* (2×), *springist* (1×), *springyn* (1×), *spryng* (1×), *spryngyn* (1×)
spūme *n.* foam, froth
spume (11×), *spumes* (1×)
°**spūming(e** *ng.* vomit; spit
spumynge (1×)
spurğe *n.* spurge, one of several plants of the genus *Euphorbia*, fam. *Euphorbiaceae*
spurge (7×)
squār(e *adj.* square
sqware (1×)
squille *n. (2)* squill: plant of the genus *Scilla*, esp. sea onion (*Urginea scilla*, fam. *Liliaceae*)
squille (5×), *squilla* (1×)
squillītik *adj.* containing or made with squill
squillitik (3×), *squillytik* (2×), *squilitik* (1×), *squilletik* (1×), *squillityk* (1×), *squilytik* (1×)
squinacī(e *n.* PATHOL. inflammation, swelling of the throat; quinsy
squinacie (3×), *squinacy* (1×)
squinance *n.* [see **squinacī(e**]
squinance (1×), *squinancie* (1×)
squīnaunt *n.* camel's hay (*Cymbopogon schoenanthus*, fam. *Poaceae*)
squinante (6×), *squinant* (3×), *squinantum* (3×), *squinaticum* (1×), *squynant* (1×)
stāble *adj.* stable
stabil (1×)
staf *n.* stick
staf (1×)
stāl(e *adj. (1)* stale
stale (2×)
stalk(e *n. (1)* stalk
stalk (1×), *stalkes* (1×)
stal(le *n.* stall
stalle (1×)
stamering(e *ag.* stammering
stameryng (1×)
stampen *v.* to pound or mash
stampe (43×), *j-stamped* (16×), *stamp* (8×), *j-stampid* (2×)
stāphis-āgre *n.* stavesacre, lice-bane (*Delphinium staphisagria*, fam. *Ranunculaceae*)
s[t]aphie (5×), *staphie* (2×), *staphi* (1×), *staphizagre* (1×), *staphyne* (1×)
stāt *n.* state
staat (2×), *statte* (1×)
staunchen *v.* to stop (blood, flow, humours)
staunche (17×), *staunchep* (6×), *j-staunchid* (4×), *staunchen* (4×), *staunchyn* (4×), *j-staunchyd* (1×),

staunchid (1×), *staunchiþ* (1×), *staunchyt* (1×)
staunching(e *ng.* stopping (of blood)
staunchyng (1×)
stēde *n. (1)* place
stede (1×)
sted-fast *adj.* firm
studefast (1×)
stēl(e *n. (3)* steel
steel (1×)
stench *n.* stench
stenche (1×), *stinche* (1×), *stincke* (1×), *stynche* (1×)
steu(e *n. (2)* steam bath, inhalation; cauldron
styue (2×), *stewe* (1×), *stwe* (1×)
steuen *v. (2)* to inhale the vapour of a boiling decoction; to bathe in a hot-air or steam bath
stuwe (1×), *styue* (1×)
sticados *n.* French lavender (*Lavandula stoechas*, fam. *Lamiaceae*)
sticados (1×), *stikades* (1×)
stich(e *n. (1)* sharp, localized pain
styches (2×), *stiche* (1×), *stiches* (1×), *styche* (1×)
stikke *n.* stick
stickes (2×), *sticke* (1×), *stikke* (1×)
stille *adj.* & *adv.* still
adj.: stille (3×), *stylle* (1×); *adv.: stille* (12×), *stylle* (1×)
stinken *v.* to stink
stinckeþ (3×), *stinken* (2×), *stinckiþ* (1×), *styncke* (1×), *stynckeþ* (1×), *stynkeþ* (1×), *stynkyn* (1×), *stynkyth* (1×)
stinking(e *ng.* & *ag.* stinking
ng.: stynckynges (2×), *stynckyncge* (1×), *stynckynge* (1×), *stynckyngge* (1×), *stynkyng* (1×); *ag.: stynckyng* (1×), *stynckynge* (1×)
stiren *v.* to stir
stere (7×), *j-sterid* (1×), *steryng* (1×), *stire* (1×)
stiring(e *ng.* movement
sterynge (1×)
stōl *n.* stool
stool (2×), *stoole* (1×)
stomak *n.* stomach
stomac (283×), *stomak* (3×), *stomakes* (2×), *stomackus* (1×), *stomake* (1×)
stomaticon *n.* MED. digestive or purgative medicine of various kinds
stomaticon (6×)
stōn *n.* stone; MED. calculus, stone
stoon (44×), *stoones* (28×), *ston* (8×), *stones* (5×), *stonys* (2×), *stoone* (1×)
stōn-crop *n.* plant of the genus *Sedum*, either stonecrop (*S. acre*, fam. *Crassulaceae*) or rock stonecrop (*S. reflexum*, fam. *C.*)
stancrop (2×)
stōnden *v. (1)* to stand
stonde (4×), *stondeþ* (3×), *stond* (2×), *stand* (1×), *standeþ* (1×), *sto[n]deþ* (1×), *stondiþ* (1×), *stood* (1×)
stōnding(e *ng.* standing; *ag.* stagnant (water)
ng.: stondyng (1×), *stondynge* (1×); *ag.: stondyng* (1×)
stōnī *adj.* made of stone
stony (1×)
stoppen *v.* (a) to stop; MED. & PHYSIOL. (b) to close the pores; (c)

to obstruct
stoppeþ (11×), *j-stopped* (11×), *j-stoppid* (8×), *stopped* (6×), *stoppe* (5×), *stoppen* (3×), *j-stoppyd* (2×), *stop* (2×), *i-stopped* (1×), *stoppeid* (1×), *stoppet* (1×), *stoppid* (1×), *stoppyd* (1×), *stoppyn* (1×)

stopping(e MED. & PHYSIOL. *ng.* obstruction; *ag.:* obstructing
ng.: stoppyng (16×), *stopping* (7×), *stoppynge* (6×), *stoppinge* (2×), *stopyng* (1×), *stopynge* (1×); *ag.: stoppyng* (1×)

storax *n.* gum or resin from the storax tree (*Styrax officinale*, fam. *Styracaceae*)
storace (6×), *storax* (3×), *storac* (1×), *storak* (1×), *storat* (1×)

stranglen *v.* to choke
strangle (1×), *strangleþ* (1×)

strangūrī(e *n.* difficulty of urination, strangury
stranguria (3×), *strangurie* (2×), *strangure* (1×), *strangury* (1×), *straungurie* (1×)

strau *n.* stalk
strees (1×)

strau-berī(e *n.* strawberry (genus *Fragaria*, fam. *Rosaceae*)
strauberiwise (1×)

strecchen *v.* to stretch
j-streiȝt (1×)

strecching(e *ng.* stretching
strechyng (1×)

streinen *v.* *(1)* to strain
streyne (2×), *streyneþ* (2×), *streineþ* (1×), *streynen* (1×)

streining(e *ng.* straining
streynyng (1×)

streinŏur *n.* strainer
streynour (1×)

streit *adj.* straight
streiȝt (3×), *streite* (1×), *streyt* (1×)

streitnes(se *n.* narrowness; **~ of brēst**, **~ of brēth**, difficulty in breathing
streitnesse (6×), *streiȝtnesse* (4×), *streytnesse* (3×)

strēm *n.* flow; stream
stremes (2×), *stremys* (2×), *streem* (1×)

streng(e *n.* strength
strencþe (3×)

streuen *v.* to sprinkle
strawe (8×), *straw* (3×), *strewyn* (1×), *strow* (1×)

strictōrī(e *n.* medicine or herb having constricting properties; compress or plaster with such effect; *adj.* having constricting properties or effects
n.: strictories (14×), *strictorie* (5×), *strictoryes* (3×), *stri-ctories* (1×), *stricto-ries* (1×); *adj.: strictorie* (7×), *strictories* (3×), *strictoryes* (1×)

strīf(e *n.* ?agitation of air or gas
strief (1×)

strōk(e *n.* stroke
strok (2×), *strokys* (1×), *strook* (1×)

strong *adj.* strong
strong (40×), *stronge* (9×), *strengure* (3×), *strenger* (2×), *strengere* (2×), *strengore* (1×)

stronglī *adv.* strongly
stronglyche (1×)

stupefactīf *n.* medicine with

anaesthetic or narcotic properties
stupefactis (1×), *stupefactyues* (1×)
stūphe *n.* MED. hot-air or steam bath; herbal decoction used in a steam bath; medicinal vapour
stufe (29×), *stufes* (4×), *stuphe* (2×)
stūphen *v.* MED. to administer a steam or hot-air bath or a medicinal vapour; to inhale the vapour of a boiling decoction
stufen (3×), *stufe* (2×), *j-stufed* (1×)
stūphing *ng.* MED. administering a steam bath or a medicinal vapour to a part of the body
stuffyng (1×), *stufyng* (1×)
stuth *n.* type of symptom, ?stopping[19]
stuth (1×)
substaunce *n.* substance
substaunce (8×)
subtīliātīve *n.* medicine having a thinning effect
subtiliatyfs (1×), *subtilyatyfs* (1×)
sufferen *v.* to suffer
suffre (4×), *suffren* (3×), *suffreþ* (2×)
sufficient *adj.* sufficient
sufficient (3×), *sufficyent* (1×)
sufficientlī *adv.* sufficiently
sufficiently (2×)
suffīsen *v.* to suffice
suffisiþ (2×), *sufficen* (1×), *suffisen* (1×), *suffiseþ* (1×), *suffyce* (1×)
suffōcāciŏoun *n.* (a) obstruction; (b) condition attributed to the rising of the uterus, with compression of the heart and lungs; **~ of the mōder**
suffocacioun (3×), *suffocacion* (1×), *suffocacyoun* (1×)
sugre *n.* (a) sugar; (b) MED. in phrases indicating combination of sugar with a distillation or petals of roses, borage, or violets: **~ of roses (borage, violet)**
sugre (78×), *sugyr* (2×), *sugere* (1×)
~ rōsēt, MED. mixture of sugar and a distillation of roses
sugre roset (9×), *sugre rooset* (3×), *suger roset* (1×)
sulphurī *adj.* sulphurous
souffry (1×)
sulphur-vīve *n.* native sulfur
suphur-vife (1×)
sumac *n.* sumac (*Rhus coriaria*, fam. *Anacardiaceae*)
sumac (12×)
superflūitē *n.* PHYSIOL. excess of humours
superfluite (2×), *superfluites* (2×)
suppōsen *v.* to suppose
suppose (2×)
suppositōrī(e *n.* MED. suppository
suppositorie (8×), *suppositories* (8×), *suppositorys* (2×), *suppo-sitorie* (1×), *suppositoris* (1×)
surfēt *n.* excess, overabundance
surfeet (1×), *surfet* (1×), *surfetes* (1×)
sustenaunce *n.* sustenance
sustenaunce (1×)
swāğen *v.* *(2)* to alleviate
swage (1×)
swalm *n.* inflammation, swelling
swalm (15×)
swalwe *n.* ZOOL. swallow

19 Different meaning in the *MED*.

swalwe (3×)
swarm *n.* swarm
swa[r]mes (1×)
swart *adj.* dark
swart (23×)
swartnes(se *n.* darkness
swartnesse (1×)
swāthel *n.* cloth binding used as a bandage
swaþel (1×), *swaþeles* (1×)
swellen *v.* PATHOL. to swell
swelleþ (7×), *swelle* (3×), *swellen* (3×), *swelliþ* (1×), *swellun* (1×), *swellyn* (1×), *swolle* (1×), *swollen* (1×)
swelling(e *ng.* & *ag.* PATHOL. swelling
ng.: swellyng (28×), *swellynge* (11×), *swelling* (6×), *swellinge* (4×), *sqwellyng* (1×), *swellinges* (1×), *swellynges* (1×), *swelynge* (1×), *swollyng* (1×); *ag.: swellyng* (1×)
swēt(e *n.* *(1)* sweat
swete (2×), *swet* (1×)
swēt(e *adj.* sweet
swete (28×), *swet* (1×)
swēten *v.* *(1)* to sweat
swete (4×), *sweteþ* (1×)
swētenes(se *n.* sweetness
sweetnesse (1×), *swetnesse* (1×)
swēting(e *ng.* sweat(ing)
swetyng (2×)
swift(e *adj.* swift
swyft (10×), *swift* (1×), *swyfttere* (1×)
swiftlī *adv.* swiftly
swiftli (1×), *swyftly* (1×)
swīn(e *n.* ZOOL. swine
swynes (12×), *swynnes* (3×), *swyn* (1×)
swolwen *v.* to swallow
swolewyd (2×), *swolwe* (2×), *swelewe* (1×), *swelwiþ* (1×), *swelwyn* (1×), *swolewe* (1×), *swolewen* (1×), *swoleweþ* (1×), *swolewiþ* (1×)
swolwing(e *ng.* swallowing
swolewynge (2×)
swōt *n.* sweat
swoot (1×), *swot* (1×)
swŏun(e *n.* loss of consciousness, swoon
swennes (1×)
swŏunen *v.* to become unconscious, to swoon
j-swounnyd (1×), *swondenn* (1×), *swonnen* (1×)

T

tail *n.* tail
tail (1×), *tayl* (1×)
tāken *v.* to take
tak (193×), *tac* (140×), *take* (75×), *j-take* (3×), *takyn* (3×), *taken* (2×), *takeþ* (2×), *takyng* (2×), *j-tak* (1×), *[tak]* (1×), *takyth* (1×)
talent *n.* desire
talent (1×)
talking(e *ng.* talking
talkyng (1×)
talou(e *n.* tallow
talwe (16×), *talow* (1×), *talowe* (1×)
tamarinde *n.* tamarind (*Tamarindus indica*, fam. *Fabaceae*)
tamarynd (1×), *tamarynde* (1×)
tansei(e *n.* common tansy

(*Tanacetum vulgare* or *Chrysanthemum v.*, fam. *Asteraceae*)
tansey (2×)
tartar *n. (1)* wine dregs
tartarum (1×)
tāsten *v.* to taste
tast (1×), *taste* (1×)
tēchen *v.* to teach
teche (6×), *techen* (2×), *techyn* (2×), *techeþ* (1×)
teien *v.* to tie
j-teyȝed (1×), *teid* (1×)
tellen *v.* to tell
j-teld (28×), *told* (14×), *j-teeld* (13×), *teld* (13×), *telle* (11×), *toold* (8×), *j-told* (5×), *j-telde* (4×), *teeld* (4×), *j-toold* (3×), *tolden* (2×), *j-teeldin* (1×), *j-tel* (1×), *jteld* (1×), *teldyn* (1×), *tellen* (1×), *teylden* (1×), *toolde* (1×)
temperāt(e *adj.* (a) MED. of a medicine, food taken as medicine: of an intermediate degree between extreme qualities; mild in effect; (b) moderate
temperat (6×), *temperad* (1×), *te[m]perat* (1×), *temporat* (1×)
temperūre *n.* PHYSIOL. proper balance of humours or qualities
temprure (1×)
temple *n. (2)* temple
temples (9×), *templis* (1×), *tempyls* (1×)
tempren *v.* to mix, to blend
tempre (45×), *tempere* (4×), *j-tempre* (2×), *j-temperid* (1×), *j-tempred* (1×), *j-temprid* (1×), *j-tempryd* (1×), *temp[r]e* (1×), *tempreþ* (1×)
tēnasmon *n.* urge to defecate but inability to do so, tenesmus
tenasmon (5×), *thenasmoun* (1×)
tenden *v. (2)* to intensify
teendiþ (1×), *tendiþ* (1×)
tender *adj.* tender
tendere (1×), *tendre* (1×)
tendernes(se *n.* tenderness
tendyrnesse (1×)
terciān *n.* & *adj.* tertian (fever)
n.: *tercian* (1×); *adj.*: *tercian* (7×), *tercyan* (2×)
terebentīne *n.* turpentine, oleoresin of terebinth (*Pistacia terebinthus*, fam. *Anacardiaceae*)
terbentyne (2×), *terebentyne* (1×)
ters *n.* penis
ters (1×)
tēsen *v.* to card
teese (1×)
tēt(e *n.* nipple; breast
tetes (2×)
thamarīke *n.* one of the shrubs of the genus *Tamarix*, prob. the common tamarisk (*T. gallica*, fam. *Tamaricaceae*)
tamarysk (1×)
thanne *adv.* then
þan (164×), *þanne* (44×)
theodoricon *n.* purgative medicine
theodoricon (1×)
thēr *adv.* there
þer (194×), *þere* (37×), *there* (1×)
thēr-abǒute(n *adv.* thereabouts
þer-a-boute (3×)
thēr-after *adv.* thereafter
þerafter (2×), *þer-after* (1×)
thēr-at *adv.* thereat
þer-at (1×), *þer-ate* (1×)

thēr-bī *adv.* thereby
þer-bie (1×), *þer-by* (1×)
therf *n.*[20] unleavened (food)
þerf (1×)
thēr-for(e *adv.* therefore
þerfore (18×), *þer-fore* (12×)
thēr-in(ne *adv.* therein
þer-inne (37×), *þerinne* (3×), *þerynne* (1×)
thēr-of *adv.* thereof
þer-of (136×), *þerof* (28×), *þereof* (2×), *þere-of* (1×)
thēr-on *adv.* thereon
þer-on (23×), *þer-oon* (3×), *þeron* (2×), *þere-on* (1×), *þer-onn* (1×)
thēr-tō *adv.* thereto
þer-to (155×), *þer-too* (8×), *þerto* (7×)
thēr-upon *adv.* thereupon
þer-up-on (1×), *þer-vp-on* (1×)
thēr-whīle *adv.* in the meantime
þer-whyle (1×)
thēr-with *adv.* therewith
þer-wiþ (36×), *þerwiþ* (18×), *þer-with* (17×), *þerwith* (12×), *þere-wiþ* (1×), *þerewiþ* (1×), *þer-wyth* (1×), *þer-wythe* (1×), *þer-wyȝþ* (1×)
thēve-thorn *n.* (a) any of several types of prickly shrubs, thornbush; (b) hawthorn (*Crataegus monogyna*, fam. *Rosaceae*)
þefe-þorn (1×)
thider *adv.* to that place, thither
þedre (2×)
thīgh *n.* thigh
þeiȝ (3×), *thies* (1×), *þiees* (1×), *þiȝes* (1×)
thik(ke *adj.* thick
þicke (69×), *thicke* (5×), *þick* (5×), *thyk* (3×), *þicker* (2×), *þikke* (2×), *thykke* (1×)
thikkenes(se *n.* thickness
þicnesse (3×)
thing *n.* thing
þinges (110×), *þing* (18×), *thynges* (10×), *þynges* (8×), *þinge* (6×), *þingus* (5×), *thinges* (4×), *þingys* (4×), *thyngis* (2×), *þyng* (2×), *þynge* (2×), *thinge* (1×), *thyng* (1×), *thyngys* (1×), *þinng* (1×), *þinngus* (1×), *þynng* (1×)
thinken *v. (2)* to think
þenke (2×), *þenkyn* (2×), *thynke* (1×)
thin(ne *adj.* thin
þinne (54×), *þynne* (9×), *thynne* (6×), *thinne* (1×), *thyn* (1×)
thinnes(se *n.* thinness
thynnesse (1×)
thinship *n.* thinness
thynschepe (2×), *þinneschipe* (2×), *þinschepe* (1×)
thirl *n.* nostril
þirles (1×)
thirst *n.* thirst
þirst (17×), *þurst* (17×), *thurst* (1×)
thirsten *v.* to suffer from thirst
a-þirst (1×), *þirsteþ* (1×), *þirstiþ* (1×)
thirstful *adj.* thirsty
þirstful (5×), *þirstfulle* (3×), *thirstful* (1×), *thristfulle* (1×), *thrust-fulle* (1×), *þristfulle* (1×), *þurstful* (1×)
thirstī *adj.* thirsty

20 Only recorded as an adjective in the *MED*.

þirsti (1×), *þirsty* (1×)
thistel *n.* common thistle (genus *Carduus*, fam. *Asteraceae*)
þistelis (1×)
thŏndring(e *ng.* thundering
þundryng (1×)
thong *n.* thong
þwonges (1×)
thorn *n.* (a) hawthorn (*Crataegus monogyna*, fam. *Rosaceae*); (b) thorn
þorn (3×), *thorn* (1×), *thornes* (1×)
thought *n.* thought
þouȝt (2×), *þowt* (1×), *þowȝt* (1×)
thoughtful *adj.* thoughtful
þouȝtful (1×)
thŏume *n.* thumb
thombe (1×), *thumbe* (1×), *þombe* (1×)
thrēd(e *n.* thread
þredis (4×), *thred* (1×)
threst(e *n.* thrust
þrist (1×)
thrēten *v. (1)* to threaten
þreteneþ (1×)
thrīce *adv.* three times, thrice
þries (2×), *iij* (1×), *thriȝes* (1×)
thristen *v.* to thrust
þristeþ (2×), *þrist* (1×)
thristing(e *ng.* constriction
þristeng (1×)
thrōte *n.* throat
þrote (23×)
thrōte-bolle *n.* Adam's apple; larynx
þrote-bolle (4×)
throuen *v. (1)* to throw
j-þrowe (1×)
thus *adv.* thus
þus (49×)
tīle *n. (2)* tile
tyyl (1×)
tīle-stōn *n.* tile, brick
tyl-stoon (3×), *tilstoon* (1×), *tiylston* (1×), *tyil-stoon* (1×), *tylestoon* (1×), *tylstone* (1×), *tylstoon* (1×)
tīme *n. (1)* thyme (genus *Thymus*, fam. *Lamiaceae*)
tyme (8×), *thime* (3×), *thyime* (1×), *thyme* (1×)
tīme *n. (2)* time
tyme (31×), *tymes* (8×), *tymys* (1×)
tin *n. (1)* tin
tynne (1×)
tinkinge *ng.* ringing sound
tynchynge (1×)
tinnen *adj.* made of tin
tinnen (1×), *tynnen* (1×)
tisane *n.* medicinal drink made from shelled barley and water
tysane (12×), *tisane* (10×)
tisik(e *n.* phthisis
tysik (14×), *tisyk* (6×), *tisik* (2×), *t[i]sik* (1×), *tjsyk* (1×), *tysyk* (1×)
titimal(le *n.* spurge, one of several plants of the genus *Euphorbia*, fam. *Euphorbiaceae*
titymalle (2×), *[t]itymalle* (1×), *tyntinalle* (1×)
tō *n.* toe
toon (2×)
tō *adv. (2)* too
to (47×), *too* (3×)
ø**Tobie** *n.* Tobias
tobie (1×)
tōbrēken *v.* to break up
to-broke (9×), *to-breke* (1×), *tobroke*

(1×), *to-broken* (1×), *tobroken* (1×), *to-brokyn* (1×)

tōgeder *adv.* together
to-gidere (172×), *to-gedere* (19×), *to-gydere* (6×), *togidere* (4×), *to-geder* (3×), *togedere* (2×), *to-gedre* (1×), *to-gidre* (1×), *togydere* (1×), *to-gydre* (1×)

tōken *n.* MED. symptom
tokenes (58×), *toknes* (40×), *tokene* (22×), *tokenys* (9×), *tokne* (9×), *token* (8×), *tokens* (6×), *tokyn* (3×), *tokyns* (3×), *to-kene* (1×), *tokenis* (1×), *toknys* (1×), *tokynnes* (1×)

tōkning(e *n.* sign
tokenyng (1×)

tŏng(e *n. (2)* tongue
tonge (35×), *tunge* (12×), *tounge* (1×)

tōrīven *v.* to tear
to-ryf (1×)

tormentil(le *n.* tormentil (*Potentilla erecta*, fam. *Rosaceae*)
turmentille (6×)

tormentīn(e *n.* [see **tormentil(le**]
turmentyne (6×), *turmentyn* (1×)

tōsten *v.* to toast
toosted (1×), *tosted* (1×)

tōswellen *v.* PATHOL. to be morbidly enlarged
to-swolle (10×), *to-swollen* (2×)

tōth *n. (1)* tooth
teeþ (48×), *tooþ* (4×)

tōth-āche *n.* toothache
tooþ-ache (3×)

touail *n.* towel
twaile (1×)

tŏuchen *v.* to touch
touche (3×), *touching* (1×)

tŏuching(e *ng.* touching
touchyng (1×), *[t]ouchynge* (1×), *towchyng* (1×)

tough *adj.* tough
touȝ (1×), *tow* (1×)

travail *n.* travail
trauayle (4×), *traueile* (3×), *trauaile* (2×)

travailen *v.* to work (hard)
trauailed (1×), *traualeid* (1×), *traueil* (1×), *traueile* (1×), *traueileþ* (1×)

travailŏus *adj.* difficult; painful
traueilouse (1×), *traueliows* (1×), *trauelouse* (1×)

trē *n.* tree
tree (22×), *tre* (6×), *trees* (5×), *[tre]* (1×)

treble *adj.* threefold
treble (1×)

trēden *v.* to tread
j-trodyn (1×)

tremblen *v.* to tremble
trembleþ (3×), *trembeleþ* (1×), *trembelyn* (1×), *tremble* (1×)

trembling(e *ng.* & *ag.* trembling
ng.: *tremblyng* (4×), *tremelyng* (1×); *ag.*: *trembelyng* (1×)

trespassen *v.* to trespass
trespasyd (1×)

trētīs(e *n.* treatise
tretys (3×)

trīacle *n.* medicine against poison
triacle (16×)

~ **dīatesserŏun**, PHARM. medicine originally consisting of four ingredients
triacle diatesseron (2×), *triacle dyatesseron* (1×)

°**trīarodon abbates** *n.* [see **dīarodon**]
triarodon abbates (1×)
triasandrī *n.* MED. electuary made of three kinds of sandalwood
triasendri (6×), *triasandry* (1×), *triasendi* (1×)
trifer sarasenica[21] *n.* MED. medicinal preparation or substance used as a mild purgative
trifera sarasenica (2×), *trifera saracenica* (1×)
trŏuble *adj.* turbid
troble (1×), *trouble* (1×)
trŏublen *v.* (a) to be turbid; (b) to disturb
troublid (1×), *troublyd* (1×)
trŏublī *adj.* turbid
troubly (1×)
turbit *n.* root of turpeth (*Ipomoea turpethum*, fam. *Convolvulaceae*)
turbith (1×), *turbithe* (1×)
turble *adj.* turbid
turbul (1×)
turnen *v.* to turn
turneþ (8×), *turne* (7×), *j-turned* (6×), *turnyng* (3×), *j-turnyd* (2×), *turned* (2×)
turning(e *ng.* turning
turnyng (6×)
turtel *n.* ZOOL. turtledove
turtyl (1×)
tūtīe *n.* tutty (crude zinc oxide obtained by smelting copper ore with zinc)
tuchie (6×), *tuchia* (3×)

21 The word *sarasenica* is not collected in the *MED*.

twīes *adv.* twice
twies (4×), *ij* (1×), *twyes* (1×)

U

uncertainlī *adv.* randomly
oncertenlyche (1×), *on-certeynlyche* (1×)
unctuŏus *adj.* oily
vnctuose (2×), *vnnctuose* (1×)
uncūrāble *adj.* incurable
vncurabil (1×), *vncurabyl* (1×)
undēfīen *v.* (*ppl.*) **undefied**, undigested
vndefized (3×), *vndefied* (1×), *vndefizeid* (1×)
underfongen *v.* to receive
vnderfongeþ (2×), *vnderfong* (1×), *vnderfonge* (1×)
undern *n.* (a) 9 a.m.; (b) midday; (c) late afternoon
vndern (1×)
understōnden *v.* to understand
vnderstond (17×), *vnderstonde* (10×), *vnderstand* (1×), *vnderstande* (1×), *vndirstondyt* (1×), *vndyr-stonde* (1×), *vunderstonde* (1×), *vundyrstand* (1×)
unēthe *adv.* rarely
vnneþe (6×), *on-neþe* (1×), *vn-eþes* (1×), *vnneþis* (1×)
ungle *n. (1)* (**ungula**) MED. morbid growth on the eye
vngula (1×)
unhēled *ppl.* unhealed
on-hillid (1×)
ūniversāl *adj.* universal
vniuersel (1×)
unkīnd(e *adj.* MED. & PHYSIOL.

harmful; unhealthy
vnkynde (4×)
unkīndelī *adj.* [see **unkīnd(e**]
vnkyndly (2×)
unmēsūrāble *adj.* immeasurable
vnmesurabil (2×), *vnmensurabil* (1×)
unmightī *adj.* unable
on-myti (1×), *on-myty* (1×), *vn-myty* (1×), *vnmyȝtty* (1×)
unnātūrāl *adj.* unnatural
vnnaturel (1×)
unrēsōnāble *adj.* unreasonable
vnresonabil (3×), *vnresonabyl* (3×), *on-resonabyl* (1×), *vn-resonabyl* (1×)
unsāvǒurī *adj.* lacking in taste
vnsauery (3×), *on-sauery* (1×), *vnsauerey* (1×)
unsāvǒurnesse *n.* absence of taste
vnsauernesse (1×)
unsēmelī *adj.* unpleasant
vnsemely (1×)
unskilful *adj.* excessive
vnskille-ful (1×)
unslekked *ppl.* not mixed with water
vnslecked (1×), *vnsleckyd* (1×)
unstāble *adj.* unstable
vnstabil (1×)
unstāblenes(se *n.* agitation
vnstabilnesse (1×)
unstoppen *v.* MED. & PHYSIOL. to unblock
vnstopped (1×)
unwashen *ppl.* not washed
on-wasche (2×), *vnwasche* (2×), *on-waische* (1×), *onwasche* (1×), *on-wassche* (1×), *on-waysche* (1×), *oon-waschen* (1×), *vn-waische* (1×), *vnwaische* (1×), *vn-waisschene* (1×), *vn-wasche* (1×), *vnwassche* (1×)
unworthī *adj.* unworthy
vnwurþi (1×)
up *adv.* up
vp (58×), *up* (12×), *vppe* (1×)
upon *adv.* above
up-on (1×), *vp-on* (1×)
upright *adv.* upright
vp-riȝt (1×), *vpriȝt* (1×)
up-sō-dǒun *adv.* upside down
vp-so-down (2×), *vp-so-doun* (1×)
upward *adv.* upwards
vpward (7×), *upward* (2×)
ūrīnāl *n.* chamber pot
vrinal (2×)
ūrīne *n.* urine
vrine (169×), *vrines* (10×), *vryne* (5×), *vrinys* (1×), *vryn* (1×)
ūse *n. (1)* use
vse (1×)
ūsen *v.* to use
vse (98×), *vsen* (76×), *vsyn* (12×), *vseþ* (3×), *vsyng* (3×), *vsed* (2×), *j-vsed* (1×), *vsist* (1×), *vsyd* (1×)

V

valeriān(e *n.* valerian (*Valeriana officinalis*, fam. *Valerianaceae*)
valerian (3×)
vanishen *v.* to vanish
vanysche (2×), *wanysche* (1×)
vein(e *n. (1)* vein
veynes (46×), *veyne* (35×), *veynis* (8×), *veynys* (8×), *veyn* (5×), *veinys* (4×), *veines* (3×), *veine* (2×), *veynne*

(1×), *[v]eynys* (1×) [see also **liver(e** *n. (1)*]

venesŏun *n.* venison (meat of a game animal)
venyson (1×)

venimŏus *adj.* venomous
venemouse (2×), *venenouse* (1×), *venymouse* (1×)

venimŏusnes *n.* capacity to injure by introducing venom
venimysnesse (1×)

ventisshinge *ng.* releasing
a-ventesyng (2×), *a-ventisynge* (1×), *a-ventysyng* (1×), *ventesyng* (1×)

ventōsitē *n.* PATHOL. flatulence
ventosite (1×)

vēr *n. (1)* spring
ver (6×), *vere* (1×)

verdegrēce *n.* MED. verdigris
vertegrece (2×), *verte-grese* (1×), *vertigrece* (1×)

verrei *adj.* true
verri (12×), *verry* (2×), *verye* (1×)

vertū *n.* virtue
vertu (7×), *vertue* (2×), *vertues* (2×)

vertūŏus *adj.* virtuous
vertues (1×)

vervein(e *n.* vervain (*Verbena officinalis*, fam. *Verbenaceae*)
verueyne (12×), *veruene* (1×)

vessel *n.* vessel
vessel (14×), *vessele* (3×), *vesselles* (1×)

vīce *n.* vice
vicys (1×)

viciŏus *adj.* vicious
vicyows (1×)

vīne *n. (1)* vine (*Vitis vinifera*, fam. *Vitaceae*)
vyne (8×), *vine* (2×)

vinegre *n.* vinegar; **swēte ~**, vinegar made from boiled sweet wine
vinegre (94×), *vynegre* (9×), *venegre* (1×), *winegre* (1×)

vīolence *n.* violence
violence (11×), *v[i]olence* (1×)

vīolent *adj.* violent
violent (13×)

vīolentlī *adv.* violently
violently (1×)

vīolet *n.* sweet violet (*Viola odorata*, fam. *Violaceae*)
violet (130×)

virğīn(e *adj.* new (wax)
vergyn (1×), *virgin* (1×)

visāğe *n.* face
visage (18×)

viscōsitē *n.* viscosity
viscosite (2×)

viscŏus *n.* viscosity; *adj.* viscous
n.: viscouse (1×); *adj.: viscouse* (25×), *viscous* (1×)

ºvitucelle *n.* type of plant
vitucelle (1×)

voice *n.* voice
vois (3×)

void(e *adj.* MED. void of humours; of the pulse: not characterised by fullness of the blood vessel
voyid (2×), *voide* (1×), *voyd* (1×)

voiden *v.* MED. to purge
voide (1×), *voidiþ* (1×)

vomen *v.* to vomit
vomeþ (5×), *vimeþ* (1×), *vomen* (1×)

voming *ng.* vomit

vomyng (1×), *vomynge* (1×)
vŏuchen (sauf) *v.* to grant
fowche saf (1×)
vulva *n.* female external genitalia, vulva
devulua (1×)

W

wākeful *adj.* wakeful
wacful (1×)
wāken *v. (1)* to be awake
wake (2×), *wakyng* (1×)
wāking(e *ng.* wakefulness
wakyng (7×), *wakynge* (3×)
wal *n. (1)* wall
walles (1×)
walken *v. (1)* to walk
walke (4×), *walken* (2×), *walkeþ* (2×)
walsh-nŏt(e *n.* walnut (*Juglans regia*, fam. *Juglandaceae*)
walsche-note (2×), *walsche-nootys* (1×)
wal-wort *n.* danewort, dwarf elder (*Sambucus ebulus*, fam. *Caprifoliaceae*)
walwort (3×)
wan *adj.* grayish; dim
wan (4×), *whan* (1×)
wāning(e *ng.* waning (of the moon)
wanyng (2×)
wār(e *adj.* aware
ware (14×), *war* (5×)
warm *adj.* warm
warm (47×), *warme* (3×)
warmen *v.* to warm
j-warmed (3×), *warm* (2×), *j-warmyd* (1×)
wart *n.* wart
werte (1×), *wrettes* (1×)
washen *v.* to wash
waische (21×), *wasche* (8×), *waisch* (4×), *j-waische* (3×), *j-waischen* (3×), *waischen* (3×), *j-waschyn* (2×), *waschen* (2×), *wassche* (2×), *j-wasche* (1×), *j-waschen* (1×), *j-waschin* (1×), *j-wassched* (1×), *j-wasschin* (1×), *j-wasschyn* (1×), *waischeþ* (1×), *waischin* (1×), *waisching* (1×), *wasch* (1×), *waschyn* (1×)
washing(e *ng.* washing
waschyng (2×), *wasching* (1×), *wasschinges* (1×), *wasschyng* (1×)
wāsten *v.* to waste, to reduce
wasted (3×), *wasteþ* (3×), *j-wastyd* (2×), *j-wasted* (1×), *wasten* (1×), *wastid* (1×), *wastyn* (1×)
wāter *n.* water
water (351×), *watere* (7×), *watur* (5×), *wateris* (2×), *watyr* (2×), *wateres* (1×), *watter* (1×)
wāter-cresse *n.* watercress (*Nasturtium officinale*, fam. *Brassicaceae*)
water-crassys (1×), *watercressum* (1×)
wāterī *adj.* watery
wateri (2×), *watery* (2×), *watri* (1×), *wattery* (1×)
wāterīnesse *n.* wateriness
watrinesse (1×), *wattrinesse* (1×)
wāter-lēche *n.* water-leech
water-leche (2×), *waterleche* (1×), *water-lechis* (1×), *waterlechis* (1×)
wāter-lilīe *n.* water lily (fam. *Nymphaeaceae*)
water-lilies (6×), *waterlilies* (3×),

water-lilie (2×), *water-lilees* (1×), *water-lilien* (1×), *water-lilyen* (1×)

wātren *v.* of the eyes: to secrete fluid
watereþ (1×), *watteryn* (1×)

wātring(e *ng.* watering
wateryng (1×)

wax *n. (1)* wax
wex (24×), *wax* (4×), *wexe* (2×)

waxen *v. (1)* to grow, to wax
wexeþ (14×), *wexe* (9×), *wexiþ* (9×), *wex* (4×), *waxen* (3×), *waxeþ* (3×), *wax* (2×), *waxyn* (2×), *wexþ* (2×), *wexyng* (2×), *j-waxe* (1×), *j-wexe* (1×), *waxyt* (1×), *wexen* (1×), *wexing* (1×), *wexinge* (1×), *wexun* (1×), *wexyn* (1×)

waxing(e *ng. (1)* & *ag. (1)* increasing in size or dimension, waxing
ng.: wexyng (3×), *wexinge* (1×), *wexynge* (1×); *ag.: wexyng* (1×)

web *n.* PATHOL. cataract
web (11×), *webbys* (3×)

wēd(e *n. (1)* weed
weed (1×)

wēder *n.* weather
weder (1×), *wederes* (1×), *wedur* (1×)

weğğe *n.* wedge
wegge (1×)

weght *n. (1)* weight
wheiȝte (5×), *weiȝte* (1×)

wei *n. (1)* way
wei (7×), *wey* (5×), *weie* (4×), *weies* (1×), *we[i]es* (1×), *weis* (1×), *weyis* (1×), *weys* (1×)

wei-brēd(e *n.* great plantain (*Plantago major*, fam. *Plantaginaceae*)
weybrode (1×)

wēk(e *n. (1)* piece of flaxen or cotton wicking
weke (1×)

wēk(e *n. (3)* week
weke (3×), *woke* (3×), *wyke* (3×), *wokes* (2×)

wel *adj.* & *adv.* well
adj.: wel (10×), *weel* (2×), *weele* (1×), *welle* (1×); *adv.: wel* (105×), *weel* (15×), *wele* (14×), *welle* (3×), *j-wel* (1×)

wel(le *n.* well
welle (1×)

welling(e *ng.* gushing
wellynge (1×)

wem *n.* PATHOL. spot, flaw in the eye
wem (2×)

wēnen *v. (2)* to believe
wene (2×)

wēpen *v.* to weep
wepyng (1×)

wēping(e *ng.* & *ag.* weeping
ng.: wepynge (2×), *wepyng* (1×); *ag.: wepyng* (1×)

wērī *adj.* weary
wery (1×)

wērīen *v.* to tire
werid (1×)

werk *n. (1)* work
werke (1×)

werken *v. (1)* to work
worche (12×), *werche* (1×), *werke* (1×), *wurche* (1×)

werking(e *ng. (1)* working
worchyng (2×), *worchynge* (1×)

wermōd(e *n.* wormwood (*Artemisia absinthium*, fam. *Asteraceae*)

wermot (54×), *wermod* (2×), *wermote* (2×), *wermode* (1×), *wirmode* (1×), *wormosede* (1×)
werst(e *adj. sup.* worst
werst (3×), *worst* (2×)
wēsaunt(e *n.* esophagus; throat
wesyng (5×), *wesynge* (3×)
west *n.* west
west (4×)
westward *adv.* westwards
westward (1×)
west-wīnd *n.* wind blowing from the west
westwynd (1×)
wēt *adj.* wet
wete (2×), *j-wet* (1×), *weet* (1×)
wēten *v.* to wet
wete (11×), *weet* (6×), *j-wet* (4×), *wet* (4×), *wetyn* (3×), *weete* (2×), *j-weet* (1×), *j-wetyn* (1×), *weten* (1×)
wether *n.* ZOOL. male sheep, ram
weþeres (3×)
whei *n.* whey
whey (3×), *wheey* (1×), *whei* (1×), *wheiȝ* (1×)
whelp *n.* puppy; cub
qwelpe (1×), *whelpe* (1×)
whēte *n.* wheat (genus *Triticum*, fam. *Poaceae*)
whete (32×), *wheete* (3×), *wete* (1×)
whet-stōn *n.* sharpening stone used for tools, whetstone
wheston (4×), *weston* (1×)
whīle *n.* while
while (12×), *whyle* (1×)
whistle *n.* whistle
whistel (1×)
whīt *n.* (a) egg white; (b) ANAT. white of the eye; *adj.* white
n.: whiȝt (19×), *whiȝte* (9×), *white* (8×), *whyte* (2×); *adj.: whiȝt* (101×), *whiȝte* (9×), *whit* (5×), *white* (5×), *whyȝt* (4×), *whyt* (3×), *whith* (1×), *whiȝ* (1×), *whiȝtas* (1×), *whiȝthe* (1×), *whyiȝt* (1×), *whyte* (1×), *whyth* (1×), *wyth* (1×)
whītish *adj.* whitish
whitysche (1×), *whytische* (1×), *whytysche* (1×)
whītnes(se *n.* whiteness
whiȝtnesse (1×)
wikked(e *adj.* wicked
wyckyd (2×)
wikkednes(se *n.* wickedness
wyckydnesse (1×)
wīld(e *adj.* wild
wyld (3×), *wilde* (2×), *wylde* (2×), *wild* (1×)
wil(le *n.* will
wille (20×), *wyl* (5×), *wil* (4×)
willed *adj.* willing
wyllyd (1×)
willen *v. (1)* will, to want
wole (73×), *wul* (19×), *wol* (14×), *wolt* (11×), *wollen* (8×), *wolen* (7×), *wulle* (6×), *wult* (5×), *wyl* (5×), *wylt* (5×), *wolde* (4×), *wold* (3×), *wilt* (2×), *wolden* (2×), *vol* (1×), *vollen* (1×), *vul* (1×), *wel* (1×), *wele* (1×), *woil* (1×), *woldest* (1×), *wol[e]* (1×), *wolle* (1×), *woold* (1×), *woolde* (1×), *w[u]l* (1×), *wylle* (1×)
wilnen *v.* to wish
wylneþ (2×)
wīnd *n.* (a) wind; (b) gas, air within the body

wynd (39×), *wyndes* (15×), *wyndys* (6×), *wynde* (3×), *wyndis* (1×)

wīndī *adj. (2)* causing flatulence, gassy

wyndy (6×), *wyndi* (2×)

wīndīnes(se *n.* excessive gas or air

wyndnesse (5×), *wyndenesse* (1×), *wyndynesse* (1×)

°**wīndish** *adj.* gassy

wyndisch (1×), *wyndysche* (1×)

wīn(e *n. (2)* wine

wyn (181×), *wyne* (1×), *wynne* (1×)

winful *adj. (1)* oriented towards material benefit

wynfulle (1×)

winter *n.* winter

wynter (15×), *wyntres* (1×), *wyntris* (1×), *wyntrys* (1×)

wīpen *v.* to wipe

wipe (1×)

wīs(e *n. (2)* manner

wyse (11×), *wise* (2×), *wysis* (1×)

wīs(e *adj.* wise

wysere (1×)

wit *n.* wit

wyt (15×), *wit* (6×), *wyttes* (5×), *wiȝt* (2×), *wyȝt* (2×), *wiȝttes* (1×), *wutes* (1×)

witen *v. (1)* to know

white (1×), *wite* (1×), *wot* (1×)

withdrauen *v.* to withdraw

whiþ-drawe (1×)

withhōlden *v.* PHYSIOL. to retain, to cause retention

with-holden (3×), *withholden* (1×), *with-holdyn* (1×), *with-hoolden* (1×), *wiþ-holdiþ* (1×), *wythe-holden* (1×)

withhōlding(e *ng.* PHYSIOL. retention of a bodily fluid or substance

withholdyng (2×), *whiþholdynge* (1×), *wi[t]h-holdyng* (1×), *with-hooldyng* (1×), *wiþ-holdyng* (1×), *wiþholdyng* (1×), *wiþ-holdynge* (1×), *wiþholdynge* (1×)

within(ne *adv.* inside

with-inne (22×)

withinne-forth *adv.* inside

with-inne-forþ (32×), *with-inneforþ* (6×), *with-inne-forþe* (5×), *with-inne-foorþ* (2×), *with-in-forþe* (1×), *with-inne-forthe* (1×), *wiþ-in-for-þe* (1×)

withŏuten *adv.* outside

with-owtyn (8×), *with-oute* (7×), *with-outen* (5×), *with-outyn* (5×), *with-owte* (3×), *with-owten* (3×), *withowtyn* (1×), *wiþ-oute* (1×), *wiþ-owtyn* (1×)

withŏuten-forth *adv.* outside

with-oute-forþ (6×), *with-outen-forþ* (5×), *with-owtyn-forþ* (5×), *with-outyn-forþ* (4×), *with-owte-forþ* (2×), *with-owten-forþ* (2×), *with-outeforþ* (1×), *with-oute-forþe* (1×), *with-out-forþ* (1×), *with-outyn-forth* (1×), *wiþouten-forþ* (1×), *wythouteforþe* (1×)

wlāten *v. (1)* (a) to loathe; (b) to become nauseated

wlateþ (4×), *wlaten* (2×), *wlate* (1×), *wlatyn* (1×)

wlāting(e *ng.* nausea

wlatinge (1×)

wō *n.* distress

wo (5×), *woo* (1×)

wōde *n. (2)* wood, forest

wodes (1×)

wōd(e *adj.* mad

wood (3×), *woode* (2×), *wode* (1×)
wōdnes(se *n.* madness
woodnesse (3×), *wodnesse* (1×)
wŏl *n. (1)* wool
wolle (13×), *wulle* (4×), *woolle* (1×)
wŏlf *n.* ZOOL. wolf
wolues (1×)
wŏllen *adj.* woollen
wollen (1×)
wōmb(e *n.* stomach; womb
wombe (62×), *womb* (2×), *womb[e]* (1×), *wombis* (1×), *wombys* (1×)
wōmbed(e *adj.* (**nēshe**) ~, not constipated
j-wombyd (1×), *wombed* (1×)
wŏmman *n.* woman
womannus (13×), *women* (12×), *woman* (8×), *womannes* (6×), *wommanus* (5×), *wymman* (4×), *wymmen* (4×), *whomen* (2×), *wymmanus* (2×), *wemman* (1×), *whimmanus* (1×), *whymmannus* (1×), *womanes* (1×), *woman[es]* (1×), *womannys* (1×), *womans* (1×), *womanus* (1×), *wommen* (1×), *wymmenus* (1×)
wŏnder *adv.* extraordinarily
wonder (1×)
wŏnderfullī *adv.* effectively
wonderefullyche (1×)
wŏnen *v. (1)* (**bēn wŏnt**) to be normally; to be present
j-wont (2×), *wont* (2×), *wount* (2×), *wunt* (1×)
wōrd *n.* word
wurdis (1×)
world *n.* world
world (1×), *wor[l]d* (1×)
wŏrm *n.* ZOOL. worm
wormes (48×), *worm* (8×), *wermes* (2×), *wurmes* (2×), *worme* (1×)
wŏrt *n. (1)* plant
wort (2×), *worten* (1×)
wŏrt *n. (2)* infusion
wortes (1×), *wortis* (1×)
worthen *v.* to turn
j-wharte (1×)
worthī *adj.* worthy
worþi (2×)
wŏund *n.* wound
wound (9×), *wounde* (6×), *woundes* (4×), *woundys* (3×)
wrappen *v.* to wrap
wrappe (2×), *wrap* (1×)
wratthe *n.* wrath, anger
wraþþe (7×), *wrath* (1×), *wraþ* (1×)
wratthful *adj.* given to anger
wrathfulle (1×)
wrēchen *v. (2)* to recover through energetic action
wretche (1×)
wresten *v.* to turn
wreestiþ (1×)
wrestler(e *n.* wrestler
wrastelers (1×)
wrestling(e *ng.* wrestling
wrastelynges (1×)
wrīen *v. (1)* to be covered
wrien (1×)
wringen *v.* to wring
wryng (9×), *wrynge* (4×), *wryngyn* (1×)
wrinkle *n.* wrinkle
wrynclus (1×)
wrinklen *v.* to wrinkle
wryncli[þ] (1×)

wrīten *v.* to write
write (2×), *wretyn* (1×), *wryte* (1×), *wryten* (1×)
wrōth *adj.* angry
wroop (1×), *wrothe* (1×)
wrōthen *v.* to become angry
wroth (1×)

X

xiloaloes *n.* wood or bark of the aloe tree (*Aquilaria agallocha*, fam. *Thymelaeaceae*)
xiloaloes (1×)
xilobalsamum *n.* wood or bark of the balsam tree (*Commiphora meccanensis* or *opobalsamum*, fam. *Burseraceae*)
xilobalsamum (2×), *xilobalȝamum* (1×), *ȝilobalsamum* (1×), *ȝilobalȝamum* (1×)
xilocassie *n.* bark from a tree, shrub, or plant of the genus *Cassia*, fam. *Fabaceae*
xilocassia (1×), *xilocassie* (1×)

Y

yelwe *adj.* yellow
ȝelwe (32×), *ȝelewe* (10×), *ȝelowe* (3×), *ȝelew* (2×), *ȝelow* (1×)
yelwenesse *n.* PATHOL. abnormal yellowness
ȝelewnesse (2×), *ȝelwnesse* (1×)
yelwish *adj.* yellowish
ȝelewysche (2×), *ȝelwysche* (2×)
yēr *n. (2)* year
ȝeer (6×), *ȝere* (6×), *ȝeere* (5×), *ȝeris* (1×)
yērd *n. (1)* garden
ȝerdys (1×)
~ **cresse**, watercress (*Lepidium sativum*, fam. *Brassicaceae*)
ȝarde-crassen (1×)
yērd *n. (2)* penis
ȝerde (36×), *ȝerd* (7×), *ȝeerde* (1×)
yēt *adv.* yet
ȝit (5×)
yēven *v.* to give
ȝif (180×), *ȝyue* (29×), *ȝeue* (23×), *ȝyf* (18×), *gyf* (3×), *j-ȝeuyn* (3×), *ȝeuyst* (3×), *ȝeuist* (2×), *ȝeuyn* (2×), *ȝeuyng* (1×), *ȝeyf* (1×), *ȝife* (1×), *ȝiue* (1×), *ȝoue* (1×), *ȝouen* (1×), *ȝouyn* (1×), *ȝyuen* (1×), *ȝyuest* (1×)
yexen *v.* (a) to hiccup; (b) to sob
shyȝynge (1×), *ȝixep* (1×), *ȝixip* (1×)
yexinge *ng.* hiccup(ping)
ȝixinge (12×), *oksynge* (1×), *ȝixynges* (1×), *ȝyxynge* (1×)
*__(y)-gloderid__ *adj.* coagulated
j-gloderid (2×), *j-glodeyd* (1×), *j-gloterid* (1×)
yicchen *v.* to itch
itche (1×), *ychche* (1×)
yicching *ng.* itch(ing)
icchyng (3×), *icchinge* (2×), *ichinge* (2×), *icching* (1×), *ichchyng* (1×), *ichynge* (1×), *itchyng* (1×), *itchynge* (1×), *jchinge* (1×), *jchynge* (1×), *yching* (1×), *ychynge* (1×), *ȝichinge* (1×)
yolk(e *n.* yolk
ȝelkes (8×), *ȝelkys* (8×), *ȝelke* (3×),

ȝel[k]es (1×)
yonderward *adv.* farther away
ȝyndurward (1×)
yŏng *adj.* young
ȝong (5×), *ȝonge* (4×), *ȝounge* (1×)
yŏngthe *n.* youth
ȝongþe (2×)
yōre *adv.* earlier
ȝore (1×)
yŏuth *n.* youth
ȝouþe (6×), *youthe* (1×), *ȝouthe* (1×)

Bibliography

Arakelian, P. G. "Punctuation in a Late Middle English Manuscript". *Neuphilologische Mitteilungen* 76/4 (1975): 614–624.

Beadle, R. and A. J. Piper, eds. *New Science out of Old Books: Studies in Manuscripts and Early Printed Books in Honour of A. I. Doyle*. Aldershot: Scolar Press, 1995.

Beaujouan, G. "Manuscrits médicaux du Moyen Âge conservés en Espagne". *Mélanges de la Casa de Velázquez* 8 (1972): 161–221.

Benskin, M. "The Letters ⟨þ⟩ and ⟨y⟩ in Later Middle English, and Some Related Matters". *Journal of the Society of Archivists* 7 (1982): 13–30.

Benson, L. D., gen. ed. *The Riverside Chaucer*. 3rd ed. Oxford: Oxford University Press, 1987.

Brock, C. H. *Dr William Hunter's Papers and Drawings in the Hunterian Collection of Glasgow University Library: A Handlist*. Cambridge: Wellcome Unit for the History of Medicine, 1990.

Brown, M. P. *A Guide to Western Historical Scripts from Antiquity to 1600*. London: The British Library, 1990.

Bullough, V. and C. Campbell. "Female Longevity and Diet in the Middle Ages". *Speculum* 55/2 (1980): 317–325.

Burke, P. *Languages and Communities in Early Modern Europe*. Cambridge: Cambridge University Press, 2004.

Calle-Martín, J. and A. Miranda-García. "Editing Middle English Punctuation. The Case of MS Egerton 2622 (ff. 136–165)". *International Journal of English Studies* 5/2 (2005): 27–44.

Calman, K. C. *Medical Education: Past, Present and Future: Handing on Learning*. Edinburgh: Churchill Livingstone Elsevier, 2007.

Cross, R. *A Handlist of Manuscripts Containing English in the Hunterian Collection, Glasgow University Library*. Glasgow: Glasgow University Library, 2004.

Dawson, W. R., ed. *A Leechbook or Collection of Medical Recipes of the Fifteenth Century*. London: Macmillan, 1934.

Derolez, A. *The Palaeography of Gothic Manuscript Books: From the Twelfth to the Early Sixteenth Century*. Cambridge: Cambridge University Press, 2003.

Díaz Vera, J. E. and R. Caballero, eds. *Textual Healing: Studies in Medieval English Medical, Scientific and Technical Texts*. Bern, Berlin, etc.: Peter Lang, 2009.

Edwards, A. S. G., V. Gillespie and R. Hanna, eds. *The English Medieval Book: Studies in Memory of Jeremy Griffiths*. London: The British Library, 2000.
Esteban-Segura, L. *G.U.L. MS Hunter 509 (ff. 1r–167v): An Edition and Philological Study*. Unpublished doctoral dissertation. Universidad de Málaga, 2008a.
——. "Hands and Script in Glasgow University Library MS Hunter 509". In *Proceedings from the 31st AEDEAN Conference*, ed. by M. J. Lorenzo Modia. A Coruña: Universidade da Coruña, 2008b, 417–432.
——. (2009a) "Punctuation Practice in G.U.L. MS Hunter 509". In Díaz Vera and Caballero 2009, 93–107.
——. "Mecanismos de formación de palabras en G.U.L. MS Hunter 509". *Interlingüística* 18 (2009b): 336–343.
——. "Dialectal Study of a Version of the Middle English Gilbertus Anglicus: The Case of G.U.L. MS Hunter 509 (ff. 14r–167v)". *English Studies. A Journal of English Language and Literature* 91/3 (2010): 256–273.
——. "Glasgow, University Library, MS Hunter 509: A Description". *Atlantis. Journal of the Spanish Association of Anglo-American Studies* 33/2 (2011a): 105–122.
——. "Suffixal Doublets in Late Middle English: *-NESS* VS *-SHIP*". *Neuphilologische Mitteilungen* 112/2 (2011b): 183–194.
——. (2011c) "Syntactic Aspects of MSS Hunter 503 and 513: Relatives and Negation". In Miranda-García and González 2011, 75–87.
——. "Editing Middle English Medical Manuscripts: The Case of Glasgow, University Library, MS Hunter 509". *Journal of English Studies* 9 (2011d): 97–108.
——. "Estudio léxico del campo de la enfermedad en un manuscrito medieval inglés (G.U.L. MS Hunter 509, fols. 1r-167v)". *ODISEA. Journal of English Studies* 12 (2011e): 273–287.
——. "Medical, Official, and Monastic Documents in Sociolinguistic Research". In J. M. Hernández-Campoy and J. C. Camilo Conde-Silvestre, eds. *The Handbook of Historical Sociolinguistics*. Oxford: Wiley-Blackwell, 2012. 140–155.
——. "Scribal Errors and Corrections in Two Versions of the Middle English Gilbertus Anglicus". In J. Martín Arista *et al.*, eds. *Convergent Approaches on Mediaeval English Language and Literature. Selected Papers from the 22nd International Conference of SELIM*. Newcastle: Cambridge Scholars, forthcoming.
Esteban-Segura, L. and T. Marqués-Aguado. "New Software Tools for the Analysis of Computerized Historical Corpora: GUL MSS Hunter 509 and

513 in the Light of *TexSEn*". In V. Gillespie and A. Hudson, eds. *Editing Medieval Texts from Britain in the Twenty-First Century*. Turnhout: Brepols, forthcoming.

Fisiak, J. and P. Trudgill, eds. *East Anglian English*. Woodbrige: D. S. Brewer, 2001.

French, R., J. Arrizabalaga, A. Cunningham and L. García-Ballester, eds. *Medicine from the Black Death to the French Disease*. Aldershot: Ashgate, 1998.

Getz, F. M. "Gilbertus Anglicus Anglicized". *Medical History* 26/4 (1982): 436–442.

——. "Charity, Translation, and the Language of Medical Learning in Medieval England". *Bulletin of the History of Medicine* 64/1 (1990): 1–17.

——, ed. *Healing and Society in Medieval England: A Middle English Translation of the Pharmaceutical Writings of Gilbertus Anglicus*. Madison: University of Wisconsin Press, 1991.

——. *Medicine in the English Middle Ages*. Princeton: Princeton University Press, 1998.

Gilbertus Anglicus. *Compendium medicinae*. Lyons: J. Saccon for V. de Portonariis, 1510.

Gottfried, R. S. *Doctors and Medicine in Medieval England, 1340–1530*. Princeton: Princeton University Press, 1986.

Grieve, H. E. P. *Examples of English Handwriting 1150–1750: With Transcripts and Translations*. Chelmsford: Essex Education Committee, 1954.

Griffiths, J. and D. Pearsall, eds. *Book Production and Publishing in Britain, 1375–1475*. Cambridge: Cambridge University Press, 1989.

Grymonprez, P., ed. *'Here men may se the vertues off herbes'*: *A Middle English Herbal* (MS. Bodley 483, ff. 57r–67v). Scripta 3. Brussels: Omirel, 1981.

Hallaert, M.-R., ed. *The 'Sekenesse of wymmen': A Middle English Treatise on Diseases in Women* (Yale Medical Library, Ms. 47 fols. 60r–71v). Scripta 8. Brussels: Omirel, 1982.

Handerson, H. E. *Gilbertus Anglicus. Medicine of the Thirteenth Century*. Cleveland: Cleveland Medical Library Association, 1918. *The Project Gutenberg eBook*, 2005 [Electronic resource available from <http://www.gutenberg.org/files /16155/16155-h/ 16155-h.htm>].

Harris, K. "Patrons, Buyers and Owners: The Evidence for Ownership, and the Rôle of Book Owners in Book Production and the Book Trade". In Griffiths and Pearsall 1989, 163–199.

Hellinga, L. and J. B. Trapp, eds. *The Cambridge History of the Book in Britain: Volume III, 1400–1557*. Cambridge: Cambridge University Press, 1999.

Henslow, G. *Medical Works of the Fourteenth Century Together with a List of Plants Recorded in Contemporary Writings, with Their Identifications*. Reprint. New York: Burt Franklin, 1972.

Hieatt, C. B. "Editing Middle English Culinary Manuscripts". In McCarren and Moffat 1998, 133–140.

Hunt, T. *Plant Names of Medieval England.* Cambridge: D. S. Brewer, 1989.

Jacobs, N. "Kindly Light or Foxfire? The Authorial Text Reconsidered". In McCarren and Moffat 1998, 3–14.

Jacquart, D. and C. Thomasset. *Sexuality and Medicine in the Middle Ages*. Trans. by M. Adamson. Cambridge: Polity Press, 1988.

James, M. R. *A Descriptive Catalogue of the Manuscripts in the Library of Pembroke College, Cambridge*. Cambridge: Cambridge University Press, 1905.

Jasin, J. "The Transmission of Learned Medical Literature in the Middle English *Liber Uricrisiarum*". *Medical History* 37/3 (1993): 313–329.

Jones, M. C. *Vernacular Literacy in Late-Medieval England: The Example of East Anglian Medical Manuscripts*. Unpublished doctoral dissertation. University of Glasgow, 2000.

Jones, P. M. 1998. "Thomas Fayreford: An English Fifteenth-Century Medical Practitioner". In French, Arrizabalaga, Cunningham and García-Ballester 1998, 156–183.

Keiser, G. R. "Serving the Needs of Readers: Textual Division in Some Late-Medieval English Texts". In Beadle and Piper 1995, 207–226.

——. *XXV. Works of Science and Information*. In *A Manual of the Writings in Middle English, 1050–1500*. Vol. 10, ed. by A. E. Hartung. New Haven: Connecticut Academy of Arts and Sciences, 1998a, 3593–3967.

——. (1998b) "Editing Scientific and Practical Writings". In McCarren and Moffat 1998, 109–122.

Ker, N. R. *William Hunter as a Collector of Medieval Manuscripts*. Glasgow: University of Glasgow, 1983.

Laing, M. and K. Williamson, eds. *Speaking in our Tongues: Proceedings of a Colloquium on Medieval Dialectology and Related Disciplines*. Woodbridge: D. S. Brewer, 1994.

Levere, T. H., ed. *Editing Texts in the History of Science and Medicine: Papers Given at the Seventeenth Annual Conference on Editorial Problems, University of Toronto, 6–7 November 1981*. London: Garland, 1982.

Lucas, P. J. "The Treatment of Language". In McCarren and Moffat 1998, 169–183.

Manzalaoui, M. A., ed. *Secretum secretorum: Nine English Versions. Volume 1: Text.* EETS O.S. 276. London: Oxford University Press, 1977.

Marqués-Aguado, T. "Punctuation Practice in the *Antidotary* in G.U.L. MS Hunter 513 (ff. 37v–96v)". *Miscelánea: A Journal of English and American Studies* 39 (2009): 55–72.

Marqués-Aguado, T., A. Miranda-García and S. González, eds. *The Middle English Ophthalmic Treatise on the Use of the Eye in G.U.L. MS Hunter 513 (ff. 1r–37r).* Málaga: Servicio de Publicaciones de la Universidad de Málaga, 2008.

Matheson, L. M., ed. *Popular and Practical Science of Medieval England.* East Lansing: Colleagues Press, 1994.

McCarren, V. P. and D. Moffat, eds. *A Guide to Editing Middle English.* Ann Arbor: University of Michigan Press, 1998.

McIntosh, A., M. L. Samuels and M. Benskin, with the assistance of M. Laing and K. Williamson. *A Linguistic Atlas of Late Mediaeval English.* 4 vols. Aberdeen: Aberdeen University Press, 1986.

MED: Kurath, H., S. M. Kuhn and R. E. Lewis, eds. *Middle English Dictionary.* Ann Arbor: University of Michigan Press, 1952–2001. Online version in *Middle English Compendium*, ed. by F. McSparran *et al.* (University of Michigan Digital Library Production Service, 2001–). <http://quod.lib.umich.edu/m/med>.

Minnis, A. J., ed. *Latin and Vernacular: Studies in Late-Medieval Texts and Manuscripts.* Cambridge: D. S. Brewer, 1989.

Minnis, A. J. and C. Brewer, eds. *Crux and Controversy in Middle English Textual Criticism.* Woodbridge: D. S. Brewer, 1992.

Minnis, A. J. and A. B. Scott, eds. *Medieval Literary Theory and Criticism c.1100–c.1375: The Commentary-Tradition.* 1988. Oxford: Clarendon Press, 1991.

Minns, E. H. "John Sperhawke D.D.". *Pembroke College Cambridge Society Annual Gazette* 23 (1949): 10–15.

Miranda-García, A. and J. Garrido-Garrido. *Text Search Engine (TexSEn).* Málaga: Servicio de Publicaciones de la Universidad de Málaga, forthcoming.

Miranda-García, A. and S. González, eds. *Benvenutus Grassus' On the Well-Proven Art of the Eye.* Practica oculorum & De probatissima arte oculorum. *Synoptic Edition and Philological Studies.* Bern, Berlin, etc.: Peter Lang, 2011.

Moorman, C. *Editing the Middle English Manuscript.* Jackson: University Press of Mississippi, 1975.

Nikolov, H. *Dictionary of Plant Names in Latin, German, English and French.* Berlin; Stuttgart: J. Cramer, 1996.

OED: Simpson, J. A. and E. S. C. Weiner, eds. *The Oxford English Dictionary. Second Edition on CD-ROM. Version 3.1*. Oxford: Oxford University Press, 2004.

Ogden, M. S., ed. *The 'Liber de diversis medicinis'* in the Thornton Manuscript (MS. Lincoln Cathedral A.5.2) EETS O. S. 207. London: Oxford University Press, 1938.

Pahta, P. and I. Taavitsainen. "Vernacularisation of Scientific and Medical Writing in Its Sociohistorical Context". In Taavitsainen and Pahta 2004, 1–22.

Parkes, M. B. *English Cursive Book Hands 1250–1500*. London: Scolar Press, 1969.

——. *Scribes, Scripts and Readers: Studies in the Communication, Presentation and Dissemination of Medieval Texts*. London; Rio Grande: Hambledon Press, 1991.

——. *Pause and Effect: An Introduction to the History of Punctuation in the West*. Hants: Scolar Press, 1992.

Pearsall, D., ed. *Manuscripts and Readers in Fifteenth Century England: The Literary Implications of Manuscript Study. Essays from the 1981 Conference at the University of York*. Woodbridge: D. S. Brewer, 1983.

——, ed. *New Directions in Later Medieval Manuscript Studies: Essays from the 1998 Harvard Conference*. Woodbridge: York Medieval Press, 2000.

Petti, A. G. *English Literary Hands from Chaucer to Dryden*. London: Edward Arnold, 1977.

Rawcliffe, C. *Medicine & Society in Later Medieval England*. Gloucestershire: Alan Sutton, 1995.

——. "Sickness and Health". In Rawcliffe and Wilson 2004, 301–326.

Rawcliffe, C. and R. Wilson, eds. *Medieval Norwich*. London: Hambledon and London, 2004.

Robbins, R. H. "Medical Manuscripts in Middle English". *Speculum* 45/3 (1970): 393–415.

Roberts, J. *Guide to Scripts Used in English Writings up to 1500*. London: The British Library, 2005.

Rubin, S. *Medieval English Medicine*. Newton Abbot: David & Charles (Holdings) Limited, 1974.

Schleissner, M. R., ed. *Manuscript Sources of Medieval Medicine: A Book of Essays*. New York: Garland, 1995.

Seymour, M. C. *et al.*, eds. *On the Properties of Things: John Trevisa's Translation of Bartholomaeus Anglicus 'De proprietatibus rerum'*. 3 vols. Oxford: Clarendon Press, 1975–1988.

Singer, P. N. *Galen: Selected Works*. Oxford: Oxford University Press, 1997.

Slack, P. 1979. "Mirrors of Health and Treasures of Poor Men: The Uses of the Vernacular Medical Literature of Tudor England". In Webster 1979, 237–273.

Taavitsainen, I. and P. Pahta. "Vernacularisation of Medical Writing in English: A Corpus-Based Study of Scholasticism". *Early Science and Medicine* 3/2 (1998): 157–185.

——, eds. *Medical and Scientific Writing in Late Medieval English*. Cambridge: Cambridge University Press, 2004.

Talbot, C. H. *Medicine in Medieval England*. London: Oldbourne, 1967.

Thorndike, L. and P. Kibre. *A Catalogue of Incipits of Mediaeval Scientific Writings in Latin*. New York: Mediaeval Academy of America, 1963.

Voigts, L. E. 1995. "Multitudes of Middle English Medical Manuscripts, or the Englishing of Science and Medicine". In Schleissner 1995, 183–195.

Voigts, L. E. and P. D. Kurtz, eds. *Scientific and Medical Writings in Old and Middle English: An Electronic Reference*. Ann Arbor: University of Michigan Press, 2000.

Voigts, L. E. and M. R. McVaugh. "A Latin Technical Phlebotomy and Its Middle English Translation". *Transactions of the American Philosophical Society* 74/2 (1984): 1–69.

Webster, C., ed. *Health, Medicine, and Mortality in the Sixteenth Century*. Cambridge: Cambridge University Press, 1979.

Young, J. and P. H. Aitken. *A Catalogue of the Manuscripts in the Library of the Hunterian Museum in the University of Glasgow*. Glasgow: Maclehose, 1908.

Late Middle English Texts

General Editors:
Antonio Miranda-García, University of Málaga (amiranda@uma.es)
& Santiago González, University of Oviedo (sigonzalez@uniovi.es)

This series is conceived to facilitate the edition of unpublished scientific treatises written in Late Middle English (late 13th century to the very early 16th century) as well as the publication of monographs dealing with their transmission, palaeographical and dialectal features, and/or their lexical, syntactic and pragmatic characteristics. The second aspect of the series seeks to favour studies specializing in linguistic variation or any of the multi-faceted aspects of the Middle English language even from a diachronic perspective.

The Late Middle English Texts series is directed towards a wide scholarly readership that includes Textual Edition, Textual Criticism and Transmission – especially on electronic and digital formats both as standalone and online –, Ecdotics, History of Science, History of the English Language and Linguistics, Late Medieval Studies, History of Cultural Artifacts and Librarianship. The chronological scope we contemplate will range approximately from the mid 1200's to the early 1500's, and will include both manuscripts , incunabula and early prints that have come down to us in English, with the occasional excursion into analogues in other languages. Editions will include codicological and language studies that will enhance the relevance of the text within the cultural transmission European framework.

The series includes both scholarly and academic editions and monograph studies with a specialised and comprehensive focus. Thematic and teaching textual anthologies will also be considered for the series. We do not aim primarily at publishing collected papers from conferences, symposia, meetings and other reunions, unless the occasion had a very relevant topic and was strongly coherent and specialised in its discussions.

Each publication is subject to a rigorous blind double peer-review system that involves at least five readers from five different institutions (Universities or Research Institutes).

1 Antonio Miranda-García & Santiago González Fernández-Corugedo
Benvenutus Grassus' On the well-proven art of the eye
Practica oculorum & De probatissima arte oculorum
524 pages / 2011 / 978-3-0343-0698-0

2 Javier Calle-Martín & Antonio Miranda-García
The Middle English Version of *De viribus herbarum*
(GUL MS Hunter 497, ff. 1r-92r)
258 pages / 2012 / 978-3-0343-0697-3

3 Laura Esteban-Segura
System of Physic
(GUL MS Hunter 509, ff. 1r-167v)
A Compendium of Mediaeval Medicine
Including the Middle English Gilbertus Anglicus
461 pages / 2012 / 978-3-0343-0077-3